ESSENTIAL OILS
DESK REFERENCE

Compiled by Essential Science Publishing

THIRD EDITION

Third Edition
Second Printing February 2005

Copyright ©2004 Essential Science Publishing
1-800-336-6308
www.essentialscience.net

ISBN 0-943685-39-7

Printed in the United States of America   10 9 8 7 6 5 4 3 2

Disclaimer: The information contained in this book is for educational purposes only.
It is not provided to diagnose, prescribe, or treat any condition of the body.
The information in this book should not be used as a substitute for
medical counseling with a health professional.
Neither the author nor publisher accepts responsibility for such use.

To all those who seek truth, light, and wisdom.
After all, it is their hearts that turn to
the information in this book.

Contents

— SECTION 1 —

— SECTION 6 —

— SECTION 7 —

— SECTION 8 —

— SECTION 9 —

Preface

Essential oils are some of the oldest and most powerful therapeutic agents known. Most people today are unaware that they have an impressive, multimillennium-long history of use in healing and anointing throughout the ancient world. Dozens of essential oils are cited repeatedly in Judeo-Christian religious texts and records show they were used to treat virtually every ailment known to man at that time. Frankincense, myrrh, lotus, cedarwood, and sandalwood oils were widely used in ancient Egyptian purification and embalming rituals. Other oils, like cinnamon, clove and lemon, were highly valued as antiseptics hundreds of years before the development of today's synthetic medicines.

With the advance of antibiotics and prescription drugs during the last century, natural therapeutic agents, especially essential oils, have been largely overlooked. Only during the last decade have essential oils begun a resurgence in popularity in the United States, as their broad-spectrum antibacterial and therapeutic action is rediscovered by many researchers and health-care professionals. No doubt part of the reason essential oils have been slow to emerge—especially in the United States—is because they were heavily extended and adulterated for commercial use, destroying their therapeutic biochemistry and making them useful only as air-freshening or flavoring compounds.

In their pure state, essential oils are some of the most concentrated natural extracts known, exhibiting significant and immediate antiviral, anti-inflammatory, antibacterial, and hormone-balancing effects. In clinical practice, they have been shown to have a profound influence on the central nervous system, helping to reduce or eliminate pain, release muscle tension and provide strong emotional uplift.

The chemical structure of an essential oil is such that it can rapidly penetrate cell membranes, travel throughout the blood and tissues, and enhance cellular function. For those health professionals who have worked regularly with quality essential oils on patients, it has become very clear that there is a powerful life force inherent in these substances, which gives them an unmatched ability to communicate and interact with cells in the human body.

For many there is no doubt that essential oils are ordained as medicines for mankind and will provide critical medical solutions in the future. They could very well be the missing link of modern health care, bringing allopathic and holistic practice together for optimal health in the 21st century.

Healthy-minded people the world over have learned the value of using high quality natural herbs. Interestingly, most therapeutic herbs can be distilled into an essential oil. The key difference is one of concentration. The essential oil can be from 100 to 10,000 times more concentrated – and therefore more potent – than the herb itself.

Even though they are many times more potent than natural herbs, essential oils--unlike prescription drugs--very rarely generate any negative side effects. This carries profound implications for those wanting to maintain or regain their health quickly AND naturally.

Sometimes the effects of administering essential oils are so dramatic that the patients themselves call it "miraculous." And while no one fully understands yet 'why' or 'how' essential oils provide such significant benefits, the fact is that they do. With pure essential oils, millions of people can find relief from disease, from infections, from pain, and even from mental difficulties. Their therapeutic potential is enormous and is only just beginning to be tapped.

Acknowledgments

We wish to acknowledge D. Gary Young, ND, for his tremendous contribution to the rebirth of essential oils in North America. One of the pioneers in researching, cultivating, and distilling essential oils in North America, he has spent decades conducting clinical research on the ability of essential oils to combat disease and improve health. He has also developed new methods of application from which thousands of people have benefitted, especially his integration of therapeutic-grade essential oils with dietary supplements and personal care products. He is certainly one of the first, if not the first, to create these types of quality products.

Growing up as a farmer and rancher in Idaho, Gary developed a passion for the land, that has driven him to become one of the leading organic growers and distillers of essential oils in North America. With over 2,000 acres of land under cultivation in the US and Europe, he has set new standards for excellence that are redefining how therapeutic-grade essential oils are produced.

Gary's long experience as a grower, distiller, researcher, and alternative care practitioner not only gives him an unsurpassed insight into essential oils but also makes him an ideal spokespersona and educator on therapeutic properties of essential oils. Gary regularly travels throughout the world lecturing on the powerful potential of essential oils and how to produce therapeutic-grade essential oils that can consistently deliver results.

Much of the material contained in this book is derived from his research, lectures, and workshops, as well as the work of other practitioners and physicians who are at the forefront of understanding the clinical potential of essential oils to treat disease. To these researchers, the publisher is deeply indebted.

1

Essential Oils: The Missing Link in Modern Medicine

Yesterday's Wisdom, Tomorrow's Destiny

Plants not only play a vital role in the ecological balance of our planet, but they have also been intimately linked to the physical, emotional, and spiritual well-being of people since the beginning of time.

The plant kingdom continues to be the subject of an enormous amount of research and discovery. At least 30 percent of prescription drugs in the United States are based on naturally occurring compounds from plants. Each year, millions of dollars are allocated to universities searching for new therapeutic agents that lie undiscovered in the bark, roots, flowers, seeds, and foliage of jungle canopies, river bottoms, forests, hillsides, and vast wilderness regions throughout the world.

As the most powerful part of the plant, essential oils and plant extracts have been woven into history since time immemorial. Essential oils have been used medicinally to kill bacteria, fungi, and viruses. They provide exquisite fragrances to balance mood, lift spirits, dispel negative emotions, and create a romantic atmosphere. They can stimulate the regeneration of tissue or stimulate nerves. They can even carry nutrients to, and oxygenate the cells.

What Is an Essential Oil?

Essential oils are aromatic volatile liquids distilled from shrubs, flowers, trees, roots, bushes, and seeds.

The chemistry of essential oils is very complex: each one may consist of hundreds of different and unique chemical compounds. Moreover, essential oils are highly concentrated and far more potent than dried herbs. The distillation process is what makes essential oils so concentrated. It often requires an entire plant or more to produce a single drop of distilled essential oil.

Essential oils are also different from vegetable oils such as corn oil, peanut oil, and olive oil. They are not greasy and do not clog the pores like many vegetable oils can.

Vegetable oils can become oxidized and rancid over time and are not antibacterial. Most essential oils, on the other hand, cannot go rancid and are powerful antimicrobials. Pressed oils and essential oils high in plant waxes such as patchouli, if not distilled properly, could go rancid after time, particularly if exposed to heat for extended periods of time.

Essential oils are substances that definitely deserve the respect of proper education. Users need to be fully versed in the chemistry and safety of the oils. However, this knowledge is not being taught at universities in the United States. There is a disturbing lack of institutional information, knowledge, and training on essential oils and the scientific approach to aromatherapy. Only in the Middle East, the Orient, and Europe, with their far longer history of using natural products and botanical extracts, can one obtain adequate instruction on the chemistry and therapy of essential oils.

The European communities have a tight framework of controls and standards concerning botanical extracts and who may administer them. Only practitioners with proper training and certification can practice aromatherapy. However, in the United States, the regulatory agencies have not recognized these disciplines or mandated the type and degree of training required to distribute and apply essential oils. This means that in the U.S. individuals can bill themselves as "aromatherapists" after a brief class in essential oils, and apply oils to people—even though they may not have the experience or training to properly understand and administer them. This may not only undermine and damage the credibility of the entire discipline of aromatherapy, but it can be dangerous to patients.

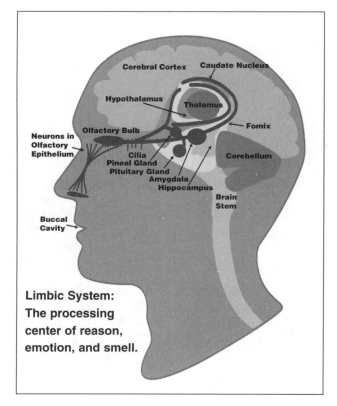

Cerebral Cortex
Caudate Nucleus
Hypothalamus
Thalamus
Olfactory Bulb
Fomix
Neurons in Olfactory Epithelium
Cilia
Cerebellum
Pineal Gland
Pituitary Gland
Amygdala
Hippocampus
Brain Stem
Buccal Cavity

Limbic System: The processing center of reason, emotion, and smell.

Essential oils are not simple substances. They are mosaics of hundreds—or even thousands—of different chemicals. Any given essential oil may contain anywhere from 80 to 300 or more different chemical constituents. An essential oil like lavender is very complex with many of its constituents occurring in minute quantities—but all contributing to the oil's therapeutic effects to some degree. To understand these constituents and their functions requires years of study.

Even though an essential oil may be labeled as "basil" and have the botanical name Ocimum basilicum, it can have widely different therapeutic actions, depending on its chemistry. For example, basil high in linalool or fenchol is primarily used for its antiseptic properties. However, basil high in methyl chavicol is more anti-inflammatory than antiseptic. A third type, basil high in eugenol, has both anti-inflammatory and antiseptic effects.

Additionally, essential oils can be distilled or extracted in different ways that have dramatic effects on their chemistry and medicinal action. Oils derived from a second or third distillation of the same plant material are obviously not going to be as potent as oils extracted during the first distillation. Also, oils that are subjected to high heat and pressure have a distinctly simpler (and inferior) profile of chemical

constituents, since excessive heat and temperature fractures and breaks down many of the delicate aromatic compounds within the oil—some of which are responsible for its therapeutic action. In addition, oils that are steam distilled are far different from those that are solvent extracted.

Of greatest concern is the fact that some oils are adulterated, engineered, or "extended" with the use of synthetic chemicals. For example, pure frankincense is often extended with colorless, odorless solvents such as diethylphthalate or dipropylene glycol. The only way to distinguish the "authentic" from the "adulterated" is to subject the essential oil to rigorous analytical testing using state-of-the-art gas chromatography, mass spectroscopy, and NMR (nuclear magnetic resonance).

However, even gas chromatography doesn't identify a natural chemical from a synthetic one. That is why it is very easy to engineer oils or extend poor quality oils to make them smell and look good.

Unfortunately, a large percentage of essential oils marketed in the United States fall in this adulterated category. When you understand the world of synthetic oils as well as low-grade oils cut with synthetic chemicals, you realize why unsuspecting people with their untrained noses don't know the difference.

Different Schools of Application

Therapeutic treatment using essential oils follows three different models or frameworks: French, German, and English.

The English model advocates diluting a small amount of essential oil in a vegetable oil and massaging the body for the purpose of relaxation and relieving stress.

The French model prescribes the ingestion and neat (undiluted) topical application of therapeutic-grade essential oils. A common form of internal use is to add a few drops of an essential oil to blue agave nectar or honey, a piece of bread, or a small amount of vegetable oil. Many French practitioners have found that taking the oils internally yields excellent benefits.

The German model focuses on inhalation of essential oils. Research has shown that the effect of fragrance and aromatic compounds on the sense of smell can exert strong effects on the brain—

especially on the hypothalamus (the hormone command center of the body) and limbic system (the seat of emotions). Some essential oils high in sesquiterpenes, such as myrrh, sandalwood, cedarwood, vetiver, melissa, and frankincense, can dramatically increase oxygenation and activity in the brain. This may directly improve the function of many systems of the body.

Together, these three models show how versatile and powerful essential oils can be. By integrating all three models with Vita Flex, auricular technique, touch therapy, spinal touch, lymphatic massage, and Raindrop Technique, the best possible results may be obtained.

In some cases, inhalation of essential oils might be preferred over topical application, if the goal is to increase growth hormone secretion, induce weight loss, or balance mood and emotions. Sandalwood, peppermint, vetiver, lavender, and white fir oils are effective for inhalation.

In other cases, however, topical application of essential oils would produce better results, particularly in the case of spinal or muscle injuries or defects. Topically applied, marjoram is excellent for muscles, lemongrass for ligaments, and wintergreen for bones. For indigestion, a drop or two of peppermint oil taken orally may be very effective. However, this does not mean that peppermint cannot produce the same results when massaged on the stomach. In some cases, all three methods of application (topical, inhalation, and ingestion) are interchangeable and may produce similar benefits.

The ability of essential oils to act on both the mind and the body is what makes them truly unique among natural therapeutic agents. The fragrance of some essential oils can be very stimulating—both psychologically and physically. The fragrance of other essential oils may be calming and sedating, helping to overcome anxiety or hyperactivity. On a physiological level, essential oils may stimulate immune function and regenerate damaged tissue. Essential oils may also combat infectious disease by killing viruses, bacteria, and other pathogens.

Probably the two most common methods of essential oil application are cold-air diffusing and neat (undiluted) topical application. Other modes of application include incorporating essential oils into the disciplines of reflexology, Vita Flex, and acu-pressure. Combining these disciplines with essential oils enhances the healing response and often produces amazing results that can not be achieved by acupuncture or reflexology alone. Just 1–3 drops of an essential oil applied to an acupuncture meridian or Vita Flex point on the hand or foot can produce results within a minute or two.

Several years ago at a university in Europe, a professor well known in the field of aromatherapy commented that anyone who claims to cure diseases using essential oils is a quack. However, there are many people who are living proof that essential oils can be used to engineer recoveries from serious illness. Essential oils have been pivotal in helping many people live pain-free after years of intense pain. Patients have also witnessed firsthand how essential oils have corrected scoliosis and even restored hearing in those who were born deaf.

For example, a woman from Palisades Park, California, developed scoliosis after surviving polio as a teenager, which was further complicated by a serious fall and a dislocated shoulder. Suffering pain and immobility for 22 years, she had traveled extensively in a fruitless search to locate a practitioner who could permanently reset her shoulder. Upon learning about essential oils, she topically applied the oils of helichrysum and wintergreen, among others, to the shoulder. Within a short time she became pain free as the shoulder relocated. She was able to raise her arm over her head for the first time in 22 years.

When one sees such dramatic recoveries, it is difficult to discredit the value and the power of essential oils and the potential they hold.

Mankind's First Medicine

For many centuries essential oils and other aromatics were used for religious rituals, the treatment of illness, and other physical and spiritual needs.

Records dating back to 4500 BC describe the use of balsamic substances with aromatic properties for religious rituals and medical applications. Ancient writings tell of scented barks, resins, spices, and aromatic vinegars, wines, and beers that were used in rituals, temples, astrology, embalming, and medicine. The evidence suggests that the people of ancient times had a greater understanding of essential oils than we have today.

The Egyptians were masters in using essential oils and other aromatics in the embalming process. Historical records describe how one of the founders of "pharaonic" medicine was the architect Imhotep, who was the Grand Vizier of King Djoser (2780 - 2720 BC). Imhotep is often given credit for ushering in the use of oils, herbs, and aromatic plants for medicinal purposes.

Many hieroglyphics on the walls of Egyptian temples depict the blending of oils and describe hundreds of oil recipes.

An ancient papyrus found in the Temple of Edfu contained medicinal formulae and perfume recipes used by alchemists and high priests in blending aromatic substances for rituals.

The Egyptians may have been the first to discover the potential of fragrance. They created various aromatic blends for both personal use and for ceremonies performed in the temples and pyramids.

Well before the time of Christ, the ancient Egyptians collected essential oils and placed them in alabaster vessels. These vessels were specially carved and shaped for housing scented oils. In 1922, when King Tut's tomb was opened, some 50 alabaster jars designed to hold 350 liters of oils were discovered. Tomb robbers had stolen nearly all of the precious oils leaving the heavy jars behind. Some of them still contained oil traces. The robbers chose oils over a literal king's ransom in gold, showing how valuable the fragrant essential oils were to this ancient civilization.

In 1817 the Ebers Papyrus, a medical scroll over 870 feet long, was discovered. Dating back to 1500 BC, the scroll included over 800 different herbal prescriptions and remedies. Other scrolls described a high success rate in treating 81 different diseases. Many of the remedies contained myrrh and honey. Myrrh is still recognized for its ability to help with infections of the skin and throat and to regenerate skin tissue. Because of its effectiveness in preventing bacterial growth, myrrh was used for embalming.

The physicians of Ionia, Attia, and Crete (ancient civilizations based in the Mediterranean Sea) came to the cities of the Nile to increase their knowledge. At this time, the school of Cos was founded and was attended by Hippocrates (460-377 BC), whom the Greeks, with perhaps some exaggeration, named the "Father of Medicine."

The Romans purified their temples and political buildings by diffusing essential oils. They also used aromatics in their steam baths to both invigorate the flesh and ward off disease.

Early History of Essential Oil Extraction

Ancient cultures found that aromatic essences or oils could be extracted from the plant by a variety of methods. One of the oldest and crudest forms of extraction was known as enfleurage. Raw plant material (usually stems, foliage, bark, or roots) was crushed and mixed with olive oil or animal fat. Other vegetable oils were also used. In the case of cedar, for example, the bark was stripped from the trunk and branches, ground into a powder, soaked with olive oil, and placed in a wool cloth. The cloth was then heated. The heat pulled the essential oil out of the bark particles into the olive oil, and the wool was pressed to extract the essential oil. Sandalwood oil was also extracted in this fashion.

Enfleurage was also used to extract essential oils from flower petals. In fact, the French word enfleurage means literally "to saturate with the perfume of flowers." For example, petals from roses or jasmine were placed in goose or goat fat. The essential oil molecules were pulled from the petals into the fat, which was then processed to separate the essential oils from the fat. This ancient technique was among the most primitive forms of essential oil extraction.

Other extraction techniques were also used. Some of these included:
• Soaking plant parts in boiling water
• Cold-pressing
• Soaking in alcohol
• Steam distillation by passing steam through the plant material and condensing the steam to separate the oil from the plant.

Many ancient cosmetic formulas were created from a base of goat fat. Ancient Egyptians formulated eyeliners, eyeshadows, and other cosmetics this way. They also stained their hair and nails with a variety of ointments and perfumes. They probably used the same aromatic oils that were used in the temples. Such temple oils were commonly poured into evaporation dishes for fragrancing the chambers associated with sacred rituals and religious rites.

Fragrance "cones" made of wax and fragrant essential oils were worn by aristocratic Egyptian women who enjoyed the oils' rich scents as the cones melted with the heat of the day.

Ancient Arabians were another early culture that developed and refined a process of distillation. They perfected the extraction of rose oils and rose water, which were popular in the Middle East during the Byzantine Empire (330 AD - 1400 AD).

Biblical and Ancient References to Essential Oils

There are over 200 references to aromatics, incense, and ointments throughout the Old and New Testaments of the Bible. Aromatics such as frankincense, myrrh, galbanum, cinnamon, cassia, rosemary, hyssop, and spikenard were used for anointing and healing the sick. In Exodus, the Lord gave the following recipe to Moses for a holy anointing oil:

Myrrh	"five hundred shekels" (about 1 gallon)
Cinnamon	"two hundred and fifty shekels"
Calamus	"two hundred and fifty shekels"
Cassia	"five hundred shekels"
Olive Oil	"an hin" (about 1 1/3 gallons)

Psalms 133:2 speaks of the sweetness of brethren dwelling together in unity: "It is like the precious ointment upon the head, that ran down the beard, even Aaron's beard: that went down to the skirts of his garments." Another scripture that refers to anointing and the overflowing abundance of precious oils is Ecclesiastes 9:8: "Let thy garments be always white; and let thy head lack no ointment."

The Bible also lists an incident where an incense offering by Aaron stopped a plague. Numbers 16:46-50 records that Moses instructed Aaron to take a censer, add burning coals and incense, and to "go quickly into the congregation to make an atonement for them: for there is a wrath gone out from the Lord; the plague is begun." The Bible records that Aaron stood between the dead and the living and the plague was stayed. It is significant that according to the biblical and Talmudic recipes for incense, three varieties of cinnamon were involved. Cinnamon is known to be highly antimicrobial, anti-infectious, and antibacterial. The incense ingredient listed as "stacte" is believed to be a sweet, myrrh-related spice, which would make it anti-infectious and antiviral as well.

The New Testament records that wise men presented the Christ child with frankincense and myrrh. There is another precious aromatic, spikenard, described in the anointing of Jesus:

And being in Bethany in the house of Simon the leper, as he sat at meat, there came a woman having an alabaster box of ointment of spikenard very precious; and she brake the box, and poured it on his head. Mark 14:3.

The anointing of Jesus is also referred to in John 12:3:

Then took Mary a pound of ointment of spikenard, very costly, and anointed the feet of Jesus, and wiped his feet with her hair: and the house was filled with the odour of the ointment.

Other Historical References

Throughout world history, fragrant oils and spices have played a prominent role in everyday life.

Napoleon is reported to have enjoyed a cologne water made of neroli and other ingredients so much that he ordered 162 bottles of it. After conquering Jerusalem, one of the things the Crusaders brought back to Europe was solidified essence of roses.

The 12th century mystic, Hildegard of Bingen, used herbs and oils extensively in healing. This Benedictine nun founded her own convent and was the author of numerous works. Her book, Physica, has more than 200 chapters on plants and their uses for healing.

The Rediscovery

The reintroduction of essential oils into modern medicine first began during the late 19th and early 20th centuries.

During World War I, the use of aromatic essences in civilian and military hospitals became widespread. One physician in France, Dr. Moncière, used essential oils extensively for their antibacterial and wound-healing properties, and developed several kinds of aromatic ointments.

René-Maurice Gattefossé, PhD, a French cosmetic chemist, is widely regarded as the father of aromatherapy. He and a group of scientists began studying essential oils in 1907.

In his 1937 book, Aromatherapy, Dr. Gattefossé told the real story of his now-famous use of lavender essential oil to heal a serious burn. The tale has assumed mythic proportions in essential oil literature. His own words about this accident are even more powerful than what has been told over the years.

Dr. Gattefossé was literally aflame—covered in burning substances—following a laboratory explosion in July, 1910. After he extinguished the flames by rolling on a grassy lawn, he wrote that "both my hands were covered with rapidly developing gas gangrene." He further reported that, "just one rinse with lavender essence stopped the gasification of the tissue. This treatment was followed by profuse sweating and healing which began the next day."

Robert B. Tisserand, editor of The International Journal of Aromatherapy, searched for Dr. Gattefossé's book for 20 years. A copy was located and Tisserand edited the 1995 reprint. Tisserand noted that Dr. Gattefossé's burns "must have been severe to lead to gas gangrene, a very serious infection."

Dr. Gattefossé shared his studies with his colleague and friend, Jean Valnet, a medical doctor practicing in Paris. Exhausting his supply of antibiotics as a physician in Tonkin, China, during World War II, Dr. Valnet began using therapeutic-grade essential oils on patients suffering battlefield injuries. To his surprise, they exerted a powerful effect in combating and counteracting infection. He was able to save the lives of many soldiers who might otherwise have died.

Two of Dr. Valnet's students, Dr. Paul Belaiche and Dr. Jean-Claude Lapraz, expanded his work. They clinically investigated the antiviral, antibacterial, antifungal, and antiseptic properties in essential oils.

Because of the work of these doctors and scientists, the healing power of essential oils is again gaining prominence.

Today, it has become evident that we have not yet found permanent solutions for dreaded diseases such as the Ebola virus, hanta virus, AIDS, HIV, and new strains of tuberculosis and influenza. Essential oils may assume an increasingly important role in combating new mutations of bacteria, viruses, and fungi. More and more researchers are undertaking serious clinical studies on the use of essential oils to combat these types of diseases.

Research conducted at Weber State University in cooperation with D. Gary Young as well as other documented research, indicates that most viruses, fungi, and bacteria cannot live in the presence of many essential oils, especially those high in phenols, carvacrol, thymol, and terpenes. This, perhaps, offers a modern explanation why the Old Testament prophet Moses used aromatic substances to protect the Israelites from the plagues that decimated ancient Egypt. It may also help us understand why a notorious group of thieves, reputed to be spice traders and perfumers, was protected from the Black Plague as they robbed the bodies of the dead during the 15th century.

A vast body of anecdotal evidence (testimonials) suggests that those who use essential oils are less likely to contract infectious diseases. Moreover, oil users who do contract an infectious illness tend to recover faster than those using antibiotics.

2

How Do Essential Oils Work?

Therapeutic-Grade Essential Oils

One of the factors that determines the purity of an oil is its chemical constituents. These constituents can be affected by a vast number of variables, including: the part(s) of the plant from which the oil was produced, soil condition, fertilizer (organic or chemical), geographical region, climate, altitude, harvesting methods, and distillation processes. For example, common thyme (Thymus vulgaris) produces several different chemotypes (biochemically unique variants within one species) depending on the conditions of its growth, climate, and altitude. One chemotype of thyme will yield an essential oil with high levels of thymol, depending on the time of year it is distilled. The later it is distilled in the growing season (ie., mid-summer or fall), the more thymol the oil will contain.

Proper cultivation assures that more specific chemotypes like Thymus vulgaris will maintain a good strain of thymol, where as with wildcrafting, you may produce linalol and eugenol thyme on the same mountainside.

An example of this was shown in studies at the University of Ege botany department in Izmir, Turkey where it was found that among Oreganum compactum plants within a 100 square foot radius, one plant would be very high in carvacrol and another would be high in another compound. Wildcrafting plants cannot guarantee the same chemotype even on the same hillside.

The key to producing a therapeutic-grade essential oil is to preserve as many of the delicate aromatic compounds within the essential oil as possible. Fragile aromatic chemicals are easily destroyed by high temperature and pressure, as well as contact with chemically reactive metals such as copper or aluminum. This is why all therapeutic-grade essential oils should be distilled in stainless steel cooking chambers at low pressure and low temperature.

The plant material should also be free of herbicides and other agrichemicals. These can react with the essential oil during distillation to produce toxic compounds. Because many pesticides are oil-soluble, they can also mix into the essential oil.

As we begin to understand the power of essential oils in the realm of personal, holistic healthcare, we will appreciate the necessity for obtaining the purest essential oils possible. No matter how costly pure essential oils may be, there can be no substitutes.

Although chemists have successfully recreated the main constituents and fragrances of some essential oils in the laboratory, these synthetic oils lack therapeutic benefits and may even carry risks. Why? Because essential oils contain hundreds of different chemical compounds, which, in combination, lend important therapeutic properties to the oil. Also, many essential oils contain molecules and isomers that are impossible to manufacture in the laboratory.

Anyone venturing into the world of therapy using essential oils must use the purest quality oils available. Inferior quality or adulterated oils most likely will not produce therapeutic results and could possibly be toxic. In Europe, a set of standards has been established that outlines the chemical profile and principal constituents that a quality essential oil should have. Known as AFNOR (Association French Normalization Organization Regulation) and ISO (International Standards Organization) standards, these guidelines help buyers differentiate between a therapeutic-grade essential oil and a lower grade oil with a similar chemical makeup and fragrance. **All of the therapeutic effects of the essential oils in this book are based on oils that have been graded according to AFNOR standards.**

Science and Application

Essential oils and human blood share several common properties: They fight infection, contain hormone-like compounds, and initiate regeneration. Working as the chemical defense mechanism of the plant, essential oils possess potent antibacterial, antifungal, and antiviral properties. They also ward off attacks by insects and animals. The ability of some essential oils to work as hormones helps them bring balance to many physiological systems of the human body. Oils like clary sage and sage that contain sclerol, for example, have an estrogenic action. Essential oils also play a role in initiating the regeneration process for the plant, the same way the blood does in the human body.

This similarity goes even deeper. Essential oils have a chemical structure that is similar to that found in human cells and tissues. This makes essential oils compatible with human protein and enables them to be readily identified and accepted by the body.

Essential oils have a unique ability to penetrate cell membranes and diffuse throughout the blood and tissues. The unique, lipid-soluble structure of essential oils is very similar to the makeup of our cell membranes. The molecules of essential oils are also relatively small, which enhances their ability to penetrate into the cells. When topically applied to the feet or elsewhere, essential oils can travel throughout the body in a matter of minutes.

The ability of some essential oils, like clove, to decrease the viscosity or thickness of the blood can also enhance circulation and immune function. Adequate circulation is vital to good health, since it affects the function of every cell and organ, including the brain.

Research indicates that when essential oils are diffused, they can increase atmospheric oxygen and provide negative ions, which in turn inhibits bacterial growth. This suggests that essential oils could play an important role in air purification and neutralizing odors. Because of their ionizing action, essential oils have the ability to break down potentially harmful chemicals and render them nontoxic.

In the human body, essential oils stimulate the secretion of antibodies, neurotransmitters, endorphins, hormones, and enzymes. Oils containing limonene have been shown to prevent and slow the progression of cancer. Other oils, like lavender, have

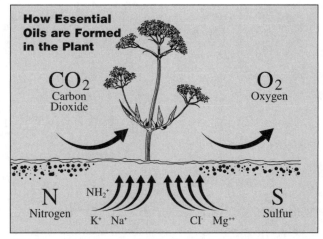

How Essential Oils are Formed in the Plant

CO_2 Carbon Dioxide

O_2 Oxygen

N Nitrogen NH_2^+ K^+ Na^+ Cl^- Mg^{++} S Sulfur

Minerals and carbons are combined with nitrogen in the soil to form amino acids in the plant. These amino acids form proteins that contribute to essential oil formation. Essential oils and amino acids like phenylalanine share a similar aromatic structure.

been shown to promote the growth of hair and increase the rate of wound healing. They increase the uptake of oxygen and ATP (adenosine triphosphate), the fuel for individual cells.

European scientists have studied the ability of essential oils to work as natural chelators, binding with heavy metals and petrochemicals and ferrying them out of the body.

Today approximately 300 essential oils are distilled or extracted, with several thousand chemical constituents and aromatic molecules identified and registered. The quantity, quality, and type of these aromatic compounds will vary depending on climate, temperature, and distillation factors. Ninety-eight percent of essential oils produced today are used in the perfume and cosmetic industry. Only about 2 percent are produced for therapeutic and medicinal applications.

Because essential oils are composites of hundreds of different chemicals, they can exert many different effects on the body. For example, clove oil can be simultaneously antiseptic and anaesthetic when applied topically. It can also be antitumoral. Lavender oil has been used for burns, insect bites, headaches, PMS, insomnia, stress, and hair growth.

Importantly, because of their complexity, essential oils do not disturb the body's natural balance or homeostasis: if one constituent exerts too strong an effect, another constituent may block or counteract it. Synthetic chemicals, in contrast, usually have only one action and often disrupt the body's homeostasis.

Using European AFNOR/ISO Standards to Identify Therapeutic-Grade Oils

As previously mentioned, one of the most reliable indicators of essential oil quality is the AFNOR (Association French Normalization Organization Regulation) or ISO certification (ISO is the International Standards Organization which has set standards for therapeutic-grade essential oils adopted from AFNOR). This standard is more stringent and differentiates true therapeutic-grade essential oils from similar oils with inferior chemistry (For more information, see Appendix A).

The AFNOR standard was written by a team headed up by the government-certified botanical chemist Hervé Casabianca, PhD, while working with several analytical laboratories throughout France.

Dr. Casabianca recognized that the primary constituents within an essential oil had to occur in certain percentages in order for the oil to be considered therapeutic. He combined his studies with research conducted by other scientists and doctors, including the Central Service Analysis Laboratory certified by the French government for essential oil analysis.

As a result, many oils that are listed as therapeutic-grade such as frankincense or lavender, can be checked to see if they do indeed meet AFNOR standards. If some constituents are too high or too low, the oils cannot be certified.

For example, the AFNOR standard for Lavandula angustifolia (true lavender) dictates that the level of linalool should range from 25 to 38 percent and the level of linalyl acetate should range between 25 and 34 percent. As long as the oil's marker compounds are within the specified ranges, it can be recognized as a therapeutic-grade essential oil.

As a general rule, if two or more marker compounds in an essential oil fall outside the prescribed percentages, the oil does not meet the AFNOR standard. It cannot be recognized as therapeutic-grade essential oil, even though it is still of relatively high quality.

What distinguishes a therapeutic-grade essential oil from an essential oil that is not therapeutic-grade or AFNOR-certified? A lavender oil produced in one region of France might have a slightly different chemistry than that grown in another region and as a result may not meet the standard. It may have

excessive camphor levels (1.0 instead of 0.5), a condition that might be caused by distilling lavender that was too green. Or the levels of lavandulol may be too low due to certain weather conditions at the time of harvest.

By comparing the gas chromatograph chemistry profile of a lavender essential oil with the AFNOR standard, you may also distinguish true lavender from various species of lavandin (hybrid lavender). Usually lavandin has high camphor levels, almost no lavandulol, and is easily identified. However, Tasmania produces a lavandin that yields an essential oil with naturally low camphor levels that mimics the chemistry of true lavender. Only by analyzing the chemical fingerprint of this Tasmanian lavandin using high resolution gas chromatography and comparing it with the AFNOR standard for genuine lavender can this hybrid lavender be identified.

Currently, there is no agency responsible for certifying that an essential oil is therapeutic grade. The only indication for a therapeutic-grade oil is if it meets AFNOR or ISO standards. **The therapeutic effects discussed in this book can only be achieved using essential oils which meet the AFNOR standards.**

In the United States, few companies use the proper analytical equipment and methods to properly analyze essential oils. Most labs use equipment best-suited for synthetic chemicals—not for natural essential oil analysis. Young Living Essential Oils uses the proper machinery and has made serious efforts to adopt the European testing standards, widely regarded as the "gold standard" for testing essential oils. In addition to operating its analytical equipment on the same standard as the European-certified laboratories, Young Living is continually expanding its analytical chemical library in order to perform more thorough chemical analysis.

Properly analyzing an essential oil by gas chromatography is a complex undertaking. The injection mixture, column diameter and length, and oven temperature must fall within certain parameters. Unless someone has gone to France and Turkey as Gary Young has and been trained in the analytical procedures of a gas chromatograph, they will not understand how to accurately test essential oils.

The column length should be at least 50 or 60 meters. However, almost all labs in the United States use a 30-meter column that is not long enough to achieve proper separation of all the

9

essential oil constituents. While 30-meter columns are adequate for analyzing synthetic chemicals and marker compounds in vitamins, minerals, and herbal extracts, they are far too short to properly analyze the complex mosaic of natural chemicals found in an essential oil.

A longer column also enables double-phased ramping, which makes it possible to identify constituents that occur in very small percentages by increasing the separation of compounds. Without a longer column, it would be extremely difficult to identify these molecules, especially if they are chemically similar to each other or a marker compound.

While gas chromatography (GC) is an excellent tool for dissecting the anatomy of an essential oil, it does have limitations. Dr. Brian Lawrence, one of the foremost experts on essential oil chemistry, has commented that sometimes it can be difficult to distinguish between natural and synthetic compounds using GC analysis. If synthetic linalyl acetate is added to pure lavender, a GC analysis cannot really tell whether that compound is synthetic or natural, only that it is linalyl acetate. Adding a chiral column can help, however, in distinguishing between synthetic and natural oils. This addition allows the chemist to identify structural varieties of the same compound.

This is why oils must be analyzed by a chemist specially trained on the interpretation of a gas chromatograph chart. The chemist examines the entire chemical fingerprint of the oil to determine its purity and potency, measuring how various compounds in the oil occur in relation to each other. If some chemicals occur in higher quantities than others, these provide important clues to determine if the oil is adulterated or pure.

Adulteration is such a major concern that every batch of essential oil that comes into Young Living must be tested at either Central Service Laboratory or the Albert Vieille Laboratory, both AFNOR-certified laboratories, by chemists licensed to test therapeutic-grade essential oils. Batches that do not meet the standards are rejected and returned.

Adulteration of essential oils will become more and more common as the supply of top-quality essential oils dwindles and demand continues to increase. These adulterated essential oils will jeopardize the integrity of aromatherapy in the United States and may put many people at risk.

Adulterated Oils and Their Dangers

Today much of the lavender oil sold in America is the hybrid called lavandin, grown and distilled in China, Russia, France, and Tasmania. It is brought into France and cut with synthetic linalyl acetate to improve the fragrance. Then propylene glycol, DEP, or DOP (solvents that have no smell and increase the volume) are added and it is sold in the United States as lavender oil.

Often lavandin is heated to evaporate the camphor and then is adulterated with synthetic linalyl acetate. Most consumers don't know the difference, and are happy to buy it for $7 to $10 per half ounce in health food stores, beauty salons, grocery and department stores, and through mail order. This is one of the reasons why it is important to know about the integrity of the company or vendor from which you purchase your essential oils.

Frankincense is another example of a commonly adulterated oil. The frankincense resin that is sold in Somalia costs between $30,000 and $35,000 per ton. A great deal of time--12 hours or more--is required to properly steam-distill this essential oil from the resin, making the oil very expensive. Frankincense oil that sells for $25 per ounce or less is cheaply distilled with gum resins, alcohol, or other solvents, leaving the essential oil laden with harmful chemicals. Sadly, when these cut, synthetic, and adulterated oils cause rashes, burns, or other irritations, people wonder why they do not get the benefit they expected and conclude that essential oils do not have much value.

Some commercial statistics show that one large, U.S. corporation uses twice as much of a particular essential oil as is naturally grown and produced in the entire world! Where are these "phantom" essential oils coming from?

In France, production of true lavender oil (Lavandula angustifolia) dropped from 87 tons in 1967 to only 12 tons in 1998. During this same period the worldwide demand for lavender oil grew over 100 percent. So where did essential oil marketers obtain enough lavender to meet the demand? They probably used a combination of synthetic and adulterated oils. There are huge chemical companies on the east coast of the U.S. that specialize in creating synthetic chemicals that mimic every common essential oil. For every kilogram of pure essential oil that is produced, it is estimated there are between 10 and 100 kilograms of synthetic oil created.

Adulterated and mislabeled essential oils present dangers for consumers. One woman who had heard of the ability of lavender oil to heal burns used "lavender oil" purchased from a local health food store when she spilled boiling water on her arm. But the pain intensified and the burn worsened, so she later complained that lavender oil was worthless for healing burns. When her "lavender" oil was analyzed, it was found to be lavandin, the hybrid lavender that is chemically very different from pure Lavandula angustifolia. Lavandin contains high levels of camphor (12-18 percent) and can itself burn the skin. In contrast, true lavender contains virtually no camphor and has burn-healing agents not found in lavandin.

Adulterated oils that are cut with synthetic extenders can be very detrimental, causing rashes, burning, and skin irritations. Petrochemical solvents, such dipropylene glycol and diethylphthalate, can all cause allergic reactions, besides being devoid of any therapeutic effects.

Some people assume that because an essential oil is "100 percent pure," it will not burn their skin. This is not true. Some pure essential oils may cause skin irritation if applied undiluted. If you apply straight oregano oil to the skin of some people, it may cause severe reddening. Citrus and spice oils, like orange and cinnamon, may also produce rashes. Even the terpenes in conifer oils, like pine, may cause skin irritation on sensitive people.

Some writers have claimed that a few compounds, when isolated from the essential oil and tested in the lab, can exert toxic effects. Even so-called "nature-identical" essential oils (structured essential oils that have been chemically duplicated using 5 to 15 of the essential oil's primary chemical compounds in synthetic form) can produce unwanted side effects or toxicities. Isolated compounds may be toxic; however pure essential oils, in most cases, are not. This is because natural essential oils contain hundreds of different compounds, some of which balance and counteract each other's effects.

Many tourists in Egypt are eager to buy local essential oils, especially lotus oil. Vendors convince the tourists that the oils are 100 percent pure, going so far as to touch a lighted match to the neck of the oil container to show that the oil is not diluted with alcohol or other petrochemical solvents. However, this test provides no reliable indicator of purity.

Many synthetic compounds can be added to an essential oil that are not flammable, including propylene glycol. Or, flammable solvents can be added to a vegetable oil base that will cause it to catch fire. Some natural essential oils high in terpenes can be flammable.

Fact or Fiction: Myths and Misinformation

Much of the published information available on essential oils should be regarded with caution. Many aromatherapy books are merely compilations of two or three other books. The content is similar, only phrased and worded differently. Because the information has been copied from sources that have never been documented, the same misinformation repeatedly surfaces.

Many aromatherapy books claim that essential oils, such as clary sage, fennel, sage, and bergamot, can trigger an abortion. Several years ago, a rumor circulated about a laboratory research project in which the uterus of a rat was turned inside out and a cold drop of clary sage oil was applied to the exposed uterine wall. When this caused a contraction of the muscle, clary sage was labeled as abortion-causing. One must ask, what would have happened if cold water had been dropped on the exposed uterus? The uterine wall would likely have contracted in response. Following this reasoning, water could be labeled as abortion-causing as well.

The truth is that to our knowledge, there has never been a single documented case that clary sage, lemon, sage, or bergamot essential oils have caused an abortion. Sclareol, a compound in clary sage, is not an estrogen, although it can mimic estrogen if there is an estrogen deficiency. If there is not an estrogen deficiency, sclareol will not create more estrogen in the body. As a rule, essential oils bring balance to the human body.

The belief that pure essential oils will not leave a stain when poured on a tissue is also unfounded. Any essential oil high in waxes will leave stains. Oils like frankincense, cedarwood, clove, ylang ylang, blue cypress, or German chamomile may also leave a noticeable residue. However, an essential oil spiked with synthetic diluents or solvent may or may not leave a stain.

The Powerful Influence of Aromas on Both Mind and Body

The fragrance of an essential oil can directly affect everything from your emotional state to your lifespan.

When a fragrance is inhaled, the odor molecules travel up the nose where they are trapped by olfactory membranes that are well protected by the lining inside the nose. Each odor molecule fits like a little puzzle piece into specific receptor cell sites that line a membrane known as the olfactory epithelium. Each one of these hundreds of millions of nerve cells is replaced every 28 days. When stimulated by odor molecules, this lining of nerve cells triggers electrical impulses to the olfactory bulb in the brain. The olfactory bulb then transmits the impulses to the gustatory center (where the sensation of taste is perceived), the amygdala (where emotional memories are stored), and other parts of the limbic system of the brain. Because the limbic system is directly connected to those parts of the brain that control heart rate, blood pressure, breathing, memory, stress levels, and hormone balance, essential oils can have profound physiological and psychological effects.

The sense of smell is the only one of the five senses directly linked to the limbic lobe of the brain, the emotional control center. Anxiety, depression, fear, anger, and joy all emanate from this region. The scent of a special fragrance can evoke memories and emotions before we are even consciously aware of it. When smells are concerned, we react first and think later. All other senses (touch, taste, hearing, and sight) are routed through the thalamus, which acts as the switchboard for the brain, passing stimuli onto the cerebral cortex (the conscious thought center) and other parts of the brain.

The limbic lobe (a group of brain structures that includes the hippocampus and amygdala located below the cerebral cortex) can also directly activate the hypothalamus. The hypothalamus is one of the most important parts of the brain, acting as our hormonal control center. It releases chemical messengers that can affect everything from sex drive to energy levels. The production of growth hormones, sex hormones, thyroid hormones, and neurotransmitters such as serotonin, are all governed by the hypothalamus. Thus, the hypothalamus is referred to as the "master gland."

Essential oils—through their fragrance and unique molecular structure—can directly stimulate the limbic lobe and the hypothalamus. Not only can the inhalation of essential oils be used to combat stress and emotional trauma, but it can also stimulate the production of hormones from the hypothalamus. This results in increased thyroid hormones (our energy hormone) and growth hormones (our youth and longevity hormone).

Essential oils may also be used to reduce appetite and produce significant reductions in weight because of their ability to stimulate the ventromedial nucleus of the hypothalamus, a section of the brain that governs our feeling of satiety or fullness following meals. In a large clinical study,[1] Alan Hirsch, MD, used fragrances, including peppermint, to trigger significant weight losses in a large group of patients who had previously been unsuccessful in any type of weight-management program. During the course of the six-month study involving over 3,000 people, the average weight loss exceeded 30 pounds. According to Dr. Hirsch, some patients actually had to be dropped from the study to avoid becoming underweight.

Another double-blind, randomized study by Hirsch[2] documents the ability of aroma to enhance libido and sexual arousal. When 31 male volunteers were subjected to the aromas of 30 different essential oils, each one exhibited a marked increase in arousal, based on measurements of brachial penile index and the measurement of both penile and brachial blood pressures. Among the scents that produced the most sexual excitement, was a combination of lavender and pumpkin fragrances. This study shows that fragrances enhance sexual desire by stimulating the amygdala, the emotional center of the brain.

In 1989, Dr. Joseph Ledoux at New York Medical University discovered that the amygdala plays a major role in storing and releasing emotional trauma.[3] From the studies of Dr. Hirsch and Dr. Ledoux the conclusion can be drawn that aromas may exert a profound effect in triggering a response from this almond-shaped neuro-structure.

1. Hirsch, AR, Inhalation of Odorants for Weight Reduction, Int J Obes, 1994, page 306
2. Alan R. Hirsch, MD, FACP, Dr. Hirsch's Guide to Scentsational Sex, Harper Collins, 1998 1993 Dec. 20;58(1-2):69-79
3. LeDoux, JE, Rationalizing Thoughtless Emotions, Insight, Sept. 1989

In studies conducted at Vienna and Berlin Universities, researchers found that sesquiterpenes, found in essential oils such as vetiver, patchouli, cedarwood, sandalwood and frankincense, can increase levels of oxygen in the brain by up to 28 percent (Nasel, 1992). Such an increase in brain oxygen may lead to a heightened level of activity in the hypothalamus and limbic systems of the brain, which can have dramatic effects on not only emotions, learning, and attitude, but also many physical processes of the body, such as immune function, hormone balance, and energy levels. High levels of sesquiterpenes also occur in melissa, myrrh, cedarwood, and clove oil.

People who have undergone nose surgery or suffer olfactory impairment may find it difficult or impossible to detect a complete odor. The same is true of people who use makeup, perfume, cologne, hair sprays, hair coloring, perms, or other products containing synthetic odors. These people may not derive the full physiological and emotional benefits of essential oils and their fragrances.

Proper stimulation of the olfactory nerves may offer a powerful and entirely new form of therapy that could be used as an adjunct against many forms of illness. Essential oils, through inhalation, may occupy a key position in this relatively unexplored frontier in medicine.

Chemical Sensitivities and Allergies

Occasionally, individuals beginning to use quality essential oils will suffer rashes or allergic reactions. This may be due to using an undiluted spice, conifer, or citrus oil, or it may be caused by an interaction of the oil with residues of synthetic, petroleum-based personal care products that have leached into the skin.

When using essential oils on a daily basis, it is imperative to avoid personal care products containing ammonium or hydrocarbon-based chemicals. These include quaternary compounds such as quaternariums and polyquaternariums. These compounds are commonly found in a variety of hand creams, mouthwashes, shampoos, antiperspirants, after-shave lotions, and hair-care products. In small concentrations they can be toxic and present the possibility of reacting with essential oils and producing chemical byproducts of unknown toxicity.

These chemicals can be fatal if ingested, especially benzalkonium chloride, which unfortunately is used in many personal care products on the market.

Other compounds that present concerns are sodium lauryl sulfate, propylene glycol—extremely common in everything from toothpaste to shampoo—and aluminum salts found in many deodorants.

Of particular concern are the potentially hazardous preservatives and synthetic fragrances that abound in virtually all modern personal-care products. Some of these include methylene chloride, methyl isobutyl ketone, and methyl ethyl ketone. These are not only toxic, but they can also react with some compounds in natural essential oils. The result can be a severe case of dermatitis or even septicemia (blood poisoning).

A classic case of a synthetic fragrance causing widespread damage occurred in the 1970s. AETT (acetylethyltetramethyltetralin) appeared in numerous brands of personal care products throughout the United States. Even after a series of animal studies revealed that it caused significant brain and spinal cord damage, the FDA refused to ban the chemical. Finally, the cosmetic industry voluntarily withdrew AFTT after allowing it to be distributed for years. How many other toxins masquerading as preservatives or fragrances are currently being used in personal care products?

Many chemicals are easily absorbed through the skin due to its permeability. One study found that 13 percent of BHT (butylated hydroxytoluene) and 49 percent of DDT (a carcinogenic pesticide) can be absorbed into the skin upon topical contact (Steinman, 1997). Once absorbed, they can become trapped in the fatty subdermal layers of skin where they can leach into the blood stream. These chemicals can remain trapped in fatty tissues underneath the skin for several months or years, where they harbor the potential of reacting with essential oils that may be topically applied later. The user may mistakenly assume that the threat of an interaction between oils and synthetic cosmetics used months before is small. However, a case of dermatitis is a possibility.

3

The Chemistry of Essential Oils

Unlike synthetic chemicals, essential oil chemicals are diverse in their effects. No two oils are alike. Some constituents, such as aldehydes found in lavender and chamomile, are antimicrobial and calming. Eugenol, found in cinnamon and clove, is antiseptic and stimulating. Ketones, found in lavender, hyssop, and patchouli, stimulate cell regeneration and liquefy mucous. Phenols, found in oregano and thyme oil, are highly antimicrobial. Sesquiterpenes, predominant in vetiver, cedarwood, and sandalwood, are soothing to inflamed tissue and can also produce profound effects on emotions and hormonal balance.

The complex chemistry of essential oils makes them ideal for killing and preventing the spread of bacteria, since microorganisms have a difficult time mutating in the presence of so many different antiseptic compounds. At the March 2000 International Symposium in Grasse, France, Dr. Bérangere Arnal-Schnebelen presented a paper showing the antibacterial properties of essential oils against several infectious agents. Spanish oregano and cinnamon essential oils tested at above 95 percent efficiency against Candida albicans, E. coli, and a Streptococcus strain. This is significant as we face life-threatening, drug-resistant viruses and bacteria.

The essential oils of ravensara, melissa, oregano, mountain savory, clove, cumin, cistus, hyssop, and frankincense are highly antibacterial and contain immune supportive properties that have been documented by many researchers, such as Daniel Pénoël, MD and Pierre Franchomme. These oils are found in varying amounts in the immune support and antimicrobial essential blends presented later in this book (see Chapter 9).

Understanding Essential Oil Chemistry

Basic Chemical Structure

The aromatic constituents of essential oils (i.e. terpenes, monoterpenes, phenols, aldehydes, etc.) are constructed from long chains of carbon and hydrogen atoms, which have a predominantly ring-like chemical structure. Links of carbon atoms form the backbone of these chains, with oxygen, hydrogen, nitrogen, sulfur, and other carbon atoms attached at various points of the chain.

Essential oils are chemically different from fatty oils (also known as fatty acids). In contrast to the simple linear carbon-hydrogen structure of fatty oils, essential oils have a far more complex ring structure and contain sulfur and nitrogen atoms that fatty oils do not have.

The terpenoids found in many essential oils are actually constructed out of the same basic building block—a five-carbon molecule known as isoprene.

When two isoprene units link together, they create a monoterpene; when three join, they create a sesquiterpene; and so on. Some of the largest molecules found in essential oils are triterpenoids, which consist of 30 carbon atoms or six isoprene

Key Chemical Constituents in Essential Oils and Their Effects		
Constituent	**Representative Oil**	**Effect**
Ketones	Sage	mucolytic
Aldehydes	Lemongrass	calming
Esters	Lavender	balancing
Ethers	Tarragon	balancing
Alcohols	Ravensara	toning
Phenols	Savory	stimulant
Terpenes	Pine	stimulant

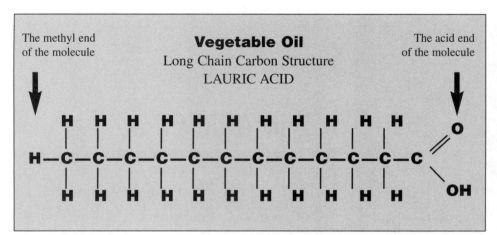

Vegetable Oil
Long Chain Carbon Structure
LAURIC ACID

The methyl end of the molecule

The acid end of the molecule

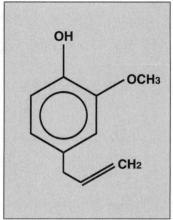

Eugenol—An aromatic molecule found in several essential oils including clove. Clove oil has been used as an antiseptic for many years.

units linked together. Carotenoids, which consist of 40 carbons or eight isoprene units, only occur in essential oils in tiny quantities because they are too heavy to be extracted via steam distillation.

Different molecules in an essential oil can exert different effects. For example, German chamomile (Matricaria recutita) contains azulene, a dark blue compound that has powerful anti-inflammatory compounds. German chamomile also contains bisobolol, a compound studied for its sedative and mood-balancing properties. There are other compounds in German chamomile that perform different functions, such as speeding up the regeneration process of tissue.

Chemotypes

A single species of plant can have several different chemotypes based on chemical composition. This means that basil (Ocimum basilicum) grown in one area might produce an essential oil with a completely different chemistry than a basil grown in another location. The plant's growing environment, such as soil pH and mineral content, can dramatically affect the plant's ultimate chemistry as well. Different chemotypes of basil are listed below:

Ocimum basilicum CT linalol fenchol
(Germany)
— antiseptic

Ocimum basilicum CT methyl chavicol
(Reunion, Comoro, or Egypt)
— anti-inflammatory

Ocimum basilicum CT eugenol (Madagascar)
— anti-inflammatory, pain-relieving

Another species of plant that occurs in a variety of different chemotypes is rosemary (Rosmarinus officinalis).

Rosmarinus officinalis CT camphor is obviously high in camphor. Camphor serves best as a general stimulant and works synergistically with other oils, such as pepper (Piper nigrum), and can be a powerful energy stimulant.

Rosmarinus officinalis CT cineol is rich in 1,8 cineol, which is used in other countries for pulmonary congestion and to help with the elimination of toxins from the liver and kidneys.

Rosmarinus officinalis CT verbenon is high in verbenon and is the most gentle of the rosemary chemotypes. It offers powerful regenerative properties and has outstanding benefits for skin care.

Thyme (Thymus vulgaris) also has several different chemotypes. Some of these are:

Thymus vulgaris CT thymol is germicidal and anti-inflammatory.

Thymus vulgaris CT linalool is anti-infectious.

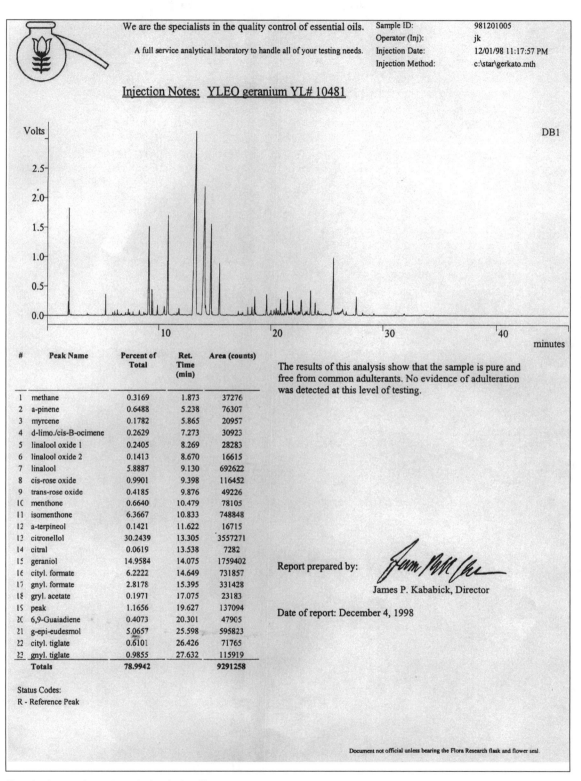

We are the specialists in the quality control of essential oils.

A full service analytical laboratory to handle all of your testing needs.

Sample ID:	981201005
Operator (Inj):	jk
Injection Date:	12/01/98 11:17:57 PM
Injection Method:	c:\star\gerkato.mth

Injection Notes: YLEO geranium YL# 10481

DB1

The results of this analysis show that the sample is pure and free from common adulterants. No evidence of adulteration was detected at this level of testing.

#	Peak Name	Percent of Total	Ret. Time (min)	Area (counts)
1	methane	0.3169	1.873	37276
2	a-pinene	0.6488	5.238	76307
3	myrcene	0.1782	5.865	20957
4	d-limo./cis-B-ocimene	0.2629	7.273	30923
5	linalool oxide 1	0.2405	8.269	28283
6	linalool oxide 2	0.1413	8.670	16615
7	linalool	5.8887	9.130	692622
8	cis-rose oxide	0.9901	9.398	116452
9	trans-rose oxide	0.4185	9.876	49226
10	menthone	0.6640	10.479	78105
11	isomenthone	6.3667	10.833	748848
12	a-terpineol	0.1421	11.622	16715
13	citronellol	30.2439	13.305	3557271
14	citral	0.0619	13.538	7282
15	geraniol	14.9584	14.075	1759402
16	cityl. formate	6.2222	14.649	731857
17	gnyl. formate	2.8178	15.395	331428
18	gryl. acetate	0.1971	17.075	23183
19	peak	1.1656	19.627	137094
20	6,9-Guaiadiene	0.4073	20.301	47905
21	g-epi-eudesmol	5.0657	25.598	595823
22	cityl. tiglate	0.6101	26.426	71765
23	gnyl. tiglate	0.9855	27.632	115919
	Totals	**78.9942**		**9291258**

Status Codes:
R - Reference Peak

Report prepared by:

James P. Kababick, Director

Date of report: December 4, 1998

Document not official unless bearing the Flora Research flask and flower seal.

Sample of a gas chromatograph chemical profile.

17

4

How to Safely Use Essential Oils

There are important guidelines to follow when using essential oils, especially if you are unfamiliar with the oils and their benefits. Many guidelines are listed below and are elaborated further throughout the chapter. However, no list of do's and don'ts can ever replace common sense. It is foolish to dive headlong into a pond when you don't know the depth of the water. The same is true when using essential oils. Start gradually, and patiently find what works best for you and your family members.

Basic Guidelines for Safe Use

1. Always keep a bottle of a pure vegetable oil handy when using essential oils. Vegetable oils dilute essential oils if they cause discomfort or skin irritation.

2. Keep bottles of essential oils tightly closed and store them in a cool location away from light. If stored properly, essential oils will maintain their potency for many years.

3. Keep essential oils out of reach of children. Treat them as you would any product for therapeutic use.

4. Essential oils rich in menthol (such as peppermint) should not be used on the throat or neck area of children under 30 months of age.

5. Angelica, bergamot, grapefruit, lemon, orange, tangerine, and other citrus oils are photosensitive and may cause a rash or dark pigmentation on skin exposed to direct sunlight or UV rays within 3-4 days after application.

6. Keep essential oils well away from the eye area and never put them directly into ears. Do not handle contact lenses or rub eyes with essential oils on your fingers. Even in minute amounts, oils with high phenol content, such as oregano, cinnamon, thyme, clove, lemongrass, and bergamot, may damage contacts and will irritate eyes.

7. Pregnant women should always consult a health care professional when starting any type of health program.

8. Epileptics and those with high blood pressure should consult their health care professional before using essential oils. Use caution with hyssop, fennel, basil, wintergreen, nutmeg, rosemary, peppermint, sage, tarragon, and tansy oils.

9. People with high blood pressure should avoid using sage and rosemary.

10. People with allergies should test a small amount of oil on an area of sensitive skin, such as the inside of the upper arm, for 30 minutes, before applying the oil on other areas.

    The bottom of the feet is one of the safest, most effective places to use essential oils.

11. Before taking GRAS (Generally Regarded As Safe, listed in Appendix B) essential oils internally, test your reactions by diluting one drop of essential oil in one teaspoon of an oil-soluble liquid like blue agave, olive oil, or rice milk. Never consume more than a few drops of diluted essential oil per day without the advice of a physician.

12. Do not add undiluted essential oils directly to bath water. Using Epsom salts or a bath gel base for all oils applied to your bath is an excellent way to disperse the oils into the bath water.

    When essential oils are put directly into bath water without a dispersing agent, they can cause serious discomfort on sensitive skin because the essential oils float, undiluted, on top of the water.

13. Keep essential oils away from open flames, sparks, or electricity. Some essential oils, including orange, fir, pine, and peppermint are potentially flammable (See Appendix J).

Before You Start

Always skin test an essential oil before using it. Each person's body is different, so apply oils to a small area first. Apply one oil or blend at a time. When layering oils that are new to you, allow enough time (3-5 minutes) for the body to respond before applying a second oil.

Exercise caution when applying essential oils to skin that has been exposed to cosmetics, personal care products, soaps, and cleansers containing synthetic chemicals. Some of them—especially petroleum-based chemicals—can penetrate and remain in the skin and fatty tissues for days or even weeks after use. Essential oils may react with such chemicals and cause skin irritation, nausea, headaches, or other uncomfortable effects.

Essential oils can also react with toxins built up in the body from chemicals in food, water, and work environment. If you experience a reaction to essential oils, it may be wise to temporarily discontinue their use and start an internal cleansing program before resuming regular use of essential oils. In addition, double your water intake while using essential oils.

You may also want to try the following alternatives to a detoxification program to determine the cause of the problem:

- Dilute 1-3 drops of essential oil to 1/2 tsp. of massage oil, vegetable mixing oil, or any pure vegetable oil, such as almond or olive. More dilution may be needed, as necessary.

CAUTION: Essential oils may sting if applied in or around the eyes. Some oils may be painful on mucous membranes unless diluted properly. Immediate dilution is strongly recommended if skin becomes painfully irritated or if oil accidentally gets into eyes. Flushing the area with a vegetable oil should minimize discomfort almost immediately. DO NOT flush with water! Essential oils are oil-soluble, not water-soluble. Water will only spread the oils over a larger surface, possibly worsening the problem.

- Reduce the number of oils used at any time.
- Use single oils or oil blends, one at a time.
- Reduce the amount of oil used.
- Reduce the frequency of application.
- Drink more purified or distilled water.
- Ask your health care professional to monitor detoxification.
- Skin-test the diluted essential oil on a small patch of skin for 30 minutes. If any redness or irritation results, dilute the area immediately with a pure vegetable or massage oil. Then cleanse with soap and water.
- If skin irritation or other uncomfortable side effects persist, discontinue using the oil on that location and apply the oils on the bottoms of the feet.

You may also want to avoid using products that contain the following ingredients to eliminate potential problems:

- Cosmetics, deodorants, and skin care products containing aluminum, petrochemicals, or other synthetic ingredients.
- Perms, hair colors or dyes, and hair sprays or gels containing synthetic chemicals. Avoid shampoos, toothpaste, mouthwash, and soaps containing synthetic chemicals such as sodium laurel sulfate, propylene glycol, or lead acetate.
- Garden sprays, paints, detergents, and cleansers containing toxic chemicals and solvents.

You can use many essential oils anywhere on the body except on the eyes and in the ears. Other oils may irritate certain sensitive tissues. See recommended dilution rates in Appendix F.

Keep all essential oils out of reach of children and only apply to children under skilled supervision. If a child or infant swallows an essential oil:

- Administer a mixture of milk, cream, yogurt, or another safe, oil-soluble liquid.
- Call a Poison Control Center or seek immediate emergency medical attention if necessary.

NOTE: If your body pH is low (meaning that your system is very acidic), you also could have a negative reaction to the oils.

Topical Application

Many oils are safe to apply directly to the skin. Lavender is safe to use on children without dilution. However, you must be sure what you are using is not lavandin labeled as lavender or genetically-altered lavender. When applying most other essential oils on children, dilute them with a carrier oil. For dilution, add 15–30 drops of essential oil to 1 oz. of a quality carrier oil as mentioned previously.

Carrier oils, such as a vegetable mixing oil, extend essential oils and provide more efficient use. When massaging, the vegetable oil helps lubricate the skin. Some excellent carrier oils include cold-pressed grapeseed, olive, wheat germ, and sweet almond oils, or a blend of any of these.

When starting an essential oil application, always apply the oil first to the bottom of the feet. This allows the body to become acclimated to the oil, minimizing the chance of a reaction. The Vita Flex foot charts (see Chapter 10) identify areas for best application. Start by applying 3–6 drops of a single or blended oil, spreading it over the bottom of each foot.

When applying essential oils to yourself, use 1–2 drops of oil on 2–3 locations twice a day. Increase to four times a day if needed. Apply the oil and allow it to absorb for 2–3 minutes before applying another oil or getting dressed (to avoid staining clothing).

As a general rule, when applying oils to yourself or another person for the first time, do not apply more than two single oils or blends at one time.

When mixing essential oil blends or diluting essential oils in a carrier oil, it is best to use containers made of glass or earthenware, rather than plastic. Plastic particles can leach into the oil and then into the skin once it is applied.

Before applying oils, wash hands thoroughly with soap and water.

Massage

Start by applying 2 drops of a single oil or blend on the skin and massaging it in. If you are working on a large area, such as the back, mix 1–3 drops of the selected essential oil into 1 tsp. of pure carrier oil (such as a vegetable mixing oil or a massage oil base).

Keep in mind that many massage oils such as olive, almond, or wheat germ oil may stain some fabrics.

Acupuncture

Licensed acupuncturists can dramatically increase the effectiveness of acupuncture by using essential oils. To start, place several drops of essential oil into the palm of your hand. Dip the acupuncture needle tip into the oil before inserting it. You can pre-mix several oils in your hand if you wish to use more than one oil.

Acupressure

When performing acupressure treatment, apply 1–3 drops of essential oil to the acupressure point with a finger. Using an auricular probe with a slender point to dispense oil can enhance the application. Start by pressing firmly and then releasing. Avoid applying pressure to any particular pressure point too long. You may continue along the acupressure points and meridians or use the reflexology or Vita Flex points as well. Once you have completed small point stimulation, massage the general area with the oil.

Warm Packs

For deeper penetration of an essential oil, use warm packs after applying oils. Dip a cloth in comfortably warm water. Wring the cloth out and place it on the location. Then cover the cloth loosely with a dry towel or blanket to seal in the heat. Allow the cloth to stand for 15–30 minutes. Remove the cloth immediately if there is any discomfort.

Cold Packs

Apply essential oils on the location, followed by cold water or ice packs when treating inflamed or swollen tissues. Frozen packages of peas or corn make excellent ice packs that will mold to the contours of the body part and will not leak. Keep the cold pack on until the swelling diminishes. For neurological problems, always use cold packs, never hot ones.

Layering

This technique consists of applying multiple oils one at a time. For example, place marjoram over a sore muscle, massage it into the tissue gently until the area is dry, and then apply a second oil, such as peppermint, until the oil is absorbed and the skin is dry. Then layer on the third oil, such as basil, and continue massaging.

Creating a Compress

- Rub 1–3 drops on the location, diluted or neat, depending on the oil used and the skin sensitivity at that location.

- Cover the location with a hot, damp towel.

- Cover the moist towel with a dry towel for 10–30 minutes, depending on individual need.

As the oil penetrates the skin, you may experience a warming or even a burning sensation, especially in areas where the greatest benefits occur. If burning becomes uncomfortable, apply a massage oil, vegetable mixing oil, or any pure vegetable oil such as olive or almond, to the location.

A second type of application is very mild and is suitable for children, or those with sensitive skin.

- Place 5–15 drops of essential oil into a basin filled with warm water.

- Water temperature should be approximately 100°F. (38°C.), unless the patient suffers neurological conditions; in this case, use cool water.

- Vigorously agitate the water and let it stand for 1 minute.

- Place a dry face cloth on top of the water to soak up oils that have floated to the surface.

- Wring out the water and apply the cloth on the location. To seal in the warmth, cover the location with a thick towel for 15–30 minutes.

Bath

Adding essential oils to bath water is challenging because oil does not mix with water. For even dispersion, mix 5–10 drops of essential oil in 1/4 cup of Epsom salts or bath gel base and then add this mixture under a running faucet. This method will help the oils disperse in the bath evenly and prevent stronger oils from stinging sensitive areas.

You can also use premixed bath gels and shampoos containing essential oils as a liquid soap in the shower or bath. Lather down with the bath gel, let it soak in, and then rinse. To maximize benefits, leave the soap or shampoo on the skin or scalp for several minutes to allow the essential oils to penetrate. You can create your own aromatic bath gels by placing 5–15 drops of essential oil in 1/2 oz. of an unscented bath gel base and then add to the bath water as described above.

Shower

Essential oils can be added to Epsom salts and used in the shower. There are special shower heads containing an attached receptacle that is filled with the essential oil/salts mixture. This allows essential oils to not only make contact with the skin, but also diffuses the fragrance of the oils into the air. The shower head receptacle can hold approximately 1/4 to 1/2 cup of bath salts.

Start by adding 5–10 drops of essential oil to 1/4 cup of bath salt. Fill the shower head receptacle with the oil/salt mixture. Make sure neither oils nor salts come in contact with the plastic seal on top of the receptacle. This should provide enough salt material for about 2–3 showers. Some shower heads have a bypass feature that allows the user to switch from aromatic salt water to regular tap water.

How to Enhance the Benefits of Topical Application

The longer essential oils stay in contact with the skin, the more likely they are to be absorbed. A high-quality lotion may be layered on top of the essential oils to reduce evaporation of the oils and enhance penetration. This may also help seal and protect cuts and wounds. Do not use ointments on burns until they are at least three days old.

Diffusing

Diffused oils alter the structure of molecules that create odors, rather than just masking them. They also increase oxygen availability, produce negative ions, and release natural ozone. Many essential oils such as lemongrass, orange, grapefruit, *Eucalyptus globulus*, tea tree, lavender, frankincense, and lemon, along with essential oil blends (Purification and Thieves), are extremely effective for eliminating and destroying airborne germs and bacteria.

A cold-air diffuser is designed to atomize a microfine mist of essential oils into the air, where they can remain suspended for several hours. Unlike aroma lamps or candles, a diffuser disperses essential oils without heating or burning, which can render the oil therapeutically less beneficial and even create toxic compounds. Burned oils may become carcinogenic. Research shows that cold air diffusing certain oils may:

- Reduce bacteria, fungus, mold, and unpleasant odors.

- Relax the body, relieve tension, and clear the mind.

- Help with weight management.

- Improve concentration, alertness, and mental clarity.

- Stimulate neurotransmitters.

- Stimulate secretion of endorphins.

- Stimulate growth hormone production and receptivity.

- Improve the secretion of IgA antibodies that fight candida.

- Improve digestive function.

- Improve hormonal balance.

- Relieve headaches.

Start by diffusing oils for 15–30 minutes a day. As you become accustomed to the oils and recognize their effects, you may increase the diffusing time to 1–2 hours per day.

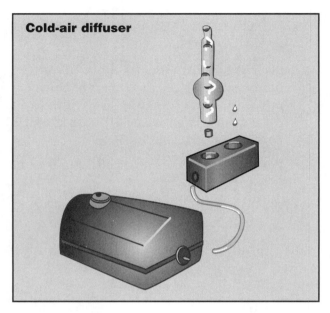

Cold-air diffuser

Place the diffuser high in the room so that the oil mist falls through the air and removes the odor-causing substances.

By connecting your diffuser to a timer, you can gain better control over the length and duration of diffusing. For some respiratory conditions, you may diffuse the oils the entire night.

Do not use more than one blend at a time in a diffuser as this may alter the smell and the therapeutic benefit. However, a single oil may be added to a blend when diffusing.

Always wash the diffuser before using a different oil blend. Use natural soap and warm or hot water.

If you don't have a diffuser, you may add several drops of essential oil to a spray bottle, add 1 cup purified water, and shake. You can use this to mist your entire house, workplace, or car.

To freshen the air, use the following essential oil blend:

- 20 drops lavender
- 10 drops lemon
- 6 drops bergamot
- 5 drops lime
- 5 drops grapefruit

Diffuse neat, or mix with 1 cup of distilled water in a spray bottle; shake well before spraying.

Other Ways to Diffuse Oils

- Add essential oils to cedar chips to make your own potpourri.

- Put scented cedar chips in closets or drawers to deodorize them.

- Place any conifer essential oil such as spruce, fir (all varieties), cedar, or pine onto each log in the fireplace. As they burn, they will disperse an evergreen smell. This method has no therapeutic benefit, however.

- Put essential oil on cotton balls and place in your car or home air vents.

- Place a bowl of water with a few drops of oil on a wood stove.

- Dampen a cloth, apply essential oils to it, and place it near the intake duct of your heating and cooling system.

Humidifier and Vaporizer

Essential oils such as peppermint, lemon, Eucalyptus radiata, Melaleuca alternifolia, and frankincense make ideal additions to humidifiers or vaporizers.*

* NOTE: Test the oil in the vaporizer or humidifier first, some essential oils may damge the plastic parts of vaporizers.

Other Uses

Inhalation

Direct

- Place 2 or more drops into the palm of your left hand, and rub clockwise with the flat palm of your right hand. Cup your hands together over the nose and mouth and inhale deeply. (Do not touch your eyes!)

- Add several drops of an essential oil to a bowl of hot (not boiling) water. Inhale the steaming vapors that rise from the bowl. To increase the intensity of the oil vapors inhaled, drape a towel over your head and bowl before inhaling.

- Apply oils to a cotton ball, tissue, or handkerchief (do not use synthetic fibers or fabric) and place it in the air vent of your car.

- Inhale directly.

Indirect or Subtle Inhalation (wearing as a perfume or cologne)

- Rub 2 or more drops of oil on your chest, neck, upper sternum, wrists, or under the nose and ears. Breathe in the fragrance throughout the day.

Vaginal Retention

For systemic health problems such as candida or vaginitis, vaginal retention is one of the best ways for the body to absorb essential oils.

- Mix 20–30 drops of essential oil in 2 tablespoons of carrier oil.

- Apply this mixture to a tampon (for internal infection) or sanitary pad (for external lesions). Insert and retain for 8 hours or overnight. Use tampons or sanitary pads made with organic cotton.

Rectal Retention

Retention enemas are the most efficient way to deliver essential oils to the urinary tract and reproductive organs. Always use a sterile syringe.

- Mix 15–20 drops of essential oil in a tablespoon of carrier oil.

- Place the mixture in a small syringe and inject into the rectum.

- Retain the mixture through the night (or longer for best results).

- Clean and disinfect the applicator after each use.

Water Distillers and Filters

You can apply oils like peppermint, lemon, clove, and cinnamon to the post-filter side of your water purifier. This will help purify the water.

Dishwashing Soap

To add fragrance or improve the antiseptic action of your liquid soap, add several drops of essential oils such as lavender, Melaleuca alternifolia, fir, spruce, pine, lemon, bergamot, and orange.

Cleaning and Disinfecting

A few drops of oil may be added to the dishwasher to help disinfect and purify. Some popular oils are pine, orange, tangerine, lemon, and peppermint, although any antibacterial oil would work well.

Painting

When painting, add 1 teaspoon of your favorite essential oil to one gallon of paint. Mix well. The oil will counteract the unpleasant smell of paint. Because essential oils are not fatty oils, they will not leave oil spots on the walls.

Laundry

Essential oils may be used to enhance the cleanliness and fragrance of your laundry. As unpleasant as it seems, dust mites live in your bedding, feeding from the dead skin cells you constantly shed. Recent research has shown that eucalyptus oil kills dust mites. To achieve effective dust mite control, add 25 drops of eucalyptus to each load, or approximately 1 tablespoon to a bottle of liquid laundry detergent.

You may also add several drops of essential oils to the rinse cycle, such as fir, spruce, juniper, lavender, cedarwood, wintergreen, or rosewood.

Instead of using toxic and irritating softening agents in the dryer, place a washcloth dampened with 10 drops of lavender, lemon, melaleuca, bergamot, or other essential oils. While the oils will not reduce static cling, they will impart a distinctive fragrance to the clothes.

Toothpick Application:

Dip end of wooden toothpick into oil and apply to mixtures when one drop of oil is too much.

Surface Cleansers: Counters, Furniture, etc.

Instead of purchasing standard household cleaners for surfaces, you can create your own natural, safe version by filling a plastic spray bottle with water and a squirt of dishwashing soap. Add 3 to 5 drops each of lavender, lemon, and pine essential oils. Shake the spray bottle well, and your homemade cleaner is ready to spray. This simple solution is extremely economical, yet it cleans and disinfects as well as any commercial cleaner.

Please keep in mind that some of the oils, if used directly, may stain some surfaces, such as linoleum.

Additional antibacterial and antiviral oils that are excellent for cleaning include cinnamon, clove, Eucalyptus globulus, thyme, juniper, Melaleuca alternifolia, spruce, lemongrass, and grapefruit.

Floors and Carpet

By combining essential oils with common household products, you can create your own nontoxic aromatic floor and carpet cleaners.

To clean non-carpeted floors, add 1/4 cup of white vinegar to a bucket of water. Then add 5–10 drops of lemon, pine, spruce, Melaleuca alternifolia, Antibacterial Blend, or another suitable oil. If the floor is especially dirty, add several drops of dishwashing soap. This will clean even the dirtiest floor.

To make a carpet freshener, add 16–20 drops of essential oils to a cup of baking soda or borax powder. Mix well and place in a covered container overnight so that the oil can be absorbed. Sprinkle over your carpet the next day and then vacuum the powder up.

You may also saturate a disposable cloth or tissue with several drops of essential oil and place it into the collecting bag of your vacuum. This will diffuse a pleasant odor as you clean. If your vacuum collects dirt into water, simply add a few drops into the water reservoir before cleaning. This refreshes both the carpet and the room.

Insecticide and Repellent: Dust Mites, Fleas, Ticks, Ants, Spiders, etc.

Many of us use synthetic chemicals to deal with insects. Single oils such as lavender, lemon, peppermint, lemongrass, cypress, Eucalyptus globulus, cinnamon, thyme, basil, citronella, and the Purification and Thieves blends (see Chapter 30), effectively repel many types of insects including mites, lice, and fleas. Peppermint placed on entryways prevents ants from entering.

If you need moth repellents for your linens and woolens, avoid toxic commercial mothballs made of naphthalene. Natural essential oils like citronella, lavender, lemongrass, Western red cedar, or rosemary can just as effectively repel moths and other insects. You can make a sachet by placing several drops of essential oil on a cotton ball. Wrap and tie this in a small handkerchief or square of cotton. Hang this cloth in storage areas or add it to your chest of linens. Refresh as often as necessary.

You can put this sachet in your bureau drawers to keep your clothes freshly scented. Lavender and rose are classic scents. For children's sleepwear, Roman chamomile is especially fragrant and relaxing. To scent stationery, stretch out an oil-scented cotton ball and place it in an envelope.

Hot Tubs and Saunas

Hot tubs, jacuzzis, and saunas act as reservoirs for germs, especially if used frequently. Lavender, cinnamon, clove, Eucalyptus globulus, thyme, lemon, or grapefruit can be used to disinfect and fragrance the water. Use 3 drops per person. For saunas, add several drops of rosemary, thyme, pine, or lavender to a spray bottle with water and then spray down the surfaces. Scented water can also be used to splash on hot sauna stones.

CAUTION: Some essential oils may damage plastic sauna/spa filters or hoses.

Deodorizing: Kitchens, Bathrooms, etc.

The kitchen and bathroom are often a source of odors and bacteria. Use the following mixtures to freshen, deodorize, and disinfect the air, work areas, cupboards, bathroom fixtures, sinks, tiles, wood-

work, carpets, etc. These blends are safe for the family and the environment.

Since essential oils separate easily from water, always shake well and keep on shaking the bottle as you use these mixtures. They will deodorize and clean the air, instead of covering the odors.

Single oils:
Rosemary CT cineol with lemon, Eucalyptus globulus, and lavender

Blends:
Lavender with Purification

Recipe #1
Mix:
- 2 drops rosemary CT cineol
- 4 drops lemon
- 3 drops Eucalyptus globulus
- 4 drops lavender with 1 quart water
- 1 cup water

Shake the mixture well and put it in a spray bottle.

Recipe #2
Mix:
- 3–4 drops lavender
- 5–6 drops Purification
- 1 cup water

Shake the mixture well and put it in a spray bottle.

Recipe #3
Mix:
- Pine with chamomile, Melaleuca alternifolia, lemongrass, or clove

Cooking

Many essential oils make excellent food flavorings. They are so concentrated that only 1–2 drops of an essential oil is equivalent to a full bottle (1–2 oz. size) of dried herbs.

As a general rule, spice oils impart a far stronger flavor than citrus oils do. For strong spice oils (such as oregano, nutmeg, cinnamon, marjoram, tarragon, wintergreen, thyme, or basil), you can dip a toothpick into the oils and stir food (after cooking) with the toothpick. This controls the amount of essential oil that is put into the food.

Cooking Tips:

- Ginger, cinnamon, clove, or nutmeg can be added to spice up gingersnap cookies. Use the toothpick application method.

- Lemon, orange, mandarin, or tangerine oil can be added to a regular sponge or bundt cake recipe.

- Peppermint or spearmint oil can be added to chocolate cake, brownie, or frosting recipes.

- Nutmeg, cinnamon, clove, or ginger oil can be used in pumpkin pie or spice cake recipes.

- Oregano, marjoram, thyme, or basil can be put in tomato sauces for spaghetti, pizza, ravioli, and lasagna recipes. Use the toothpick method of application.

- Lemon, clove, orange, mandarin, or peppermint oil can be added to enhance the flavor of puddings and fruit pies. Add 1–2 drops for 4–8 servings.

- Lavender, Roman chamomile, orange, tangerine, lemon, peppermint, wintergreen, and melissa can be used to make herbal teas. Mix 2 drops essential oil with 1 tsp. of blue agave nectar and stir into a cup of warm water.

- Lemon, orange, mandarin, tangerine, or peppermint can be mixed into a cool refreshing drink. Mix several drops of essential oil with 1 tsp. of blue agave nectar and add to a pitcher of cold water.

- Cinnamon, clove, lavender, basil, German or Roman chamomile, or lemon can be used to flavor blue agave nectar. Warm the blue agave until it becomes a thin liquid, then stir in your favorite oil.

Some oils that can be used as spices are: basil, cinnamon, clove, fennel, ginger, lemon, marjoram, nutmeg, oregano, peppermint, rosemary CT cineol, sage, spearmint, tarragon, coriander, grapefruit, mandarin, orange, wintergreen, black pepper, and thyme.

For a recipe that serves 6–10 people, add 1–2 drops of an oil and stir in after cooking and just before serving, so the oil does not evaporate.

Internal and Oral Use as a Dietary Supplement

All essential oils that are Generally Regarded As Safe (GRAS) or certified as Food Additives (FA) by the FDA may be safely taken internally as dietary supplements (See GRAS and FA lists in Appendix B). But ingesting essential oils should only be done under the direction of a knowledgeable health professional.

In fact, many oils are actually more effective when taken orally in very small amounts. Essential oils should always be diluted in vegetable oil, blue agave nectar or rice milk prior to ingestion. More or less dilution may be required, depending on how strong the oil is. More potent oils, such as cinnamon, oregano, lemongrass, and thyme, will require far more dilution than relatively mild oils, and very mild oils like lavender or lemon may not need any dilution at all.

As a general rule, dilute 1 drop of essential oil in 1 tsp. of blue agave nectar or in at least 4 ounces of a beverage.

Usually no more than 2 or 3 drops should be ingested at one time (during any 4–8 hour period). Because essential oils are so concentrated, 1–2 drops are often sufficient to achieve significant benefits.

Essential oils should not be given as dietary supplements to children under six years of age. Parents should exercise caution before orally administering essential oils to any child, and again, oils should always be diluted prior to ingestion.

Essential oils are extremely concentrated, so they should be kept out of reach of infants and children. If a large quantity of oil is ingested at one time (more than 5 drops), contact your health care physician and a Poison Control Center immediately.

5

Producing Therapeutic-Grade Essential Oils

Organic Herb Farming

The key to producing oils that are of genuine therapeutic quality starts with the proper cultivation of the herbs in the field.

- Plants should be grown on virgin land uncontaminated by chemical fertilizers, pesticides, fungicides, or herbicides. They should also be grown away from nuclear plants, factories, interstates, highways, and heavily-populated cities, if possible.

- Because robust, healthy plants produce higher quality essential oils, the soil should be nourished with enzymes, minerals, and organic mulch. The mineral content of the soil is crucial to the proper development of the plant, and soils that lack minerals result in plants that produce inferior oils.

- Land and crops should be watered with deep-well, reservoir, or watershed water. Mountain stream water is best because of its purity and high mineral content. Municipally treated water or secondary run-off water from residential and commercial areas can introduce undesirable chemical residues into the plant and the essential oil.

- Different varieties of plants produce different qualities of oils. Only those plants that produce the highest quality essential oil should be selected.

- The timing of the harvest is one of the most important factors in the production of therapeutic-grade oils. If the plants are harvested at the wrong time of the season or even at the incorrect time of day, they may distill into a substandard essential oil. In some instances, changing harvest time, by even a few hours, can make a huge difference. For example, German chamomile harvested in the morning will produce an oil with far more azulene (a powerful anti-inflammatory compound) than chamomile harvested in the late afternoon.

- Other factors that should be taken into consideration during the harvest include the amount of dew on the leaves, the percentage of plant in bloom, and weather conditions during the two weeks prior to harvest.

- To prevent herbs from drying out prior to being distilled, distillers should be located as close to the field as possible. Transporting herbs to distillers hundreds or thousands of miles away heightens the risk of exposure to pollutants, dust, mold, and petrochemical residues.

Steam Distillation

Essential oils can be extracted from the plant by a variety of methods, including solvent extraction, carbon-dioxide extraction, and steam distillation. Steam distillation actually takes three forms. The first uses just water, where plant material is placed in boiling water. The rising steam and oils are captured and then separated. Clove oil is distilled this way. There is also a combination water/steam method where boiling water and steam are pushed through and around the plant matter (this is how nutmeg essential oil is distilled). The final method is straight steam, where steam is pushed through the plant material, picking up the essential oils. Lavender is distilled this way.

In each of these processes, as the steam rises, it ruptures the oil membranes in the plant and releases the essential oil. The steam, carrying the essential oil molecules, rises to a condenser, where the oil-steam mixture condenses and reliquefies. As the steam condenses back to water, the lighter essential

Distillation

The temperature and pressure levels during steam distillation can enhance or destroy the value of the oil. The operator of the distiller must have a full understanding of the value of essential oils in order to produce quality oils. If the pressure or temperature is too high, it may change the molecular structure of the fragrance molecule, altering the chemical constituents. For example, the distilling process for lavender should not exceed three pounds of pressure, and the temperature should not exceed 245° F.

oil collects and floats on the top. This mixture is then sent to a separator where the oil is separated from the water. The remaining water is referred to as hydrosol or floral water.

There are many variants in steam distillation. Subtle differences in equipment and processing conditions can translate into huge differences in essential oil quality. The size and material of the cooking chamber, the type of condenser and separator, and the degree of temperature and pressure can all have a huge impact on the oil. Distillation is as much a science as it is an art. If the pressure or temperature is too high, or if the cooking chambers are constructed from reactive materials, the oil may not be therapeutic grade.

Vertical steam distillation offers the greatest potential for protecting the therapeutic benefits and quality of essential oils. In ancient distillation, low pressure (5 pounds or lower) and low temperature were extremely important to produce the therapeutic benefits. Marcel Espieu, president of the Lavender Growers Association in Southern France, has long maintained that the best oil quality can only be produced when the pressure is zero pounds during distillation.

Temperature also has a distinct effect. At certain temperatures, the oil fragrance, as well as the chemical constituents, become altered. High pressures and high temperatures seem to cause a harshness in the oil. Even the oil pH and the electrical polarity are greatly affected.

For example, cypress requires a minimum of 24 hours of distillation at 265° F and 5 pounds of pressure to extract most of the therapeutically-active constituents. If distillation time is cut by only two hours, 18 to 20 constituents will be missing from the resulting oil.

However, most commercial cypress oil is distilled for only 2 hours and 15 minutes! This short distillation time allows the producer to cut costs and produces a cheaper oil, since money is saved on the fuel needed to generate the steam. It also causes less wear and tear on equipment. Sadly, it results in an oil with little or no therapeutic value.

Pressure/Temperature Chart for Distilling Several Therapeutic-Grade Essential Oils

Essential Oil	Starting Material	Oil Production	Optical Rotation	Pressure in pounds	Distilling Temp.	Distilling Time
Cypress	2000 lb	1 lb	24	0	220	24 hrs.
Pine	1000 lb	1 lb	2	0	180	8 hrs.
Myrtle	500 kl	1 kl	22	1-2	200	7-9 hrs.
Palmarosa	600 kl	1 kl	6	2	200	4 hrs.
Lemongrass	650 kl	17.5 kl	0	5	230	2.75 hrs.
Citronella	150 lb	1 lb	0	5	225	4.5 hrs.
Rosewood	500 kl	1 kl	-4	30	287	3 hrs.
Cinnamon	1300 lb	5 oz	0	5	225-235	9-24 hrs.
Clove	450 kl	5 lit	0	10	229	18 hrs.
Eucalyptus globulus	250 lb	1 lb	5	5	225	3-18 hrs.
Melaleuca alternifolia	1000 lb	10-15 lb	3	3	218	2-3 hrs.
Geranium	500 lb	6 lb	-8	1.2	200	1-3 hrs.

In France, lavender produced commercially is often distilled for only 15 to 20 minutes at 155 pounds of pressure with a steam temperature approaching 350° F. Although this high temperature, high pressure oil costs less to produce and is easily marketed, it is of poor quality. It retains few, if any, of the therapeutic properties of high-grade lavender distilled at zero pounds of pressure for a minimum of 1 hour and 15 minutes.

In many large commercial operations, distillers introduce chemicals into the steam distillation process to increase the volume of oil produced. Chemical trucks may even pump solvents directly into the boiler water. This expands oil production by as much as 18 percent. These chemicals inevitably leach into the distilling water and mix with the essential oil, fracturing the molecular structure of the oil and altering both its fragrance and therapeutic value. These chemicals remain in the oil after it is sold because it is impossible to completely separate them from the oil.

Another way that essential oil producers increase the quantity of the oil extracted is through redistillation. This refers to the repeated distillation of the plant material to maximize the volume of oil by using second, third, and fourth stages of steam distillation. Each successive distillation generates a weaker and less potent essential oil. Such essential oils are also degraded due to prolonged exposure to water and heat used in the redistillation process. This water can hydrolize or oxidize the oil and begin to chemically break down the constituents responsible for its aroma and therapeutic properties.

Combining Traditional Steam Distillation with Modern Technology

Few people appreciate how chemically complex essential oils are. They are rich tapestries of literally hundreds of chemical components, some of which— even in small quantities—contribute important therapeutic benefits. The key to preserving as many as possible of these delicate aromatic constituents is to steam-distill plant material in small batches using low pressure and low heat. This is the traditional method of distillation that has been used for centuries in Europe but is being abandoned in favor of high-volume pressure cookers designed to operate at over 400° F and use over 50 pounds of pressure.

Different Forms of Essential Oil Production

Expressed oils are pressed from the rind of fruits, such as grapefruit, lemon, lime, mandarin, orange, and tangerine. Rich in terpene alcohols, expressed oils are not technically "essential oils," even though they are highly regarded for their therapeutic properties. Expressed oils should only be obtained from organically grown crops, since pesticide residues can become highly concentrated in the oil.

Steam distillation is the oldest and traditional method of extraction. Plant material is inserted into a cooking chamber, and steam is passed through it. After the steam is collected and condensed, it is run through a separator to collect the oil.

Solvent-extraction involves the use of oil-soluble solvents, such as hexane, dimethylenechloride, and acetone.

Absolutes are technically not "essential oils" but are "essences." They are obtained from the grain alcohol extraction of a concrete, which is the solid waxy residue that is derived from the extraction of plant materials, usually flower petals. This method of extraction is used primarily for botanicals where the fragrance and therapeutic parts of the plant can only be unlocked using solvents. Jasmine and neroli are extracted this way.

Even more important, the cooking chamber where the plants are distilled should be constructed of a non-reactive metal, preferably stainless steel, to reduce the possibility of the essential oil being chemically altered by more reactive metals such as aluminum or copper.

No solvents or synthetic chemicals should be used or added to the water used to generate steam because they might jeopardize the integrity of the essential oil. Even the addition of chemicals to water used in a closed-loop, heat-exchange system of the condenser can be risky, since there is no guarantee that they will be completely isolated from the essential oil. It is unfortunate that many essential oils distilled commercially are processed using boiler water laden with chemicals and descaling agents.

Absolutely no pesticides, herbicides, fungicides, or agricultural chemicals of any kind should be used in the cultivation of herbs earmarked for distillation. These chemicals—even in minute quantities—can react with the essential oil and degrade its purity and quality and render it therapeutically less effective. During distillation, pesticide residue leaches out of the plant material, with the extracted essential oil.

Essential Oil Production

Producing pure essential oils is very costly. It often requires several hundred or even thousands of pounds of raw plant material to produce a single pound of essential oil. For example, it can take 2–3 tons of melissa plant material to produce one pound of melissa oil. Its extremely low yield explains why it sells for $9,000 to $15,000 per kilo. It takes 5,000 pounds of rose petals to produce approximately one pint of rose oil. It is not difficult to understand why these oils are so expensive.

The vast majority of oils are produced for the perfume industry, which is only interested in their aromatic qualities. High pressure, high temperatures, and the use of chemical solvents are used in this distillation process to produce greater quantities of oil in a shorter time. To most people, these oils carry a pleasant aroma, but they lack true therapeutic properties. Many of the important chemical constituents necessary to produce therapeutic results are either flashed off with the high heat or are not released from the plant material.

A Summary of the Benefits of Therapeutic-Grade Essential Oils

1. Essential oils are small enough in molecular size that they can quickly penetrate the tissues of the skin.

2. Essential oils are lipid-soluble and are capable of penetrating cell membranes, even if the membranes have hardened because of an oxygen deficiency. According to Jean Valnet, MD, essential oils can affect every cell of the body within 20 minutes and are then metabolized like other nutrients.

3. Essential oils, according to researchers at the University of Vienna, stimulate blood flow, which increases oxygen and nutrient delivery.

4. Essential oils are some of the most powerful known antioxidants as determined by the ORAC test developed at Tufts University.

5. Essential oils are antibacterial, antifungal, anti-infectious, antimicrobial, antiparasitic, antiviral, and antiseptic. Some essential oils have been shown to destroy all tested bacteria and viruses.

6. Essential oils may detoxify the cells and blood in the body.

7. Essential oils containing sesquiterpenes have the ability to pass the blood-brain barrier.

8. Essential oils are aromatic, and when diffused, may provide air purification by:

   - Increasing ozone and negative ions in the area.

   - Eliminating odors from cooking, bacteria, mold, animals, and other sources.

   - Filling the air with a fresh, aromatic scent.

9. Essential oils promote emotional, physical, and spiritual well-being.

6

Single Oils

This section describes over 80 single essential oils, including botanical information, therapeutic and traditional uses, chemical constituents of each oil, extraction method, cautions, and application instructions.

How to be Sure Your Essential Oils are Therapeutic Grade

How can you be sure that your essential oils are of therapeutic grade? Start by asking the following questions from your essential oil and supplier:

Are the fragrances delicate, rich, and organic? Do they "feel" natural? Do the aromas vary from batch to batch as an indication that they are painstakingly distilled in small batches rather than industrially processed on a large scale?

Does your supplier subject each batch of essential oils through multiple chemical analyses to test for purity and therapeutic quality? Are these tests performed by independent labs?

Does your supplier grow and distill its own organically grown herbs?

Are the distillation facilities part of the farm where the herbs are grown (so oils are freshly distilled), or do herbs wait days to be processed and lose potency?

Does your supplier use low pressure and low temperature to distill essential oils so as to preserve all of their fragile chemical constituents? Are the distillation cookers fabricated from costly food-grade stainless steel alloys to reduce the likelihood of the oils chemically reacting with metal?

Does your supplier personally inspect the fields and distilleries where the herbs are grown and distilled? Do they verify that no synthetic or harmful solvents or chemicals are being used?

Do your essential oils meet AFNOR or ISO standards?

How many years has your supplier been doing all of this?

How to Maximize the Shelf Life of Your Essential Oils

The highest quality essential oils are bottled in dark glass. The reason for this is two-fold: glass is more stable than plastic and does not "breathe" the same way plastic does. Also, the darkness of the glass protects the oil from light that may chemically alter or degrade it over time.

After using an essential oil, keep the lid tightly sealed. Bottles that are improperly sealed can result in the loss of some of the lighter, lower-molecular-weight parts of the oil. In addition, over time, oxygen in the air reacts with and oxidizes the oil.

Essential oils should be stored away from light, especially sunlight—even if they are already stored in amber glass bottles. The darker the storage conditions, the longer your oil will maintian its orginal chemistry and quality.

Store essential oils in a cool location. Excessive heat can derange the molecular structure of the oil the same way ultraviolet light can.

Diluting Essential Oils

Most essential oils (EO) require dilution with a vegetable oil (VO) when being used either internally or externally. The amount of dilution depends on the essential oil. For example, oregano will require four times as much dilution as that of Roman chamomile. For more information on specific usage instructions for each essential oil, please see the preface to Chapter 28 "Personal Usage Guide" as well as Appendices E and T.

In this chapter the following abbreviations will be used to signify common dilutions: "Dilute 1 part EO with 1 part VO." In all cases, "EO" means Essential Oil and "VO" means Vegetable Oil. Vegetable Oils such the V6 Vegetable Oil Complex are specifically formulated to dilute essential oils and have a long shelf life (over two years) without going rancid.

Angelica *(Angelica archangelica)*

Botanical Family: Apiaceae or Umbelliferae (parsley family)

Plant Origin: France, Belgium

Extraction Method: Steam distilled from root.

Key Constituents:
Limonene (60-70%)
Alpha Pinene (5-8%
Alpha and Beta Phellandrene (3-6%)

Historical Data: Known as the "holy spirit root" or the "oil of angels" by the Europeans, angelica's healing powers were so strong that it was believed to be of divine origin. From the time of Paracelsus, it was credited with the ability to protect from the plague. The stems were chewed during the plague of 1660 to prevent infection. When burned, the seeds and roots were thought to purify the air.

Medical Properties: Anticoagulant, relaxant

USES: Throat/lung infections, indigestion, menstrual problems/PMS.

Fragrant Influence: assisting in the release of pent-up negative feeling and restores memories to the point of origin before trauma or anger was experienced.

Application: Dilute 1 part EO with 1 part VO; (1) apply 1-2 drops on location, (2) chakras/vitaflex points, (3) directly inhale, (4) diffuse (see Appendices E and T)

Avoid applying to skin that will be exposed to direct sunlight or UV light within 72 hours.

Found In: Awaken, Forgiveness, Grounding, Harmony, Live With Passion, and Surrender.

Anise *(Pimpinella anisum)*

Botanical Family: Umbelliferae (parsley family)

Plant Origin: Turkey

Extraction Method: Steam distillation from the seeds (fruit).

Key Constituents:
Trans-Anethol (85-95%)
Methyl Chavicol (2-4%)

ORAC: 333,700 µTE/100g

History: Listed in Dioscorides' De Materia Medica (A.D. 78), Europe's first authoritive guide to medicines, that became the standard reference work for herbal treatments for over 1,700 years.

Medical Properties: Digestive stimulatnt, anti-coagulant, anesthetic/analgesic, antioxidant, diuretic, antitumoral.

USES: Arthritis/rheumatism, cancer.

Application: Dilute 1 part EO with 1 part VO; (1) apply 1-2 drops on location, (2) chakras/vitaflex points, (3) directly inhale, (4) diffuse, or (5) take as dietary supplemnt (see Appendices E and T)

Fragrant Influence: Opens emotional blocks and recharges vital energy.

Found In: Awaken, Di-Tone, Dream Catcher.

Selected Research:

Ghelardini C, Galeotti N, Mazzanti G. "Local anaesthetic activity of monoterpenes and phenylpropanes of essential oils." *Planta Med.* 2001 Aug;67(6):564-6.

Chainy GB, Manna SK, Chaturvedi MM, Aggarwal BB. "Anethole blocks both early and late cellular responses transduced by tumor necrosis factor: effect on NF-kappaB, AP-1, JNK, MAPKK and apoptosis." *Oncogene.* 2000 Jun 8;19(25):2943-50.

Balsam Fir, Idaho *(Abies balsamea)*

Botanical Family: Pinaceae (pine)

Plant Origin: Bonner's Ferry, Idaho

Extraction Method: Steam distilled from needles.

Key Constituents:
Alpha-Pinene (28-49%)
Beta Pinene (14-24%)
Camphene (13-20%)
Limonene (13-20%)

ORAC: 20,500 µTE/100g

Historical Data: The fir tree—a tree commonly used as a christmas tree today—has been prized through the ages for its medicinal effects and ability to heal respiratory conditions and muscular and rheumatic pain.

Medical Properties: Anticoagulant, anti-inflammatory

USES: Throat/lung/sinus infections, fatigue. arthritis/rheumatism, urinary tract infections, scoliosis/lumbago/sciatica.

Fragrant Influence: Grounding, stimulating to the mind, and relaxing to the body.

Application: Dilute 1 part EO with 1 part VO; (1) apply 2-4 drops on location or use neat in Raindrop Technique, (2) chakras/vitaflex points, (3) directly inhale, (4) diffuse, or (5) take as dietary supplemnt (see Appendices E and T)

Bible References: (see additional Bible references in Appendix D)

2 Samuel 6:5—"And David and all the house of Israel played before the Lord on all manner of [instruments made of] fir wood, even on harps, and on psalteries, and on timbrels, and on cornets, and on cymbals."

1 Kings 5:8—"And Hiram sent to Solomon, saying, I have considered the things which thou sentest to me for: [and] I will do all thy desire concerning timber of cedar, and concerning timber of fir."

1 Kings 5:10—"So Hiram gave Solomon cedar trees and fir trees [according to] all his desire."

Found In: En-R-Gee, Grounding, Into The Future, Sacred Mountain.

Basil *(Ocimum basilicum)*

Botanical Family: Lamiaceae or Labiatae (mint)

Plant Origin: Egypt, India, Utah, France

Extraction Method: Steam distilled from leaves, stems, and flowers.

Key Constituents:
Methylchavicol (estragol) (40-80%)
Linalol (10-50%)
1,8 Cineole (1-7%)
Eugenol (1-10%)

ORAC: 54,000 µTE/100g

Historical Data: Used extensively in traditional Asian Indian medicine, basil's name is derived from "basileum," the Greek name for king. In the 16th century, the powdered leaves were inhaled to treat migraines and chest infections. The Hindu people put basil sprigs on the chests of the dead to protect them from evil spirits. Italian women wore basil to attract possible suitors. It was listed in Hildegard's Medicine, a compilation of early German medicines by highly-regarded Benedictine herbalist Hildegard of Bingen (1098-1179).

Medical Properties: Powerful antispasmodic, antiviral, antibacterial, anti-inflammatory, muscle relaxant.

USES: Migraines, throat/lung infections, insect bites

Fragrant Influence: Fights mental fatigue.

Application: Dilute 1 part EO with 1 part VO; (1) apply 2-4 drops on location, temples, neck (2) chakras/vitaflex points (crown of head, forehead, heart, and navel), (3) directly inhale, (4) diffuse, or (5) take as dietary supplement (see Appendices E and T)

Avoid use if epileptic.

Found In: Aroma Siez, Clarity, M-Grain.

Selected Research:

Fyfe L., et al. "Inhibition of *Listeria monocytogenes* and *Salmonella enteriditis* by combinations of plant oils and derivatives of benzoic acid: the development of synergistic antimicrobial combinations." *Int J Antimicrob Agents.* 1997;9(3):195-9.

Wan J, et al. "The effect of essential oils of basil on the growth of *Aeromonas hydrophila* and *Pseudomonas fluorescens*." *J Appl Microbiol.* 1998;84(2):152-8.

Lachowicz KJ, et al. "The synergistic preservative effects of the essential oils of sweet basil (*Ocimum basilicum* L.) against acid-tolerant food microflora." *Lett Appl Microbiol.* 1998;26(3):209-14.

Elgayyar M, et al., Antimicrobial activity of essential oils from plants against selected pathogenic and saprophytic microorganisms. *J Food Prot.* 2001 Jul;64(7):1019-24.

Bay Laurel (see *Laurus nobilis*)

Bergamot (*Citrus bergamia*)

Botanical Family: Rutaceae (citrus)

Plant Origin: Italy, Ivory Coast

Extraction Method: Pressed from the rind, rectified and void of terpenes. Also produced by solvent extraction or vacuum distillation.

Key Constituents:
Limonene (30-45%)
Linaly Acetate (22-36%)
Linalol (3-15%)
Gamma-Terpinene (6-10%)
Beta-Pinene (5.5-9.5%)

Historical Data: It is believed that Christopher Columbus brought bergamot to Bergamo in Northern Italy from the Canary Islands. A mainstay in traditional Italian medicine, bergamot has been used in the Middle East for hundreds of years for skin conditions associated with an oily complexion. Bergamot is responsible for the distinctive flavor of the renowned Earl Grey Tea, and was used in the first genuine eau de cologne.

Medical Properties: Calming, hormonal support, antibacterial, antidepressant.

USES: Agitation, depression, anxiety, intestinal parasites, insomnia, viral infections (Herpes, cold sores).

Fragrant Influence: Relieves anxiety; mood-lifting qualities.

Application: Dilute 1 part EO with 1 part VO; (1) apply 1-2 drops on location, (2) chakras/vitaflex points, (3) directly inhale, (4) diffuse, or (5) take as dietary supplement (see Appendices E and T).

Cautions: Avoid applying to skin that will be exposed to sunlight or UV light within 72 hours.

Found In: Awaken, Clarity, Dream Catcher, Forgiveness, Gentle Baby, Harmony, Joy, and White Angelica.

Cajeput (*Melaleuca leucadendra*)

Botanical Family: Myrtaceae (myrtle)

Key Constituents:
Eucalyptol (50-65%)
Alpha-Terpineol (7-13%)
Limonene (3-8%)
Alpha Pinene (1-3%)

ORAC: 37,600 µTE/100g

Historical Data: Traditionally used in Malaysia and other Indonesian islands, for respiratory/throat infections, headaches, rheumatism, toothache, skin conditions, and sore muscles. Cajeput derives its name from the Malaysian word for white tree.

Medical Properties: Antibacterial, antiparasitic, antispasmodic, anti-inflammatory, analgesic

USES: Throat/lung/sinus infections, urinary tract infections, coughs, intestinal problems.

Application: Dilute 1 part EO with 1 part VO; (1) apply on location, (2) chakras/vitaflex points, (3) directly inhale, or (4) diffuse (see Appendices E and T).

Caution: Do not use synthetic cajeput, as it could cause further blistering and skin eruption.

Cardamom *(Elettaria cardamomum)*

Botanical Family: Zingiberaceae (ginger)

Key Constituents:
Alpha Terpinyl Acetate (45-55%)
1,8 Cineol (Eucalyptol) (16-24%)
Linalol (4-7%)
Linalyl Acetate (3-7%)
Limonene (1-3%)

ORAC: 36,500 μTE/100g

Historical Data: Called "Grains of Paradise" since the Middle Ages, it has been used medicinally by Indian healers for millennia. One of the most prized spices in ancient Greece and Rome, cardamom was cultivated by the king of Babylon around the seventh century B.C.

It is mentioned in one of the oldest known medical records, Ebers Papyrus (dating from sixteenth century BC) an ancient Egyptian list of 877 prescriptions and recipes.

Medical Properties: Antispasmodic (neuro-muscular), expectorant, antiparasitc (worms)

USES: lung/sinus infection, indigestion, senility, headaches.

Fragrant Influence: Uplifting, refreshing, and invigorating.

Application: Dilute 1 part EO with 1 part VO; (1) apply 2-4 drops on location, stomach, solar plexus, or thighs, (2) chakras/vitaflex points, (3) directly inhale, (4) diffuse, or (5) take as 4 drops as dietary supplement (see Appendices E and T).

Found In: Clarity.

Carrot Seed *(Duacus carota)*

Botanical Family: Apiaceae (Ubelliferae)

Plant Origin: Native to Europe, Asia and North Africa

Extraction Method: Steam distilled from dried seeds

Key Constituents:
Carotol (30-40%)
Alpha Pinene (12-16%)
Trans Beta Caryophyllene (6-10%)
Caryophyllene Oxide (3-5%)

Historical Data: Traditionally used for kidney and digestive disorders and to relieve liver congestion.

Medical Properties: Antiparasitic, antiseptic, depurative, diuretic, vasodilatory

USES: Skin conditions (eczema, oily skin, psoriasis, wrinkles), water retention, liver problems.

Application: Dilute 1 part EO with 1 part VO; (1) apply 1-2 drops on location, (2) chakras/vitaflex points, or (3) take as dietary supplement (see Appendices E and T).

Selected Research:

Friedman M, Henika PR, Mandrell RE. "Bactericidal activities of plant essential oils and some of their isolated constituents against Campylobacter jejuni, Escherichia coli, Listeria monocytogenes, and Salmonella enterica." *J Food Prot.* 2002 Oct;65(10):1545-60.

Cassia *(Cinnamomum cassia)*

Botanical Family: Lauraceae (laurel)

Plant Origin: China

Extraction Method: Steam distilled from bark. NOTE: While its aroma is similar to cinnamon, cassia is chemically and physically quite different.

Key Constituents:
Trans-Cinnamaldehyde (70-88%)
Trans-O-Methoxycinnamaldehyde (3-15%)
Coumarine (1.5-4%)
Cinnamyl Acetate (0-6%)

ORAC: 15,170 µTE/100g

Historical Data: Rich Biblical history. Mentioned in one of the oldest known medical records, Ebers Papyrus (dating from sixteenth century BC) an ancient Egyptian list of 877 prescriptions and recipes.

Medical Properties: Anti-inflammatory (COX2 inhibitor), antifungal, antibacterial, antiviral, anticoagulant

USES: Cataracts, fungal infections (ringworm, candida), atherosclerosis, arterosclerosis.

Application: Dilute 1 part EO with 4 parts VO; (1) apply 1-2 drops on location, (2) chakras/vitaflex points, (3) diffuse, or (4) take as dietary supplement (see Appendices E and T).

Caution: May irritate the nasal membranes if inhaled directly from diffuser or bottle.

Found In: Exodus II.

Bible References: (See additional Bible references in Appendix D.)

Exodus 30:23,24,25—Take thou also unto thee principal spices, of pure myrrh five hundred shekels, and of sweet cinnamon half so much, even two hundred and fifty shekels, and of sweet calamus two hundred and fifty shekels, And of **cassia** five hundred shekels, after the shekel of the sanctuary, and of oil olive an hin: And thou shalt make it an oil of holy ointment, an ointment compound after the art of the apothecary: it shall be an holy anointing oil.

Psalm 45:8—All thy garments smell of myrrh, and aloes, and **cassia**, out of the ivory palaces, whereby they have made thee glad.

Selected Research:

Lee HS. "Inhibitory activity of Cinnamomum cassia bark-derived component against rat lens aldose reductase." *J Pharm Pharm Sci.* 2002 Sep-Dec;5(3):226-30.

Walsh SE, et al., "Activity and mechanisms of action of selected biocidal agents on Gram-positive and -negative bacteria." *J Appl Microbiol.* 2003;94(2):240-7.

Lee HS, Kim BS, Kim MK. "Suppression effect of Cinnamomum cassia bark-derived component on nitric oxide synthase." *J Agric Food Chem.* 2002 Dec 18;50(26):7700-3.

Huss U, et al., "Screening of ubiquitous plant constituents for COX-2 inhibition with a scintillation proximity based assay." *J Nat Prod.* 2002 Nov;65(11):1517-21.

Friedman M, Henika PR, Mandrell RE. "Bactericidal activities of plant essential oils and some of their isolated constituents against Campylobacter jejuni, Escherichia coli, Listeria monocytogenes, and Salmonella enterica." *J Food Prot.* 2002 Oct;65(10):1545-60.

Lee HS, Ahn YJ. "Growth-Inhibiting Effects of Cinnamomum cassia Bark-Derived Materials on Human Intestinal Bacteria." *J Agric Food Chem.* 1998 Jan 19;46(1):8-12.

Inouye S, Yamaguchi H, Takizawa T. "Screening of the antibacterial effects of a variety of essential oils on respiratory tract pathogens, using a modified dilution assay method." *J Infect Chemother.* 2001 Dec;7(4):251-4.

Canadian Red Cedar *(Thuja plicata)* (distilled from bark)

Botanical Family: Cupressaceae (Cypress)

Plant Origin: Canada

Extraction Method: Steam distilled from bark and sawdust.

Key Constituents:
Alpha-thujone (70-85%)
Beta-thujone (5-9%)
Sabinene (2-5%)

Historical Data: It was used traditionally by the Native American Indians to help them enter a higher spiritual realm. They used it to stimulate the scalp and as an antimicrobial and antiseptic agent.

Medical Properties: Antifungal, antibacterial, hair follicle stimulator, antiparasitic, and insect repellent.

USES: balding/thinning hair, fungal infections, digestive/intestinal problems.

Application: Dilute 1 part EO with 1 part VO; (1) apply 1-2 drops on location, (2) chakras/vitaflex points, (3) directly inhale, or (4) diffuse (see Appendices E and T).

Cautions: Temporary skin discoloration may occur.

Cedar, Western Red *(Thuja plicata)* (distilled from leaves)

Botanical Family: Cupressaceae

Plant Origin: Utah, Idaho

Extraction Method: Steam distilled from leaves and branches.

Key Constituents:
Alpha Thujone (70-80%)
Beta Thujone (4-7%)
Alpha Pinene (2-4%)
Sabinene (2-4%)

Historical Data: This oil is different from Canadian red ceder which is distlled from the bark of the same plant, Thuja plicata. This oil is not red in color, because it is derived from leaves.

Medical Properties: Antiseptic

USES: Throat/lung infections, urinary tract infections

Application: Dilute 1 part EO with 1 part VO; (1) apply 1-2 drops on location, (2) chakras/vitaflex points, (3) directly inhale, (4) diffuse, or (5) add to woodchips or place in closets/dressers to repel insects (see Appendices E and T).

Cedarwood *(Cedrus atlantica)*

Botanical Family: Pinaceae (pine)

Plant Origin: Morocco, USA. *Cedrus atlantica* is the species most closely related to the biblical Cedars of Lebanon.

Extraction Method: Steam distilled from bark.

Key Constituents:
Alpha-Himachalene (10-20%)
Beta-Himachalene (35-55%)
Gamma-Himachalene (8-15%)
Delta-Cadinene (2-6%)

ORAC: 169,000 μTE/100g

Historical Data: Throughout antiquity, cedarwood has been used in medicines. The Egyptians used it for embalming the dead. It was used as both a traditional medicine and incense in Tibet.

Medical Properties: Combats hair loss (alopecia areata), antibacterial, lymphatic stimulatant.

USES: Hair loss, arteriosclerosis, ADHD, skin problems (acne, eczema)

Fragrant Influence: Stimulates the limbic region of the brain (the center of emotions) stimulates the pineal gland, which releases melatonin. Terry Friedmann MD found in clinical tests that this oil was able to successfully treat ADD and ADHD (attention deficit disorders) in children. It is recognized for its calming, purifying properties.

Application: (1) Apply on location, (2) chakras/vitaflex points, (3) directly inhale, (4) diffuse, or (5) take as dietary supplement (see Appendices E and T).

Bible References: (See additional Bible references in Appendix D**).**

Leviticus 14:4—"Then shall the priest command to take for him that is to be cleansed two birds alive and clean, and cedar wood, and scarlet, and hyssop."

Leviticus 14:6—"As for the living bird, he shall take it, and the cedar wood, and the scarlet, and the hyssop, and shall dip them and the living bird in the blood of the bird [that was] killed over the running water."

Leviticus 14:49—"And he shall take to cleanse the house two birds, and cedar wood, and scarlet, and hyssop."

Found In: Brain Power, Grounding, Inspiration, Into The Future, Live With Passion, Sacred Mountain, and SARA.

Selected Research:

Hay IC, et al. "Randomized trial of aromatherapy. Successful treatment for alopecia areata." *Arch Dermatol.* 1998;134(11):1349-52.

Friedman M, Henika PR, Mandrell RE. "Bactericidal activities of plant essential oils and some of their isolated constituents against Campylobacter jejuni, Escherichia coli, Listeria monocytogenes, and Salmonella enterica." *J Food Prot.* 2002 Oct;65(10):1545-60.

Celery Seed *(Apium graveolens)*

Botanical Family: Apiaceae (Umbelliferae)

Plant Origin: Europe

Extraction Method: Steam distilled from dried seeds

Key Constituents:
Limonene (60-75%)
Alpha and Beta Selinene (14-20%)
Sednenolide (4-7%)

ORAC: 30,300 µTE/100g

Medical Properties: Antibacterial, antioxidant, antirheumatic, digtesive aid, diuretic, liver protectant.

Historical Data: Long recognized as helpful in digestion, liver cleansing, and urinary tract support. Also said to increase milk flow in nursing mothers.

Medical Properties: Liver protectant.

USES: Arthritis/rheumatism, digestive problems, liver problems/hepatitis

Application: Dilute 1 part EO with 1 part VO; (1) apply on location or (2) take as dietary supplement (see Appendices E and T).

Found In: JuvaCleanse

Selected Research:

Friedman M, Henika PR, Mandrell RE. "Bactericidal activities of plant essential oils and some of their isolated constituents against Campylobacter jejuni, Escherichia coli, Listeria monocytogenes, and Salmonella enterica." *J Food Prot.* 2002 Oct;65(10):1545-60.

Zheng GQ, et al., "Chemoprevention of benzo[a]pyrene-induced forestomach cancer in mice by natural phthalides from celery seed oil." *Nutr Cancer.* 1993;19(1):77-86.

Chamomile (German) *(Matricaria recutita)*

Botanical Family: Asteraceae or Compositae (daisy)

Plant Origin: Utah, Egypt, Hungary

Extraction Method: Steam distilled from flowers.

Chemical Constituents:
Chamazulene (2-5%)
Bisabolol Oxide A (32-42%)
Trans-Beta-Farnesene (18-26%)
Bisbolol Oxide B (3-6%)
Bisbolone Oxide A (3-6%)
Cis Spiro Ether (4-8%)

ORAC: 218,600 µTE/100g

Historical Data: Listed in Dioscorides' De Materia Medica (A.D. 78), Europe's first authoritive guide to medicines, that became the standard reference work for herbal treatments for over 1,700 years.

Medical Properties: Powerful antioxidant, (inhibits lipid peroxidation), antitumoral, anti-inflammatory, relaxant, anesthetic. Promotes digestion, liver, and gallbladder health.

USES: Hepatitis/fatty liver, arteriosclerosis, insomnia, nervous tension, arthritis, carpal tunnel syndrome, skin problems (acne, eczema, scar tissue).

Fragrant Influence: Dispels anger, stabilizes emotions, and helps release emotions linked to the past. Soothes and clears the mind.

Application: (1) Apply 2-4 drops on location, (2) chakras/vitaflex points, (3) directly inhale, (4) diffuse, or (5) take as dietary supplement (see Appendices E and T).

Found In: EndoFlex, Surrender, Gentle Baby, JuvaFlex, Motivation

Selected Research:

Burns E, et al., "The use of aromatherapy in intrapartum midwifery practice an observational study." *Complement Ther Nurs Midwifery*. 2000 Feb;6(1):33-4.

Rekka E, et al., "Synthesis of new azulene derivatives and study of their effect on lipid peroxidation and lipoxygenase activity." *Chem Pharm Bull* (Tokyo). 2002 Jul;50(7):904-7.

Rekka EA, Kourounakis AP, Kourounakis PN. "Investigation of the effect of chamazulene on lipid peroxidation and free radical processes." *Res Commun Mol Pathol Pharmacol*. 1996 Jun;92(3):361-4.

Hernandez-Ceruelos A, Madrigal-Bujaidar E, de la Cruz C. "Inhibitory effect of chamomile essential oil on the sister chromatid exchanges induced by daunorubicin and methyl methanesulfonate in mouse bone marrow." *Toxicol Lett*. 2002 Sep 5;135(1-2):103-110.

Brehm-Stecher BF, Johnson EA. "Sensitization of Staphylococcus aureus and Escherichia coli to antibiotics by the sesquiterpenoids nerolidol, farnesol, bisabolol, and apritone." *Antimicrob Agents Chemother*. 2003 Oct;47(10):3357-60.

Chamomile (Roman) *(Chamaemelum nobile)*

Botanical Family: Asteraceae or Compositae (daisy)

Plant Origin: Utah, Egypt

Extraction Method: Steam distilled from flowers.

Key Constituents:
Isobutyl Angelate + Isamyl Methacrylate (30-45%)
Isoamyl Angelate (12-22%)
Methyl Allyl Angelate (6-10%)
Isobutyl n-butyrate (2-9%)
2-Methyl Butyl Angelate (3-7%)

ORAC: 240 µTE/100g

Historical Data: Used in Europe for skin regeneration. For centuries, mothers have used chamomile to calm crying children, combat digestive and liver ailments, and relieve toothaches.

Medical Properties: Relaxant, antispasmodic, anti-inflammatory, antiparasitic, nerve regenerative, anesthetic, detoxifies blood and liver.

USES: Relieves restlessness, anxiety, ADHD. depression, insomnia, skin conditions (acne, dermatitis, eczema).

Fragrant Influence: Because it is calming and relaxing, it can combat depression, insomnia, and stress. It minimizes anxiety, irritability, and nervousness. It may also dispel anger, stabilize the emotions, and help to release emotions that are linked to the past.

Application: (1) Apply 2-4 drops on location, ankles, or wrists (2) chakras/vitaflex points, (3) directly inhale, (4) diffuse, or (5) take as dietary supplement (see Appendices E and T)

Found In: Awaken, Clarity, Forgiveness, Gentle Baby, Harmony, Joy, JuvaFlex, Motivation, M-Grain, and Surrender.

Cinnamon Bark *(Cinnamomum verum)*

Botanical Family: Lauraceae (laurel)

Plant Origin: Sri Lanka, Madagascar, India

Extraction Method: Steam distilled from bark.
Key Constituents:
Trans-Cinnamaldehyde (40-50%)
Eugenol (20-30%)
Beta-Caryophyllene (3-8%)
Linalol (3-7%)

ORAC: 10,340 µTE/100g

History: Listed in Dioscorides' De Materia Medica (A.D. 78), Europe's first authoritive guide to medicines, that became the standard reference work for herbal treatments for over 1,700 years.

Cinnamon was reputed to be part of the "Marseilles Vinegar" or "Four Thieves Vinegar" used by grave-robbing bandits to protect themselves during the 15th century plague.

Medical Properties: Anti-inflammatory (COX2 inhibitor), powerfully antibacterial, antiviral, antifungal, anticoagulant, circulatory stimulant, stomach protectant (ulcers), antiparasitic (worms)

USES: Cardiovascular disease, infectious diseases, viral infections (Herpes etc), digestive complaints, ulcers, and warts

Fragrant Influence: Thought to attract wealth.

Application: Dilute 1 part EO with 4 parts VO; (1) apply 1-2 drops on location, (2) chakras/vitaflex points, (3) diffuse, or (4) take as dietary supplement (see Appendices E and T).

Cautions: May irritate the nasal membranes if inhaled directly from diffuser or bottle.

Found In: Abundance, Christmas Spirit, Exodus II, Gathering, Magnify Your Purpose, and Thieves.

Bible Reference: (See additional Bible references in Appendix D)

Exodus 30:23—"Take thou also unto thee principal spices, of pure myrrh five hundred shekels, and of sweet cinnamon half so much, even two hundred and fifty shekels, and of sweet calamus two hundred and fifty shekels…"

Proverbs 7:17—"I have perfumed my bed with myrrh, aloes, and cinnamon."

Song of Solomon 4:14—"Spikenard and saffron; calamus and cinnamon, with all trees of frankincense; myrrh and aloes, with all the chief spices:"

Selected Research:

Tantaoui-Elaraki A, et al. "Inhibition of growth and aflatoxin production in *Aspergillus parasiticus* by essential oils of selected plant materials." *J Environ Pathol Toxicol Oncol.* 1994;13(1):67-72.

Capasso R, Pinto L, Vuotto ML, Di Carlo G. "Preventive effect of eugenol on PAF and ethanol-induced gastric mucosal damage." *Fitoterapia.* 2000 Aug;71 Suppl 1:S131-7.

Lee HS, Kim BS, Kim MK. "Suppression effect of Cinnamomum cassia bark-derived component on nitric oxide synthase." *J Agric Food Chem.* 2002 Dec 18;50(26):7700-3.

Huss U, et al., "Screening of ubiquitous plant constituents for COX-2 inhibition with a scintillation proximity based assay." *J Nat Prod.* 2002 Nov;65(11):1517-21.

Pessoa LM, et al., "Anthelmintic activity of essential oil of Ocimum gratissimum Linn. and eugenol against Haemonchus contortus." *Vet Parasitol.* 2002 Oct 16;109(1-2):59-63.

Friedman M, Henika PR, Mandrell RE. "Bactericidal activities of plant essential oils and some of their isolated constituents against Campylobacter jejuni, Escherichia coli, Listeria monocytogenes, and Salmonella enterica." *J Food Prot.* 2002 Oct;65(10):1545-60.

Benencia F, Courreges MC. "In vitro and in vivo activity of eugenol on human herpes virus." *Phytother Res.* 2000 Nov;14(7):495-500.

Inouye S, Uchida K, Yamaguchi H. "In-vitro and in-vivo anti-Trichophyton activity of essential oils by vapour contact." *Mycoses.* 2001 May;44(3-4):99-107.

Inouye S, Yamaguchi H, Takizawa T. "Screening of the antibacterial effects of a variety of essential oils on respiratory tract pathogens, using a modified dilution assay method." *J Infect Chemother.* 2001 Dec;7(4):251-4.

Tantaoui-Elaraki A, Beraoud L. "Inhibition of growth and aflatoxin production in Aspergillus parasiticus by essential oils of selected plant materials." *J Environ Pathol Toxicol Oncol.* 1994;13(1):67-72.

Cistus *(Cistus ladanifer)*

(known also as *Labdanum*)

Botanical Family: Cistaceae

Plant Origin: France, Spain

Extraction Method: Steam distilled from branches.

Key Constituents:
Alpha Pinene (40-60%)
Camphene (2-5%)
Bornyl Acetate (3-6%)
Trans-Pinocarveol (3-6%)

ORAC: 3,860 µTE/100g

Historical Data: Cistus is also known as "rock rose" and has been studied for its effects on the regeneration of cells.

Medical Properties: Antiviral, antibacterial, antihemorrhagic, anti-inflammatory, supports sympathetic nervous system, immune stimulant.

USES: Hemorrhages, arthritis

Fragrant Influence: Calming to the nerves, elevates the emotions.

Application: (1) Apply 2-4 drops on location, (2) chakras/vitaflex points, (3) directly inhale, (4) diffuse, or (5) take as 4 drops as dietary supplement (see Appendices E and T).

Found In: ImmuPower.

Citronella *(Cymbopogon nardus)*

Botanical Family: Poaceae or Gramineae (grasses)

Plant Origin: Sri Lanka, Philippines, Egypt

Extraction Method: Steam distilled from leaves.

Key Constituents:
Geraniol (18-30%)
Limonene (5-10%)
Trans-Methyl Isoeugenol (4-10%)
Geranyl Acetate (5-10%)
Borneol (3-8%)

ORAC: 312,000 µTE/100g

Historical Data: Use by various cultures to treat intestinal parasites, menstrual problems, and as a stimulant. Historically used to sanitize and deodorize surfaces. Enhanced insect repelling properties when combined with cedarwood.

Medical Properties: Powerful antioxidant, antibacterial, antifungal, insect-repellent, anti-inflammatory, antispasmodic, antiparasitic (worms), relaxant

USES: Respiratory infections, muscle/nerve pain, digestive/intestinal problems, anxiety, skin problems (acne, eczema, oily skin), skin-penetration enhancer.

Fragrant Influence: Refreshing and uplifting.

Application: Dilute 1 part EO with 1 part VO; (1) apply 2-4 drops on location, (2) chakras/vitaflex points, (3) directly inhale, (4) diffuse, or (5) take as dietary supplement (see Appendices E and T).

Found In: Purification

Selected Research:

Mutalik S, Udupa N. Effect of some penetration enhancers on the permeation of glibenclamide and glipizide through mouse skin. Pharmazie. 2003 Dec;58(12):891-4.

Kumaran AM, et al., Geraniol, the putative anthelmintic principle of Cymbopogon martinii. Phytother Res. 2003 Sep;17(8):957.

Carnesecchi S, et al., "Geraniol, a component of plant essential oils, sensitizes human colon cancer cells to 5-fluorouracil treatment." *IARC Sci Publ.* 2002;156:407-9.

Carnesecchi S, et al., "Perturbation by geraniol of cell membrane permeability and signal transduction pathways in human colon cancer cells." *J Pharmacol Exp Ther.* 2002 Nov;303(2):711-5.

Umezu T, et al., "Anticonflict effects of rose oil and identification of its active constituents." *Life Sci.* 2002 Nov 22;72(1):91-102.

Choi HS, Song HS, Ukeda H, Sawamura M. "Radical-scavenging activities of citrus essential oils and their components: detection using 1,1-diphenyl-2-picrylhydrazyl." *J Agric Food Chem.* 2000 Sep;48(9):4156-61.

Citrus Hystrix

Botanical Family: Rutaceae

Plant Origin: Indochina, Malaysia

Extraction Method: Steam distilled from leaves

Key Constituents:
Citronnellal (65-80%)
Linalol (3-6%)
Citronnellol (2-5%)
Isopulegol ((2-4%)

ORAC: 69,200 µTE/100g

Historical Data: Studies at Kinki University in Japan found that it has strong anti-inflammatory properties. Other research has shown that it combats depression.

Medical Properties: Anti-inflammatory, anti-depressant, relaxant. Rich in citronellal which possesses calmative properties.

USES: Stress, anxiety, trauma

Application: (1) Apply on location, (2) chakras/vitaflex points, (3) directly inhale, (4) diffuse, or (5) take as dietary supplement (see Appendices E and T).

Cautions: Avoid applying to skin that will be exposed to sunlight or UV light within 72 hours.

Found In: Trauma Life

Clary Sage *(Salvia sclarea)*

Botanical Family: Lamiaceae or Labiatae (mint)

Plant Origin: Utah, France

Extraction Method: Steam distilled from flowering plant.

Key Constituents:
Linalyl Acetate (56-78%)
Linalol (7-24%)
Germacrene D (2-12%)
Sclareol (.4-3%)

ORAC: 221,000 µTE/100g

Historical Data: Recent medical data indicates that it naturally raises estrogen and progesterone levels.

Medical Properties: Anticoagulant, antioxidant, antidiabetic, estrogen-like, antifungal, antispasmodic, relaxant, cholesterol-reducing, antitumoral, anesthetic

USES: Leukemia, menstrual problems/PMS, hormonal imbalance, insomnia, circulatory problems, high cholesterol.

Fragrant Influence: Enhances one's ability to dream and is very calming and stress-relieving.

Application: Dilute 1 part EO with 1 part VO; (1) apply on location, feet, ankles, wrists, (2) chakras/vitaflex points, (3) directly inhale, (4) diffuse, or (5) take as dietary supplement (see Appendices E and T).

Found In: Dragon Time, Into The Future, and Live With Passion.

Selected Research:

Dimas K, et al., "The effect of sclareol on growth and cell cycle progression of human leukemic cell lines." *Leuk Res.* 1999 Mar;23(3):217-34.

Yasui K, "Synthesis of manool-related labdane diterpenes as platelet aggregation inhibitors." *Chem Pharm Bull* (Tokyo). 1993 Oct;41(10):1698-707.

Burns E, et al., "The use of aromatherapy in intrapartum midwifery practice an observational study." *Complement Ther Nurs Midwifery.* 2000 Feb;6(1):33-4.

Clove *(Syzygium aromaticum)*

Botanical Family: Myrtaceae (myrtle)

Plant Origin: Madagascar, Spice Islands

Extraction Method: Steam distilled from bud and stem.

Key Constituents:
Eugenol (75-87%)
Eugenol Acetate (8-15%)
Beta-Carophyllene (2-7%)

ORAC: 1,078,700 µTE/100g

Historical Data: The people on the island of Ternate were free from epidemics until the 16th century, when Dutch conquerors destroyed the clove trees that flourished on the islands. Many of the islanders died from the epidemics that followed.

Cloves were reputed to be part of the "Marseilles Vinegar" or "Four Thieves Vinegar" used by grave-robbing bandits to protect themselves during the 15th century plague.

Clove was listed in Hildegard's Medicine, a compilation of early German medicines by highly-regarded Benedictine herbalist Hildegard of Bingen (1098-1179).

Healers in Chinia and India have used clove buds since ancient times as part of their treatments.

Eugenol, clove's principal constituent, was used in the dental industry for years to numb gums.

Courmont et al. demonstrated that a solution of .05% eugenol from clove oil was sufficient to kill the tuberculosis bacillus (Gattefossé, 1990).

Medical Properties: Anti-aging, antitumoral, antimicrobial, antifungal, antiviral, analgesic/anesthetic, antioxidant, anticoagulant, anti-inflammatory, stomach protectant (ulcers), antiparasitic (worms), anticonvulsant.

USES: Anti-aging, cardiovacular disease, arthritis/ rheumatism, hepatitis, intestinal parasites/ infections, throat/ sinus/lung infections, cataracts, ulcers, lice, toothache, acne.

Fragrant Influence: A mental stimulant; encourages sleep, stimulates dreams, and creates a sense of protection and courage.

Application: Dilute 1 part EO with 4 parts VO; (1) apply 2-4 drops on location, gums, or mouth, (2) chakras/vitaflex points, (3) diffuse, or (4) take as dietary supplement (see Appendices E and T).

For tickling cough, put a drop on back of tongue.

Cautions: Anticoagulant properties can be enhanced when combined with Warfarin, aspirin, etc.

Found In: Abundance, En-R-Gee, ImmuPower, Longevity, Melrose, PanAway, and Thieves.

Selected Research:

Nishijima H, et al. "Mechanisms mediating the vasorelaxing action of eugenol, a pungent oil, on rabbit arterial tissue." *Jpn J Pharmacol.* 1999 Mar;79(3):327-34.

Jayashree T, et al. "Antiaflatoxigenic activity of eugenol is due to inhibition of lipid peroxidation." *Lett Appl Microbiol.* 1999; 28(3):179-83.

Wie MB, et al. "Eugenol protects neuronal cells from excitotoxic and oxidative injury in primary cortical cultures." *Neurosci Lett.* 1997: 4;225(2):93-6.

Capasso R, et al., "Preventive effect of eugenol on PAF and ethanol-induced gastric mucosal damage." *Fitoterapia.* 2000 Aug;71 Suppl 1:S131-7.

Lahlou S, et al., "Cardiovascular Effects of Eugenol, a Phenolic Compound Present in Many Plant Essential Oils, in Normotensive Rats." *J Cardiovasc Pharmacol.* 2004 Feb;43(2):250-257.

Mutalik S, Udupa N. "Effect of some penetration enhancers on the permeation of glibenclamide and glipizide through mouse skin." *Pharmazie.* 2003 Dec;58(12):891-4.

Olasupo NA, et al., "Activity of natural antimicrobial compounds against Escherichia coli and Salmonella enterica serovar Typhimurium." *Lett Appl Microbiol.* 2003; 37(6):448-51.

Miyazawa M, Hisama M. "Antimutagenic activity of phenylpropanoids from clove (Syzygium aromaticum)." *J Agric Food Chem.* 2003 Oct 22;51(22):6413-22.

Yang YC, Lee SH, Lee WJ, Choi DH, Ahn YJ. "Ovicidal and adulticidal effects of Eugenia caryophyllata bud and leaf oil compounds on Pediculus capitis." *J Agric Food Chem.* 2003 Aug 13;51(17):4884-8.

Ingvast-Larsson JC, Axen VC, Kiessling AK. "Effects of isoeugenol on in vitro neuromuscular blockade of rat phrenic nerve-diaphragm preparations." *Am J Vet Res.* 2003 Jun;64(6):690-3.

Kim SS, et al., "Eugenol suppresses cyclo-oxygenase-2 expression in lipopolysaccharide-stimulated mouse macrophage RAW264.7 cells." *Life Sci.* 2003 Jun 6;73 (3):337-48.

Nadin G, Goel BR, Yeung CA, Glenny AM. "Pulp treatment for extensive decay in primary teeth." *Cochrane Database Syst Rev.* 2003;(1):CD003220.

Kim EH, Kim HK, Ahn YJ. "Acaricidal activity of clove bud oil compounds against Dermatophagoides farinae and Dermatophagoides pteronyssinus (Acari: Pyroglyphidae)." *J Agric Food Chem.* 2003 Feb 12;51(4):885-9.

Lee HS. "Inhibitory activity of Cinnamomum cassia bark-derived component against rat lens aldose reductase." *J Pharm Pharm Sci.* 2002 Sep-Dec;5(3):226-30.

Huss U, et al., "Screening of ubiquitous plant constituents for COX-2 inhibition with a scintillation proximity based assay." *J Nat Prod.* 2002 Nov;65(11):1517-21.

Pessoa LM, et al., "Anthelmintic activity of essential oil of Ocimum gratissimum Linn. and eugenol against Haemonchus contortus." *Vet Parasitol.* 2002 Oct 16;109(1-2):59-63.

Friedman M, Henika PR, Mandrell RE. "Bactericidal activities of plant essential oils and some of their isolated constituents against Campylobacter jejuni, Escherichia coli, Listeria monocytogenes, and Salmonella enterica." *J Food Prot.* 2002 Oct;65(10):1545-60.

Sayyah M, Valizadeh J, Kamalinejad M. "Anticonvulsant activity of the leaf essential oil of Laurus nobilis against pentylenetetrazole- and maximal electroshock-induced seizures." Phytomedicine. 2002 Apr;9(3):212-6.

Lee KG, Shibamoto T. "Inhibition of malonaldehyde formation from blood plasma oxidation by aroma extracts and aroma components isolated from clove and eucalyptus." *Food Chem Toxicol.* 2001 Dec;39(12):1199-204.

Vazquez BI, Fente C, Franco CM, Vazquez MJ, Cepeda A. "Inhibitory effects of eugenol and thymol on Penicillium citrinum strains in culture media and cheese." *Int J Food Microbiol.* 2001 Jul 20;67(1-2):157-63.

Atsumi T, et al., "Reactive oxygen species generation and photo-cytotoxicity of eugenol in solutions of various pH." *Biomaterials.* 2001 Jun;22(12):1459-66.

Benencia F, Courreges MC. "In vitro and in vivo activity of eugenol on human herpesvirus." *Phytother Res.* 2000 Nov;14 (7):495-500.

Teissedre PL, Waterhouse AL. "Inhibition of oxidation of human low-density lipoproteins by phenolic substances in different essential oils varieties." *J Agric Food Chem.* 2000 Sep;48(9):3801-5.

Vidhya N, Devaraj SN. "Antioxidant effect of eugenol in rat intestine." *Indian J Exp Biol.* 1999 Dec;37(12):1192-5.

Ahmed M, et al., "Analgesic principle from Abutilon indicum." *Pharmazie.* 2000 Apr;55(4):314-6.

Kelm MA, Nair MG, Strasburg GM, DeWitt DL. "Antioxidant and cyclooxygenase inhibitory phenolic compounds from Ocimum sanctum Linn." *Phytomedicine.* 2000 Mar;7(1):7-13.

Nishijima H, et al., "Mechanisms mediating the vasorelaxing action of eugenol, a pungent oil, on rabbit arterial tissue." *Jpn J Pharmacol.* 1999 Mar;79(3):327-34.

Jayashree T, Subramanyam C. "Antiaflatoxigenic activity of eugenol is due to inhibition of lipid peroxidation." *Lett Appl Microbiol.* 1999 Mar;28(3):179-83.

Rao M, Kumar MM, Rao MA. "In vitro and in vivo effects of phenolic antioxidants against cisplatin-induced nephrotoxicity." *J Biochem* (Tokyo). 1999 Feb;125(2):383-90.

Uchida M, Nakajin S, Toyoshima S, Shinoda M. "Antioxidative effect of sesamol and related compounds on lipid peroxidation." *Biol Pharm Bull.* 1996 Apr;19(4):623-26.

Zhao ZS, O'Brien PJ. "The prevention of CCl4-induced liver necrosis in mice by naturally occurring methylenedioxybenzenes." *Toxicol Appl Pharmacol.* 1996 Oct;140 (2):411-21.

Nagababu E, Lakshmaiah N. "Inhibition of xanthine oxidase-xanthine-iron mediated lipid peroxidation by eugenol in liposomes." *Mol Cell Biochem.* 1997 Jan;166(1-2):65-71.

Nagababu E, Sesikeran B, Lakshmaiah N. "The protective effects of eugenol on carbon tetrachloride induced hepatotoxicity in rats." *Free Radic Res.* 1995 Dec;23(6):617-27.

Reddy AC, Lokesh BR. "Effect of curcumin and eugenol on iron-induced hepatic toxicity in rats." *Toxicology.* 1996 Jan 22;107(1):39-45.

Zheng GQ, Kenney PM, Lam LK. "Sesquiterpenes from clove (Eugenia caryophyllata) as potential anticarcinogenic agents." *J Nat Prod.* 1992 Jul;55(7):999-1003.

"Inhibitory effect of eugenol on non-enzymatic lipid peroxidation in rat liver mitochondria." *Biochem Pharmacol.* 1992 Jun 9;43(11):2393-400.

Combava

(See CITRUS HYSTRIX)

Coriander *(Coriandrum sativum)*

Botanical Family: Apiaceae or Umbelliferae (parsley)

Plant Origin: Russia, India

Extraction Method: Steam distilled seeds.

Chemical Constituents:
Linalol (65-78%)
Alpha-Pinene (3-7%)
Camphor (4-6%)
Gamma-Terpinene (2-7%)
Limonene (2-5%)
Geranyl Acetate (1-3.5%)
Geraniol (0.5-3%)

ORAC: 298,300 µTE/100g

Historical Data: Coriander seeds were found in the ancient Egyptian tomb of Ramses II. This oil has been researched at Cairo University for its effects in lowering glucose and insulin levels and supporting pancreatic function. It has also been studied for its effects in strengthening the pancreas.

Medical Properties: Anti-inflammatory, sedative, analgesic

USES: Diabetes, arthritis, intestinal problems.

Fragrant Influence: Soothing and calming.

Application: Dilute 1 part EO with 1 part VO; (1) apply 2-4 drops on location, (2) chakras/vitaflex points, (3) directly inhale, (4) diffuse, or (5) take as dietary supplement (see Appendices E and T).

Selected Research:

Delaquis PJ, et al., "Antimicrobial activity of individual and mixed fractions of dill, cilantro, coriander and eucalyptus essential oils." *Int J Food Microbiol.* 2002 Mar 25;74(1-2):101-9.

Elgayyar M, et al., "Antimicrobial activity of essential oils from plants against selected pathogenic and saprophytic microorganisms." *J Food Prot.* 2001 Jul;64(7):1019-24.

Cumin *(Cuminum cyminum)*

Botanical Family: Apiaceae or Umbelliferae (parsley)

Plant Origin: Egypt

Extraction Method: Steam distilled from seeds.

Key Constituents:
Cuminaldehyde (16-22%)
Gamma-Terpinene (16-22%)
Beta-Pinene (12-18%)
Para-Mentha-1,3 &1,4-dien-7-al (25-35%)
Para-Cymene (3-8%)

ORAC: 82,400 µTE/100g

Historical Data: The Hebrews used cumin as an antiseptic for circumcision.

Medical Properties: Antitumoral, anti-inflammatory, antioxidant, antiviral, digestive aid, liver protectant, immune stimulant

USES: Cancer, infectious disease, digestive problems.

Application: Dilute 1 part EO with 1 part VO; (1) apply 1-2 drops on location, (2) chakras/vitaflex points, (3) directly inhale, (4) diffuse, or (5) take as dietary supplement (see Appendices E and T).

Found In: ImmuPower, ParaFree, and Protec.

Selected Research:

Ramakrishna Rao R, Platel K, Srinivasan K. "In vitro influence of spices and spice-active principles on digestive enzymes of rat pancreas and small intestine." *Nahrung.* 2003 Dec;47(6):408-12.

Singh G, et al., "Studies on essential oils: part 10; antibacterial activity of volatile oils of some spices." *Phytother Res.* 2002 Nov;16(7):680-2.

Dhandapani S, et al., "Hypolipidemic effect of Cuminum cyminum L. on alloxan-induced diabetic rats." *Pharmacol Res.* 2002 Sep;46(3):251-5.

Krishnakantha TP, Lokesh BR. "Scavenging of superoxide anions by spice principles." *Indian J Biochem Biophys.* 1993 Apr;30(2):133-4.

Reddy AC, Lokesh BR. "Studies on spice principles as antioxidants in the inhibition of lipid peroxidation of rat liver microsomes." *Mol Cell Biochem.* 1992 Apr;111(1-2):117-24.

Banerjee S, et al., "Influence of certain essential oils on carcinogen-metabolizing enzymes and acid-soluble sulfhydryls in mouse liver." *Nutr Cancer.* 1994;21(3):263-9.

Tantaoui-Elaraki A, Beraoud L. "Inhibition of growth and aflatoxin production in Aspergillus parasiticus by essential oils of selected plant materials." *J Environ Pathol Toxicol Oncol.* 1994;13(1):67-72.

Cypress *(Cupressus sempervirens)*

Botanical Family: Cupressaceae (cypress)

Plant Origin: France, Spain

Extraction Method: Steam distilled from branches.

Key Constituents:
Alpha-Pinene (40-65%)
Beta-Pinene (0.5-3%)
Delta-3-Carene (12-25%)
Limonene (1.8-5%)
Cedrol (0.8-7%)
Myrcene (1-3.5%)
Manoyle Oxide

Iso-pimaradiene
Karahanaenone

ORAC: 24,300 µTE/100g

Historical Data: Cypress is one of the oils most used for the circulatory system.

Medical Properties: Improves circulation and strengthens blood capillaries; anti-infectious, antispasmodic

USES: Diabetes, circulatory disorders; cancer (Jean Valnet, M.D.)

Fragrant Influence: Eases the feeling of loss and creates a sense of security and grounding. Also helps heal emotional trauma.

Application: Dilute 1 part EO with 1 part VO; (1) apply 2-4 drops on location or massaging toward center of body, (2) chakras/vitaflex points, (3) directly inhale, (4) diffuse, or (5) take as dietary supplement (see Appendices E and T).

Bible Reference:

Isaiah 44:14—"He heweth him down cedars, and taketh the cypress and the oak, which he strengtheneth for himself among the trees of the forest: he planteth an ash, and the rain doth nourish it."

Found In: Aroma Life, Aroma Siez, and R.C.

Selected Research:

Karkabounas S, et al., Effects of Cupressus sempervirens cone extract on lipid parameters in Wistar rats. In Vivo. 2003 Jan-Feb;17(1):101-3.

Cypress, Blue *(Callitris intratropica)*

Botanical Family: Cypressaceae

Plant Origin: Australia

Extraction Method: Steam distillation from the leaves and wood of the tree.

Key Constituents:
Alpha, Beta, Gamma Eudesmols (18-30%)
Guaiol (8-18%)
Bulnesol (5-15%)
Alpha, Beta and Delta Selinenes (5-10%)

ORAC: 73,100 µTE/100g

Historical Data: Blue cypress in ancient times was used for incense, perfume and embalming.

Medical Properties: Anti-inflammatory, anti-viral

USES: Viral infections (Herpes simplex, herpes zoster, cold sores, human papilloma virus etc.).

Application: (1) apply 2-4 drops on location, (2) chakras/vitaflex points, (3) directly inhale, or (4) diffuse (see Appendices E and T).

Found In: Australian Blue

Dill *(Anethum graveolens)*

Botanical Family: Apiaceae or Umbelliferae (parsley).

Plant Origin: Austria, Hungary

Extraction Method: Steam distilled from whole plant.

Key Constituents:
Carvone (30-45%)
Limonene (15-25%)
Alpha- and Beta-Phellandrenes (20-35%)

ORAC: 35,600 µTE/100g

Historical Data: The dill plant is mentioned in the Papyrus of Ebers from Egypt (1550 BC). Roman gladiators rubbed their skin with dill before each match. Listed in Dioscorides' De Materia Medica (A.D. 78), Europe's first authoritive guide to medicines, that became the standard reference work for herbal treatments for over 1,700 years. It was listed in Hildegard's Medicine, a compilation of early German medicines by highly-regarded Benedictine herbalist Hildegard of Bingen (1098-1179).

Medical Properties: Antidiabetic, Antispasmodic, antibacterial, expectorant, pancreatic stimulant, insulin/blood sugar regulator.

USES: Diabetes, digestive problems, liver deficiencies

Fragrant Influence: Calms the autonomic nervous system and, when diffused with Roman chamomile, combats ADHD.

Application: Dilute 1 part EO with 1 part VO; (1) apply 2-4 drops on location or abdomen,

(2) chakras/vitaflex points, (3) directly inhale, (4) diffuse, or (5) take as dietary supplement (see Appendices E and T).

Selected Research:

Lis-Balchin M, Hart S. A preliminary study of the effect of essential oils on skeletal and smooth muscle in vitro. J Ethnopharmacol. 1997 Nov;58(3):183-7.

Delaquis PJ, et al., Antimicrobial activity of individual and mixed fractions of dill, cilantro, coriander and eucalyptus essential oils. Int J Food Microbiol. 2002 Mar 25;74(1-2):101-9.

Elemi *(Canarium luzonicum)*

Botanical Family: Burseraceae (frankincense)

Plant Origin: Philippines

Extraction Method: Steam distilled from the gum of the tree.

Key Constituents:
Limonene (40-72%)
Alpha-Phellandrene (10-24%)
Sabinene (3-8%)
Elemol (1-25%)

Historical Data: Elemi has been used in Europe for hundreds of years in salves for skin and is included in celebrated healing ointments, such as *baum paralytique*. Used by a 17th century physician, J. J. Wecker, on the battle wounds of soldiers, elemi belongs to the same botanical family as frankincense (*Boswellia carteri*) and myrrh (*Commiphora myrrha*). The Egyptians used elemi for embalming, and subsequent cultures used it for skin care.

Medical Properties: Antispasmodic, anti-inflammatory

USES: Muscle/nerve pain, skin problems (scars, acne, wrinkles).

Fragrant Influence: Its fragrance is very conducive toward meditation.

Application: (1) Apply 2-4 drops on location, (2) chakras/vitaflex points, (3) directly inhale, or (4) diffuse (see Appendices E and T).

Eucalyptus Citriodora *(Eucalyptus citriodora)*

Botanical Family: Myrtaceae (myrtle)

Plant Origin: China

Extraction Method: Steam distilled from leaves.

Key Constituents:
Citronellal (75-85%)
Neo-isopulegol + Isopulegol (0-10%)

ORAC: 83,000 µTE/100g

Historical Data: Traditionally used to perfume linen closets and as an insect repellent.

Medical Properties: Analgesic, antiviral, antibacterial, antifungal, expectorant, and insecticidal

USES: Fungal infections (ringworm, Candida), respiratory infections, viral infections (Herpes, shingles)

Application: Dilute 1 part EO with 1 part VO; (1) apply 2-4 drops on location, (2) chakras/vitaflex points, (3) directly inhale, or (4) diffuse (see Appendices E and T).

Found In: R.C.

Selected Research:

Silva J, et al., Analgesic and anti-inflammatory effects of essential oils of Eucalyptus. J Ethnopharmacol. 2003 Dec;89(2-3):277-83.

Ohno T, et al., Antimicrobial activity of essential oils against Helicobacter pylori. Helicobacter. 2003 Jun;8(3):207-15.

Ramsewak RS, In vitro antagonistic activity of monoterpenes and their mixtures against 'toe nail fungus' pathogens. Phytother Res. 2003 Apr;17(4):376-9.

Low D, Rawal BD, Griffin WJ. Antibacterial action of the essential oils of some Australian Myrtaceae with special references to the activity of chromatographic fractions of oil of Eucalyptus citriodora. Planta Med. 1974 Sep;26(2):184-5.

Eucalyptus Dives *(Eucalyptus dives)*

Botanical Family: Myrtaceae (myrtle)

Plant Origin: Australia, Brazil

Extraction Method: Steam distilled from leaves.

Key Constituents:
Alpha- and Beta-Phellandrene (23-30%)
Piperitone (35-45%)
Para-Cymene (6-10%)
Alpha-Thujen (2-6%)
Terpinene-4-ol (3-6%)

Medical Properties: Mucolytic, diuretic, antibacterial

USES: Hypertension, throat/lung infections.

Application: Dilute 1 part EO with 1 part VO; (1) apply 2-4 drops on location, (2) chakras/vitaflex points, or (3) diffuse (see Appendices E and T)

Selected Research:

Delaquis PJ, et al., Antimicrobial activity of individual and mixed fractions of dill, cilantro, coriander and eucalyptus essential oils. Int J Food Microbiol. 2002 Mar 25;74(1-2):101-9.

Eucalyptus Globulus *(Eucalyptus globulus)*

Botanical Family: Myrtaceae (myrtle)

Plant Origin: Australia, Brazil

Extraction Method: Steam distilled from leaves.

Key Constituents:
1,8 Cineole (58-80%)
Alpha Pinene (10-22%)
Limonene (1-8%)
Para-Cymene (1-5%)
Trans-Pinocarveol (1-5%)
Aromadendrene (1-5%)
Globulol (0.5-1.5%)

ORAC: 2,400 µTE/100g

Historical Data: For centuries, Australian Aborigines used the disinfecting leaves to cover wounds. Shown by laboratory tests to be a powerful antimicrobial agent, *E. globulus*

contains a high percentage of eucalyptol (a key ingredient in many antiseptic mouth rinses). Often used for the respiratory system, eucalyptus has been investigated for its powerful insect repellent effects (Trigg, 1996). Eucalyptus trees have been planted throughout parts of North Africa to successfully block the spread of malaria. According to Jean Valnet, M.D., a solution of 2 percent eucalyptus oil sprayed in the air will kill 70 percent of airborne staph bacteria. Some doctors still use solutions of eucalyptus oil in surgical dressings.

Medical Properties: Expectorant, mucolytic, antimicrobial, antibacterial, antifungal, antiviral, anti-aging.

USES: Respiratory/sinus infections, decongestant, rheumatism/arthritis.

Fragrant Influence: It promotes health, well-being, purification, and healing.

Application: Dilute 1 part EO with 1 part VO; (1) apply 2-4 drops on location, (2) chakras/vitaflex points, (3) directly inhale, (4) diffuse, or (5) take as dietary supplement (see Appendices E and T).

Found In: R.C.

Selected Research:

Tovey ER, et al. "A simple washing procedure with eucalyptus oil for controlling house dust mites and their allergens in clothing and bedding." *J Allergy Clin Immunol.* 1997; 100(4):464-6.

Weyers W, et al. "Skin absorption of volatile oils. Pharmacokinetics." *Pharm Unserer Zeit.* 1989;18(3):82-6.

Zanker KS, et al. "Evaluation of surfactant-like effects of commonly used remedies for colds." *Respiration.* 1980;39(3):150-7.

Lee KG, Shibamoto T. Inhibition of malonaldehyde formation from blood plasma oxidation by aroma extracts and aroma components isolated from clove and eucalyptus. Food Chem Toxicol. 2001 Dec;39(12):1199-204.

Eucalyptus Polybractea (*Eucalyptus polybractea*)

Botanical Family: Myrtaceae (myrtle)

Plant Origin: Australia

Extraction Method: Steam distilled from leaves.

Key Constituents:
1,8 Cineole (Eucalyptol) (60-80%)
Limonene (1-5%)
Para-Cymene (1-5%)
Alpha-Pinene (1-5%)

Medical Properties: antiviral, antibacterial, anti-inflammatory, expectorant, mucolytic, and insect repellent.

USES: Acne, urinary tract/bladder infections, viral infections (Herpes)

Application: Dilute 1 part EO with 1 part VO; (1) Apply 2-4 drops on location, (2) chakras/vitaflex points, (3) directly inhale, (4) diffuse or put in humidifier, or (5) take as dietary supplement (see Appendices E and T).

Eucalyptus Radiata (*Eucalyptus radiata*)

Botanical Family: Myrtaceae (myrtle)

Plant Origin: Australia

Extraction Method: Steam distilled from leaves.

Key Constituents:
Eucalyptol (60-75%)
Alpha Terpineol (5-10%)
Limonene (4-8%)
Alpha Pinene (2-6%)

Medical Properties: Antibacterial, antiviral, expectorant, anti-inflammatory.

USES: Respiratory/sinus infections, viral infections, (Fights Herpes simplex when combined with bergamot).

Application: Dilute 1 part EO with 1 part VO; (1) apply 2-4 drops on location, (2) chakras/vitaflex points, (3) directly inhale, (4) diffuse or put in humidifier (see Appendices E and T).

Found In: R.C., Raven, and Thieves

Fennel (*Foeniculum vulgare*)

Botanical Family: Apiaceae or Umbelliferae (parsley)

Plant Origin: Australia, Spain

Extraction Method: Steam distilled from the crushed seeds.

Key Constituents:
Trans-Anethol (60-80%)
Fenchone + Linalol (12-16%)
Alpha-Pinene (3-5%)
Methyl Chavicol (2-5%)

ORAC: 238,400 μTE/100g

Historical Data: Believed to ward off evil spirits and to protect against spells cast by witches during medieval times. Sprigs were hung over doors to fend off evil phantasms. For hundreds of years, fennel seeds have been used as a digestive aid and to balance menstrual cycles. It is mentioned in one of the oldest known medical records, Ebers Papyrus (dating from sixteenth century BC) an ancient Egyptian list of 877 prescriptions and recipes.

It was listed in Hildegard's Medicine, a compilation of early German medicines by highly-regarded Benedictine herbalist Hildegard of Bingen (1098-1179).

Medical Properties: Anti-inflammatory, antitumoral, estrogen-like, digestive aid, antiparasitic (worms) antiseptic, antispasmodic, analgesic, increases metabolism.

USES: Cancer, obesity, arthritis/rheumatism, urinary tract infection, fluid retention, intestinal parasites, menstrual problems/ PMS, digestive problems.

Application: Dilute 1 part EO with 1 part VO; (1) apply 2-4 drops on location, (2) chakras/vitaflex points, (3) directly inhale, (4) diffuse, or (5) take as dietary supplement (see Appendices E and T).

Cautions: Avoid using if epileptic.

Found In: Di-Tone, Dragon Time, JuvaFlex, and Mister.

Selected Research: Fyfe L, et al. "Inhibition of *Listeria monocytogenes* and *Salmonella enteriditis* by combinations of plant oils and derivatives of benzoic acid: the development of synergistic antimicrobial combinations." *Int J Antimicrob Agents.* 1997;9(3):195-9.

Lis-Balchin M, Hart S. A preliminary study of the effect of essential oils on skeletal and smooth muscle in vitro. J Ethnopharmacol. 1997 Nov;58(3):183-7.

Chainy GB, Manna SK, Chaturvedi MM, Aggarwal BB. Anethole blocks both early and late cellular responses transduced by tumor necrosis factor: effect on NF-kappaB, AP-1, JNK, MAPKK and apoptosis. Oncogene. 2000 Jun 8;19(25):2943-50.

Haze S, Sakai K, Gozu Y. et al., Effects of fragrance inhalation on sympathetic activity in normal adults. Jpn J Pharmacol. 2002 Nov;90(3):247-53.

Fir, Douglas (*Pseudotsuga menziesii*)

Botanical Family: Abietaceae

Plant Origin: Idaho

Extraction Method: Steam-distilled

Chemical Constituents:
Alpha Pinene (25-40%)
Beta Pinene (7-15%)
Limonene (6-11%)
Bornyl Acetate (8-15%)

ORAC: 69,000 μTE/100g

Medical Properties: Antitumoral, antioxidant, anti-fungal

USES: Respiratory/sinus infections.

Application: Dilute 1 part EO with 1 part VO; (1) apply 2-4 drops on location, (2) chakras/vitaflex points, (3) directly inhale, or (4) diffuse (see Appendices E and T).

Found In: Evergreen Essence.

Fir, Idaho Balsam (*Abies balsamea*)

(See BALSAM FIR, IDAHO)

Fir, White (Abies grandis)

Botanical Family: Abietaceae

Plant Origin: Idaho

Extraction Method: Steam-distilled

Key Constituents:
Alpha Pinene (8-12%)
Beta Pinene (20-30%)
Camphene (7-15%)
Bornyl Acetate (11-16%)
Delta Cadinene (2-7%)

ORAC: 47,900 µTE/100g

Medical Properties: Anti-tumoral, anti-cancerous, anti-oxidant

USES: Respiratory infections, anti-fungal.

Application: Dilute 1 part EO with 1 part VO; (1) apply 2-4 drops on location, (2) chakras/vitaflex points, (3) directly inhale, or (4) diffuse (see Appendices E and T).

Found In: Evergreen Essence

Fleabane, Canadian (Conyza canadensis)

Botanical Family: Asteraceae or Compositae (daisy)

Plant Origin: Canada

Extraction Method: Steam distilled from stems, leaves, and flowers.

Key Constituents:
Limonene (60-75%)
Cis Alpha Bergamotene (5-11%)
Trans Beta Ocimene (3-7%)

ORAC: 26,700 µTE/100g

Medical Properties: Stimulates liver and pancreas, anti-aging (stimulates growth hormone), antirheumatic, antispasmodic, vasodilating, reduces blood pressure.

USES: Hypertension, hepatitis, accelerated aging.

Application: Dilute 1 part EO with 1 part VO; (1) apply 2-4 drops on location, (2) chakras/vitaflex points, (3) directly inhale, (4) diffuse, or (5) take as dietary supplement (see Appendices E and T).

Frankincense (Boswellia carteri)

Botanical Family: Burseraceae (Frankincense)

Plant Origin: Somalia

Extraction Method: Steam distilled from gum/resin.

Key Constituents:
Alpha-Pinene (28-49%)
Limonene (10-16%)
Sabinene (3-7%)
Myrcene (8-12%)
Beta Caryophyllene (3-7%)
Alpha Thuyene (4-8%)
Paracymene (2-5%)

ORAC: 630 µTE/100g

Historical Data: Also known as "olibanum," or "Oil from Lebanon" the name frankincense is derived from the Medieval French word for "real incense." Frankincense is considered the "holy anointing oil" in the Middle East and has been used in religious ceremonies for thousands of years. It was well known during the time of Christ for its anointing and healing powers and was one of the gifts given to Christ at His birth. "Used to treat every conceivable ill known to man," frankincense was valued more than gold during ancient times, and only those with great wealth and abundance possessed it. It is mentioned in one of the oldest known medical records, Ebers Papyrus (dating from sixteenth century BC) an ancient Egyptian list of 877 prescriptions and recipes.

Medical Properties: Antitumoral, immuno-stimulant, antidepressant, muscle relaxing.

USES: Depression, cancer, respiratory infections, inflammation, immune-stimulating.

Fragrant Influence: Increases spiritual awareness, promotes meditation, improves attitude and uplifts spirits.

Frankincense contains sesquiterpenes which stimulate the limbic system of the brain (the center of memory and emotions) and the hypothalamus, pineal and pituitary glands. The hypothalamus is the master gland of the human body, producing many vital hormones including thyroid and growth hormone.

Application: (1) Apply 2-4 drops on location, (2) chakras/vitaflex points, (3) directly inhale, (4) diffuse, or (5) take as dietary supplement (see Appendices E and T).

Found In: Abundance, Acceptance, Brain Power, Exodus II, Forgiveness, Gathering, Harmony, Humility, ImmuPower, Inspiration, Into The Future, Wisdom, Trauma Life, and Valor.

Bible References: There are over 52 references to frankincense (considering that "incense" is translated from the Hebrew/Greek "frankincense" and is referring to the same oil). (See additional Bible references in Appendix D)

Exodus 30:34—"And the Lord said unto Moses, Take unto thee sweet spices, stacte, and onycha, and galbanum; these sweet spices with pure frankincense: of each shall there be a like weight:"

Leviticus 2:1—"And when any will offer a meat offering unto the Lord, his offering shall be of fine flour; and he shall pour oil upon it, and put frankincense thereon:"

Leviticus 2:2—"And he shall bring it to Aaron's sons the priests: and he shall take thereout his handful of the flour thereof, and of the oil thereof, with all the frankincense thereof; and the priest shall burn the memorial of it upon the altar, to be an offering made by fire, of a sweet savour unto the Lord:"

Selected Research:

Michie, C.A., et al. "Frankincense and myrrh as remedies in children." *J R Soc Med.* 1991;84(10):602-5.

Wang, L.G., et al. "Determination of DNA topoisomerase II activity from L1210 cells--a target for screening antitumor agents." Chung Kuo Yao Li Hsueh Pao. 1991;12(2):108-14.

Lis-Balchin M, Hart S. A preliminary study of the effect of essential oils on skeletal and smooth muscle in vitro. J Ethnopharmacol. 1997 Nov;58(3):183-7.

Crowell PL.Prevention and therapy of cancer by dietary monoterpenes. J Nutr. 1999 Mar;129(3):775S-778S.

Galbanum *(Ferula gummosa)*

Botanical Family: Apiaceae or Umbelliferae (parsley)

Plant Origin: Iran

Extraction Method: Steam distilled from resin derived from stems and branches.

Key Constituents:
Alpha-Pinene (5-21%)
Beta-Pinene (40-70%)
Delta-3-Carene (2-16%)
Myrcene (2.5-3.5%)
Sabinene (0.3-3%0

ORAC: 26,200 µTE/100g

Historical Data: Mentioned in Egyptian papyri and the Old Testament (Exodus 30:34) it was esteemed for its medicinal and spiritual properties. Dioscorides, an ancient Roman historian, records that galbanum was used for its antispasmodic, diuretic, and pain-relieving properties.

Medical Properties: Antiseptic, analgesic, and light antispasmodic, anti-inflammatory, circulatory stimulant, anticonvulsant.

USES: Digestive problems (diarrhea), nervous tension, rheumatism, skin conditions (scar tissue, wrinkles)

Fragrant Influence: Harmonic and balancing, amplifies spiritual awareness and meditation. When combined with frankincense or sandalwood, the frequency rises dramatically.

Application: (1) apply 2-4 drops on location, (2) chakras/vitaflex points, (3) directly inhale, (4) diffuse, or (5) take as dietary supplement (see Appendices E and T)

Found In: Exodus II and Gathering.

Bible Reference: Exodus 30:34—"And the Lord said unto Moses, Take unto thee sweet spices, stacte, and onycha, and galbanum; these sweet spices with pure frankincense: of each shall there be a like weight:"

Selected Research:

Vaziri A. Antimicrobial action of galbanum. Planta Med. 1975 Dec;28(4):370-3.

Sayyah M, Mandgary A, Kamalinejad M. Evaluation of the anticonvulsant activity of the seed acetone extract of Ferula gummosa Boiss. against seizures induced by pentylenetetrazole and electroconvulsive shock in mice. J Ethnopharmacol. 2002 Oct;82(2-3):105-9.

Sadraei H, et al., Spasmolytic activity of essential oil and various extracts of Ferula gummosa Boiss. on ileum contractions. Phytomedicine. 2001 Sep;8(5):370-6.

Geranium *(Pelargonium graveolens)*

Botanical Family: Geraniaceae

Plant Origin: Egypt, India

Extraction Method: Steam distilled from the leaves.

Key Constituents:
Citronellol + Nerol (35-50%)
Citronnellyl Formate (9-15%)
Geraniol (5-10%)
6,9-Guaiadene (4-8%)
Isomenthone (4-8%)

Historical Data: Geranium has been used for centuries for regenerating and healing skin conditions.

Medical Properties: Antispasmodic, antioxidant, antitumoral, anti-inflammatory, hemostatic (stops bleeding), antibacterial, antifungal, improves blood flow, liver and pancreas stimulant, dilates bile ducts for liver detoxification. Helps cleanse oily skin; revitalizes skin cells.

USES: Hepatitis/fatty liver (Jean Valnet, M.D), Skin conditions (dermatitis, eczema, psoriasis, acne, vitiligo), fungal infections (ringworm), viral infections (Herpes, shingles), hormone imbalances, circulatory problems (improves blood flow), menstrual problems/PMS.

Fragrant Influence: Helps release negative memories and eases nervous tension. It balances the emotions, lifts the spirit, and fosters peace, well-being, and hope.

Application: (1) Apply 2-4 drops on location, (2) chakras/vitaflex points, (3) directly inhale, (4) diffuse, or (5) take as dietary supplement (see Appendices E and T).

Found In: Acceptance, Awaken, Clarity, EndoFlex, Envision, Forgiveness, Gathering, Gentle Baby, Harmony, Humility, Joy, JuvaFlex, Release, SARA, Trauma Life, and White Angelica.

Selected Research:

Lis-Balchin, M., et al. "Antimicrobial activity of Pelargonium essential oils added to a quiche filling as a model food system." *Lett Appl Microbiol.* 1998;27(4):207-10.

Lis-Balchin, M., et al. "Comparative antibacterial effects of novel Pelargonium essential oils and solvent extracts." *Lett Appl Microbiol.* 1998;27(3):135-41.

Fang, H.J., et al. "Studies on the chemical components and anti-tumour action of the volatile oils from Pelargonium graveoleus." *Yao Hsueh Hsueh Pao.* 1989;24(5):366-71.

Thompson JD, et al., QualitativE and Tuantitative variation in monoterpene co-occurrence and composition in the essential oil of Thymus vulgaris chemotypes. J Chem Ecol. 2003 Apr;29(4):859-80.

Carnesecchi S, et al., Geraniol, a component of plant essential oils, sensitizes human colon cancer cells to 5-fluorouracil treatment. IARC Sci Publ. 2002;156:407-9.

Carnesecchi S, et al., Perturbation by geraniol of cell membrane permeability and signal transduction pathways in human colon cancer cells. J Pharmacol Exp Ther. 2002 Nov;303(2):711-5.

Choi HS, Song HS, Ukeda H, Sawamura M. Radical-scavenging activities of citrus essential oils and their components: detection using 1,1-diphenyl-2-picrylhydrazyl. J Agric Food Chem. 2000 Sep;48(9):4156-61.

Dorman HJ, Deans SG. Antimicrobial agents from plants: antibacterial activity of plant volatile oils. J Appl Microbiol. 2000 Feb;88(2):308-16.

Ginger *(Zingiber officinale)*

Botanical Family: Zingiberaceae (ginger)

Plant Origin: China

Extraction Method: Steam distilled from root.

Key Constituents:
Zingiberene + Alpha-Selinene (25-40%)
Beta-Sesquiphellandrene +
  Delta-Cadinene (7-14%)
Beta-Phellandrena +
  1,8 Cineol + Limonene (8-15%)
AR Curcumene (5-11%)

ORAC: 99,300 µTE/100g

Historical Data: Traditionally used to combat nausea. Women in the West African country of Senegal weave belts of ginger root to restore their mates' sexual potency.

Medical Properties: Anti-inflammatory, anticoagulant, digestive aid, anesthetic, expectorant.

USES: Rheumatism/arthritis, digestive disorders, respiratory infections/congestion, muscular aches/pains, nausea.

Fragrant Influence: Gentle, stimulating, endowing physical energy, and courage.

Application: Dilute 1 part EO with 1 part VO; (1) apply 2-4 drops on location, (2) chakras/vitaflex points, (3) directly inhale, (4) diffuse, or (5) take as dietary supplement (see Appendices E and T).

Cautions: Anticoagulant properties can be enhanced when combined with Warfarin, aspirin, etc.

Found In: Abundance, Di-Tone, Magnify Your Purpose, and Live With Passion.

Selected Research:

Martins AP, Essential oil composition and antimicrobial activity of three Zingiberaceae from S.Tome e Principe. Planta Med. 2001 Aug;67(6):580-4.

Nurtjahja-Tjendraputra E, et al., Effective anti-platelet and COX-1 enzyme inhibitors from pungent constituents of ginger. Thromb Res. 2003;111(4-5):259-65.

Baliga MS, Jagetia GC, Rao SK, Babu K. Evaluation of nitric oxide scavenging activity of certain spices in vitro: a preliminary study.Nahrung. 2003 Aug;47(4):261-4.

Kirana C, et al., Antitumor activity of extract of Zingiber aromaticum and its bioactive sesquiterpenoid zerumbone. Nutr Cancer. 2003;45(2):218-25.

Ippoushi K, et al., [6]-Gingerol inhibits nitric oxide synthesis in activated J774.1 mouse macrophages and prevents peroxynitrite-induced oxidation and nitration reactions. Life Sci. 2003 Nov 14;73(26):3427-37.

Goldenrod *(Solidago canadensis)*

Botanical Family: Asteraceae

Plant Origin: Canada

Extraction Method: Steam distilled.

Key Constituents:
Germacrene D (22-35%)
Alpha-Pinene (10-18%)
Myrcene (8-15%0
Sabinene (5-11%)
Limonene (6-12%)

ORAC: 61,900 µTE/100g

Historical Data: The genus name, solidago, comes from the Latin solide, which means 'to make whole'. During the Boston Tea Party, when English tea was dumped into Boston Harbor, Colonists drank goldenrod tea instead, which gave it the nickname 'Liberty Tea'.

Medical Properties: Diuretic, anti-inflammatory, anti-hypertensive, liver stimulant

USES: Hypertension, liver congestion, hepatitis/fatty liver, circulatory conditions, urinary tract/bladder conditions

Application: Dilute 1 part EO with 1 part VO; (1) apply 2-4 drops on location or compress, (2) chakras/vitaflex points, (3) directly inhale, (4) diffuse, or (5) take as dietary supplement (see Appendices E and T).

Selected Research:

Yarnell E. Botanical medicines for the urinary tract. World J Urol. 2002 Nov;20(5):285-93. Epub 2002 Oct 17.

Grapefruit *(Citrus paradisi)*

Botanical Family: Rutaceae (citrus)

Plant Origin: California. (Grapefruit is a hybrid between *Citrus maxima* and *Citrus sinensis*.)

Extraction Method: Cold pressed from rind.

Key Constituents:
Limonene (88-95%)
Myrcene (1-4%)

ORAC: 22,600 µTE/100g

Medical Properties: Antitumoral, metabolic stimulant, antiseptic, detoxifying, diuretic, fat-dissolving, cleansing for kidneys, lymphatic and vascular system, antidepressant. Rich in limonene, which has been extensively studied for its ability to combat tumor growth in over 50 clinical studies.

USES: Alzheimers, fluid retention. depression, obesity, liver disorders, anxiety, cellulite

Fragrant Influence: Refreshing and uplifting. A 1995 Mie University study found that citrus fragrances boosted immunity, induced relaxation, and reduced depression.

Application: Dilute 1 part EO with 1 part VO; (1) apply 2-4 drops on location, (2) chakras/vitaflex points, (3) directly inhale, (4) diffuse, or (5) take as dietary supplement (see Appendices E and T).

Cautions: Avoid applying to skin that will be exposed to sunlight or UV light within 24 hours.

Found In: Citrus Fresh

Selected Research:

Haze S, Sakai K, Gozu Y. et al., Effects of fragrance inhalation on sympathetic activity in normal adults. Jpn J Pharmacol. 2002 Nov;90(3):247-53.

Miyazawa M, Tougo H, Ishihara M. Inhibition of acetylcholinesterase activity by essential oil from Citrus paradisi. Nat Prod Lett. 2001;15(3):205-10.

Niijima A, Nagai K. Effect of olfactory stimulation with flavor of grapefruit oil and lemon oil on the activity of sympathetic branch in the white adipose tissue of the epididymis. Exp Biol Med (Maywood). 2003 Nov;228(10):1190-2.

Wattenberg LW, et al., Inhibition of carcinogenesis by some minor dietary constituents. Princess Takamatsu Symp. 1985;16:193-203.

Alderman GG, Marth EH. Inhibition of growth and aflatoxin production of Aspergillus parasiticus by citrus oils. Z Lebensm Unters Forsch. 1976 Apr 28;160(4):353-8.

Fisher JF et al., A new coumarin from grapefruit peel oil. Tetrahedron. 1967 Jun;23(6):2523-8.

Crowell PL.Prevention and therapy of cancer by dietary monoterpenes. J Nutr. 1999 Mar;129(3):775S-778S.

Komori T, et al., Application of fragrances to treatments for depression. Nihon Shinkei Seishin Yakurigaku Zasshi. 1995 Feb;15(1):39-42. Japanese.

Helichrysum *(Helichrysum italicum)*

Botanical Family: Asteraceae or Compositae (daisy)

Plant Origin: Yugoslavia, Corsica

Extraction Method: Steam distilled from flower.

Key Constituents:
Neryl Acetate (25-35%)
Gamma Curcuneme (9-15%)
Limonene (8-13%)
Neryl Propionate (3-7%)
Alpha Pinene (3-8%)
Beta-Caryophyllene (1-5%)
Linalol (1-4%)
Nerol (2-5%)

ORAC: 1,700 µTE/100g

Medical Properties: Anticoagulant, anesthetic, anticoagulant, antispasmodic, antiviral, liver protectant / detoxifier / stimulant, chelates chemicals and toxins. regenerates nerves.

USES: Herpes virus, Arteriosclerosis, atherosclerosis, hypertension, blood clots, liver disorders, circulatory disorders, skin conditions (eczema, psoriasis scar tissue, varicose veins)

Fragrant Influence: Uplifting to the subconscious.

Application: (1) Apply 2-4 drops on location, temple, forehead, back of neck, or outside of ear (2) chakras/vitaflex points, (3) directly inhale, (4) diffuse, or (5) take as dietary supplement (see Appendices E and T).

Found In: JuvaCleanse

Selected Research:

Nostro A, et al., Evaluation of antiherpesvirus-1 and genotoxic activities of Helichrysum italicum extract. New Microbiol. 2003 Jan;26(1):125-8.

Sala A, Anti-inflammatory and antioxidant properties of Helichrysum italicum. J Pharm Pharmacol. 2002 Mar;54(3):365-71.

Schinella GR, et al., Antioxidant activity of anti-inflammatory plant extracts. Life Sci. 2002 Jan 18;70(9):1023-33.

Hyssop *(Hyssopus officinalis)*

Botanical Family: Lamiaceae or Labiatae (mint)

Plant Origin: France, Hungary

Extraction Method: Steam distilled from stems/leaves.

Key Constituents:
Beta Pinene (13.5-23%)
Sabinene (2-3%)
Pinocamphone (5.5-17.5%)
Iso-Pinochamphone (34.5-50%)
Gemacrene D (2-3%)
Limonene (1-4%)

ORAC: 20,900 µTE/100g

Historical Data: While there is some uncertainty that *Hyssopus officinalis* is the same species of plant as the hyssop referred to in the Bible, there is no question that *H. officinalis* has been used medicinally for almost a millennium for its antiseptic properties. It has also been used for opening the respiratory system.

Medical Properties: Mucolytic, decongestant, anti-inflammatory, regulates lipid metabolism, antiviral, antibacterial, antiparasitic

USES: Respiratory infections/congestion, parasites (expelling worms), viral infections, circulatory disorders

Fragrant Influence: Stimulates creativity and meditation.

Application: Dilute 1 part EO with 1 part VO; (1) apply 2-4 drops on location, (2) chakras/vitaflex points, (3) directly inhale, (4) diffuse, or (5) take as dietary supplement (see Appendices E and T).

Cautions: Avoid use if epileptic.

Found In: Exodus II, Harmony, ImmuPower, Relieve It, and White Angelica.

Bible References: (see additional Bible references in Appendix D).

Exodus 12:22— "And ye shall take a bunch of hyssop, and dip it in the blood that is in the bason, and strike the lintel and the two side posts with the blood that is in the bason; and none of you shall go out at the door of his house until the morning."

Leviticus 14:4—"Then shall the priest command to take for him that is to be cleansed two birds alive and clean, and cedar wood, and scarlet, and hyssop:"

Leviticus 14:6—"As for the living bird, he shall take it, and the cedar wood, and the scarlet, and the hyssop, and shall dip them and the living bird in the blood of the bird that was killed over the running water:"

Selected Research:

Lu M, et al., Muscle relaxing activity of Hyssopus officinalis essential oil on isolated intestinal preparations. Planta Med. 2002 Mar;68(3):213-6.

Jasmine Absolute (*Jasminum officinale*)

Botanical Family: Oleaceae (olive)

Plant Origin: India

Extraction Method: Absolute extraction from flower. Jasmine is actually an "essence" not an essential oil. The flowers must be picked at night to maximize fragrance.

NOTE: One pound of jasmine oil requires about 1,000 pounds of jasmine or 3.6 million fresh unpacked blossoms. The blossoms must be collected before sunrise, or much of the fragrance will have evaporated. The quality of the blossoms may also be compromised if they are crushed. A single pound of pure jasmine oil may cost between $1,200 to $4,500. In contrast, synthetic jasmine oils can be obtained for $3.50 per pound, but they do not possess the same therapeutic qualities as the pure oil.

Key Constituents:
Benzyl Acetate (18-28%)
Benzyl Benzoate (14-21%)
Linalol (3-8%)
Phytol (6-12%)
Isophytol (3-7%)
Squalene (3-7%)

Historical Data: Nicknamed as the "queen of the night" and "moonlight of the grove." For centuries, women have treasured jasmine for its beautiful, seductive fragrance.

Medical Properties: Uplifting, antidepressant, stimulating, antibacterial.

USES: Anxiety, depression, menstrual problems/PMS, skin problems (eczema, wrinkles, greasy), frigidity.

Fragrant Influence: Uplifting, counteracts hopelessness, nervous exhaustion, anxiety, depression, indifference, and listlessness. University researchers in Japan found that diffusing certain aromas in an office environment dramatically improved mental accuracy and concentration. Diffused lemon resulted in 54 percent fewer errors, jasmine 33 percent fewer errors, and lavender 20 percent fewer errors. When aromas were diffused during test taking, scores increased by as much as 50 percent.

Application: (1) Apply 2-4 drops on location, (2) chakras/vitaflex points, (3) directly inhale, or (4) diffuse (see Appendices E and T).

Found In: Awaken, Clarity, Dragon Time, Forgiveness, Gentle Baby, Harmony, Inner Child, Into The Future, Joy, Live With Passion, and Sensation.

Selected Research:

Friedman M, Henika PR, Mandrell RE. Bactericidal activities of plant essential oils and some of their isolated constituents against Campylobacter jejuni, Escherichia coli, Listeria monocytogenes, and Salmonella enterica. J Food Prot. 2002 Oct;65(10):1545-60.

Juniper (*Juniperus osteosperma* and *J. scopulorum*)

Botanical Family: Cupressaceae (cypress)

Plant Origin: Utah

Extraction Method: Steam distilled from berries, branches, and twigs.

Key Constituents:
Alpha-pinene (20-40%)
Sabinene (3-18%)
Myrcene (1-6%)
Camphor (10-18%)
Limonene (3-8%)
Bornyl Acetate (12-20%)
Terpinene-4-ol (3-8%)

ORAC: 250 μTE/100g

Historical Data: Bundles of juniper berries were hung over doorways to ward off witches during medieval times. It has been used for centuries as a diuretic. Until recently, French hospital wards burned sprigs of juniper and rosemary to protect from infection.

Medical Properties: Antiseptic, digestive cleanser/stimulant, purifying, detoxifying, increases circulation through the kidneys and promotes excretion of toxins, promotes nerve regeneration.

USES: Skin conditions (acne, eczema), liver problems, urinary/bladder infections, fluid retention

Fragrant Influence: Juniper evokes feelings of health, love, and peace and may help to elevate one's spiritual awareness.

Application: Dilute 1 part EO with 1 part VO; (1) apply 2-4 drops on location, (2) chakras/vitaflex points, (3) directly inhale, (4) diffuse, or (5) take as dietary supplement (see Appendices E and T).

Found In: Di-Tone, Dream Catcher, En-R-Gee, Grounding, Hope, and Into the Future

Bible Reference:

Job 30:45—"Who cut up mallows by the bushes, and juniper roots for their meat."

Selected Research:

Takacsova M, et al. "Study of the antioxidative effects of thyme, sage, juniper and oregano." *Nahrung*. 1995;39(3):241-3.

Laurus Nobilis *(Laurus nobilis-Bay Laurel)*

Botanical Family: Lauraceae

Plant Origin: France

Extraction Method: Steam distilled from leaves.

Key Constituents:
Alpha-Pinene (4-10%)
Beta-Pinene (3-8%)
Sabinene (4-12%)
Linalol (4-16%)
1,8 Cineol(Eucalyptol) (35-50%)
Eugenol + Terpenyl Acetate (10-18%)

ORAC: 98,900 µTE/100g

Historical Data: Both the leaves and the black berries were also used to alleviate indigestion, and loss of appetite. During the Middle Ages, it was used for angina, migraine, heart palpitations, and liver and spleen complaints.

Medical Properties: Antimicrobial, expectorant, mucolytic, antibacterial (Staph, Strep, *E. coli*), antifungal (Candida), anticoagulant, anticonvulsant

USES: Nerve regeneration, arthritis (rheumatoid), and oral infections (gingivitis), respiratory infections, viral infections.

Application: Dilute 1 part EO with 1 part VO; (1) apply 2-4 drops on location or abdomen, (2) chakras/vitaflex points, (3) directly inhale, (4) diffuse, or (5) take as dietary supplement (see Appendices E and T).

Found In: Di-Tone, Dream Catcher, En-R-Gee, Grounding, Hope, and Into the Future.

Selected Research:

Sayyah M, Valizadeh J, Kamalinejad M. Anticonvulsant activity of the leaf essential oil of Laurus nobilis against pentylenetetrazole- and maximal electroshock-induced seizures. Phytomedicine. 2002 Apr;9(3):212-6.

Lavandin *(Lavandula* x *hybrida)*

Botanical Family: Lamiaceae or Labiatae (mint)

Key Constituents:
Linalyl acetate (28-35%)
Linalol (30-38%)
Camphor (5-12%)
Limonene + 1,8 Cineol (Eucalyptol) (2-8%)
Borneol (2-6%)
Terpinene-4-ol (2-7%)
Lavandulyl Acetate (1-5%)

Historical Data: Also known as *Lavandula* x *intermedia*, lavandin is a hybrid plant developed by crossing true lavender with spike lavender or aspic (*Lavandula latifolia*). It has been used to sterilize the animal cages in veterinary clinics and hospitals throughout Europe.

Medical Properties: Antibacterial, antifungal

USES: Lavandin is a stronger antiseptic than Lavandula officinialis. Its greater penetrating qualities make it well suited to help with respiratory, circulatory, and muscular conditions.

Fragrant Influence: Similar calming effects as lavender.

Application: (1) Apply 2-4 drops on location, (2) chakras/vitaflex points, (3) directly inhale, or (4) diffuse (see Appendices E and T).

Cautions: Avoid using for burns; instead use lavender.

Found In: Purification, Release.

Lavender (*Lavandula angustifolia*)

Botanical Family: Lamiaceae or Labiatae (mint)

Plant Origin: Utah, Idaho, France

Extraction Method: Steam distilled from flowering top.

Key Constituents:
Linalyl Acetate (24-45%)
Linalol (25-38%)
Cis-beta-Ocimene (4-10%)
Trans-beta Ocimene (1.5-6%)
Terpinene-4-ol (2-6%)

ORAC: 360 µTE/100g

Historical Data: The French scientist René Gattefossé was the first to discover lavender's ability to promote tissue regeneration and speed wound healing when he severely burned his arm in a laboratory accident. Today, lavender is one of the few essential oils to still be listed in the British Pharmacopoeia.

Medical Properties: Antiseptic, antifungal, analgesic, antitumoral, anticonvulsant, vasodilating, relaxant, anti-inflammatory, reduces blood fat/cholesterol, combats excess sebum on skin.

USES: Respiratory infections, high blood pressure, arteriosclerosis, menstrual problems/PMS, skin conditions (perinial repair, acne, eczema, psoriasis, scarring stretch marks), burns, hair loss, insomnia, nervous tension,

Fragrant Influence: Calming, relaxing, and balancing, both physically and emotionally. University researchers in Japan found that diffusing certain aromas in an office environment dramatically improved mental accuracy and concentration. Diffused lemon resulted in 54 percent fewer errors, jasmine 33 percent fewer errors, and lavender 20 percent fewer errors. When aromas were diffused during test taking, scores increased by as much as 50 percent. Has been documented to improve concentration and mental acuity.

University of Miami researchers found that inhalation of lavender oil increased beta waves in the brain, suggesting heightened relaxation. It also reduced depression and improved cognitive performance (Diego et al., 1998). A 2001 Osaka Kyoiku University study found that lavender reduced mental stress and increased alertness (Motomura et al., 2001).

Application: (1) Apply 2-4 drops on location, (2) chakras/vitaflex points, (3) directly inhale, (4) diffuse, or (5) take as dietary supplement (see Appendices E and T).

Cautions: True lavender is often extended with hybrid lavender or synthetic linalol and linalyl acetate.

Found In: Aroma Siez, Brain Power, Dragon Time, Envision, Forgiveness, Gathering, Gentle Baby, Harmony, Mister, Motivation, M-Grain, R.C., SARA, Surrender, and Trauma Life.

Selected Research:

Larrondo JV, et al. "Antimicrobial activity of essences from labiates." *Microbios*. 1995; 82(332):171-2.

Guillemain J, et al. "Neurodepressive effects of the essential oil of *Lavandula angustifolia* Mill." *Ann Pharm Fr*. 1989;47(6):337-43.

Kim HM, et al. "Lavender oil inhibits immediate-type allergic reaction in mice and rats." *J Pharm Pharmacol*. 1999;51(2):221-6.

Siurin SA. Effects of essential oil on lipid peroxidation and lipid metabolism in patients with chronic bronchitis. Klin Med (Mosk). 1997;75(10):43-5.

Nikolaevskii VV, et al., Effect of essential oils on the course of experimental atherosclerosis, Patol Fiziol Eksp Ter. 1990 Sep-Oct;(5):52-3.

Holmes C, et al., Lavender oil as a treatment for agitated behaviour in severe dementia: a placebo controlled study. Int J Geriatr Psychiatry. 2002 Apr;17(4):305-8.

Inouye S, Uchida K, Yamaguchi H. In-vitro and in-vivo anti-Trichophyton activity of essential oils by vapour contact. Mycoses. 2001 May;44(3-4):99-107.

Morris N. The effects of lavender (Lavendula angustifolium) baths on psychological well-being: two exploratory randomised control trials. Complement Ther Med. 2002 Dec;10(4):223-8.

Louis M, Kowalski SD. Use of aromatherapy with hospice patients to decrease pain, anxiety, and depression and to promote an increased sense of well-being. Am J Hosp Palliat Care. 2002 Nov-Dec;19(6):381-6.

Cornwell S, Dale A. Lavender oil and perineal repair. Mod Midwife. 1995 Mar;5(3):31-3.

Yamada K, Mimaki Y, Sashida Y. Anticonvulsive effects of inhaling lavender oil vapour. Biol Pharm Bull. 1994 Feb;17(2):359-60.

Ghelardini C, et al., Local anaesthetic activity of the essential oil of Lavandula angustifolia. Planta Med. 1999 Dec;65(8):700-3.

Motomura N, Sakurai A, Yotsuya Y. Reduction of mental stress with lavender odorant. Percept Mot Skills. 2001 Dec;93(3):713-8.

Ledum (Ledum groenlandicum)

Botanical Family: Ericaceae

Plant Origin: North America

Extraction Method: Steam distilled.

Key Constituents:
Limonene (20-35%)
Cis- and Trans-Paramenth1(7)
   8 Diene 8-ol (12-17%)
Cis- and Trans-Paramenthatriene
   1,3,8 (8-15%)

Historical Data: Known colloquially as "Labrador tea", ledum is a strongly aromatic herb that has been used for centuries in folk medicine. The native people of Eastern Canada used this herb for tea, as a general tonic, and to treat a variety of kidney-related problems. Ledum has helped protect the native people of North America against scurvy for more than 5,000 years. The Cree used it for fevers and colds.

Medical Properties: Anti-inflammatory, anti-tumoral, antibacterial, diuretic, liver-protectant

USES: Liver problems/hepatitis/fatty liver, obesity, water retention

Application: (1) Apply 2-4 drops on location, (2) chakras/vitaflex points, (3) directly inhale, (4) diffuse, or (5) take as dietary supplement (see Appendices E and T).

Found In: Raven, R.C., JuvaCleanse, JuvaFlex

Lemon (Citrus limon)

Botanical Family: Rutaceae (citrus)

Plant Origin: California, Italy

Extraction Method: Cold pressed from rind. It takes 3,000 lemons to produce a kilo of oil.

Key Constituents:
Limonene (59-73%)
Gamma-Terpinene (6-12%)
Beta-Pinene (7-16%)
Alpha-Pinene (1.5-3%)
Sabinene (1.5-3%)

ORAC: 660 µTE/100g

Historical Data: Research by Jean Valnet, M.D., showed that vaporized lemon oil can kill meningococcus bacteria in 15 minutes, typhoid bacilli in one hour, *Staphylococcus aureus* in two hours, and *Pneumococcus* bacteria within three hours. Even a 0.2% solution of lemon oil can kill diphtheria bacteria in 20 minutes and inactivate tuberculosis bacteria. Lemon oil has been widely used in skin care to cleanse skin and reduce wrinkles and combat acne. Lemon has shown to have antidepressant effects in research done by Komori, et al., 1995.

Medical Properties: Antitumoral, antiseptic, improves microcirculation, and immune stimulant (increases white blood cells), improves memory, relaxation. Rich in limonene, which has been extensively studied for its ability to combat tumor growth in over 50 clinical studies.

USES: Circulatory problems, arteriosclerosis, obesity, parasites, urinary tract infections, varicose veins, anxiety, hypertension, digestive problems, acne.

Fragrant Influence: It promotes clarity of thought and purpose with a fragrance is invigorating, enhancing, and warming. University researchers in Japan found that diffusing certain aromas in an office environment dramatically improved mental accuracy and concentration. Diffused lemon resulted in 54 percent fewer errors, jasmine 33 percent fewer errors, and lavender 20 percent fewer errors. When aromas were diffused during test taking, scores increased by as much as 50 percent.

A 1995 Mie University study found that citrus fragrances boosted immunity, induced relaxation, and reduced depression.

Application: Dilute 1 part EO with 1 part VO; (1) apply 2-4 drops on location, (2) chakras/vitaflex points, (3) directly inhale, (4) diffuse, or (5) take as dietary supplement (see Appendices E and T).

Cautions: Avoid applying to skin that will be exposed to sunlight or UV light within 24 hours.

Found In: Awaken, Citrus Fresh, Clarity, Forgiveness, Gentle Baby, Harmony, Joy, Raven, Surrender, and Thieves.

Selected Research:

Lu XG, et al., D-limonene induces apoptosis of gastric cancer cells. Zhonghua Zhong Liu Za Zhi. 2003 Jul;25(4):325-7.

Nishino H et al. Cancer Chemoprevention by Phytochemicals and their Related Compounds. Asian Pac J Cancer Prev. 2000;1(1):49-55.

Parija T, Das BR. Involvement of YY1 and its correlation with c-myc in NDEA induced hepatocarcinogenesis, its prevention by d-limonene. Mol Biol Rep. 2003 Mar;30(1):41-6.

Uedo N, et al., Inhibition by D-limonene of gastric carcinogenesis induced by N-methyl-N'-nitro-N-nitrosoguanidine in Wistar rats. Cancer Lett. 1999 Apr 1;137(2):131-6.

Hakim IA, Harris RB, Ritenbaugh C. Citrus peel use is associated with reduced risk of squamous cell carcinoma of the skin. Nutr Cancer. 2000;37(2):161-8.

Asamoto M, et al., Mammary carcinomas induced in human c-Ha-ras proto-oncogene transgenic rats are estrogen-independent, but responsive to d-limonene treatment. Jpn J Cancer Res. 2002 Jan;93(1):32-5.

Guyton KZ, Kensler TW. Prevention of liver cancer. Curr Oncol Rep. 2002 Nov;4(6):464-70.

Bradlow HL, Sepkovic DW. Diet and breast cancer. Ann N Y Acad Sci. 2002 Jun;963:247-67.

Niijima A, Nagai K. Effect of olfactory stimulation with flavor of grapefruit oil and lemon oil on the activity of sympathetic branch in the white adipose tissue of the epididymis. Exp Biol Med (Maywood). 2003 Nov;228(10):1190-2.

Wattenberg LW, et al., Inhibition of carcinogenesis by some minor dietary constituents. Princess Takamatsu Symp. 1985;16:193-203.

Alderman GG, Marth EH. Inhibition of growth and aflatoxin production of Aspergillus parasiticus by citrus oils. Z Lebensm Unters Forsch. 1976 Apr 28;160(4):353-8.

Crowell PL.Prevention and therapy of cancer by dietary monoterpenes. J Nutr. 1999 Mar;129(3):775S-778S.

Komori T, et al., Application of fragrances to treatments for depression. Nihon Shinkei Seishin Yakurigaku Zasshi. 1995 Feb;15(1):39-42. Japanese.

Lemongrass *(Cymbopogon flexuosus)*

Botanical Family: Poaceae or Gramineae (grasses)

Plant Origin: India, Guatemala

Extraction Method: Steam distilled from leaves.

Key Constituents:
Geranial (35-45%)
Geraniol (5-10%)
Neral (25-40%)
Trans-beta-Caryophyllene (2-6%)

ORAC: 1,780 µTE/100g

Historical Data: Lemongrass is used for purification and digestion. Research was published in *Phytotherapy Research* on topically applied lemongrass for its powerful antifungal properties.

Medical Properties: Antifungal, antibacterial, antiparasitic, anti-inflammatory, regenerates connective tissues and ligaments, dilates blood vessels, improves circulation, promotes lymph flow.

USES: Bladder infection, respiratory/sinus infection, digestive problems, parasites, torn ligaments/muscles, fluid retention, varicose veins, Salmonella.

Fragrant Influence: Promotes psychic awareness and purification.

Application: Dilute 1 part EO with 4 parts VO; (1) apply 1-2 drops on location, (2) chakras/vitaflex points, (3) directly inhale, (4) diffuse, or (5) take as dietary supplement (see Appendices E and T).

Found In: Di-Tone, En-R-Gee, Inner Child, and Purification.

Selected Research:

Pattnaik S, et al. "Antibacterial and antifungal activity of ten essential oils in vitro." *Microbios.* 1996;86(349):237-46.

Inouye S, Yamaguchi H, Takizawa T. Screening of the antibacterial effects of a variety of essential oils on respiratory tract pathogens, using a modified dilution assay method. J Infect Chemother. 2001 Dec;7(4):251-4.

Lorenzetti BB, et al. "Myrcene mimics the peripheral analgesic activity of lemongrass tea." *J Ethnopharmacol.* 1991;34(1):43-8.

Elson CE, et al. "Impact of lemongrass oil, an essential oil, on serum cholesterol." *Lipids.* 1989;24(8):677-9.

Friedman M, Henika PR, Mandrell RE. Bactericidal activities of plant essential oils and some of their isolated constituents against Campylobacter jejuni, Escherichia coli, Listeria monocytogenes, and Salmonella enterica. J Food Prot. 2002 Oct;65(10):1545-60.

Venturini ME, Blanco D, Oria R. In vitro antifungal activity of several antimicrobial compounds against Penicillium expansum. J Food Prot. 2002 May;65(5):834-9.

Inouye S, Uchida K, Yamaguchi H. In-vitro and in-vivo anti-Trichophyton activity of essential oils by vapour contact. Mycoses. 2001 May;44(3-4):99-107.

Lime *(Citrus auantifolia)*

Botanical Family: Rutaceae

Plant Origin: Native to South Asia

Extraction Method: Cold expression from the peel of the unripe fruit

Key Constituents:
Limonene & Eucalyptol (50-60%)
Gamma Terpinene (10-15%)
Beta Pinene (8-12%)
Alpha Pinene (2-5%)

ORAC: 26,200 µTE/100g

Historical Data: Primarily used in skin care, and in supporting and strengthening the respiratory and immune systems.

Medical Properties: Antirheumatic, antiviral, antibacterial

USES: Skin conditions (acne, herpes), insect bites, respiratory problems.

Application: Dilute 1 part EO with 1 part VO; (1) apply 1-2 drops on location, (2) chakras/vitaflex points, (3) directly inhale, (4) diffuse, or (5) take as dietary supplement (see Appendices E and T).

Cautions: Avoid applying to skin that will be exposed to sunlight or UV light within 48 hours.

Selected Research:

Crowell PL. Prevention and therapy of cancer by dietary monoterpenes. J Nutr. 1999 Mar;129(3):775S-778S.

Limette

(See CITRUS HYSTRIX)

Mandarin *(Citrus reticulata)*

Botanical Family: Rutaceae (citrus)

Plant Origin: Madagascar, Italy, China

Extraction Method: Cold pressed from rind.

Key Constituents:
Limonene (65-75%)
Gamma-Terpinene (16-22%)
Alpha-Pinene (2-3%)
Beta-Pinene (1.2-2%)
Myrcene (1.5-2%)

ORAC: 26,500 µTE/100g

Historical Data: This fruit was traditionally given to Imperial Chinese officials named the Mandarins.

Medical Properties: Light antispasmodic, digestive tonic (digestoid), antifungal, and stimulates gallbladder. Rich in limonene, which has been extensively studied for its ability to combat tumor growth in over 50 clinical studies.

USES: Digestive problems, fluid retention, insomnia, anxiety, intestinal problems, skin problems (congested and oily skin, scars, acne), stretch marks (when combined with either jasmine, lavender, sandalwood, and/or frankincense).

Fragrant Influence: It is appeasing, gentle, and promotes happiness.

Application: Dilute 1 part EO with 1 part VO; (1) apply 2-4 drops on location, (2) chakras/vitaflex points, (3) directly inhale, (4) diffuse, or (5) take as dietary supplement (see Appendices E and T).

Cautions: Avoid applying to skin that will be exposed to sunlight or UV light within 24 hours.

Found In: Citrus Fresh, Joy, Awaken, Dragon Time.

Selected Research:

A 1995 Mie University study found that citrus fragrances boosted immunity, induced relaxation, and reduced depression.

Komori T, et al., Application of fragrances to treatments for depression. Nihon Shinkei Seishin Yakurigaku Zasshi. 1995 Feb;15(1):39-42. Japanese

Marjoram *(Origanum majorana)*

Botanical Family: Lamiaceae or Labiatae (mint)

Plant Origin: France

Extraction Method: Steam distilled from leaves.

Key Constituents:
Terpinene-4-ol (25-35%)
Gamma-Terpinene (12-20%)
Linalol +Cis-4-Thujanol (3-8%)
Alpha-Terpinene (6-13%)
Alpha-Terpineol (2-6%)
Sabinene (2-6%)

ORAC: 130,900 µTE/100g

Historical Data: Marjoram was known as the "herb of happiness" to the Romans and "joy of the mountains" to the Greeks. It was believed to increase longevity. Listed in Dioscorides' De Materia Medica (A.D. 78), Europe's first authoritive guide to medicines, that became the standard reference work for herbal treatments for over 1,700 years. It was listed in Hildegard's Medicine, a compilation of early German medicines by highly-regarded Benedictine herbalist Hildegard of Bingen (1098-1179).

Medical Properties: Antibacterial, antifungal, vasodilator, lowers blood pressure, promotes intestinal peristalsis, expectorant, mucolytic

USES: Arthritis/rheumatism, muscle/nerve pain, headaches, circulatory disorders, respiratory infections, menstrual problems/PMS, fungal infections (ringworm, shingles, sores, spasms, and fluid retention.

Fragrant Influence: Assists in calming the nerves.

Application: Dilute 1 part EO with 1 part VO; (1) apply 2-4 drops on location, (2) chakras/vitaflex points, (3) directly inhale, (4) diffuse, or (5) take as dietary supplement (see Appendices E and T).

Found In: Aroma Life, Aroma Siez, Dragon Time, M-Grain, and R.C.

Melaleuca Alternifolia

(See TEA TREE)

Melaleuca Ericifolia *(Melaleuca ericifolia)*

Botanical Family: Myrtaceae (myrtle)

Plant Origin: Australia

Key Constituents:
Alpha-Pinene (5-10%)
1,8 Cineol + Beta Phellandrene (18-28%)
Alpha-Terpineol (1-5%)
Para-Cymene (1-6%)
Linalol (34-45%)
Aromadendrene (2-6%)

ORAC: 61,100 µTE/100g

Medical Properties: Powerful antibacterial, antifungal, antiviral, antiparasitic, anti-inflammatory

USES: Herpes virus, respiratory/sinus infections

Application: Dilute 1 part EO with 1 part VO; (1) apply 2-4 drops on location, temples, wrists, throat, face, or chest (2) chakras/vitaflex points, (3) directly inhale, (4) diffuse, or (5) take as dietary supplement (see Appendices E and T).

Selected Research:

Stablein JJ, Bucholtz GA, Lockey RF. Melaleuca tree and respiratory disease. Ann Allergy Asthma Immunol. 2002 Nov;89 (5):523-30.

Farag RS, et al., Chemical and biological evaluation of the essential oils of different Melaleuca species. Phytother Res. 2004 Jan;18(1):30-5.

Melissa *(Melissa officinalis)*

Botanical Family: Lamiaceae or Labiatae (mint)

Plant Origin: Utah, Idaho, France

Extraction Method: Steam distilled from leaves and flowers.

Key Constituents:
Geranial (25-35%)
Neral (18-28%)
Beta Caryophyllene (12-19%)

ORAC: 134,300 µTE/100g

Historical Data: Anciently, melissa was used for nervous disorders and many different ailments dealing with the heart or the emotions. It was also used to promote fertility. Melissa was the main ingredient in Carmelite water, distilled in France since 1611 by the Carmelite monks. Dr. Dietrich Wabner, a professor at the Technical University of Munich, reported that a one-time application of true melissa oil led to complete remission of Herpes Simplex lesions.

Medical Properties: Anti-inflammatory, antiviral, relaxant, hypotensive

USES: Viral infections (herpes etc), depression, anxiety, insomnia.

Fragrant Influence: Brings out gentle characteristics within people. It is calming and uplifting and balances emotions. It removes emotional blocks and instills a positive outlook on life.

Application: (1) Apply 2-4 drops on location, (2) chakras/vitaflex points, (3) directly inhale, (4) diffuse, or (5) take as dietary supplement (see Appendices E and T).

Found In: Brain Power, Forgiveness, Hope, Humility, Live With Passion, White Angelica

Selected Research: Yamasaki K, et al. "Anti-HIV-1 activity of herbs in Labiatae." *Biol Pharm Bull.* 1998;21(8):829-33.

Larrondo JV, et al. "Antimicrobial activity of essences from labiates." *Microbios.* 1995;82 (332):171-2.

Kucera LS, et al. "Antiviral activities of extracts of the lemon balm plant." *Ann NY Acad Sci.* 1965 Jul 30;130(1):474-82.

Sadraei H, Ghannadi A, Malekshahi K. Relaxant effect of essential oil of Melissa officinalis and citral on rat ileum contractions. Fitoterapia. 2003 Jul;74(5):445-52.

Radonic A, Milos M. "Chemical composition and in vitro evaluation of antioxidant effect of free volatile compounds from Satureja montana L." *Free Radic Res.* 2003 Jun;37(6):673-9.

Mountain Savory *(Satureja montana)*

Botanical Family: Lamiaceae or Labiatae

Plant Origin: France

Extraction Method: Steam distilled from flowering plant.

Key Constituents:
Carvacrol (22-35%)
Thymol (14-24%)
Gamma-Terpinene (8-15%)
Carvacrol Methyl Ether (4-9%)
Beta-Caryophyllene (3-7%)

ORAC: 11,300 µTE/100g

Historical Data: Mountain savory has been used historically as a general tonic for the body.

Medical Properties: Strong antibacterial, antifungal, antiviral, antiparasitic, immune stimulant, anti-inflammatory

USES: Viral infections (Herpes, HIV, etc), scoliosis/lumbago/back problems

Fragrant Influence: Revitalizes and stimulates the nervous system. It is a powerful energizer and motivator.

Application: Dilute 1 part EO with 4 parts VO; (1) apply 2-4 drops on location, (2) chakras/vitaflex points, (3) diffuse, or (4) take as dietary supplement (see Appendices E and T).

Found In: ImmuPower, Surrender

Selected Research:

Yamasaki K, et al. "Anti-HIV-1 activity of herbs in Labiatae." *Biol Pharm Bull.* 1998; 21(8):829-33.

Panizzi L, et al. "Composition and antimicrobial properties of essential oils of four Mediterranean Lamiaceae." *J Ethnopharmacol.* 1993;39(3):167-70.

Mugwort *(Artemisia vulgaris)*

Botanical Family: Asteraceae (Daisy family)

Plant Origin: Canada

Extraction Method: Steam distilled from leaves and roots

Key Constituents:
Sabinene (9-14%)
Myrcene (20-25%)
Limonene & Beta Phellandrene (1-5%)
Alpha- and Beta-Thujone (8-12%)
Germacrene D (4-8%)

Historical Data: Used by Chinese in moxibustion. Was worn to protect against evil spirits in 14th century England. Introduced by the Portuguese to the French in the 1800's where it became known as a cure for blindness and other diseases. Has been placed under pillows to produce vivid dreams.

Medical Properties: Antibacterial, antifungal, antiparasitic, gastrointestinal regulator

USES: Intestinal complaints, worm infestations, headaches, muscle spasms, circulatory problems, menstrual problems/ PMS, dysentery, gout

Application: Dilute 1 part EO with 1 part VO; (1) apply 1-2 drops on location, (2) chakras/vitaflex points, (3) diffuse, or (4) take as dietary supplement (see Appendices E and T).

Found In: Comfortone, Inspiration

Selected Research:

Friedman M, Henika PR, Mandrell RE. Bactericidal activities of plant essential oils and some of their isolated constituents against Campylobacter jejuni, Escherichia coli, Listeria monocytogenes, and Salmonella enterica. J Food Prot. 2002 Oct;65(10):1545-60.

Myrrh *(Commiphora myrrha)*

Botanical Family: Burseraceae (Frankincense)

Plant Origin: Somalia

Extraction Method: Steam distilled from gum/resin.

Key Constituents:
Lindestrene (30-45%)
Curzerene (17-25%)
Furanoendesma-1,3-diene (4-8%)
Methoxyfuronogermacrene (5-9%)
Beta- and Gamma-Elemenes (3-6%)

ORAC: 379,800 µTE/100g

Historical Data: It is mentioned in one of the oldest known medical records, Ebers Papyrus (dating from sixteenth century BC) an ancient Egyptian list of 877 prescriptions and recipes. The Arabian people used myrrh for many skin conditions, such as chapped and cracked skin and wrinkles. It was listed in Hildegard's Medicine, a compilation of early German medicines by highly-regarded Benedictine herbalist Hildegard of Bingen (1098-1179).

Medical Properties: Powerful antioxidant, antitumoral, anti-inflammatory, antiviral, antiparasitic, analgesic/ anesthetic

USES: Diabetes, cancer, hepatitis, fungal infections (Candida, ringworm, eczema), tooth/gum infections, skin conditions (chapped, cracked, wrinkles, stretch marks)

Fragrant Influence: Promotes spiritual awareness and is uplifting. It contains sesquiterpenes which stimulate the limbic system of the brain (the center of memory and emotions) and the hypothalamus, pineal and pituitary glands. The hypothalamus is the master gland of the human body, producing many vital hormones including thyroid and growth hormone.

Application: (1) Apply 2-4 drops on location, (2) chakras/vitaflex points, (3) directly inhale, (4) diffuse, or (5) take as dietary supplement (see Appendices E and T).

Found In: Abundance, Exodus II, Hope, Humility, Wisdom, and White Angelica.

Bible References: (see additional Bible references in Appendix D).

Genesis 37:25—"And they sat down to eat bread: and they lifted up their eyes and looked, and behold, a company of Ishmelites came from Gilead with their camels bearing spicery and balm and myrrh, going to carry it down to Egypt."

Genesis 43:11—"And their father Israel said unto them, If it must be so now, do this; take of the best fruits in the land in your vessels, and carry down the man a present, a little balm, and a little honey, spices, and myrrh, nuts, and almonds:"

Exodus 30:23—"Take thou also unto thee principal spices, of pure myrrh five hundred shekels, and of sweet cinnamon half so much, even two hundred and fifty shekels, and of sweet calamus two hundred and fifty shekels,"

Selected Research:

Tipton DA, In vitro cytotoxic and anti-inflammatory effects of myrrh oil on human gingival fibroblasts and epithelial cells. Toxicol In Vitro. 2003 Jun;17(3):301-10.

Al-Awadi FM, et al. "Studies on the activity of individual plants of an antidiabetic plant mixture." *Acta Diabetol Lat.* 1987;24(1):37-41.

Dolara P, et al. "Analgesic effects of myrrh." *Nature.* 1996 Jan 4;379(6560):29.

Michie CA, et al. "Frankincense and myrrh as remedies in children." *J R Soc Med.* 1991;84(10):602-5.

Anderson C, et al., Evaluation of massage with essential oils on childhood atopic eczema. Phytother Res. 2000 Sep;14(6):452-6.

al-Harbi MM, et al., Anticarcinogenic effect of Commiphora molmol on solid tumors induced by Ehrlich carcinoma cells in mice. Chemotherapy. 1994 Sep-Oct;40(5):337-47.

Qureshi S, et al., Evaluation of the genotoxic, cytotoxic, and antitumor properties of Commiphora molmol using normal and Ehrlich ascites carcinoma cell-bearing Swiss albino mice. Cancer Chemother Pharmacol. 1993;33(2):130-8.

Dolara P, Corte B. Local anaesthetic, antibacterial and antifungal properties of sesquiterpenes from myrrh. Planta Med. 2000 May;66(4):356-8.

Myrtle *(Myrtus communis)*

Botanical Family: Myrtaceae (myrtle)

Plant Origin: Tunisia, Morocco

Extraction Method: Steam distilled from leaves.

Key Constituents:
Alpha Pinene (45-60%)
1,8 Cineol (Eucalyptol) (17-27%)
Limonene (5-11%)
Linalol (2-5%)

ORAC: 25,400 µTE/100g

Historical Data: Myrtle has been researched by Dr. Daniel Pénoël for normalizing hormonal imbalances of the thyroid and ovaries, as well as balancing the hypothyroid. It has also been researched for its soothing effects on the respiratory system.

Medical Properties: Antimutagenic, liver stimulant, liver stimulant, prostate and thyroid stimulant sinus/lung decongestant, antispasmodic

USES: Thyroid problems, throat/lung/sinus infections, prostate problems, (acne, blemishes, bruises, oily skin, psoriasis, etc.), muscle spasms

Fragrant Influence: Elevating and euphoric.

Application: Dilute 1 part EO with 1 part VO; (1) apply 2-4 drops on location, (2) chakras/vitaflex points, (3) directly inhale, (4) diffuse or put in humidifier, or (5) take as dietary supplement (see Appendices E and T).

Found In: EndoFlex, Inspiration, Mister, Purification, and R.C.

Bible Reference: (see additional Bible references in Appendix D).

Nehemiah 8:15—"And that they should publish and proclaim in all their cities, and in Jerusalem, saying, Go forth unto the mount, and fetch olive branches, and pine branches, and myrtle branches, and palm branches, and branches of thick trees, to make booths, as it is written."

Isaiah 41:19—"I will plant in the wilderness the cedar, the shittah tree, and the myrtle, and the oil tree; I will set in the desert the fir tree, and the pine, and the box tree together:"

Isaiah 55:13—"Instead of the thorn shall come up the fir tree, and instead of the brier shall come up the myrtle tree: and it shall be to the Lord for a name, for an everlasting sign that shall not be cut off."

Selected Research:

Hayder N, et al., Antimutagenic activity of aqueous extracts and essential oil isolated from Myrtus communis. Pharmazie. 2003 Jul;58(7):523-4.

Monti D, et al., Effect of different terpene-containing essential oils on permeation of estradiol through hairless mouse skin. Int J Pharm. 2002 Apr 26;237(1-2):209-14.

Neroli Absolute *(Citrus aurantium)*

Botanical Family: Rutaceae (citrus)

Plant Origin: Morocco, Tunisia

Extraction Method: Absolute extraction from flowers of the orange tree.

Key Constituents:
Linalol (28-44%)
Limonene (9-18%)
Beta-Pinene (7-17%)
Linalyl Acetate (3-15%)
Trans-Ocimene (3-8%)
Alpha Terpineol (2-5.5%)
Trans-Nerolidol (1-5%)
Myrcene (1-4%)

Medical Properties: Antiparasitic, digestive tonic, antidepressive, and hypotensive (lowers blood pressure).

Historical Data: Highly regarded by the ancient Egyptians for its ability to heal the mind, body, and spirit.

Medical Properties: Antidepressant, antihypertensive, stimulates skin cell regeneration.

USES: Hypertension, anxiety, depression, hysteria, insomnia, skin conditions (scars, stretch marks, thread veins, wrinkles).

Fragrant Influence: A natural relaxant used to treat depression and anxiety. It strengthens and stabilizes the emotions and uplifts and inspires the hopeless, encouraging confidence, courage, joy, peace, and sensuality. It brings everything into focus at the moment.

Application: Dilute 1 part EO with 1 part VO; (1) apply 2-4 drops on location, (2) chakras/vitaflex points, (3) directly inhale, or (4) diffuse (see Appendices E and T).

Found In: Acceptance, Awaken, Humility, Inner Child, Live With Passion, and Present Time.

Niaouli *(Melaleuca quinquenervia)*

Botanical Family: Myrtaceae (myrtle)

Plant Origin: Australia

Extraction Method: Steam distilled from leaves and twigs.

Key Constituents:
1,8 Cineole + Limonene (55-70%)
Alpha-Pinene (7-15%)
Beta-Pinene (2-6%)
Viridiflorol (2-6%)

ORAC: 18,600 µTE/100g

Medical Properties: Male hormone-like, anti-inflammatory, antibacterial, antiviral, and antiparasitic (amoeba and parasites in the blood), vasodilating, skin penetration enhancer (hormones)

USES: Hypertension, urinary tract/bladder infections, respiratory/sinus infections and allergies.

Application: Dilute 1 part EO with 1 part VO; (1) apply 2-4 drops on location, (2) chakras/vitaflex points, (3) directly inhale, or (4) diffuse (see Appendices E and T).

Found In: Melrose

Selected Research:

Monti D, et al., Effect of different terpene-containing essential oils on permeation of estradiol through hairless mouse skin. Int J Pharm. 2002 Apr 26;237(1-2):209-14.

Groppo FC, et al., Antimicrobial activity of garlic, tea tree oil, and chlorhexidine against oral microorganisms. Int Dent J. 2002 Dec;52(6):433-7.

Stablein JJ, Bucholtz GA, Lockey RF. Melaleuca tree and respiratory disease. Ann Allergy Asthma Immunol. 2002 Nov;89 (5):523-30.

Nutmeg *(Myristica fragrans)*

Botanical Family: Myristicaceae

Plant Origin: Tunisia, Indonesia

Extraction Method: Steam distilled from fruits and seeds.

Key Constituents:
Sabinene (14-29%)
Beta-Pinene (13-18%)
Alpha-Pinene (15-28%)
Limonene (2-7%)
Gamma-Terpinene (2-6%)
Terpinene-4-ol (2-6%)
Myristicine (5-12%)

ORAC: 158,100 µTE/100g

Historical Data: It was listed in Hildegard's Medicine, a compilation of early German medicines by highly-regarded Benedictine herbalist Hildegard of Bingen (1098-1179).

Recently the University of Ibadan revealed that nutmeg has potent anti-inflammatory and anticoagulant action.

Medical Properties: Anti-inflammatory, anticoagulant, antiseptic, antiparasitic, analgesic, liver protectant, stomach protectant (ulcers) and circulatory stimulant, adrenal stimulant, muscle relaxing, increases production of growth hormone/melatonin.

USES: Rheumatism/arthritis, cardiovascular disease, hypertension, hepatitis, ulcers, digestive disorders, antiparasitic, nerve pain, fatigue/exhaustion

Application: Dilute 1 part EO with 2 parts VO; (1) apply 1-2 drops on location, (2) chakras/vitaflex points, (3) directly inhale, (4) diffuse, or (5) take as dietary supplement (see Appendices E and T).

Found In: EndoFlex, En-R-Gee, and Magnify Your Purpose.

Selected Research:

OA Olajide et al., Biological effects of Myristica fragrans (nutmeg) extract. Phytother Res. 1999 Jun;13(4):344-5.

Valero M, Salmeron MC. Antibacterial activity of 11 essential oils against Bacillus cereus in tyndallized carrot broth. Int J Food Microbiol. 2003 Aug 15;85(1-2):73-81.

Ramsewak RS, et al., In vitro antagonistic activity of monoterpenes and their mixtures against 'toe nail fungus' pathogens. Phytother Res. 2003 Apr;17(4):376-9.

Morita T, et al., Hepatoprotective effect of myristicin from nutmeg (Myristica fragrans) on lipopolysaccharide/d-galactosamine-induced liver injury. J Agric Food Chem. 2003 Mar 12;51(6):1560-5.

Grover JK, et al., Pharmacological studies on Myristica fragrans--antidiarrheal, hypnotic, analgesic and hemodynamic (blood pressure) parameters. Methods Find Exp Clin Pharmacol. 2002 Dec;24(10):675-80.

Capasso R, Pinto L, Vuotto ML, Di Carlo G. Preventive effect of eugenol on PAF and ethanol-induced gastric mucosal damage. Fitoterapia. 2000 Aug;71 Suppl 1:S131-7.

Ram A, et al., Hypolipidaemic effect of Myristica fragrans fruit extract in rabbits.J Ethnopharmacol. 1996 Dec;55(1):49-53.

Lis-Balchin M, Hart S. A preliminary study of the effect of essential oils on skeletal and smooth muscle in vitro. J Ethnopharmacol. 1997 Nov;58(3):183-7.

Rashid A, Misra DS. Antienterotoxic effect of Myristica fragrans (nutmeg) on enterotoxigenic Escherichia coli. Indian J Med Res. 1984 May;79:694-6.

Sherry CJ, Burnett RE. Enhancement of ethanol-induced sleep by whole oil of nutmeg. Experientia. 1978 Apr 15;34(4):492-3.

Dietz WH Jr, Stuart MJ. Nutmeg and prostaglandins. N Engl J Med. 1976 Feb 26;294(9):503.

Banerjee S, et al., Influence of certain essential oils on carcinogen-metabolizing enzymes and acid-soluble sulfhydryls in mouse liver. Nutr Cancer. 1994;21(3):263-9.

Dorman HJ, Deans SG. Antimicrobial agents from plants: antibacterial activity of plant volatile oils. J Appl Microbiol. 2000 Feb;88(2):308-16.

Orange *(Citrus sinensis)*

Botanical Family: Rutaceae (citrus)

Plant Origin: USA, South Africa, Italy, China

Extraction Method: Cold pressed from rind.

Chemical Constituents:
Limonene (85-96%)
Myrcene (0.5-3%)

ORAC: 1,890 µTE/100g

Medical Properties: Antitumoral, relaxant, anticoagulant, circulatory stimulant. Rich in limonene, which has been extensively studied for its ability to combat tumor growth in over 50 clinical studies.

USES: Arteriosclerosis, hypertension, cancer, insomnia, and complexion (dull and oily), fluid retention, and wrinkles.

Fragrant Influence: Uplifting and antidepressant. A 1995 Mie University study found that citrus fragrances boosted immunity, induced relaxation, and reduced depression.

Application: Dilute 1 part EO with 1 part VO; (1) apply 2-4 drops on location, (2) chakras/vitaflex points, (3) directly inhale, (4) diffuse, or (5) take as dietary supplement (see Appendices E and T).

Cautions: Avoid applying to skin that will be exposed to sunlight or UV light within 24 hours.

Found In: Abundance, Christmas Spirit, Citrus Fresh, Envision, Harmony, Inner Child, Into The Future, Peace & Calming, and SARA.

Selected Research:

Lu XG, et al., D-limonene induces apoptosis of gastric cancer cells. Zhonghua Zhong Liu Za Zhi. 2003 Jul;25(4):325-7.

Nishino H et al. Cancer Chemoprevention by Phytochemicals and their Related Compounds. Asian Pac J Cancer Prev. 2000;1(1):49-55.

Parija T, Das BR. Involvement of YY1 and its correlation with c-myc in NDEA induced hepatocarcinogenesis, its prevention by d-limonene. Mol Biol Rep. 2003 Mar;30(1):41-6.

Bodake HB, Panicker KN, Kailaje VV, Rao KV. Chemopreventive effect of orange oil on the development of hepatic preneoplastic lesions induced by N-nitrosodiethylamine in rats: an ultrastructural study. Indian J Exp Biol. 2002 Mar;40(3):245-51.

Uedo N, et al., Inhibition by D-limonene of gastric carcinogenesis induced by N-methyl-N'-nitro-N-nitrosoguanidine in Wistar rats. Cancer Lett. 1999 Apr 1;137(2):131-6.

Hakim IA, Harris RB, Ritenbaugh C. Citrus peel use is associated with reduced risk of squamous cell carcinoma of the skin. Nutr Cancer. 2000;37(2):161-8.

Asamoto M, et al., Mammary carcinomas induced in human c-Ha-ras proto-oncogene transgenic rats are estrogen-independent, but responsive to d-limonene treatment. Jpn J Cancer Res. 2002 Jan;93(1):32-5.

Guyton KZ, Kensler TW. Prevention of liver cancer.Curr Oncol Rep. 2002 Nov;4(6):464-70.

Bradlow HL, Sepkovic DW. Diet and breast cancer. Ann N Y Acad Sci. 2002 Jun;963:247-67.

Wattenberg LW, et al., Inhibition of carcinogenesis by some minor dietary constituents. Princess Takamatsu Symp. 1985;16:193-203.

Alderman GG, Marth EH. Inhibition of growth and aflatoxin production of Aspergillus parasiticus by citrus oils. Z Lebensm Unters Forsch. 1976 Apr 28;160(4):353-8.

Crowell PL.Prevention and therapy of cancer by dietary monoterpenes. J Nutr. 1999 Mar;129(3):775S-778S.

Komori T, et al., Application of fragrances to treatments for depression. Nihon Shinkei Seishin Yakurigaku Zasshi. 1995 Feb;15(1):39-42. Japanese

Oregano *(Origanum compactum)*

Botanical Family: Lamiaceae or Labiatae (mint)

Plant Origin: Utah, Turkey, France

Extraction Method: Steam distilled from leaves and flowers.

Key Constituents:
Carvacrol (60-75%)
Gamma-Terpinene (3.5-8.5%)
Para-Cymene (5.5-9%)
Beta Caryophyllene (2-5%)
Myrcene (1-3%)
Thymol (0-5%)

ORAC: 15,300 µTE/100g

Historical Data: Listed in Hildegard's Medicine, a compilation of early German medicines by highly-regarded Benedictine herbalist Hildegard of Bingen (1098-1179).

Medical Properties: Anti-aging, powerful antiviral, antibacterial, antifungal, antiparasitic, anti-inflammatory, immune stimulant.

USES: Arthritis/rheumatism respiratory infectious diseases, infections/tuberculosis, digestive problems.

Fragrant Influence: Creates a feeling of security.

Application: Dilute 1 part EO with 4 parts VO; (1) apply 1-2 drops on location or neat as Raindrop Technique, (2) chakras/vitaflex points, (3) diffuse, or (4) take as dietary supplement, (see Appendices E and T).

Caution: May irritate the nasal membranes if inhaled directly from diffuser or bottle.

Found In: ImmuPower

Selected Research:

Friedman M, Henika PR, Mandrell RE. Bactericidal activities of plant essential oils and some of their isolated constituents against Campylobacter jejuni, Escherichia coli, Listeria monocytogenes, and Salmonella enterica. J Food Prot. 2002 Oct;65(10):1545-60.

Papageorgiou G, et al., Effect of dietary oregano oil and alpha-tocopheryl acetate supplementation on iron-induced lipid oxidation of turkey breast, thigh, liver and heart tissues. J Anim Physiol Anim Nutr (Berl). 2003 Oct;87(9-10):324-35.

Elgayyar M, et al., Antimicrobial activity of essential oils from plants against selected pathogenic and saprophytic microorganisms. J Food Prot. 2001 Jul;64(7):1019-24.

Tantaoui-Elaraki A, Beraoud L. Inhibition of growth and aflatoxin production in Aspergillus parasiticus by essential oils of selected plant materials. J Environ Pathol Toxicol Oncol. 1994;13(1):67-72.

Dorman HJ, Deans SG. Antimicrobial agents from plants: antibacterial activity of plant volatile oils. J Appl Microbiol. 2000 Feb;88(2):308-16.

Palmarosa *(Cymbopogon martinii)*

Botanical Family: Poaceae or Gramineae (grasses)

Plant Origin: India, Conoros

Extraction Method: Steam distilled from leaves.

Key Constituents:
Geraniol (70-85%)
Geranyl Acetate (6-10%)
Linalol (3-7%)

ORAC: 127,800 µTE/100g

Historical Data: A relative of lemongrass, palmarosa was used in temple incense by the ancient Egyptians..

Medical Properties: Antibacterial, antifungal, antiviral, supports heart and nervous system, stimulates new skin cell growth, regulates sebum production in skin.

USES: Fungal infections/Candida, cardiovascular/ circulatory diseases, digestive problems, skin problems (acne, eczema)

Fragrant Influence: Creates a feeling of security. It also helps to reduce stress and tension and promotes recovery from nervous exhaustion.

Application: Dilute 1 part EO with 1 part VO; (1) apply 2-4 drops on location, (2) chakras/vitaflex points, (3) directly inhale, (4) diffuse, or (5) take as dietary supplement (see Appendices E and T).

Found In: Awaken, Clarity, Forgiveness, Gentle Baby, Harmony, Joy.

Selected Research:

Friedman M, Henika PR, Mandrell RE. Bactericidal activities of plant essential oils and some of their isolated constituents against Campylobacter jejuni, Escherichia coli, Listeria monocytogenes, and Salmonella enterica. J Food Prot. 2002 Oct;65(10):1545-60.

Kumaran AM, et al., Geraniol, the putative anthelmintic principle of Cymbopogon martinii. Phytother Res. 2003 Sep;17(8):957.

Prashar A, et al., Antimicrobial action of palmarosa oil (Cymbopogon martinii) on Saccharomyces cerevisiae. Phytochemistry. 2003 Jul;63(5):569-75

Carnesecchi S, et al., Geraniol, a component of plant essential oils, sensitizes human colon cancer cells to 5-fluorouracil treatment. IARC Sci Publ. 2002;156:407-9.

Carnesecchi S, et al., Perturbation by geraniol of cell membrane permeability and signal transduction pathways in human colon cancer cells. J Pharmacol Exp Ther. 2002 Nov;303(2):711-5.

Umezu T, et al., Anticonflict effects of rose oil and identification of its active constituents. Life Sci. 2002 Nov 22;72(1):91-102.

Choi HS, Song HS, Ukeda H, Sawamura M. Radical-scavenging activities of citrus essential oils and their components: detection using 1,1-diphenyl-2-picrylhydrazyl. J Agric Food Chem. 2000 Sep;48(9):4156-61.

Patchouli *(Pogostemon cablin)*

Botanical Family: Lamiaceae or Labiatae (mint)

Plant Origin: Indonesia, India

Extraction Method: Steam distilled from flowers.

Key Constituents:
Patchoulol (25-35%)
Alpha-Bulnesene (14-20%)
Alpha-Guaiene + Seychellene (15-25%)
Alpha-Patchoulene (5-9%)

ORAC: 49,400 µTE/100g

Medical Properties: Relaxant, digestive aid, anti-inflammatory, antimicrobial, prevents wrinkles/chapped skin, relieves itching.

USES: Hypertension, skin conditions (eczema, acne), fluid retention, Listeria infection

Application: (1) apply 2-4 drops on location, (2) chakras/vitaflex points, (3) directly inhale, (4) diffuse, or (5) take as dietary supplement (see Appendices E and T)

Fragrant Influence: A relaxant that clarifies thoughts, allowing the discarding of jealousies, obsessions, and insecurities.

Found In: Abundance, Di-Tone, Magnify Your Purpose, Live With Passion, Peace & Calming

Selected Research:

Friedman M, Henika PR, Mandrell RE. Bactericidal activities of plant essential oils and some of their isolated constituents against Campylobacter jejuni, Escherichia coli, Listeria monocytogenes, and Salmonella enterica. J Food Prot. 2002 Oct;65(10):1545-60.

Haze S, Sakai K, Gozu Y. et al., Effects of fragrance inhalation on sympathetic activity in normal adults. Jpn J Pharmacol. 2002 Nov;90(3):247-53.

Pepper, Black *(Piper nigrum)*

Botanical Family: Piperaceae

Plant Origin: Madagascar, Egypt, India

Extraction Method: Steam distilled from berries.

Key Constituents:
Beta Caryophyllene (25-35%)
Limonene (8-12%)
Sabinene (5-10%)
Alpha and Beta Pinenes (10-15%)

ORAC: 79,700 µTE/100g

Historical Data: Used by the Egyptians in mummification as evidenced by the discovery of black pepper in the nostrils and abdomen of Ramses II. Indian monks ate several black peppercorns a day to to give them endurance during their arduous travels. In ancient times pepper was as valuable as gold or silver. When the barbarian Goth tribes of Europe vanquished Rome in 410 AD, they demanded 3,000 pounds of pepper as well as other valuables as a ransom. Traditional Chinese healers used pepper to treat cholera, malaria, and digestive problems.

Medical Properties: Analgesic, stimulates metabolism, antifungal

USES: Obesity, arthritis. digestive problems, fatigue, nerve/muscle pain, fungal infections

Fragrant Influence: Stimulating, energizing and empowering. A 2002 study found that fragrance inhalation of pepper oil induced a 1.7-fold increase in plasma adrenaline concentration (Haze et al.).

Application: Dilute 1 part EO with 1 part VO; (1) apply 2-4 drops on location, (2) chakras/vitaflex points, (3) directly inhale, (4) diffuse, or (5) take as dietary supplement (see Appendices E and T).

Found In: Dream Catcher, En-R-Gee, and PanAway.

Selected Research: Unnikrishnan MC, et al. "Tumour reducing and anticarcinogenic activity of selected spices." *Cancer Lett.* 1990;51(1):85-9.

Haze S, Sakai K, Gozu Y. et al., Effects of fragrance inhalation on sympathetic activity in normal adults. Jpn J Pharmacol. 2002 Nov;90(3):247-53.

Tantaoui-Elaraki A, Beraoud L. Inhibition of growth and aflatoxin production in Aspergillus parasiticus by essential oils of selected plant materials. J Environ Pathol Toxicol Oncol. 1994;13(1):67-72.

Dorman HJ, Deans SG. Antimicrobial agents from plants: antibacterial activity of plant volatile oils. J Appl Microbiol. 2000 Feb;88(2):308-16.

Haze S, Sakai K, Gozu Y. Effects of fragrance inhalation on sympathetic activity in normal adults. Jpn J Pharmacol. 2002 Nov;90(3):247-53.

Peppermint (*Mentha piperita*)

Botanical Family: Lamiaceae or Labiatae (mint)

Plant Origin: North America

Extraction Method: Steam distilled from leaves, stems, and flower buds.

Key Constituents:
Menthol (34-44%)
Menthone (12-20%)
Menthofurane (4-9%)
1.8 Cineol (Eucalyptol) (2-5%)
Pulegone (2-5%)
Menthyl Acetate (4-10%)

ORAC: 37,300 µTE/100g

Historical Data: Reputed to be part of the "Marseilles Vinegar" or "Four Thieves Vinegar" used by grave-robbing bandits to protect themselves during the 15th century plague. A highly regarded digestive stimulant. Jean Valnet, M.D., used peppermint to treat liver and respiratory diseases.

Medical Properties: Anti-inflammatory, antitumoral, antiparasitic (worms), antibacterial, antiviral, antifungal, gallbladder/digestive stimulant, pain-relieving, pain-reliever, curbs appetite.

USES: Rheumatism/arthritis, respiratory infections (pneumonia, tuberculosis, etc), obesity, viral infections (Herpes simplex, herpes zoster, cold sores, human papilloma virus etc.), fungal infections/Candida, digestive problems, headaches, nausea, skin conditions (itchy skin, varicose veins, eczema, psoriasis, dermatitis), scoliosis/lumbago/back problems.

Fragrant Influence: Purifying and stimulating to the conscious mind. Dr. William N. Dember of the University of Cincinnati found that inhaling peppermint oil increased the mental accuracy by 28 percent

Alan Hirsch, M.D. researched peppermint's stimulation of the brain's satiety center (ventromedial nucleus of the hypothalamus) to curb appetite.

When inhaled, it improves/restores sense of taste by stimulating the trigeminal nerve. University of Kiel researchers found that peppermint blocked headache pain in a double-blind placebo-controlled cross-over study.

Application: Dilute 1 part EO with 2 parts VO; (1) apply 1-2 drops on location, abdomen, temples (2) chakras/vitaflex points, (3) directly inhale, (4) diffuse, or (5) take as dietary supplement (see Appendices E and T).

To improve concentration, alertness, and memory, place 1-2 drops on the tongue. Inhale 5-10 times a day to curb appetite.

Cautions: Avoid contact with eyes, mucus membranes, sensitive skin, or fresh wounds or burns. Do not apply to infants younger than 18 months of age.

Found In: Aroma Siez, Clarity, Di-Tone, M-Grain, Mister, PanAway, R.C., Raven, and Relieve It.

Selected Research:

Gobel H, et al. "Effect of peppermint and eucalyptus oil preparations on neurophysiological and experimental algesimetric headache parameters." *Cephalalgia.* 1994; 14(3):228-34.

Juergens UR, Stober M, Vetter H. The anti-inflammatory activity of L-menthol compared to mint oil in human monocytes in vitro: a novel perspective for its therapeutic use in inflammatory diseases. Eur J Med Res. 1998 Dec 16;3(12):539-45.

Samman MA, et al. "Mint prevents shamma-induced carcinogenesis in hamster cheek pouch." *Carcinogenesis.* 1998;19(10):1795-801.

Schuhmacher A, Reichling J, Schnitzler P. Virucidal effect of peppermint oil on the enveloped viruses herpes simplex virus type 1 and type 2 in vitro. Phytomedicine. 2003;10(6-7):504-10.

Samarth RM, et al., Mentha piperita (Linn) leaf extract provides protection against radiation induced alterations in intestinal mucosa of Swiss albino mice. Indian J Exp Biol. 2002 Nov;40(11):1245-9.

Mimica-Dukic N, et al., Antimicrobial and antioxidant activities of three Mentha species essential oils. Planta Med. 2003 May;69(5):413-9.

Edris AE, Farrag ES. Antifungal activity of peppermint and sweet basil essential oils and their major aroma constituents on some plant pathogenic fungi from the vapor phase. Nahrung. 2003 Apr;47(2):117-21.

Shkurupii VA, et al., Efficiency of the use of peppermint (Mentha piperita L) essential oil inhalations in the combined multi-drug therapy for pulmonary tuberculosis. Probl Tuberk. 2002;(4):36-9.

Iscan G, et al., Antimicrobial screening of Mentha piperita essential oils. J Agric Food Chem. 2002 Jul 3;50(14):3943-6.

Imai H, et al., Inhibition by the essential oils of peppermint and spearmint of the growth of pathogenic bacteria. Microbios. 2001;106 Suppl 1:31-9.

Petitgrain *(Citrus aurantium)*

Botanical Family: Rutaceae (citrus)

Plant Origin: Italy

Extraction Method: Steam distilled from leaves and twigs.

Key Constituents:
Linalyle Acetate (40-55%)
Linalol (15-30%)
Alpha Terpineol (3.5-7.5%)
Geranyl Acetate (2-5%)
Geraniol (2-4.5%)

ORAC: 73,600 µTE/100g

Historical Data: Petitgrain derives its name from the extraction of the oil, which at one time was from the green unripe oranges when they were still about the size of a cherry.

Medical Properties: Antispasmodic, anti-inflammatory, relaxant, re-establish nerve equilibrium

USES: Insomnia, anxiety, muscle spasms.

Fragrant Influence: Uplifting and refreshing to the senses; it clears confusion, reduces mental fatigue and depression. Stimulates the mind and improves memory.

Application: Dilute 1 part EO with 1 part VO; (1) apply 2-4 drops on location, (2) chakras/vitaflex points, (3) directly inhale, or (4) diffuse (see Appendices E and T).

Pine *(Pinus sylvestris)*

Botanical Family: Pinaceae (pine)

Plant Origin: Austria, Russia, Canada

Extraction Method: Steam distilled from needles.

Key Constituents:
Alpha Pinene (55-70%)
Beta Pinene (3-8%)
Limonene (5-10%)
Delta 3 Carene (6-12%)

Historical Data: Pine was first investigated by Hippocrates, the father of Western medicine, for its benefits to the respiratory system. In 1990, Dr. Pénoël and Dr. Franchomme described pine oil's antiseptic properties in their medical textbook. Pine is used in massage for stressed muscles and joints. It shares many of the same properties as *Eucalyptus globulus*, and the action of both oils is enhanced when blended. Native Americans stuffed mattresses with pine needles to repel lice and fleas. It was used to treat lung infections and even added to baths to revitalize those suffering from mental or emotional fatigue.

Medical Properties: Hormone-like, antidiabetic, cortisone-like, antiseptic, hormone-like, lymphatic stimulant

USES: Throat/lung/sinus infections, rheumatism/arthritis, skin parasites, urinary tract infection

Fragrant Influence: Relieves anxiety and revitalizes mind, body, and spirit.

Application: Dilute 1 part EO with 1 part VO; (1) apply 2-4 drops on location, (2) chakras/vitaflex points, (3) directly inhale, or (4) diffuse (see Appendices E and T).

Cautions: Avoid oils adulterated with turpentine, a low-cost, but potentially hazardous filler.

Found In: Grounding and R.C.

Bible Reference: Nehemiah 8:15—"And that they should publish and proclaim in all their cities, and in Jerusalem, saying, Go forth unto the mount, and fetch olive branches, and pine branches, and myrtle branches, and palm branches, and branches of thick trees, to make booths, as it is written."

Isaiah 41:19—"I will plant in the wilderness the cedar, the shittah tree, and the myrtle, and the oil tree; I will set in the desert the fir tree, and the pine, and the box tree together:"

Isaiah 60:13—"The glory of Lebanon shall come unto thee, the fir tree, the pine tree, and the box together, to beautify the place of my sanctuary; and I will make the place of my feet glorious."

Ravensara *(Ravensara aromatica)*

Botanical Family: Lauraceae

Plant Origin: Madagascar

Extraction Method: Steam distilled from branches.

Key Constituents:
Limonene + Eucalyptol (50-65%)
Sabinene (6-12%)
Alpha-Terpineol (5-11%)
Alpha Pinene (4-9%)
Beta-Pinene (1-5%)

ORAC: 890 µTE/100g

Historical Data: Ravensara is referred to by the people of Madagascar as "the oil that heals." It is antimicrobial and supporting to the nerves and respiratory system.

Medical Properties: Antitumoral, antiviral, antibacterial.

USES: Herpes virus/viral infections, throat/lung infections, hepatitis, shingles, cancer, pneumonia.

Application: (1) Apply 2-4 drops on location, (2) chakras/vitaflex points, (3) directly inhale, or (4) diffuse (see Appendices E and T).

Found In: ImmuPower and Raven.

Selected Research:

Raharivelomanana PJ, Terrom GP, Bianchini JP, Coulanges Study of the antimicrobial action of various essential oils extracted from Malagasy plants. II: Lauraceae. Arch Inst Pasteur Madagascar. 1989;56(1):261-71.

Rosalina

(See MELALEUCA ERICIFOLIA)

Rose (*Rosa damascena*)

Botanical Family: Rosaceae

Plant Origin: Bulgaria, Turkey

Extraction Method: Therapeutic-grade oil is steam distilled from flower (a two-part process). NOTE: The Bulgarian *Rosa damascena* (high in citronellol) is very different from Morrocan *Rosa centifolia* (high in phenyl ethanol). They have different colors, aromas, and therapeutic actions.

Key Constituents:
Geraniol (12-28%)
Citronellol (34-44%)
Nerol (6-9%)
Phenylethylic Alcohol (0-2%)

ORAC: 160,400 μTE/100g

Historical Data: Rose has been used for the skin for thousands of years. The Arab physician, Avicenna, was responsible for first distilling rose oil, eventually authoring an entire book on the healing attributes of the rose water derived from the distillation of rose. Throughout much of ancient history, the oil was produced by enfleurage, a process of pressing the petals along with a vegetable oil to extract the essence. Today, however, almost all rose oils are solvent extracted.

Medical Properties: Anti-inflammatory, relaxant, reduces scarring, anti-ulcer

USES: Hypertension, anxiety, viral infections (Herpes simplex), skin conditions (scarring, wrinkles), ulcers

Fragrant Influence: Its beautiful fragrance is intoxicating and aphrodisiac-like. It helps bring balance and harmony, allowing one to overcome insecurities. It is stimulating and elevating to the mind, creating a sense of well-being.

Application: (1) Apply 2-4 drops on location, (2) chakras/vitaflex points, (3) directly inhale, (4) diffuse, or (5) take as dietary supplement (see Appendices E and T).

Found In: Envision, Forgiveness, Gathering, Gentle Baby, Humility, Harmony, Joy, SARA, Trauma Life, and White Angelica.

Selected Research:

Sysoev NP "The effect of waxes from essential-oil plants on the dehydrogenase activity of the blood neutrophils in mucosal trauma of the mouth." *Stomatologiia* 1991;70(1):12-3.

Mahmood N, et al. "The anti-HIV activity and mechanisms of action of pure compounds isolated from Rosa damascena." *Biochim Biophys Res Commun.* 1996;229(1):73-9.

Umezu T, et al., Anticonflict effects of rose oil and identification of its active constituents. Life Sci. 2002 Nov 22;72(1):91-102.

Haze S, Sakai K, Gozu Y. et al., Effects of fragrance inhalation on sympathetic activity in normal adults. Jpn J Pharmacol. 2002 Nov;90(3):247-53.

Boyanova L, Neshev G. Inhibitory effect of rose oil products on Helicobacter pylori growth in vitro: preliminary report. J Med Microbiol. 1999 Jul;48(7):705-6.

Rosemary (*Rosmarinus officinalis* CT cineol)

Botanical Family: Labiatae

Plant Origin: France, U.S.

Extraction Method: Steam distilled from leaves.

Key Constituents:
1,8 Cineol (Eucalyptol) (38-55%)
Alpha-Pinene (9-14%)
Beta-Pinene (4-9%)
Camphor (5-15%)
Camphene (2.5-6%)
Borneol (1.5-5%)
Limonene (1-4%)

ORAC: 330 μTE/100g

Historical Data: Rosemary was part of the "Marseilles Vinegar" or "Four Thieves Vinegar" used by grave-robbing bandits to protect themselves during the 15th century plague. The name of the oil is derived from the Latin words for dew of the sea (ros + marinus). According to folklore history, rosemary originally had white flowers; however, they turned red after the Virgin Mary laid her cloak on the bush. Since the time of ancient Greece (about 1000 BC), rosemary was burnt as incense. Later cultures believed that it warded off devils, a practice that eventually became adopted by the sick who then burned rosemary to protect against infection.

It was listed in Hildegard's Medicine, a compilation of early German medicines by highly-regarded Benedictine herbalist Hildegard of Bingen (1098-1179).

Until recently, French hospitals used rosemary to disinfect the air.

Medical Properties: Liver-protecting, anti-tumoral, antifungal, antibacterial, antiparasitic, enhances mental clarity/ concentration.

USES: Infectious disease, liver conditions/ hepatitis, throat/lung infections, hair loss (alopecia areata), impaired memory/ Alzheimers

Fragrant Influence: Helps overcome mental fatigue and improves mental clarity and focus. University of Miami scientists found that inhaling rosemary boosted alertness, eased anxiety, and amplified analytic and mental ability.

Application: Dilute 1 part EO with 1 part VO; (1) apply 2-4 drops on location, (2) chakras/vitaflex points, (3) directly inhale, (4) diffuse, or (5) take as dietary supplement (see Appendices E and T).

Found In: Clarity, En-R-Gee, JuvaFlex, Melrose, Purity, and Thieves.

Selected Research:

Larrondo JV, et al. "Antimicrobial activity of essences from labiates." *Microbios*. 1995; 82(332):171-2.

Panizzi L, et al. "Composition and antimicrobial properties of essential oils of four Mediterranean Lamiaceae." *J Ethnopharmacol*. 1993;39(3):167-70.

Diego MA, et al. "Aromatherapy positively affects mood, EEG patterns of alertness and math computations." *Int J Neurosci*. 1998; 96(3-4):217-24.

Moss M, Cook J, Wesnes K, Duckett P. Aromas of rosemary and lavender essential oils differentially affect cognition and mood in healthy adults. Int J Neurosci. 2003 Jan;113(1):15-38.

Fahim FA, et al., Allied studies on the effect of Rosmarinus officinalis L. on experimental hepatotoxicity and mutagenesis. Int J Food Sci Nutr. 1999 Nov;50(6):413-27.

Tantaoui-Elaraki A, Beraoud L. Inhibition of growth and aflatoxin production in Aspergillus parasiticus by essential oils of selected plant materials. J Environ Pathol Toxicol Oncol. 1994;13(1):67-72.

Rosewood *(Aniba rosaeodora)*

Botanical Family: Lauraceae

Plant Origin: Brazil

Extraction Method: Steam distilled from wood.

Key Constituents:
Linalol (70-90%)
Alpha-Terpineol (2-7%)
Alpha-Copaene (trace-3%)
1,8 Cineole (Eucalyptol) (trace-3%)
Geraniol (0.5-2.5%)

ORAC: 113,200 µTE/100g

Medical Properties: antibacterial, antiviral, antiparasitic, antifungal, stimulant, improves skin elasticity.

USES: Fungal infections/Candida, skin conditions (eczema, psoriasis)

Fragrant Influence: Empowering and emotionally stabilizing.

Application: (1) Apply 2-4 drops on location, (2) chakras/vitaflex points, (3) directly inhale, (4) diffuse, or (5) take as dietary supplement (see Appendices E and T).

Found In: Acceptance, Awaken, Clarity, Forgiveness, Gentle Baby, Harmony, Humility, Inspiration, Joy, Magnify Your Purpose, Sensation, Valor, and White Angelica.

Sage *(Salvia officinalis)*

Botanical Family: Lamiaceae or Labiatae (mint)

Plant Origin: Spain, Croatia, France

Extraction Method: Steam distilled from leaves and flowers.

Key Constituents:

Alpha-Thuyone (18-43%)
Beta-Thuyone (3-8.5%)
1,8 Cineole (Eucalyptol) (5.5-13%)
Camphor (4.5-24.5%)
Camphene (1.5-7%)
Alpha-Pinene (1-6.5%)
Alpha-Humulene (0-12%) α β.

ORAC: 14,800 µTE/100g

Historical Data: Known as "herba sacra" or sacred herb by the ancient Romans, sage's name, *Salvia,* is derived from the word for "salvation." Sage has been used in Europe for oral infections and skin conditions. It has been recognized for its benefits of strengthening the vital centers and supporting metabolism.

Medical Properties: Antitumoral, hormone regulating, estrogen-like, antifungal, antiviral, circulatory stimulant, gallbladder stimulant

USES: Menstrual problems/PMS, estrogen, progesterone, and testosterone deficiencies, liver problems.

Fragrant Influence: Mentally stimulating and helps combat despair and mental fatigue. Sage strengthens the vital centers of the body, balancing the pelvic chakra where negative emotions from denial and abuse are stored.

Application: Dilute 1 part EO with 1 part VO; (1) apply 2-4 drops on location, (2) chakras/vitaflex points, (3) directly inhale, (4) diffuse, or (5) take as dietary supplement (see Appendices E and T).

Cautions: Avoid if epileptic.

Found In: EndoFlex, Envision, Magnify Your Purpose, and Mister.

Selected References:

Gali-Muhtasib HU, Affara NI. Chemopreventive effects of sage oil on skin papillomas in mice. Phytomedicine. 2000 Apr;7(2):129-36.

Sandalwood *(Santalum album)*

Botanical Family: Santalaceae (sandalwood)

Plant Origin: Indonesia, India

Extraction Method: Steam distilled from wood.

Key Constituents:

Alpha-Santalol (47-55%)
Beta-Santalol (19-23%)

ORAC: 160 µTE/100g

Historical Data: Used for centuries in Ayurvedic medicine for skin revitalization, yoga, and meditation. Listed in Dioscorides' De Materia Medica (A.D. 78), Europe's first authoritive guide to medicines, that became the standard reference work for herbal treatments for over 1,700 years.

Recent research at Brigham Young University documented its ability to inhibit many types of cancer cells.

Medical Properties: Antitumoral, antiviral, immune stimulant

USES: Cancer, viral infections (Herpes simplex, herpes zoster, cold sores, human papilloma virus etc.), skin conditions (acne, wrinkles, scars)

Fragrant Influence: Enhances deep sleep, may help remove negative programming from the cells. It is high in sesquiterpenes that stimulate the pineal gland and the limbic region of the brain, the center of emotions. The pineal gland is responsible for releasing melatonin, a powerful immune stimulant and antitumoral agent.

Application: (1) Apply 2-4 drops on location, (2) chakras/vitaflex points, (3) directly inhale, (4) diffuse, or (5) take as dietary supplement (see Appendices E and T).

Found In: Acceptance, Brain Power, Dream Catcher, Forgiveness, Gathering, Harmony, Inner Child, Inspiration, Magnify Your Purpose, Live With Passion, Release, Wisdom, Trauma Life, and White Angelica.

Selected References:

Benencia F, et al. "Antiviral activity of sandalwood oil against herpes simplex viruses-1 and -2." *Phytomedicine.* 1999;6(2):119-23

Dwivedi C, et al. "Chemopreventive effects of sandalwood oil on skin papillomas in mice." *Eur J Cancer Prev.* 1997;6(4):399-401.

Spearmint *(Mentha spicata)*

Botanical Family: Lamiaceae or Labiatae (mint)

Plant Origin: Utah

Extraction Method: Steam distilled from leaves.

Key Constituents:
Carvone (45-55%)
Cis-Dihydrocarvone (5-10%)
Limonene (15-25%

ORAC: 540 µTE/100g

Medical Properties: Increase metabolism, anti-inflammatory, antiseptic, mucolytic, gallbladder stimulant, digestive aid.

USES: Obesity, intestinal/digestive disorders, hepatitis

Fragrant Influence: Opens and releases emotional blocks and bring about a feeling of balance and a lasting sense of well-being.

Application: Dilute 1 part EO with 2 parts VO; (1) apply 2-4 drops on location, (2) chakras/vitaflex points, (3) directly inhale, (4) diffuse, or (5) take as dietary supplement (see Appendices E and T).

Found In: Citrus Fresh, EndoFlex

Selected Research:

Imai H, et al., Inhibition by the essential oils of peppermint and spearmint of the growth of pathogenic bacteria. Microbios. 2001;106 Suppl 1:31-9.

Spikenard *(Nardostachys jatamansi)*

Botanical Family: Valerianaceae

Plant Origin: India

Extraction Method: Steam distilled from roots.

Key Constituents:
Calarene (22-35%)
Beta-Ionene (4-8%)
Beta-Maaliene (4-9%)
Aristoladiene (3-7%)

ORAC: 54,800 µTE/100g

Historical Data: Highly regarded in India as a medicinal herb. It was the one of the most precious oils in ancient times, used only by priests, kings, or high initiates. References in the New Testament describe how Mary of Bethany used a salve of spikenard to anoint the feet of Jesus before the Last Supper. According to Dietrich Gumbel, Ph.D. it strengthens heart and improves circulation.

Medical Properties: Antibacterial, antifungal, anti-inflammatory, relaxant, immune stimulant

USES: Insomnia, menstrual problems/PMS, heart arrhythmias, nervous tension.

Fragrant Influence: Relaxing, soothing, and helps nourish and regenerate the skin.

Application: (1) Apply 2-4 drops on location, (2) chakras/vitaflex points, (3) directly inhale, (4) diffuse, or (5) take as dietary supplement (see Appendices E and T).

Found In: Exodus II and Humility

Bible References: (see additional Bible references in Appendix D).

Song Of Solomon 1:12—"While the king sitteth at his table, my spikenard sendeth forth the smell thereof."

Song Of Solomon 4:13—"Thy plants are an orchard of pomegranates, with pleasant fruits; camphire, with spikenard,"

Song Of Solomon 4:14—"Spikenard and saffron; calamus and cinnamon, with all trees of frankincense; myrrh and aloes, with all the chief spices:"

Selected Research:

Friedman M, Henika PR, Mandrell RE. Bactericidal activities of plant essential oils and some of their isolated constituents against Campylobacter jejuni, Escherichia coli, Listeria monocytogenes, and Salmonella enterica. J Food Prot. 2002 Oct;65(10):1545-60.

Spruce (Picea mariana)

Botanical Family: Pinaceae (pine)

Plant Origin: Canada

Extraction Method: Steam distilled from leaves, needles, and twigs.

Key Constituents:
Bornyl Acetate (18-28%)
Camphene (17-25%)
Alpha Pinene (12-19%)
Beta Pinene (4-8%)
Delta-3-Carene (5-10%)
Limonene (2-7%)
Santene (1-5%)
Tricyclene (1-5%)

Historical Data: The Lakota Indians used spruce to strengthen their ability to communicate with the Great Spirit.

Medical Properties: Antispasmodic, antiparasitic, antiseptic, anti-inflammatory, hormone-like, cortisone-like; immune stimulant.

USES: Arthritis/rheumatism, fungal infections (Candida), sinus/respiratory infections, sciatica/lumbago

Fragrant Influence: Release emotional blocks, bringing about a feeling of balance.

Application: Dilute 1 part EO with 1 part VO; (1) apply 2-4 drops on location, (2) chakras/vitaflex points, (3) directly inhale, (4) diffuse, or (5) take as dietary supplement (see Appendices E and T)

Found In: Abundance, Christmas Spirit, Envision, Gathering, Grounding, Harmony, Hope, Inner Child, Inspiration, Motivation, Present Time, R.C., Relieve It, Sacred Mountain, Surrender, Wisdom, Trauma Life, Valor, and White Angelica.

Tamanu (Calophyllum inophyllum) (NOT an essential oil, but rather a fatty acid)

Botanical Family: Bintangor

Plant Origin: Tahiti

Extraction Method: Extracted by a cold pressed method from the nut of the Polynesian Tamanu tree.

Key Constituents: (all of these constituents are fatty acid compounds--NOT essential oil compounds)
Oleic acid (35-39%)
Linoleic Acid (30-35%)
Palmitic Acid (12-14%)
Stearic Acid (12-14%)

Historical Data: The natives of Tahiti believed tamanu oil was "sacred" gift of nature. The Tahitian women used the oil as a moisturizing natural cosmetic on their faces and bodies. It was also used as sunburn protection.

Medical Properties: Used on scalp for healthy hair. When mixed with helichrysum it is affective on burns and wounds. Also the oil is used for a natural sunscreen.

Application: Dilute 1 part EO with 1 part VO; (1) apply 2-4 drops on location or (2) take as dietary supplement (see Appendices E and T).

Tangerine (Citrus nobilis)

Botanical Family: Rutaceae (citrus)

Plant Origin: USA, South Africa

Extraction Method: Cold pressed from rind.

Key Constituents:
Limonene (85-93%)
Beta-Phellandrene+Cis-Beta-Ocimene(2-5%)
Myrcene (1-4%)

Medical Properties: Antitumoral, relaxant, relaxant, antispasmodic, digestive aid, circulatory enhancer. Rich in limonene, which has been extensively studied for its ability to combat tumor growth in over 50 clinical studies.

USES: Obesity, anxiety, insomnia, irritability, liver problems, digestive problems, parasites, fluid retention.

Fragrant Influence: Promotes happiness, calming, helps with anxiety and nervousness. A 1995 Mie University study found that citrus fragrances boosted immunity, induced relaxation, and reduced depression.

Application: Dilute 1 part EO with 1 part VO; (1) apply 2-4 drops on location, (2) chakras/vitaflex points, (3) directly inhale, (4) diffuse, or (5) take as dietary supplement (see Appendices E and T)

Found In: Citrus Fresh, Dream Catcher, Inner Child, Peace & Calming.

Selected Research:

Wattenberg LW, et al., Inhibition of carcinogenesis by some minor dietary constituents. Princess Takamatsu Symp. 1985;16:193-203.

Alderman GG, Marth EH. Inhibition of growth and aflatoxin production of Aspergillus parasiticus by citrus oils. Z Lebensm Unters Forsch. 1976 Apr 28;160(4):353-8.

Crowell PL. Prevention and therapy of cancer by dietary monoterpenes. J Nutr. 1999 Mar;129(3):775S-778S.

Komori T, et al., Application of fragrances to treatments for depression. Nihon Shinkei Seishin Yakurigaku Zasshi. 1995 Feb;15(1):39-42. Japanese

Tansy, Blue (*Tanacetum annuum*)

Botanical Family: Asteraceae or Compositae (daisy)

Plant Origin: Morocco, France

Extraction Method: Steam distilled from leaves and flowers.

Key Constituents:
Camphor (10-17%)
Sabinene (10-17%)
Beta-Pinene (5-10%)
Myrcene (7-13%)
Alpha-Phellandrene (5-10%)
Para-Cymene (3-8%)
Chamazulene (3-6%)

ORAC: 68,800 µTE/100g

Medical Properties: Anti-inflammatory, analgesic /anesthetic, anti-itching, relaxant, hormone-like

Application: Dilute 1 part EO with 1 part VO; (1) apply 2-4 drops on location, (2) chakras/vitaflex points, (3) directly inhale, or (4) diffuse (see Appendices E and T)

Found In: Acceptance, Dream Catcher, JuvaFlex, Peace & Calming, Release, SARA, Valor

Tansy, Idaho (*Tanacetum vulgare*)

Botanical Family: Asteraceae or Compositae (daisy)

Plant Origin: Idaho, Washington

Extraction Method: Steam distilled from leaves.

Key Constituents:
Beta Thujone (65-80%)
Camphor (3-8%)
Sabinene (1-4%)
Germacrene D (3-7%)

Historical Data: This antimicrobial oil has been used extensively as an insect repellent. According to E. Joseph Montagna's P.D.R. on herbal formulas, it may help numerous skin conditions and tone the entire system.

Medical Properties: Analgesic, anticoagulant, immune stimulant, insect repellent

USES: Arteriosclerosis, hypertension, arthritis/rheumatism

Application: Dilute 1 part EO with 1 part VO; (1) apply 2-4 drops on location, (2) chakras/vitaflex points, (3) directly inhale, or (4) diffuse (see Appendices E and T)

Cautions: If pregnant or under a doctor's care, consult your physician.

Found In: ImmuPower, Into The Future

Tarragon *(Artemisia dracunculus)*

Botanical Family: Asteraceae or Compositae (daisy)

Plant Origin: Slovenia, France

Extraction Method: Steam distilled from leaves.

Key Constituents:
Methyl Chavicol (Estragole) (68-80%)
Trans-Beta Ocimene (6-12%)
Cis-Beta-Ocimene (6-12%)
Limonene (2-6%)

ORAC: 37,900 µTE/100g

Medical Properties: Antispasmodic, anti-inflammatory, antifermentation, antiparasitic, digestive aid.

USES: Instestinal disorders, urinary tract infection, nausea, menstrual problems/PMS.

Application: Dilute 1 part EO with 1 part VO; (1) apply 2-4 drops on location, (2) chakras/vitaflex points, or (3) take as dietary supplement (see Appendices E and T)

Cautions: Avoid use if epileptic.

Found In: Di-Tone

Tea Tree *(Melaleuca alternifolia)*

Botanical Family: Myrtaceae (myrtle)

Plant Origin: Australia

Extraction Method: Steam distilled from leaves.

Key Constituents:
Gamma Terpinene (10-28%)
Alpha-Terpinene (5-13%)
1,8 Cineole (Eucalyptol) (0-15%)
Alpha-Terpineol (1.5-8%)
Para-Cymene (0.5-12%)
Terpinenol-4 (30-45%)
Limonene (0.5-4%)
Aromadendrene (trace-7%)
Delta-Cadinene (trace-8%)
Alpha Pinene (1-6%)

Historical Data: Highly regarded as an antimicrobial and antiseptic essential oil. It has high levels of terpinen-4-ol.

Medical Properties: Powerful antibacterial, antifungal, antiviral, antiparasitic, anti-inflammatory

USES: Fungal infections (Candida, ringworm), sinus/lung infections), tooth/gum disease, water retention/hypertension, skin conditions (acne, sores)

Fragrant Influence: Promotes cleansing and purity.

Application: Dilute 1 part EO with 1 part VO; (1) apply 2-4 drops on location, (2) chakras/vitaflex points, (3) directly inhale, (4) diffuse, or (5) take as dietary supplement (see Appendices E and T).

Found In: Melrose, Purification

Selected Research:

Syed TA, et al. "Treatment of toenail onychomycosis with 2% butenafine and 5% *Melaleuca alternifolia* (tea tree) oil in cream." *Trop Med Int Health.* 1999;4(4):284-7.

Hammer KA, et al. "In vitro susceptibilities of lactobacilli and organisms associated with bacterial vaginosis to *Melaleuca alternifolia* (tea tree) oil." Antimicrob Agents Chemother. 1999;43(1):196.

Concha JM, et al. 1998 William J. Stickel Bronze Award. "Antifungal activity of *Melaleuca alternifolia* (tea-tree) oil against various pathogenic organisms." *J Am Podiatr Med Assoc.* 1998;88(10):489-92.

Groppo FC, et al., Antimicrobial activity of garlic, tea tree oil, and chlorhexidine against oral microorganisms. Int Dent J. 2002 Dec;52(6):433-7.

Stablein JJ, Bucholtz GA, Lockey RF. Melaleuca tree and respiratory disease. Ann Allergy Asthma Immunol. 2002 Nov;89(5): 523-30.

Thyme *(Thymus vulgaris* CT thymol*)*

Botanical Family: Lamiaceae or Labiatae (mint)

Plant Origin: Utah, Idaho, France

Extraction Method: Steam distilled from leaves, stems, and flowers.

Key Constituents:
Thymol (37-55%)
Para-cymene (14-28%)
Gamma-Terpinene (4-11%)
Linalol (3-6.5%)
Carvacrol (0.5-5.5%)
Myrcine (1-2.8%)

ORAC: 15,960 μTE/100g

Historical Data: It is mentioned in one of the oldest known medical records, Ebers Papyrus (dating from sixteenth century BC) an ancient Egyptian list of 877 prescriptions and recipes. The Egyptians used thyme for embalming. Listed in Dioscorides' De Materia Medica (A.D. 78), Europe's first authoritative guide to medicines, that became the standard reference work for herbal treatments for over 1,700 years.

Thyme was listed in Hildegard's Medicine, a compilation of early German medicines by highly-regarded Benedictine herbalist Hildegard of Bingen (1098-1179).

Medical Properties: Anti-aging, Highly anti-microbial, antifungal, antiviral, antiparasitic.

USES: Infectious diseases, cardiovascular disease, Alzheimers disease, hepatitis.

Fragrant Influence: It may be beneficial in helping to overcome fatigue and exhaustion after illness.

Application: Dilute 1 part EO with 4 parts VO; (1) apply 1-2 drops on location, (2) chakras/vitaflex points, (3) diffuse, or (4) take as dietary supplement (see Appendices E and T).

Caution: May irritate the nasal membranes if inhaled directly from diffuser or bottle.

Found In: Longevity.

Selected Research:

Panizzi L, et al. "Composition and antimicrobial properties of essential oils of four Mediterranean Lamiaceae." *J Ethnopharmacol.* 1993;39 (3):167-70.

Youdim KA, Deans SG. Dietary supplementation of thyme (Thymus vulgaris L.) essential oil during the lifetime of the rat: its effects on the antioxidant status in liver, kidney and heart tissues. Mech Ageing Dev. 1999 Sep 8;109(3):163-75.

Youdim KA, et al. "Beneficial effects of thyme oil on age-related changes in the phospholipid C20 and C22 polyunsaturated fatty acid composition of various rat tissues." *Biochim Biophys Acta.* 1999;1438(1):140-6.

Youdim KA, Deans SG. Effect of thyme oil and thymol dietary supplementation on the antioxidant status and fatty acid composition of the ageing rat brain. Br J Nutr. 2000 Jan;83(1):87-93.

Inouye S, et al. "Antisporulating and respiration- inhibitory effects of essential oils on filamentous fungi." Mycoses. 1998;41(9-10):403-10.

Friedman M, Henika PR, Mandrell RE. Bactericidal activities of plant essential oils and some of their isolated constituents against Campylobacter jejuni, Escherichia coli, Listeria monocytogenes, and Salmonella enterica. J Food Prot. 2002 Oct;65(10):1545-60.

Venturini ME, Blanco D, Oria R. In vitro antifungal activity of several antimicrobial compounds against Penicillium expansum. J Food Prot. 2002 May;65(5):834-9.

Inouye S, Yamaguchi H, Takizawa T. Screening of the antibacterial effects of a variety of essential oils on respiratory tract pathogens, using a modified dilution assay method. J Infect Chemother. 2001 Dec;7(4):251-4.

Lee KG, Shibamoto T. Inhibition of malonaldehyde formation from blood plasma oxidation by aroma extracts and aroma components isolated from clove and eucalyptus. Food Chem Toxicol. 2001 Dec;39(12):1199-204.

Vazquez BI, Fente C, Franco CM, Vazquez MJ, Cepeda A. Inhibitory effects of eugenol and thymol on Penicillium citrinum strains in culture media and cheese. Int J Food Microbiol. 2001 Jul 20;67(1-2):157-63.

Teissedre PL, Waterhouse AL. Inhibition of oxidation of human low-density lipoproteins by phenolic substances in different essential oils varieties. J Agric Food Chem. 2000 Sep;48(9):3801-5.

Inouye S, Uchida K, Yamaguchi H. In-vitro and in-vivo anti-Trichophyton activity of essential oils by vapour contact. Mycoses. 2001 May;44(3-4):99-107.

Tantaoui-Elaraki A, Beraoud L. Inhibition of growth and aflatoxin production in Aspergillus parasiticus by essential oils of selected plant materials. J Environ Pathol Toxicol Oncol. 1994;13(1):67-72.

Dorman HJ, Deans SG. Antimicrobial agents from plants: antibacterial activity of plant volatile oils. J Appl Microbiol. 2000 Feb;88(2):308-16.

Tsuga *(Tsuga canadensis)*

Botanical Family: Pinaceae

Plant Origin: Canada

Extraction Method: Steam distilled from needles and twigs of the conifer tree commercially known as hemlock.

Key Constituents:
Alpha- and Beta-Pinenes (18-25%)
Camphene (12-18%)
Limonene + Beta Phellandrene (3-7%)
Bornyl Acetate (28-38%)
Tricyclene (4-8%)
Myrcene (1-3%)

ORAC: 7,100 µTE/100g

Medical Properties: Analgesic, antirheumatic, blood cleanser, stimulant

USES: Respiratory conditions, kidney/urinary infections, skin conditions, venereal diseases.

Application: Dilute 1 part EO with 1 part VO; (1) apply 2-4 drops on location, (2) chakras/vitaflex points, (3) directly inhale, (4) diffuse, or (5) take as dietary supplement (see Appendices E and T).

Valerian *(Valeriana officinalis)*

Botanical Family: Valerianaceae

Plant Origin: Belgium, Croatia, France

Extraction Method: Steam distilled from root.

Key Constituents:
Bornyl Acetate (32-44%)
Camphene + Alpha-Fenchene (24-34%)
Alpha-Pinene (4-8%)
Beta-Pinene (2-6%)
Isobicycolgermacrenol (3-6%)
Myrtenyl Acetate (1-5%)

ORAC: 6,200 µTE/100g

Historical Data: During the last three decades, valerian has been clinically investigated for its tranquilizing properties. Researchers have pinpointed the sesquiterpenes valerenic acid and valerone as the active constituents that exerts a calming effect on the central nervous system. The German Commission E have pronounced valerian to be an effective treatment for restlessness and for sleep disturbances resulting from nervous conditions. insomnia, indigestion, migraine, restlessness, and tension.

Medical Properties: Sedative and tranquilizing to the central nervous system.

USES: Insomnia, anxiety

Fragrant Influence: Calming, relaxing, grounding, and emotionally balancing.

Application: (1) Apply 2-4 drops on location, (2) chakras/vitaflex points, (3) directly inhale, (4) diffuse, or (5) take as dietary supplement (see Appendices E and T).

Found In: Trauma Life

Selected Research:

Wagner J, et al. "Beyond benzodiazepines: alternative pharmacologic agents for the treatment of insomnia." *Ann Pharmacother.* 1998;32(6):680-91.

Vetiver *(Vetiveria zizanioides)*

Botanical Family: Poaceae or Gramineae (grasses)

Plant Origin: Haiti, India

Extraction Method: Steam distilled from root.

Key Constituents:
Alpha Vetivone (3-6%)
Beta Vetivone (3-6%)
Khusenol (6-11%)
Isovalencenol (11-15%)
Nootkatone (2-5%)
Khusimone (3-6%)

ORAC: 74,300 µTE/100g

Historical Data: It is well known for its anti-inflammatory properties and traditionally used for arthritic symptoms.

Medical Properties: Antiseptic, antispasmodic, relaxant, circulatory stimulant

USES: ADHD, anxiety, rheumatism/arthritis, depression (including postpartum), insomnia, skin care (oily, aging, acne, wrinkles).

Fragrant Influence: Psychologically grounding, calming, and stabilizing. It helps us cope with stress and recover from emotional trauma. Terry Friedmann MD found in clinical tests that this oil was able to successfully treat ADD and ADHD (attention deficit disorders) in children.

Application: (1) Apply 2-4 drops on location, (2) chakras/vitaflex points, (3) directly inhale, (4) diffuse, or (5) take as dietary supplement (see Appendices E and T).

Wintergreen *(Gaultheria Procumbens)*

Botanical Family: Ericaceae

Plant Origin: China

Extraction Method: Steam distilled from leaves.

Key Constituent:
Methyl Salicylate (90+%)

ORAC: 101,800 µTE/100g

Historical Data: Leaves have been chewed to increase respiratory capacity by Native Americans when running long distances and performing difficult labor. Settlers in early America had their children chew the leaves for several weeks each spring to prevent tooth decay. Wintergreen was used as a substitute for Black Tea during the Revolutionary War.

Medical Properties: Anticoagulant, antispasmodic, anti-inflammatory, vasodilator, analgesic/anesthetic, reduces blood pressure.

USES: Arthritis/rheumatism, muscle/nerve pain, hypertension, arteriosclerosis, hepatitis/fatty liver

Fragrant Influence: It stimulates and increases awareness in all levels of the sensory system.

Application: Dilute 1 part EO with 2 parts VO; (1) apply 1-2 drops on location, (2) chakras/vitaflex points, (3) directly inhale, (4) diffuse, or (5) take as dietary supplement (see Appendices E and T).

Cautions: Avoid use if epileptic. Anticoagulant properties can be enhanced when used with Warfarin or aspirin.

Found In: PanAway, Raven

Selected Research:

Ichiyama RM, et al., Effects of topical analgesics on the pressor response evoked by muscle afferents. Med Sci Sports Exerc. 2002 Sep;34(9):1440-5.

Battino M, In vitro antioxidant activities of mouthrinses and their components. J Clin Periodontol. 2002 May;29(5):462-7.

Charles CH, et al., Effect of an essential oil-containing dentifrice on dental plaque microbial composition. Am J Dent. 2000 Sep;13(Spec No):26C-30C.

Yu D et al., Caries inhibition efficacy of an antiplaque/antigingivitis dentifrice. Am J Dent. 2000 Sep;13(Spec No):14C-17C.

Joss JD, LeBlond RF. Potentiation of warfarin anticoagulation associated with topical methyl salicylate. Ann Pharmacother. 2000 Jun;34(6):729-33.

Trautmann M, Peskar BM, Peskar BA. Aspirin-like drugs, ethanol-induced rat gastric injury and mucosal eicosanoid release. Eur J Pharmacol. 1991 Aug 16;201(1):53-8.

Yarrow, Blue *(Achillea millefolium)*

Botanical Family: Asteraceae or Compositae (daisy)

Plant Origin: Utah

Extraction Method: Steam distilled from flowering top.

Key Constituents:
Chamazulene (12-19%)
Trans-Beta-Caryophyllene (4-8%)
Germacrene D (4-8%)
Camphor (4-9%)
Sabinene (3-7%)
Beta-Pinene (3-7%)
1,8 Cineol (Eucalyptol) (2-6%)

ORAC: 55,900 µTE/100g

Historical Data: The Greek Achilles, hero of the Trojan War, was said to have used the yarrow herb to help cure the injury to his Achilles tendon. Yarrow was considered sacred by the Chinese, who recognized the harmony of the Yin and Yang energies within it. It has been said that the fragrance of yarrow makes possible the meeting of heaven and earth. Yarrow was used by Germanic tribes for the treatment of battle wounds.

Medical Properties: Anti-inflammatory, hormone-like, combats scarring, prostate support

USES: Prostate problems, menstrual problems/PMS, varicose veins.

Fragrant Influence: Balancing highs and lows, both external and internal, yarrow simultaneously inspires and grounds us. Useful during meditation and supportive to intuitive energies. Reduces confusion and ambivalence.

Application: Dilute 1 part EO with 1 part VO; (1) apply 2-4 drops on location, (2) chakras/vitaflex points, (3) directly inhale, or (4) diffuse (see Appendices E and T).

Found In: Dragon Time, Mister

Ylang Ylang *(Cananga odorata)*

Botanical Family: Annonaceae (custard-apple)

Plant Origin: Commores, Indonesia, Philippines

Extraction Method: Steam distilled from flowers. Flowers are picked early in the morning to maximize oil yield. The highest quality oil is drawn from the first distillation and is known as ylang ylang complete. The last distillation, known as the tail, is of inferior quality and is called "cananga."

Key Constituents:
Germacrene D (15-20%)
Alpha Farnesene (8-12%)
Benzyl Acetate (9-15%)
Benzyl Benzoate (3-6%)
Linalol (6-10%)
Methyl Paracresol (5-9%)
Isoeugenol (3-5%)
Cinnamyl acetate (3-5%)

ORAC: 130,000 µTE/100g

Historical Data: Ylang ylang means "flower of flowers." The flowers have been used to cover the beds of newlywed couples on their wedding night. Traditionally used in hair formulas to promote thick, shiny, lustrous hair.

Medical Properties: Antispasmodic, vaso-dilating, antidiabetic, anti-inflammatory, antiparasitic, regulates heartbeat.

USES: Cardiac arrhythmia, cardiac problems, anxiety, hypertension, depression, hair loss, intestinal problems

Fragrant Influence: Balances male-female energies, enhances spiritual attunement, combats anger, low self-esteem, and increases focus of thoughts, filters out negative energy. Restores confidence and peace.

Application: Dilute 1 part EO with 1 part VO; (1) apply 2-4 drops on location, (2) chakras/vitaflex points, (3) directly inhale, (4) diffuse, or (5) take as dietary supplement (see Appendices E and T).

Found In: Aroma Life, Awaken, Clarity, Dream Catcher, Forgiveness, Gathering, Gentle Baby, Grounding, Harmony, Humility, Inner Child, Into The Future, Joy, Motivation, Peace & Calming, Present Time, Release, Sacred Mountain, SARA, Sensation, White Angelica

7

Essential Waters

Essential waters (hydrosols) are exquisite aromatic water extracts derived from herbs that have been steam distilled to produce essential oils. They have properties that are similar to those of the essential oil, but in lower concentrations. They are gentle, fragrant, and suitable for all ages.

Many essential waters are rehydrating, nurturing, and protective to the skin. They are also uniquely uplifting, calming, soothing, relaxing, and restorative.

Caution: DO NOT SPRAY DIRECTLY INTO EARS OR EYES.

How to Use:

1. Diffuse in cool mist diffuser.
2. Spray into the air to freshen the home or office.
3. Spray in an airplane or other enclosed environment to sanitize stale air.
4. Spray on face to energize, and overcome fatigue and drowsiness.
5. Drink undiluted or diluted to taste with water or juice.
6. Spray on animals to deter pests.
7. Spray on plants to deter pests.

Clary Sage Essential Water

Supports the cells and hormones. It contains natural sclareol, which stimulates the body's production of estrogen. It may also help with headaches, dry skin, or coughs.

Idaho Tansy Essential Water

Brings mental uplift, a positive attitude, and a general feeling of well-being. It is antimicrobial and supports the cleansing of the lymphatic system.

Lavender Essential Water

Soothing to the skin and calming. Spray on skin or mist in air to promote sleep.

Melissa Essential Water

Exquisitely relaxing and uplifting. It is used to treat herpes sores. In lab tests, it has been shown to be antimicrobial against *Streptococcus haemolytica*, which can colonize in the throat and esophagus.

Peppermint Essential Water

Uplifting, energizing, cooling, refreshing, and soothing to digestion.

8

Blends

This section describes specific blends that were formulated after years of research for both physical and emotional health. Each of these blends is formulated to maximize the synergistic effect between various oil chemistries and harmonic frequencies. When chemistry and frequency coincide, noticeable physical, spiritual, and emotional benefits can be attained.

It is important to remember that essential oils may be irritating to those with sensitive skin. Avoid eye contact. In case of accidental contact, put a few drops of any pure vegetable oil (ie., V-6 Vegetable Oil Complex) in the eye and call your doctor if necessary. Avoid using water to dilute or rinse.

Abundance

Increases the attraction of abundance and success. It enhances the frequency of the energy field that surrounds us through stimulation of the somatides. Somatides transmit frequency from the cells to the environment when stimulated through fragrance and thoughts. This frequency creates the "law of attraction," a harmonic magnetic energy field around oneself.

When focusing on issues of abundance and inhaling this oil, a memory link to the RNA template is created where memory is blueprinted and permanently transcribed.

Ingredients:

Myrrh *(Commiphora myrrha)* possessed the frequency of wealth according to legends and is referenced throughout the Old and New Testaments ("A bundle of myrrh is my well-beloved unto me... " Song of Solomon 1:13). It was also part of a formula the Lord gave to Moses (Exodus 30:22-27). It was used traditionally in the royal palaces by the queens during pregnancy and birthing.

Cinnamon Bark *(Cinnamomum verum)* is the oil of wealth from the Orient and part of the formula the Lord gave to Moses (Exodus 30:22-27). It was regarded by the emperors of China and India to have great value; their wealth was measured by the amount of oil they possessed. It was believed to attract wealth and abundance.

Frankincense *(Boswellia carteri)* was valued more than gold during ancient times, and only those with great wealth and abundance possessed it. It is considered a holy anointing oil in the Middle East and has been used in religious ceremonies for thousands of years. Frankincense contains sesquiterpenes which stimulate and elevate the mind, overcoming stress and despair.

Patchouli *(Pogostemon cablin)* is used by East Indians to fragrance their clothing and homes to attract abundance. Legends say that patchouli represented money and those who possessed it were considered wealthy.

Orange *(Citrus sinensis)* brings joy, peace, and happiness to those who possess it.

Clove *(Syzygium aromaticum)* is an oil from the Orient associated with great abundance; those who possessed it were considered wealthy.

Ginger *(Zingiber officinale)* was highly prized in ancient times. It amplifies the law of attraction.

Spruce *(Picea mariana)* was traditionally, believed to possess the frequency of prosperity.

Application:
Dilute 1 part EO to 1 part vegetable oil.
Possible sun/skin sensitivity.

Diffuse, directly inhale, or add 2-4 drops to bath water. Apply 1 to 2 drops over heart, on wrists, neck, and temples. Put 2 drops on a wet cloth and put in clothes dryer. Put 4-8 drops on a cotton ball and locate on vents.

Use Release first to release emotions that prevent us from receiving abundance. Follow with Acceptance, Envision, Into the Future, Joy, Magnify Your Purpose, Motivation, Valor, or Live with Passion.

Acceptance

Stimulates the mind, compelling it to open and accept new things in life, allowing one to reach a higher potential. It also helps to overcome procrastination and denial.

Ingredients:

Neroli *(Citrus aurantium)* was used by the ancient Egyptians for healing the mind, body, and spirit. It is stabilizing and strengthening to the emotions, promoting peace, confidence, and awareness. It brings everything into focus.

Sandalwood *(Santalum album)* is high in sesquiterpene compounds which stimulate the pineal gland and the limbic region of the brain, the center of emotions and memory. Used traditionally in yoga and meditation.

Blue Tansy *(Tanacetum annuum)* helps cleanse the liver and lymphatic system helping to overcome anger and negative emotions. Promotes a feeling of self-control.

Rosewood *(Aniba rosaeodora)* is high in linalool, which has a relaxing, empowering effect.

Geranium *(Pelargonium graveolens)* helps balance hormones and discharge toxins from the liver, where fear and anger are stored.

Frankincense *(Boswellia carteri)* is considered a holy anointing oil and has been used in religious ceremonies for thousands of years. It stimulates the limbic part of the brain, which elevates the mind, helping to overcome stress and despair.

Carrier Oil: Almond oil.

Application:
Diffuse or add 1-2 drops to bath water. Apply over heart and thymus, on wrists, behind ears, on neck and temples.

Aroma Life

Improves cardiovascular, lymphatic, and circulatory systems. Lowers high blood pressure and reduces stress.

Ingredients:

Helichrysum *(Helichrysum italicum)* improves circulation and reduces blood viscosity. It is anticoagulant, regulates cholesterol, stimulates liver cell function, and reduces plaque deposits from the veins and arteries.

Ylang Ylang *(Cananga odorata)* used traditionally to balance heart function and treat tachycardia (rapid heart beat) and high blood pressure. Combats insomnia.

Marjoram *(Origanum majorana)* helps regenerate smooth muscle tissue, and assists in relieving muscle spasms. it calms nervous tension. Has diuretic-like action.

Cypress *(Cupressus sempervirens)* improves circulation and lymphatic drainage. It reduces edema and water retention. It strengthens the vascular system.

Carrier Oil: Sesame seed oil.

Application:
Diffuse, directly inhale, or add 2-4 drops to bath water. Apply 1 to 2 drops over heart and along spine from first to fourth thoracic vertebrae (which correspond to the cardiopulmonary nerves). Dilute 1:15 with vegetable oil for a full-body massage.

Aroma Siez

An advanced complex of anti-inflammatory, muscle-relaxing essential oils that promote circulation and treat spasmed, tight, inflamed, aching muscles resulting from injury, fatigue, or stress. It also relieves headaches.

Ingredients:

Basil *(Ocimum basilicum)* combats muscle spasms and inflammation. It is relaxing to both striated and smooth muscles (involuntary muscles such as the heart and digestive system).

Cypress *(Cupressus sempervirens)* is antibacterial, antimicrobial, antiseptic, and improves circulation and lymphatic drainage. It reduces edema and water retention. It strengthens the vascular system.

Marjoram *(Origanum majorana)* helps regenerate smooth muscle tissue, and assists in relieving spasms, sprains, bruises, migraine headaches and calming the nerves. It is antibacterial and antiseptic.

Lavender *(Lavandula angustifolia)* relieves muscle spasms/sprains/pains, headaches, inflammation, anxiety, burns, and skin conditions (psoriasis) preventing scarring, and stretch marks. It is hypotensive, anti-infectious, anticoagulant.

Peppermint *(Mentha piperita)* has powerful pain-blocking, anti-inflammatory, and antispasmodic properties. A 1994 double-blind, placebo-controlled, randomized cross-over study at the University of Kiel in Germany found that peppermint oil had a significant analgesic effect (Gobel et al., 1994).

Application:
Dilute 1 part EO to 1 part vegetable oil.
Possible skin sensitivity.

Apply on location to sore muscles, ligaments or areas of poor circulation. Use with Raindrop Technique.

Australian Blue

Includes a rare Australian aromatic called blue cypress, a part of the aboriginal pharmacopoeia for thousands of years. Distilled from the wood of *Callitris intratropica*, the Northern Cypress Pine, it has antiviral properties. Its aromatic influence uplifts and inspires while simultaneously grounding and stabilizing.

Ingredients:

Blue Cypress *(Callitris intratropica)* contains guaiol and guaiazulene, strong anti-inflammatory and antiviral compounds. Oral traditions indicate that the aboriginal Tiwi people of northern Australia used resins from the bark of blue cypress as a skin wash for sores and cuts. It's also used to relieve pain and repel insects.

Ylang Ylang *(Cananga odorata)* increases relaxation; balances male and female energies. It also restores confidence and equilibrium.

Cedarwood *(Cedrus atlantica)* is high in sesquiterpenes, which can stimulate the limbic part of the brain, the center of emotions and memory. It stimulates the pineal gland, which releases melatonin, thereby improving thoughts, cognition, and memory.

Blue Tansy *(Tanacetum annuum)* is anti-inflammatory and helps cleanse the liver and lymphatic system. Emotionally, it combats anger and negative emotions and promotes a feeling of self-control.

White Fir *(Abies grandis)* is antimicrobial, antiseptic, antiarthritic, and stimulating. It supports the body and reduces the symptoms of arthritis, rheumatism, bronchitis, coughs, sinusitis. It creates a feeling of grounding, anchoring, and empowerment.

Application:
Possible skin sensitivity

Diffuse, directly inhale, or add 2-4 drops to bath water. Apply 1 to 2 drops on wrists, neck, temples, or foot VitaFlex points. Dilute 1:15 with vegetable oil for a full-body massage.

Awaken

Enhances inner self knowledge in order to make desirable transitions assisting to reach one's highest potential. Stimulates the creativity of the right brain, amplifying the function of pineal and pituitary glands in balancing the energy centers of the body.

Ingredients:

Joy produces a uplifting, magnetic energy that brings joy to the heart. It inspires romance and helps overcome grief and depression.

Forgiveness helps release negative memories. It helps people move past emotional barriers, enabling them to achieve higher awareness and compelling them to forgive and let go.

Present Time has an empowering fragrance, which gives a feeling of being "in the moment." One can only go forward and progress when in the present time.

Dream Catcher helps open the mind and enhance dreams and visualization, promoting greater potential for realizing your dreams and staying on your path. It also protects you from negative dreams that might cloud your vision.

Harmony promotes physical and emotional healing by bringing about a harmonic balance to the energy centers of the body. It reduces stress and creates a feeling of well-being.

Carrier Oil: Almond oil.

Application:

Diffuse, directly inhale, or add 2-4 drops to bath water. Apply 1 to 2 drops over heart, on wrists, neck, temples, or foot VitaFlex points. Dilute 1:15 with vegetable oil for a full-body massage. Put 2 drops on a wet cloth and put in clothes dryer. Put 4-8 drops on cotton ball and locate on vents. For clearing allergies, rub over sternum.

Believe

Helps to release the unlimited potential everyone possesses, making it possible to more fully experience health, happiness and vitality.

Ingredients:

Idaho Balsam Fir *(Abies balsamea)* opens emotional blocks and recharges vital energy.

Rosewood *(Aniba rosaeodora)* is high in linalool, which has a relaxing, empowering effect.

Frankincense (Boswellia carteri) is considered a holy anointing oil in the Middle East and has been used in religious ceremonies for thousands of years. Stimulates the limbic part of the brain, elevating the mind and helping to overcome stress and despair. It is used in European medicine to combat depression.

Application:

Dilute 1 part EO to 1 part vegetable oil. Possible skin sensitivity.

Diffuse, directly inhale, or add 2-4 drops to bath water. Apply 1 to 2 drops over heart, on wrists, neck, temples, or foot VitaFlex points. Dilute 1:15 with vegetable oil for a full-body massage. Put 2 drops on a wet cloth and put in clothes dryer. Put 4-8 drops on cotton ball and locate on vents.

Brain Power

Promotes deep concentration and channels physical energy into mental energy. It also increases mental potential and clarity, and long-term use may retard the aging process. Many of the oils in this blend are high in sesquiterpene compounds that increase activity in the pineal, pituitary, and hypothalamus glands and thereby increase output of growth hormone and melatonin. The oils also help dissolve petrochemicals that plug the receptor sites, clearing the brain fog that people experience due to exposure to synthetic petrochemicals in food, skin and hair care products, and air.

Ingredients:

Frankincense (Boswellia carteri) stimulates the limbic part of the brain, which elevates the mind, helping to overcome stress and despair. It is used in European medicine to combat depression.

Sandalwood *(Santalum album)* is high in sesquiterpene compounds which stimulate the pineal gland and the limbic region of the brain, the center of our emotions and memory. Used traditionally in yoga and meditation.

Melissa *(Melissa officinalis)* stimulates the limbic part of the brain, the emotional center of memories.

Cedarwood *(Cedrus atlantica)* is high in sesquiterpenes, which can stimulate the limbic part of the brain, the center of emotions and memory. It stimulates the pineal gland, which releases melatonin, thereby improving thoughts, cognition, and memory.

Blue Cypress *(Callitris intratropica)* improves circulation and increases the flow of oxygen to the brain, stimulating the amygdala, pineal gland, pituitary gland, and hypothalamus.

Lavender *(Lavandula angustifolia)* has been documented to improve concentration and mental acuity. University of Miami researchers found that inhalation of lavender oil increased beta waves in the brain, suggesting heightened relaxation. It also reduced depression and improved cognitive performance (Diego et al., 1998). A 2001 Osaka Kyoiku University study found that lavender reduced mental stress and increased alertness (Motomura et al., 2001).

Helichrysum *(Helichrysum italicum)* helps improve circulation and stimulate optimum nerve function. Enhances awareness and cognition and helps release feelings of anger, that allows one to gain focus and concentration.

Application:
Possible skin sensitivity.

Diffuse, directly inhale, or add 2-4 drops to bath water. Apply 1 to 2 drops on neck, throat, temples, neck, or under nose. Apply 1 or 2 drops with a finger on insides of cheeks in mouth. Put 2 drops on a wet cloth and put in clothes dryer. Put 4-8 drops on cotton ball and locate on vents.

Chivalry

Harkening back to stories of gallant knights of old, Chivalry instills respect, honor and integrity. It empowers you to higher ideals and instills courage.

Ingredients:

Valor balances energies to instill courage, confidence, and self-esteem. It helps the body self-correct its balance and alignment.

Joy produces a uplifting, magnetic energy that brings joy to the heart. It inspires romance and helps overcome grief and depression.

Harmony promotes physical and emotional healing by bringing about a harmonic balance to the energy centers of the body. It reduces stress and creates a feeling of well-being.

Gratitude fosters a humility, strength and open-mindedness.

Carrier Oil: Almond oil.

Application:
Possible sun/skin sensitivity.

Diffuse, directly inhale, or add 2-4 drops to bath water. Apply 1 to 2 drops over heart, on wrists, neck, temples, or foot VitaFlex points. Dilute 1:15 with vegetable oil for a full-body massage. Put 2 drops on a wet cloth and put in clothes dryer. Put 4-8 drops on cotton ball and locate on vents.

Christmas Spirit

A purifying blend of evergreen, citrus, and spice, reminiscent of winter holidays, that brings joy, peace, happiness, and security.

Ingredients:

Orange *(Citrus sinensis)* is elevating to the mind and body, bringing joy and peace.

Cinnamon Bark *(Cinnamomum verum)* is the oil of wealth from the Orient and part of the formula the Lord gave Moses (Exodus 30:22-27). Emperors of China and India measured their wealth partly by the amount of cinnamon they possessed. Traditionally, it was thought to have a frequency that attracted wealth and abundance. It is highly antiviral, antifungal, and antibacterial.

Spruce *(Picea mariana)* helps the respiratory and nervous systems. It is anti-infectious, anti-septic, and anti-inflammatory. Its aromatic influences help to open and release emotional blocks, bringing about a feeling of balance and grounding. Traditionally, spruce oil was believed to possess the frequency of prosperity.

Application:
Dilute 1 part EO to 1 part vegetable oil.
Possible sun/skin sensitivity.

Diffuse, directly inhale, or add 2-4 drops to bath water. Apply 1 to 2 drops over heart, on wrists, neck, temples, or foot VitaFlex points. Dilute 1:15 with vegetable oil for a full-body massage. Put 2 drops on a wet cloth and put in clothes dryer. Put 4-8 drops on cotton ball and locate on vents. Add to cedar chips for dresser drawers.

Citrus Fresh

Stimulates the right brain, to amplify creativity and well-being and eradicate anxiety. Works well as an air purifier. University researchers in Japan found that diffusing a citrus fragrance in an office environment improved mental accuracy and concentration by 54 percent.

Ingredients:

Orange *(Citrus sinensis)* is elevating to the mind and body, bringing joy and peace. It is high in limonene which prevents DNA damage. Has anticoagulant properties.

Tangerine *(Citrus nobilis)* contains esters and aldehydes that are sedating and calming, combating anxiety and nervousness. It is high in limonene which prevents DNA damage.

Lemon *(Citrus limon)* an antiseptic that is rich in limonene, which has been extensively studied for its ability to combat tumor growth in over 50 clinical studies. It increases microcirculation, which may improve vision.

Mandarin *(Citrus reticulata)* has sedative and slightly hypnotic properties, mandarin combats insomnia, stress and irritability. It is high in limonene which prevents DNA damage. Has anticoagulant properties.

Grapefruit *(Citrus paradisi)* decongesting and fat-dissolving. It is high in limonene which prevents DNA damage. Has anticoagulant properties.

Spearmint *(Mentha spicata)* oil helps support the respiratory, glandular, and nervous systems. With its hormone-like activity, it helps open and release emotional blocks and bring about a feeling of balance. It is antispasmodic, anti-infectious, antiparasitic, antiseptic, and anti-inflammatory. It has also been used to increase metabolism to burn fat.

Application:
Dilute 1 part EO to 1 part vegetable oil.
Possible sun/skin sensitivity.

Diffuse, directly inhale, or add 2-4 drops to bath water. Apply 1 to 2 drops on edge of ears, wrists, neck, temples, or foot VitaFlex points. Dilute 1:15 with vegetable oil for a full-body massage. Put 2 drops on a wet cloth and put in clothes dryer. Put 4-8 drops on cotton ball and locate on vents.

Clarity

Promotes a clear mind and amplifies mental alertness. Improves mental activity and vitality, and increases energy when overly tired.

Ingredients:

Cardamom *(Elettaria cardamomum)* is uplifting, refreshing, and invigorating. It may be beneficial for clearing confusion. In a study done by Dember, et al., 1995, cardamom was found to enhance performance accuracy.

Rosemary *(Rosmarinus officinalis* CT cineol*)* helps overcome mental fatigue, stimulating memory and opening the conscious mind. University of Miami scientists found that inhaling rosemary boosted alertness, eased anxiety, and amplified analytic and mental ability.

Peppermint *(Mentha piperita)* Dr. William N. Dember of the University of Cincinnati found that inhaling peppermint oil increased the mental accuracy by 28 percent.

Basil *(Ocimum basilicum)* alleviates mental fatigue and muscle spasms.

Bergamot *(Citrus bergamia)* is simultaneously uplifting and calming, with a unique ability to relieve anxiety, stress, and tension.

Geranium *(Pelargonium graveolens)* is antispasmodic, relaxant, anti-inflammatory, and uplifting.

Jasmine *(Jasminum officinale)* is stimulating to the mind and improves concentration.

Lemon *(Citrus limon)* is stimulating and invigorating. A 1995 Mie University study found that citrus fragrances boosted immunity, induced relaxation, and reduced depression.

Palmarosa *(Cymbopogon martinii)* is stimulating and revitalizing, enhancing both the nervous and cardiovascular system.

Roman Chamomile *(Chamaemelum nobile)* combats restlessness, tension, insomnia. It purges toxins from liver where anger is stored.

Rosewood *(Aniba rosaeodora)* is high in linalool, which has a relaxing, empowering effect.

Ylang Ylang *(Cananga odorata)* helps bring about a sense of relaxation.

Application:
Dilute 1 part EO to 1 part vegetable oil.
Possible sun/skin sensitivity.

Diffuse, directly inhale, or add 2-4 drops to bath water. Apply 1 to 2 drops on edge of ears, wrists, neck, temples, or foot Vitaflex points (brain = large toe).

Add Brain Power, lemon, or peppermint to enhance effects.

Di-Tone

Relieves digestive problems including indigestion, heartburn, and bloating. Combats candida and parasite infestation.

Ingredients:

Tarragon *(Artemisia dracunculus)* is antiseptic and combats intestinal parasites and urinary tract infection. It is antispasmodic, anti-inflammatory, anti-infectious, and prevents fermentation.

Ginger *(Zingiber officinale)* has been traditionally used to combat nausea and and gastro-intestinal fermentation. It is antispasmodic and antiseptic and combats indigestion.

Juniper *(Juniperus osteosperma* and *J. scopulorum)* works as a powerful detoxifier and cleanser and amplifies kidney function.

Anise *(Pimpinella anisum)* is antispasmodic, antiseptic, stimulates and increases bile flow. Combats spastic colitis, indigestion, and intestinal pain.

Fennel *(Foeniculum vulgare)* is antiseptic and stimulating to the gastrointestinal system. It is antispasmodic, antiseptic, and used for flatulence and nausea. It promotes digestion and prevents fermentation.

Patchouli *(Pogostemon cablin)* is powerful digestive aid that combats nausea.

Peppermint *(Mentha piperita)* is one of the most highly regarded herbs for improving digestion and combating parasites. It relaxes the smooth muscles of the intestinal tract and promotes peristalsis. It kills bacteria, yeasts, fungi, and mold.

Lemongrass *(Cymbopogon flexuosus)* has been documented to have powerful antifungal properties. It is a vasodilating, anti-inflammatory, and improves digestion.

Application:
Dilute 1 part EO to 1 part vegetable oil.
Possible skin sensitivity.

Massage or place as a compress on the stomach. Apply to Vita Flex points on feet/ankles. Take 1 capsule size 0 twice day or as needed.

Dragon Time

Relieves PMS symptoms and menstrual discomforts including cramping and irregular periods. Combats mood swings and headaches caused by hormonal imbalance.

Ingredients:

Clary Sage *(Salvia sclarea)* balances the hormones. It contains natural sclareol, a phytoestrogen that mimics estrogen function. It helps with menstrual cramps, PMS, and circulatory problems.

Yarrow *(Achillea millefolium)* balances hormones and reduces inflammation.

Lavender *(Lavandula angustifolia)* is relaxant that combats anxiety, headaches and PMS symptoms.

Jasmine *(Jasminum officinale)* is used for muscle spasms, frigidity, depression, and nervous exhaustion.

Fennel *(Foeniculum vulgare)* is antiseptic and antispasmodic. It has estrogen-like activity and hormone-like activity.

Marjoram *(Origanum majorana)* relieves muscle spasm and calms nerves. It relieves menopause symptoms as well as painful periods.

Application:
Dilute 1 part EO to 1 part vegetable oil.
Possible skin sensitivity.

Diffuse, directly inhale, or add 2-4 drops to bath water. Apply 1 to 2 drops on wrists, neck, temples, or foot VitaFlex points. Dilute 1:15 with vegetable oil for a full-body massage. Apply as a hot compress over lower abdomen, across lower back, or on location of pain.

Dream Catcher

Opens the mind to enhance dreams and visualizations, promoting greater potential for realizing your dreams and staying on your path. It also protects you from negative dreams that might cloud your vision.

Ingredients:

Sandalwood *(Santalum album)* is high in sesquiterpene compounds which stimulate the pineal gland and the limbic region of the brain, the center of our emotions and memory. Used traditionally in yoga and meditation.

Blue Tansy (*Tanacetum annuum*) helps to overcome anger and negative emotions promoting a feeling of self-control.

Juniper *(Juniperus osteosperma* and *J. scopulorum)* elevates spiritual awareness to create feelings of love and peace.

Bergamot *(Citrus bergamia)* is simultaneously uplifting and calming, with a unique ability to relieve anxiety, stress, and tension.

Anise *(Pimpinella anisum)* is antispasmodic, antiseptic, stimulates the increase of bile from the liver.

Tangerine *(Citrus nobilis)* combats anxiety and nervousness. A 1995 Mie University study found that the application of citrus fragrance to depressive patients made it possible to markedly reduce doses of antidepressants. Researchers also found that citrus fragrances boosted immunity.

Ylang Ylang *(Cananga odorata)* increases relaxation; balances male and female energies. It also restores confidence and equilibrium.

Pepper, Black *(Piper nigrum)* stimulates the endocrine system and increases energy.

Application:
Dilute 1 part EO to 1 part vegetable oil. Possible sun/skin sensitivity.

Diffuse, directly inhale, or add 2-4 drops to bath water (most effective before and during sleep). Apply on forehead, ears, throat, under nose, eyebrows, and base of neck. Use during meditation, in sweat lodges.

Note: If unpleasant dreams occur, continue to use since subconscious memories and thoughts will still need to be resolved. Hold on to your dreams and visualize them into reality. It may be helpful to write down your dreams upon arising.

EndoFlex

Amplifies metabolism and vitality, and creates hormonal balance.

Ingredients:

Spearmint *(Mentha spicata)* used to increase metabolism to burn fat. With its hormone-like activity, it supports the nervous and glandular systems. Spearmint is antispasmodic, antiseptic, and anti-inflammatory.

Myrtle *(Myrtus communis)* helps normalize hormonal imbalances of the thyroid and ovaries. It helps the respiratory system with chronic coughs and tuberculosis. Myrtle is suitable to use for coughs and chest complaints with children, and may support immune function in fighting cold, flu, and infectious disease.

Nutmeg *(Myristica fragrans)* supports the adrenal glands for increased energy. It is powerfully stimulating and energizing.

German Chamomile *(Matricaria recutita)* is highly anti-inflammatory and liver-protecting.

Geranium *(Pelargonium graveolens)* assists in balancing hormones. It is antispasmodic, relaxant, anti-inflammatory, antibacterial, antifungal, and stimulates the liver and pancreas.

Sage *(Salvia officinalis)* strengthens the vital centers. The Lakota Indians used sage for purification, healing and to dispel negative emotions.

Carrier Oil: Sesame seed oil.

Application:
Diffuse, directly inhale, or add 2-4 drops to bath water. Apply over lower back, thyroid, kidneys, liver, feet, glandular areas, and foot Vita Flex points.

En-R-Gee

Increases vitality, circulation, and alertness in the body.

Ingredients:

Clove *(Syzygium aromaticum)* a powerful general stimulant.

Juniper *(Juniperus osteosperma* and *J. scopulorum)* detoxifies and cleanses and improves nerve and kidney function. It elevates spiritual awareness.

Fir *(Abies alba)* is stimulating and empowering.

Pepper, Black *(Piper nigrum)* stimulates the endocrine system and increases energy.

Nutmeg *(Myristica fragrans)* supports the adrenal glands for increased energy. It is powerfully stimulating and energizing.

Rosemary *(Rosmarinus officinalis* CT cineol) helps overcome mental fatigue, stimulating memory and opens the conscious mind. University of Miami scientists found that inhaling rosemary boosted alertness, eased anxiety, and amplified analytic and mental ability.

Lemongrass *(Cymbopogon flexuosus)* increases blood circulation and vasodilation.

Application:

Dilute 1 part EO to 2 parts vegetable oil. Possible sun/skin sensitivity.

Diffuse, directly inhale, or add 2-4 drops to bath water. Apply 1 to 2 drops to wrists, temples, back of neck, behind ears, or foot Vita Flex points. Use with Raindrop Technique. Put 2 drops on a wet cloth and put in clothes dryer. Put 4-8 drops on cotton ball and locate on vents.

Enhance effects by rubbing En-R-Gee on feet and Awaken on temples.

Envision

Renews faith in the future, stimulates creative and intuitive abilities, and amplifies emotional fortitude to achieve your goals and dreams. It helps reawaken internal drive and independence and overcome the fear of experiencing new dimensions.

Ingredients:

Sage *(Salvia officinalis)* strengthens the vital centers. The Lakota Indians used sage for purification, healing and to dispel negative emotions.

Geranium *(Pelargonium graveolens)* helps release negative memories, thereby opening and elevating the mind.

Orange *(Citrus sinensis)* is elevating to the mind and body. A 1995 Mie University study documented the ability of citrus fragrances to combat depression and boost immunity.

Rose *(Rosa damascena)* possesses the highest frequency of the oils. It creates a sense of balance, harmony, and well-being and elevates the mind. Rose creates a magnetic energy that attracts love and brings joy to the heart.

Lavender *(Lavandula angustifolia)* has been documented to improve concentration and mental acuity. University of Miami researchers found that inhalation of lavender oil increased beta waves in the brain, suggesting heightened relaxation. It also reduced depression and improved cognitive performance (Diego et al., 1998). A 2001 Osaka Kyoiku University study found that lavender reduced mental stress and increased alertness (Motomura et al., 2001).

Spruce *(Picea mariana)* helps to open and release emotional blocks, bringing about a feeling of balance and grounding. Traditionally, spruce oil was believed to possess the frequency of prosperity.

Application:

Diffuse, directly inhale, or add 2-4 drops to bath water. Apply 1 to 2 drops on edge of ears, wrists, neck, temples, or foot VitaFlex points. Put 2 drops on a wet cloth and put in clothes dryer. Put 4-8 drops on cotton ball and locate on vents.

Evergreen Essence

Similar to Sacred Mountain, it is spiritually uplifting with deep and longlasting emotional influences. Dispels depression and melancholy.

Ingredients:

Spruce *(Picea mariana)* helps to open and release emotional blocks, creating a feeling of balance and grounding. Traditionally, spruce oil was believed to possess the frequency of prosperity.

Fir *(Abies alba)* antiseptic, antiarthritic, and stimulating. It creates a feeling of grounding, anchoring, and empowerment.

Pine *(Pinus sylvestris)* helps reduce stress, relieve anxiety, and energize the entire body.

Cedarwood *(Cedrus atlantica)* is high in sesquiterpenes, which can stimulate the limbic part of the brain, the center of emotions and memory. It stimulates the pineal gland, which releases melatonin, thereby improving thoughts, cognition, and memory.

Also contains: Colorado Blue Spruce, Ponderosa Pine, Red Fir, Black Pine, Piñon Pine, Lodge Pole Pine

Application:

Dilute 1 part EO to 1 part vegetable oil. Possible skin sensitivity.

Diffuse, directly inhale, or add 2-4 drops to bath water. Apply 1 to 2 drops on edge of ears, wrists, neck, temples, or foot VitaFlex points. Dilute 1:15 with vegetable oil for a full-body massage. Put 2 drops on a wet cloth and put in clothes dryer. Put 4-8 drops on cotton ball and locate on vents.

Exodus II

Some researchers believe that these aromatics were used by Moses to protect the Israelites from a plague. Modern science shows that these oils contain immune-stimulating and antimicrobial compounds. Because of the complex chemistry of essential oils, it is very difficult for viruses and bacteria to mutate and acquire resistance to them.

Ingredients:

Cassia *(Cinnamomum cassia)* is anti-infectious, antibacterial, and anticoagulant. It was part of the formula the Lord gave Moses (Exodus 30:22-27) for the holy anointing oil.

Hyssop *(Hyssopus officinalis)* is anti-inflammatory, antiparasitic, anti-infectious, and decongestant.

Frankincense *(Boswellia carteri)* is considered a holy anointing oil in the Middle East. It stimulates the hypothalamus to amplify immunity. Research at Ponce University shows that it inhibit breast cancer and enhances DNA repair. In ancient times, it was well-known for its healing powers, and was reportedly used to treat every conceivable ill.

Spikenard *(Nardostachys jatamansi)* was used by Mary of Bethany to anoint the feet of Jesus. Strengthens immunity and hypothalmus function.

Galbanum *(Ferula gummosa)* prized for healing since Biblical times. (And the Lord said unto Moses, Take unto thee sweet spices, stacte, and onycha, and galbanum; sweet spices with pure frankincense: Exodus 30:34).

Myrrh *(Commiphora myrrha)* is antimicrobial oil and antimutagenic. It is referenced in the Old and New Testaments (*A bundle of myrrh is my well-beloved unto me... Song of Solomon 1:13*). Its' high levels of sesquiterpenes stimulate the hypothalamus and the pituitary and amplify immune response.

Cinnamon Bark *(Cinnamomum verum)* is part of the formula the Lord gave Moses (Exodus 30:22-27). It is antibacterial, antiparasitic, antiviral, and antifungal. Researchers, including J. C. Lapraz, M.D., found that viruses could not live in the presence of cinnamon oil.

Calamus *(Acorus calamus)* is part of the formula the Lord gave Moses (Exodus 30:22-27). It is antispasmodic, anti-inflammatory (gastrointestinal).

Carrier Oil: Olive oil.

Application:

Dilute 1 part EO to 4 parts vegetable oil. Possible skin sensitivity.

Diffuse, directly inhale, or add 2-4 drops to bath water. Apply 1 to 2 drops on ears, wrists, foot Vita Flex points, or along spine raindrop-style. Put 4-8 drops on cotton ball and locate on vents. Add 2 drops to a wet cloth and put in clothes dryer.

Forgiveness

Helps one to release hurt feelings, insults, and negative emotions. Also helps release negative memories, allowing one to move past emotional barriers and attain higher awareness, assisting them to forgive and let go.

Ingredients:

Rose *(Rosa damascena)* has the highest frequency among essential oils. It creates a sense of balance, harmony, and well-being and elevates the mind. It creates a magnetic energy that attracts love and brings joy to the heart.

Melissa *(Melissa officinalis)* brings out gentleness. It is calming and balancing to the emotions, affecting the limbic part of the brain, the emotional center of memories.

Helichrysum *(Helichrysum italicum)* helps release feelings of anger, promoting forgiveness.

Angelica *(Angelica archangelica)* helps to calm emotions and to bring memories back to the point of origin before trauma or anger was experienced, helping to let go negative feelings.

Frankincense (Boswellia carteri) is considered a holy anointing oil in the Middle East and has been used in religious ceremonies for thousands of years. Stimulates the limbic part of the brain, elevating the mind and helping to overcome stress and despair.

Sandalwood *(Santalum album)* is high in sesquiterpene compounds which stimulate the pineal gland and the limbic region of the brain, the center of emotions and memory. Used traditionally in yoga and meditation.

Lavender *(Lavandula angustifolia)* is relaxing and grounding. University of Miami researchers found that inhalation of lavender oil increased beta waves in the brain, suggesting heightened relaxation. It also reduced depression and improved cognitive performance (Diego et al., 1998). A 2001 Osaka Kyoiku University study found that lavender reduced mental stress and increased alertness (Motomura et al., 2001).

Bergamot *(Citrus bergamia)* is simultaneously uplifting and calming, with a unique ability to relieve anxiety, stress, and tension.

Geranium *(Pelargonium graveolens)* assists in balancing hormones, with antidepressant, uplifting, and tension-relieving properties.

Jasmine *(Jasminum officinale)* has therapeutic effects, both emotional and physical.

Lemon *(Citrus limon)* is stimulating and invigorating, promoting a deep sense of well-being. A 1995 Mie University study found that citrus fragrances boosted immunity, induced relaxation, and reduced depression.

Palmarosa *(Cymbopogon martinii)* it is stimulating and revitalizing, enhancing both the nervous and cardiovascular system.

Roman Chamomile *(Chamaemelum nobile)* combats restlessness, tension, and opens mental blocks.

Rosewood *(Aniba rosaeodora)* is high in linalool, which has a relaxing, empowering effect.

Ylang Ylang *(Cananga odorata)* increases relaxation; balances male and female energies. It also restores confidence and equilibrium.

Carrier Oil: Sesame seed oil.

Application:
Possible sun/skin sensitivity.

Diffuse, directly inhale, or add 2-4 drops to bath water. Apply 1 to 2 drops behind ears, on wrists, neck, temples, navel, solar plexus, or heart. Dilute 1:15 with vegetable oil for a full-body massage. Put 4-8 drops on cotton ball and locate on vents.

Gathering

This blend was created to help us overcome the bombardment of chaotic energy that alters our focus and takes us off our path toward higher achievements. Galbanum, a favorite oil of Moses, has a strong effect when blended with frankincense and sandalwood in gathering our emotional and spiritual thoughts, helping us to achieve our potential. These oils helps increase the oxygen around the pineal and pituitary gland, bringing greater harmonic frequency to receive the communication we desire. This blend helps bring people together on a physical, emotional, and spiritual level for greater focus and clarity. It helps one stay focused, grounded, and clear in gathering one's potential for self-improvement.

Ingredients:

Galbanum *(Ferula gummosa)* was used for both medicinal and spiritual purposes. When combined with frankincense and sandalwood, its frequency increases dramatically. (And the Lord said unto Moses, Take unto thee sweet spices, stacte, and onycha, and galbanum; sweet spices with pure with frankincense: Exodus 30:34).

Frankincense (Boswellia carteri) is considered a holy anointing oil in the Middle East and has been used in religious ceremonies for thousands of years. Stimulates the limbic part of the brain, elevating the mind and helping to overcome stress and despair. It is used in European medicine to combat depression.

Sandalwood *(Santalum album)* is high in sesquiterpene compounds which stimulate the pineal gland and the limbic region of the brain, the center of emotions and memory. Used traditionally in yoga and meditation.

Rose *(Rosa damascena)* has the highest frequency among essential oils. It creates a sense of balance, harmony, and well-being and elevates the mind. It creates a magnetic energy that attracts love and brings joy to the heart.

Lavender *(Lavandula angustifolia)* is relaxant and grounding and improves concentration and mental acuity. University of Miami researchers found that inhalation of lavender oil increased beta waves in the brain, suggesting heightened relaxation. It also reduced depression and improved cognitive performance (Diego et al., 1998). A 2001 Osaka Kyoiku University study found that lavender reduced mental stress and increased alertness (Motomura et al., 2001).

Cinnamon Bark *(Cinnamomum verum)* is the oil of wealth from the Orient and part of the formula the Lord gave to Moses (Exodus 30:22-27). It has been traditionally used to release malice or spite.

Spruce *(Picea mariana)* helps to open and release emotional blocks, creating a feeling of balance and grounding. Traditionally, spruce oil was believed to possess the frequency of prosperity.

Ylang Ylang *(Cananga odorata)* increases relaxation; balances male and female energies. It also restores confidence and equilibrium.

Geranium *(Pelargonium graveolens)* stimulates nerves and assists in balancing hormones. Its' aromatic influence helps release negative memories, thereby opening and elevating the mind.

Application:

Dilute 1 part EO to 1 part vegetable oil. Possible skin sensitivity.

Diffuse, directly inhale, or add 2-4 drops to bath water. Apply 1 to 2 drops on edge of ears, wrists, neck, or temples. Dilute 1:15 with vegetable oil for a full-body massage. Put 2 drops on a wet cloth and put in clothes dryer. Put 4-8 drops on cotton ball and locate on vents.

Use Forgiveness on navel, Sacred Mountain on crown (to clear negative attitudes), Valor on crown or feet, Three Wise Men on crown, Clarity on temples, and Dream Catcher.

Gentle Baby

Comforting, soothing, relaxing, and beneficial for reducing stress during pregnancy. It helps reduce stretch marks and scar tissue and rejuvenates the skin, improving elasticity and reducing wrinkles. It is particularly soothing to dry, chapped skin and diaper rash.

Ingredients:

Palmarosa *(Cymbopogon martinii)* combats candida, rashes, and scaly and flaky skin. It stimulates new cell growth, as it moisturizes and promotes healing. It is antimicrobial.

Geranium *(Pelargonium graveolens)* has been used for centuries for skin care. It revitalizes tissue and nerves and has relaxant, anti-inflammatory, anti-infectious effects.

Roman Chamomile *(Chamaemelum nobile)* combats restlessness, insomnia, muscle tension, and inflammation.

Rose *(Rosa damascena)* promotes healthy skin, reduces scarring, and promotes elasticity.

Lavender *(Lavandula angustifolia)* is known as the universal oil. It is beneficial for skin conditions, such as burns, rashes, and psoriasis and prevents scarring and stretch marks.

Rosewood *(Aniba rosaeodora)* is soothing and nourishing to the skin, enhancing skin elasticity, and is antibacterial and antifungal.

Ylang Ylang *(Cananga odorata)* increases relaxation; balances male and female energies. It also restores confidence and equilibrium.

Bergamot *(Citrus bergamia)* is simultaneously uplifting and calming, with a unique ability to relieve anxiety, stress, and tension.

Jasmine *(Jasminum officinale)* is beneficial for dry, greasy, irritated, or sensitive skin.

Lemon *(Citrus limon)* increases microcirculation and lymphatic function. Its fragrance is stimulating, invigorating and antidepressant (Komori, et al., 1995).

Application:
Dilute 1 part EO to 1 part vegetable oil.
Possible sun sensitivity.

Diffuse or apply on location for dry, chapped skin or diaper rash. Apply over mother's abdomen, on feet, lower back, face, and neck areas. Dilute with vegetable oil for body massage and for applying on baby's skin.

For Pregnancy and Delivery: Use for massage throughout entire pregnancy for relieving stress and anxiety, and to prevent scarring and creating serenity. Massage on the perineum to help it stretch for easier birthing.

Gratitude

This delightful blend is designed to elevate, soothe and bring relief to the body while helping to foster a grateful attitude. It is also nourishing and supportive to the skin. The New Testament tells us that on one occasion Christ healed 10 lepers (Luke 17:12-19, but only one returned to express his thanks. This blend embodies the spirit of that one and only grateful leper.

Ingredients:

Idaho Balsam Fir *(Abies balsamea)* opens emotional blocks and recharges vital energy.

Frankincense (Boswellia carteri) is considered a holy anointing oil in the Middle East and has been used in religious ceremonies for thousands of years. Stimulates the limbic part of the brain,

elevating the mind and helping to overcome stress and despair. It is used in European medicine to combat depression.

Myrrh *(Commiphora myrrha)* is referenced throughout the Old and New Testaments constituting a part of a holy anointing formula given Moses (Exodus 30:22-27). It has one of the highest levels of sesquiterpenes, a class of compounds that can stimulate the hypothalamus, pituitary, and amygdala, the control center for emotions and hormone release in the brain.

Galbanum *(Ferula gummosa)* was used for both medicinal and spiritual purposes. It is antimicrobial and supporting to the body. When combined with frankincense and sandalwood, its frequency increases dramatically. (And the Lord said unto Moses, Take unto thee sweet spices, stacte, and onycha, and galbanum; sweet spices with pure with frankincense: Exodus 30:34).

Ylang Ylang *(Cananga odorata)* increases relaxation; balances male and female energies. It also restores confidence and equilibrium.

Rosewood *(Aniba rosaeodora)* is soothing and nourishing to the skin, enhancing skin elasticity, and is antibacterial and antifungal.

Application:
Possible skin sensitivity.

Diffuse, directly inhale, or add 2-4 drops to bath water. Apply 1 to 2 drops behind ears, on wrists, base of neck, temples, or base of spine. Put 4-8 drops on cotton ball and locate on vents.

Grounding

Creates a feeling of solidity and balance. It stabilizes and grounds us in order to cope constructively with reality. When we're hurting emotionally, we may wish to leave this physical existence. When this happens, it is easy to make poor choices that lead to unhealthy relationships and unwise business decisions. We seek to escape because we do not have anchoring or awareness to know how to deal with our emotions.

Ingredients:

Spruce *(Picea mariana)* helps to open and release emotional blocks, creating a feeling of balance and grounding.

White Fir *(Abies alba)* creates a feeling of grounding, anchoring, and empowerment.

Ylang Ylang *(Cananga odorata)* increases relaxation; balances male and female energies. It also restores confidence and equilibrium.

Pine *(Pinus sylvestris)* helps reduce stress, relieve anxiety, and energize the entire body.

Cedarwood *(Cedrus atlantica)* is high in sesquiterpenes, which can stimulate the limbic part of the brain, the center of emotions and memory. It stimulates the pineal gland, which releases melatonin, thereby improving thoughts, cognition, and memory.

Angelica *(Angelica archangelica)* helps to bring memories back to the point of origin before trauma or anger was experienced, helping us to release negative feelings.

Juniper *(Juniperus osteosperma* and *J. scopulorum)* elevates spiritual awareness creating feelings of love and peace.

Application:
Dilute 1 part EO to 1 part vegetable oil.
Possible sun/skin sensitivity.

Diffuse, directly inhale, or add 2-4 drops to bath water. Apply 1 to 2 drops behind ears, on wrists, base of neck, temples, or base of spine. Put 4-8 drops on cotton ball and locate on vents.

Harmony

Promotes physical and emotional healing by creating a harmonic balance to the energy centers of the body. It is beneficial in reducing stress and amplifying well-being. It is also uplifting and elevating to the mind creating a positive attitude.

Ingredients:

Hyssop *(Hyssopus officinalis)* is very balancing for emotions.

Spruce *(Picea mariana)* helps to open and release emotional blocks, creating a feeling of balance and grounding. Traditionally, spruce oil was believed to possess the frequency of prosperity.

Lavender *(Lavandula angustifolia)* a relaxant that helps overcome insomnia, headaches, and anxiety.

Geranium *(Pelargonium graveolens)* stimulates nerves and assists in balancing hormones. Its aromatic influence helps release negative memories, thereby opening and elevating the mind.

Frankincense (Boswellia carteri) stimulates the limbic part of the brain, elevating the mind and helping to overcome stress and despair. It is used in European medicine to combat depression.

Ylang Ylang *(Cananga odorata)* increases relaxation; balances male and female energies. It also restores confidence and equilibrium.

Sandalwood *(Santalum album)* is high in sesquiterpenes, which stimulate the pineal gland and the limbic region of the brain, the center of our emotions. Used traditionally in yoga, and meditation.

Angelica *(Angelica archangelica)* helps to bring memories back to the point of origin before trauma or anger was experienced, helping us to release negative feelings.

Rose *(Rosa damascena)* has the highest frequency among essential oils. It creates a sense of balance, harmony, and well-being and elevates the mind. It creates a magnetic energy that attracts love and brings joy to the heart.

Orange *(Citrus sinensis)* is elevating to the mind and body. A 1995 Mie University study documented the ability of citrus fragrances to combat depression and boost immunity.

Bergamot *(Citrus bergamia)* is simultaneously uplifting and calming, with a unique ability to relieve anxiety, stress, and tension.

Sage Lavender *(Salvia lavandulifolia)* is high in limonene which prevents DNA damage.

Jasmine *(Jasminum officinale)* is uplifting and relieves anxiety and hopelessness.

Palmarosa *(Cymbopogon martinii)* is stimulating and revitalizing, enhancing both the nervous and cardiovascular system.

Roman Chamomile *(Chamaemelum nobile)* combats restlessness, tension, insomnia. It purges toxins from liver where anger is stored.

Rosewood *(Aniba rosaeodora)* is high in linalool, which has a relaxing, empowering effect.

Application:
Dilute 1 part EO to 1 part vegetable oil.
Possible sun sensitivity.

Diffuse, directly inhale, or add 2-4 drops to bath water. Apply 1 to 2 drops on edge of ears, wrists, neck, temples, over heart, on areas of poor circulation, and on energy centers of body. Dilute 1:15 with vegetable oil for a full-body massage. Put 4-8 drops on cotton ball and locate on vents. Add 2 drops to a wet cloth and put in clothes dryer.

Highest Potential

Combines powerful emotional blends with the most exotic essential oil aromas, jasmine and ylang ylang and potent Biblical oils of frankincense, galbanum, cedarwood and sandalwood.

Helps you gather your possibilities and achieve your highest potential. This blend harmonizes several grounding, calming, inspiring and empowering essential oils into one easy-to-use blend. Biochemist R. W. Moncrieff wrote that ylang ylang "soothes and inhibits anger born of frustration," removing roadblocks and opening new vistas. The uplifting fragrance of jasmine spurs creativity while the lavender (in Gathering) clears the thought processes.

Ingredients:

Australian Blue uplifts and inspires, while also grounding and stabilizing.

Gathering collects our emotional and spiritual thoughts and helps overcome the bombardment of chaotic energy that alters our focus and takes us off our path toward higher achievements.

Jasmine Absolute (*Jasminum officinale*) is exhilarating to the mind and emotions, helping to unlock past blocks.

Ylang Ylang (*Cananga odorata*) increases relaxation; balances male and female energies. It also restores confidence and equilibrium.

Application:
Dilute 1 part EO to 1 part vegetable oil.
Possible sun/skin sensitivity.

Diffuse, directly inhale, or add 2-4 drops to bath water. Apply 1 to 2 drops on edge of ears, wrists, neck, or temples. Put 2 drops on a wet cloth and put in clothes dryer. Put 4-8 drops on cotton ball and locate on vents.

Hope

Hope is essential in order to go forward in life. Hopelessness can cause a loss of vision of goals and dreams. This blend helps to reconnect with a feeling of strength and grounding, restoring hope for tomorrow. It helps overcome suicidal depression.

Ingredients:

Melissa (*Melissa officinalis*) brings out gentleness. It is calming and balancing to the emotions, affecting the limbic part of the brain, the emotional center of memories.

Spruce (*Picea mariana*) opens and releases emotional blocks, creating a feeling of balance and grounding. Traditionally, it was believed to possess the frequency of prosperity.

Juniper (*Juniperus osteosperma* and *J. scopulorum*) elevates spiritual awareness and creates feelings of love and peace.

Myrrh (*Commiphora myrrha*) is referenced throughout the Old and New Testaments constituting a part of a holy anointing formula given Moses (Exodus 30:22-27). It has one of the highest levels of sesquiterpenes, a class of compounds that can stimulate the hypothalamus, pituitary, and amygdala, the control center for emotions and hormone release in the brain.

Carrier Oil: Almond oil.

Application:
Possible skin sensitivity.

Diffuse, directly inhale, or add 2-4 drops to bath water. Apply 1 to 2 drops on edge of ears, wrists, neck, or temples. Put 4-8 drops on cotton ball and locate on vents.

Humility

Having humility and forgiveness helps us to heal ourselves and our earth (Chronicles 7:14). Humility is an integral ingredient in obtaining forgiveness and needed for a closer relationship with God. Through the frequency and fragrance of this blend, you may arrive at a place where healing can begin.

Ingredients:

Frankincense (Boswellia carteri) is considered a holy anointing oil in the Middle East and has been used in religious ceremonies for thousands of years. Stimulates the limbic part of the brain, elevating the mind and helping to overcome stress and despair.

Rose *(Rosa damascena)* possesses the highest frequency of the oils. It creates a sense of balance, harmony, and well-being and elevates the mind.

Rosewood *(Aniba rosaeodora)* is high in linalool, which has a relaxing, empowering effect.

Ylang Ylang *(Cananga odorata)* increases relaxation; balances male and female energies. It also restores confidence and equilibrium.

Geranium *(Pelargonium graveolens)* helps release negative memories, thereby opening and elevating the mind.

Melissa *(Melissa officinalis)* brings out gentleness. It is calming and balancing to the emotions, affecting the limbic part of the brain, the emotional center of memories.

Spikenard *(Nardostachys jatamansi)* was highly prized at the time of Christ and was used by Mary of Bethany to anoint the feet of Jesus. It stimulates the limbic part of the brain, tapping emotional memories.

Myrrh *(Commiphora myrrha)* is referenced throughout the Bible and was part of a holy anointing formula given Moses (Exodus 30:22-27). It is high in sesquiterpenes, a class of compounds that can stimulate the hypothalamus, pituitary, and amygdala, the control center for emotions and hormone release in the brain.

Neroli *(Citrus aurantium)* was used by the ancient Egyptians for healing the mind, body, and spirit. It is stabilizing and strengthening to the emotions, promoting peace, confidence, and awareness. It brings everything into focus.

Carrier Oil: Sesame seed oil.

Application:

Diffuse, directly inhale, or add 2-4 drops to bath water. Apply 1 to 2 drops over heart, on neck, or temples. Put 2 drops on a wet cloth and put in clothes dryer. Put 4-8 drops on cotton ball and locate on vents.

ImmuPower

Strengthens immunity and DNA repair in the cells. It is strongly antiseptic and anti-infectious.

Ingredients:

Cistus *(Cistus ladanifer),* enhances immunity and immune cell regeneration. It is anti-infectious, antiviral, and antibacterial.

Frankincense *(Boswellia carteri)* stimulates the hypothalamus and pituitary to amplify immunity.

Oregano *(Origanum compactum)* is one of the most powerful antimicrobial essential oils. Laboratory research as Weber State University showed it to have a 99 percent kill rate against *in vitro* colonies of *Streptococcus pneumoniae*, a microorganism responsible for many kinds of lung and throat infections. This oil is antiviral, antibacterial, antifungal, and antiparasitic.

Idaho Tansy *(Tanacetum vulgare)* is antiviral, anti-infectious, antibacterial, and fights cold and flu and infections. According to E. Joseph Montagna's *Herbal Desk Reference*, tansy tones the entire body.

Cumin *(Cuminum cyminum)* amplifies immunity and DNA repair. It is antiseptic and antibacterial.

Clove *(Syzygium aromaticum)* is a powerful antioxidant that is one of the most antimicrobial and antiseptic of all essential oils. Prevents cellular DNA damage.

Hyssop *(Hyssopus officinalis)* has anti-inflammatory and antiviral properties and is antiparasitic, mucolytic, decongestant, and anti-infectious.

Ravensara *(Ravensara aromatica)* is referred to by the people of Madagascar as the oil that heals. It is antiseptic, anti-infectious, antiviral, antibacterial, antifungal.

Mountain Savory *(Satureja montana)* is immune stimulating, antiviral, antibacterial, antifungal, antiparasitic.

Application:

Dilute 1 part EO to 4 parts vegetable oil. Possible skin sensitivity.

Diffuse/humidify, directly inhale, or add 2-4 drops to bath water. Apply around navel, chest, temples, wrists, under nose, or foot Vitaflex points. Use with Raindrop Technique. Dilute 1:15 with vegetable oil for body massage. Add 2 drops to a wet cloth and put in clothes dryer. Put 4-8 drops on cotton ball and locate on vents.

Alternate with Thieves and Exodus II. To enhance effects add rosewood, melissa, oregano, clove, cistus, frankincense, or mountain savory.

Inner Child

When children are abused, they become disconnected from their inner child, or identity, which causes confusion. This fractures personality and creates problems in the early- to mid- adult years, often mislabeled as a mid-life crisis. This fragrance stimulates memory response and help one reconnect with the inner-self or identity. This is one of the first steps to finding emotional balance.

Ingredients:

Orange *(Citrus sinensis)* is elevating to the mind and body and brings joy and peace. A 1995 Mie University study documented the ability of citrus fragrances to combat depression and boost immunity.

Tangerine *(Citrus nobilis)* contains esters and aldehydes that are sedating and calming, helping with anxiety and nervousness.

Jasmine *(Jasminum officinale)* is stimulating to the mind and improves concentration.

Ylang Ylang *(Cananga odorata)* increases relaxation; balances male and female energies. It also restores confidence and equilibrium.

Sandalwood *(Santalum album)* is high in sesquiterpene compounds which stimulate the pineal gland and the limbic region of the brain, the center of emotions and memory. Used traditionally in yoga and meditation.

Spruce *(Picea mariana)* opens and releases emotional blocks, fostering a sense of balance and grounding. Traditionally, it was believed to possess the frequency of prosperity.

Lemongrass *(Cymbopogon flexuosus)* increases blood circulation and uplifts the spirit.

Neroli *(Citrus aurantium)* was used by the ancient Egyptians for healing the mind, body, and spirit. It is stabilizing and strengthening to the emotions, promoting peace, confidence, and awareness. It brings everything into focus.

Application:

Dilute 1 part EO to 1 part vegetable oil. Possible sun sensitivity.

Diffuse, directly inhale, or add 2-4 drops to bath water. Apply 1 to 2 drops on edge of ears, wrists, neck, or temples. Dilute 1:15 with vegetable oil for body massage. Add 2 drops to a wet cloth and put in clothes dryer. Put 4-8 drops on cotton ball and locate on vents.

Inspiration

Creates a feeling of being wrapped in a cocoon of spiritual quietness. These oils were traditionally used by the Native Americans to enhance spirituality, prayer and inner awareness. Inspiration brings us closer to our spiritual connection.

Ingredients:

Frankincense (Boswellia carteri) stimulates the limbic part of the brain, elevating the mind and helping to overcome stress and despair. It is used in European medicine to combat depression.

Cedarwood *(Cedrus atlantica)* is high in sesquiterpenes, which can stimulate the limbic part of the brain, the center of emotions and memory. It stimulates the pineal gland, which releases melatonin, thereby improving thoughts, cognition, and memory.

Spruce *(Picea mariana)* opens and releases emotional blocks, fostering a sense of balance and grounding. Traditionally, it was believed to possess the frequency of prosperity.

Rosewood *(Aniba rosaeodora)* is high in linalool, which has a relaxing, empowering effect.

Sandalwood *(Santalum album)* is high in sesquiterpene compounds which stimulate the pineal gland and the limbic region of the brain, the center of emotions and memory. Used traditionally in yoga and meditation.

Myrtle *(Myrtus communis)* is energizing and inspiring.

Mugwort *(Artemisia vulgaris)* is a European herb known for its antiseptic properties. Avoid during pregnancy.

Application:

Possible skin sensitivity.

Diffuse, directly inhale, or add 2-4 drops to bath water. Apply 1 to 2 drops on edge of ears, wrists, neck, temples, crown of head, bottom of feet, or along spine. Add 2 drops to a wet cloth and put in clothes dryer. Put 4-8 drops on cotton ball and locate on vents.

Into the Future

Helps one leave the past behind in order to progress with vision and excitement. So many times we find ourselves settling for mediocrity and sacrificing our own potential and success because of fear of the unknown and the future. This blend inspires determination and a pioneering spirit and creates a strong emotional feeling of being able to reach one's potential.

Ingredients:

Frankincense *(Boswellia carteri)* is considered a holy anointing oil in the Middle East and has been used in religious ceremonies for thousands of years. It stimulates the limbic part of the brain, which elevates the mind, helping to overcome stress and despair. It is used in European medicine to combat depression.

Clary Sage *(Salvia sclarea)* enhances circulation and hormone balance.

Jasmine *(Jasminum officinale)* is exhilarating to the mind and emotions, unlocking past blocks.

Juniper *(Juniperus osteosperma* and *J. scopulorum)* elevates spiritual awareness and creates feelings of love and peace.

White Fir *(Abies alba)* creates a feeling of grounding, anchoring, and empowerment.

Orange *(Citrus sinensis)* is elevating to the mind and body and brings joy and peace. A 1995 Mie University study documented the ability of citrus fragrances to combat depression and boost immunity.

Cedarwood *(Cedrus atlantica)* is high in sesquiterpenes, which can stimulate the limbic part of the brain, the center of emotions and memory. It stimulates the pineal gland, which releases melatonin, thereby improving thoughts, cognition, and memory.

Ylang Ylang *(Cananga odorata)* increases relaxation; balances male and female energies. It also restores confidence and equilibrium.

Idaho Tansy *(Tanacetum vulgare)* is antiviral, anti-infectious, antibacterial, and fights colds, flu, and infections. According to E. Joseph Montagna's PDR on herbal formulas, tansy helps skin problems, strengthen the kidneys, heart, joints, digestive system.

White Lotus *(Nymphaea lotus)* has been found to have anticancerous and strong immune supporting properties.

Carrier Oil: Almond Oil

Application:

Possible sun/skin sensitivity.

Diffuse, directly inhale, or add 2-4 drops to bath water. Apply 1 to 2 drops on edge of ears, over heart, on wrists, neck, or temples. Dilute 1:15 with vegetable oil for body massage. Put 4-8 drops on cotton ball and locate on vents.

Joy

Produces a magnetic energy to bring joy to the heart. It inspires romance and helps overcome grief and depression.

Ingredients:

Rose *(Rosa damascena)* has the highest frequency among essential oils. It creates a sense of balance, harmony, and well-being and elevates the mind. It creates a magnetic energy that attracts love and brings joy to the heart.

Bergamot *(Citrus bergamia)* balances hormones, calms emotions, and relieves anxiety, stress, and tension.

Mandarin *(Citrus reticulata)* has hypnotic properties and combats insomnia, stress and irritability.

Ylang Ylang *(Cananga odorata)* increases relaxation; balances male and female energies. It also restores confidence and equilibrium.

Lemon *(Citrus limon)* is stimulating and invigorating, promoting a deep sense of well-being. A 1995 Mie University study found that citrus fragrances boosted immunity, induced relaxation, and reduced depression.

Geranium *(Pelargonium graveolens)* stimulates the nerves and helps release negative memories so that joy can be attained.

Jasmine *(Jasminum officinale)* exudes an exquisite fragrance that revitalizes spirits.

Palmarosa *(Cymbopogon martinii)* it is stimulating and revitalizing, enhancing both the nervous and cardiovascular system.

Roman Chamomile *(Chamaemelum nobile)* combats restlessness, tension, insomnia. It purges toxins from liver where anger is stored.

Rosewood *(Aniba rosaeodora)* is high in linalool, which has a relaxing, empowering effect.

Application:
Dilute 1 part EO to 1 part vegetable oil. Possible sun/skin sensitivity.

Diffuse/humidify, directly inhale, or add 2-4 drops to bath water. Apply over heart, thymus, temples, and wrists. Dilute 1:15 with vegetable oil for a full-body massage. Put 2 drops on a wet cloth and put in clothes dryer. Put 4-8 drops on cotton ball and locate on vents.

Juva Cleanse

The liver is the body's largest internal organ and major detoxifier for the body. Even the toxins in the air we breathe are filtered by the liver, including chemicals from aerosol cleaners, paint, bug sprays, etc. But, even filters need cleaning. The essential oils of ledum, celery seed, and helichrysum have long been known for their liver cleansing properties. JuvaCleanse was clinically tested in 2003 for removing mercury from body tissues.

A 2003 study conducted by Roger Lewis MD at the Young Life Research Clinic in Provo, Utah evaluated the efficacy of helichrysum, ledum, and celery seed in treating cases of advanced Hepatitis C. In one case of a male age 20 diagnosed with a Hepatitis C viral count of 13,200. After taking two capsules (approx. 750 mg each) of a blend of helichrysum, ledum, and celery seed (JuvaCleanse) per day for a month with no other intervention, patients showed that viral counts dropped to 2,580, an over 80 percent reduction.

Ingredients:

Helichrysum *(Helichrysum italicum)* regenerates tissue and improves circulation. It stimulates liver cell function and removes plaque from the veins and arteries.

Celery Seed *(Apium graveolens)* is a powerful liver cleanser.

Ledum *(Ledum groenlandicum)* shown in clinical studies to protect the liver and improve bile function.

Application:
Apply over liver or on foot Vita Flex points. Use with Raindrop Technique.

Take one capsule size 0 once a day.

JuvaFlex

Supports liver and lymphatic detoxification. Anger and hate are stored in the liver, creating toxicity and leading to sickness and disease. JuvaFlex helps break addictions to coffee, alcohol, drugs, and tobacco.

Ingredients:

Geranium *(Pelargonium graveolens)* improves bile flow from the liver. It is antispasmodic and improves liver, pancreas, and kidneys function.

Rosemary *(Rosmarinus officinalis)* is antiseptic and antimicrobial. It balances the endocrine system.

Roman Chamomile *(Chamaemelum nobile)* is anti-inflammatory and expels toxins from the liver. Strengthens liver function.

Fennel *(Foeniculum vulgare)* is antiseptic and stimulating to the circulatory system. Increases bile flow and hepatocyte function.

Helichrysum *(Helichrysum italicum)* regenerates tissue and improves circulation. It stimulates liver cell function and removes plaque from the veins and arteries.

Blue Tansy *(Tanacetum annuum)* helps cleanse the liver and lymphatic system. It is anti-inflammatory.

Carrier Oil: Sesame seed oil.

Application:

Apply over liver area, foot Vita Flex points, raindrop-style along spine, or use in compress.

Lady Sclareol

Designed to be worn as an exquisite fragrance, this blend is also rich in phytoestrogens. It enhances the feminine nature by improving mood and raising estrogen levels. May provide relief for PMS symptoms.

Ingredients:

Rosewood *(Aniba rosaeodora)* is high in linalool, which has a relaxing empowering effect.

Vetiver *(Vetiveria zizanioides)* is psychologically grounding and stabilizing. It has been shown to help with concentration and coping with stress. Its anti-inflammatory qualities can help with joint and muscle pain.

Geranium *(Pelargonium graveolens)* helps release negative memories, opening and elevating the mind. It has been used for centuries for skin care. It revitalizes tissue and nerves and has relaxant, anti-inflammatory, anti-infectious effects.

Orange *(Citrus sinensis)* is elevating to the mind and body. A 1995 Mie University study documented the ability of citrus fragrances to combat depression and boost immunity.

Clary Sage *(Salvia sclarea)* balances the hormones. It contains natural sclareol, a phytoestrogen that mimics estrogen function. It helps with menstrual cramps, PMS, and circulatory problems.

Ylang Ylang *(Cananga odorata)* balances male and female energies, increases relaxation and restores confidence and equilibrium.

Sandalwood *(Santalum album)* is high in sesquiterpenes, which stimulate the pineal gland and the limbic region of the brain, the center of our emotions. Used traditionally in yoga and meditation.

Sage Lavender *(Salvia lavandulifolia)* is high in limonene which prevents DNA damage.

Jasmine Absolute *(Jasminum officinale)* is used for muscle spasms, frigidity, depression and nervous exhaustion. It is stimulating to the mind and improves concentration.

Idaho Tansy *(Tanacetum vulgare)* is antiviral, anti-infectious, antibacterial and fights cold and flu infections. According to E. Joseph Montagna's *Herbal Desk Reference*, tansy may help skin problems; and strengthens the kidneys, heart, joints and digestive system.

Application:

For topical or aromatic use as a perfume, apply 2-4 drops to Vita Flex points on the ankles or at the clavicle notch. May be applied to the abdomen for relieve of premenstrual discomfort.

Legacy

Ingredients:

Angelica *(Angelica archangelica)*, balsam fir *(Abies balsamea)*, basil *(Ocimum basilicum)*, bergamot *(Citrus bergamia)*, black pepper *(Piper nigrum)*, blue tansy *(Tanacetum annuum)*, buplevere *(Bupleurum fruticosum)*, cajeput *(Melaleuca leucadendra)*, cardamom *(Elettaria cardamomum)*, carrot seed *(Daucus carota)*, Canadian red cedar *(Thuja plicata)*, cedar leaf *(Thuja occidentalis)*, cedarwood *(Cedrus atlantica)*, cinnamon bark *(Cinnamomum verum)*, cistus *(Cistus ladanifer)*, citronella *(Cymbopogon nardus)*, clary sage *(Salvia sclarea)*, clove *(Syzygium aromaticum)*, coriander *(Coriandrum sativum)*, cumin *(Cuminum cyminum)*, cypress *(Cupressus sempervirens)*, dill *(Anethum graveolens)*, Douglas fir *(Pseudotsuga menziesii)*, elemi *(Canarium luzonicum)*, *Eucalyptus citriodora*, *Eucalyptus dives*, *Eucalyptus globulus*, *Eucalyptus polybractea*, *Eucalyptus radiata*, fennel *(Foeniculum vulgare)*, fir *(Abies alba)*, fleabane *(Conyza canadensis)*, frankincense *(Boswellia carteri)*, galbanum *(Ferula gummosa)*, geranium *(Pelargonium graveolens)*, German chamomile *(Matricaria recutita)*, ginger *(Zingiber officinale)*, goldenrod

(Solidago canadensis), grapefruit *(Citrus paradisi),* helichrysum *(Helichrysum italicum),* Tsuga *(Tsuga canadensis),* hyssop *(Hyssopus officinalis),* Idaho tansy *(Tanacetum vulgare),* jasmine *(Jasminum officinale),* juniper *(Juniperus osteosperma* and *J. scopulorum), Laurus nobilis,* lavender *(Lavendula angustifolia),* ledum *(Ledum groenlandicum),* lemon *(Citrus limon),* lemongrass *(Cymbopogon flexuosus),* lime *(Citrus aurantiifolia),* mandarin *(Citrus reticulata),* marjoram *(Origanum majorana), Melaleuca alternifolia, Melaleuca ericifolia,* melissa *(Melissa officinalis),* mountain savory *(Satureja montana),* myrrh *(Commiphora myrrha),* myrtle *(Myrtus communis),* neroli *(Citrus aurantium),* nutmeg *(Myristica fragrans),* orange *(Citrus sinensis),* oregano *(Origanum compactum),* palmarosa *(Cymbopogon martinii),* patchouli *(Pogostemon cablin),* peppermint *(Mentha piperita),* petitgrain *(Citrus aurantium),* pine *(Pinus sylvestris),* ravensara *(Respiratory Ravensara aromatica),* Roman chamomile *(Chamaemelum nobile),* rose *(Rosa damascena),* rose hip *(Rosa canina),* rosemary *(Rosemarinus officinalis),* rosemary verbenon *(Rosemarinus officinalis* CT verbenon), rosewood *(Aniba rosaeodora),* sage *(Salvia officinalis),* sandalwood *(Santalum album),* spearmint *(Mentha spicata),* spikenard *(Nardostachys jatamansi),* spruce *(Picea mariana),* tangerine *(Citrus nobilis),* tarragon *(Artemisia dracunculus),* thyme *(Thymus vulgaris* linalol CT), thyme linalol *(Thymus vulgaris),* valerian *(Valeriana officinalis),* vetiver *(Vetiveria zizanioides),* vitex *(Vitex negundo),* white fir *(Abies grandis),* wintergreen *(Gaultheria procumbens),* yarrow *(Achillea millefolium),* and ylang ylang *(Cananga odorata).*

Application:

Dilute 1 part EO to 4 parts vegetable oil. Possible sun/skin sensitivity.

Diffuse/humidify, directly inhale, or add 2-4 drops to bath water. Apply to bottom of feet or temples, neck, wrists, or ears. Put 4-8 drops on cotton ball and locate on vents. Add 2 drops to a wet cloth and put in clothes dryer.

Live with Passion

Stimulates enduring passion by stimulating the limbic region of the brain. One of the reasons people fail to be successful in business, work, or personal accomplishment, is due to lack of passion. It has often been said that the lack of passion is a source of disease in the body.

Ingredients:

Melissa *(Melissa officinalis)* brings out gentleness. It is calming and balancing to the emotions, affecting the limbic part of the brain, the emotional center of memories.

Helichrysum *(Helichrysum italicum)* helps release feelings of anger, promoting forgiveness.

Clary Sage *(Salvia sclarea)* enhances circulation and hormone balance.

Cedarwood *(Cedrus atlantica)* is high in sesquiterpenes, which can stimulate the limbic part of the brain (the center of our emotions), and has been used by American Indians to enhance spiritual awareness.

Angelica *(Angelica archangelica)* helps to bring memories back to the point of origin before trauma or anger was experienced, helping us to release negative feelings.

Ginger *(Zingiber officinale)* is energizing and uplifting.

Neroli *(Citrus aurantium)* was used by the ancient Egyptians for healing the mind, body, and spirit. It is stabilizing and strengthening to the emotions, promoting peace, confidence, and awareness. It brings everything into focus.

Sandalwood *(Santalum album)* is high in sesquiterpene compounds which stimulate the pineal gland and the limbic region of the brain, the center of our emotions and memory. Used traditionally in yoga and meditation.

Patchouli *(Pogostemon cablin)* reestablishes mental and emotional equilibrium while energizing the mind.

Jasmine *(Jasminum officinale)* exudes an exquisite fragrance that revitalizes spirits.

Application:

Possible sun/skin sensitivity.

Diffuse/humidify, directly inhale, or add 2-4 drops to bath water. Apply over heart, thymus, temples, ears, or wrists. Dilute 1:15 with vegetable oil for body massage. Put 4-8 drops on cotton ball and locate on vents. Add 2 drops to a wet cloth and put in clothes dryer.

Longevity

Contains the highest antioxidant and DNA-protecting essential oils. When taken as a dietary supplement, Longevity promotes longevity and prevents premature aging. (See Longevity Oil Capsules in the Supplement section).

ORAC: 1,511,025μTE/L

Ingredients:

Clove *(Syzygium aromaticum)* has the highest known antioxidant power as measured by ORAC (oxygen radical absorbent capacity), a test developed by USDA researchers at Tufts University. It is anticoagulant and one of the most antimicrobial and antiseptic of all essential oils. Prevents cellular DNA damage.

Thyme CT Thymol *(Thymus vulgaris* CT thymol*)* has been shown in studies to dramatically boost glutathione levels in the heart, liver, and brain. It also prevents lipid peroxidation or degradation of the fats found in many vital organs. The oxidation of fats in the body is directly linked to accelerated aging

Orange *(Citrus sinensis)* contains over 90 percent d-limonene, one of the most powerful anticancer compounds studied in recent years, the subject of over 50 peer-reviewed research papers published in leading medical journals throughout the world.

Frankincense *(Boswellia carteri)* has been shown in research at Ponce University to combat cellular mutations and combat chemotherapy-resistant cancers.

Application:

Dilute 1 part EO to 4 parts vegetable oil.
Possible sun/skin sensitivity.

Take one capsule size 00 once or twice a day.

M-Grain

Relieves pain from both headaches and severe migraine headaches. It is anti-inflammatory and antispasmodic.

Ingredients:

Marjoram *(Origanum majorana)* is anti-inflammatory and is used to treat sore and aching muscles. It relieves muscle spasms and migraine headaches and calms nerves.

Lavender *(Lavandula angustifolia)* is anti-inflammatory and antispasmodic. High in aldehydes and esters, it combats insomnia, stress, and nervous tension.

Peppermint *(Mentha piperita)* has powerful pain-blocking, anti-inflammatory, and anti-spasmodic properties. A 1994 double-blind, placebo-controlled, randomized cross-over study at the University of Kiel in Germany found that peppermint oil had a significant analgesic effect, effectively blocking headache pain (Gobel et al., 1994).

Basil *(Ocimum basilicum)* combats muscle spasms and inflammation. It is relaxing to both striated and smooth muscles (involuntary muscles such as the heart and digestive system).

Roman Chamomile *(Chamaemelum nobile)* is a strong anti-inflammatory with antispasmodic effects.

Helichrysum *(Helichrysum italicum)* is a powerful anaesthetic and analgesic. It quenches pain and inflammation and reduces muscle spasms.

Application:

Dilute 1 part EO to 1 part vegetable oil.
Possible skin sensitivity.

Diffuse, directly inhale, or add 2-4 drops to bath water. Apply on brain stem, forehead, crown, shoulders, back of neck, temples, and foot Vita Flex points. Put 4-8 drops on cotton ball and locate on vents.

Magnify Your Purpose

Stimulates the endocrine system and creates energy flow to the right hemisphere of the brain, activating creativity, motivation, and focus. This helps bring about commitment to purpose, magnifying your desire and pure intentions until they become reality.

Ingredients:

Sandalwood *(Santalum album)* is high in sesquiterpene compounds which stimulate the pineal gland and the limbic region of the brain, the center of emotions and memory. Used traditionally in yoga and meditation.

Nutmeg *(Myristica fragrans)* supports the adrenal glands for increased energy. It is powerfully stimulating and energizing.

Patchouli *(Pogostemon cablin)* is strongly grounding and centering. Very high sesquiterpenes that stimulate the limbic center of the brain. It reestablishes mental and emotional equilibrium and energizes the mind.

Rosewood *(Aniba rosaeodora)* is high in linalool, which has a relaxing, empowering effect.

Cinnamon Bark *(Cinnamomum verum)* is the oil of wealth from the Orient and part of the formula the Lord gave Moses (Exodus 30:22-27). It has a frequency that attracts wealth and abundance.

Ginger *(Zingiber officinale)* is energizing and uplifting.

Sage *(Salvia officinalis)* strengthens the vital centers. The Lakota Indians used sage for purification, healing and to dispel negative emotions.

Application:
Dilute 1 part EO to 1 part vegetable oil. Possible skin sensitivity.

Diffuse/humidify, directly inhale, or add 2-4 drops to bath water. Apply on heart, thymus, temples, ears, or wrists. Put 4-8 drops on cotton ball and locate on vents. Add 2 drops to a wet cloth and put in clothes dryer.

Melrose

A strong topical antiseptic that cleans and disinfects cuts, scrapes, burns, rashes, and bruised tissue. It helps regenerate damaged tissue and reduces inflammation. When diffused it dispels odors.

Ingredients:

Melaleuca *(Melaleuca alternifolia)* is antiseptic, antibacterial, antifungal, antiparasitic, anti-inflammatory.

Naouli *(Melaleuca quinquenervia)* is anti-infectious, antiparasitic, and antibacterial.

Rosemary *(Rosmarinus officinalis* CT cineol*)* is antiseptic, antifungal, and antimicrobial.

Clove *(Syzygium aromaticum)* is one of the most antimicrobial and antiseptic of all essential oils. It is antifungal, antiviral, anti-infectious, and antibacterial.

Application:
Dilute 1 part EO to 1 part vegetable oil. Possible skin sensitivity.

Diffuse/humidify, directly inhale, or add 2-4 drops to bath water. Apply to broken skin, cuts, scrapes, burns, rashes, and infection. Follow with rose ointment to keep wound and oils sealed in. Put 1 to 2 drops on a piece of cotton and place in the ear for earaches.

Mister

Helps to decongest the prostate and promote greater male hormonal balance.

Ingredients:

Yarrow *(Achillea millefolium)* is a prostate decongestant and hormone balancer. It is anti-inflammatory.

Sage *(Salvia officinalis)* has been used in Europe for hair loss. It strengthens vital centers, relieves depression and mental fatigue.

Myrtle *(Myrtus communis)* helps normalize hormonal imbalances of the thyroid and sex glands.

Fennel *(Foeniculum vulgare)* has hormone-like activity and is stimulating to the circulatory, cardiovascular and respiratory systems.

Lavender *(Lavandula angustifolia)* is antispasmodic, hypotensive, anti-inflammatory, anti-infectious, and an anticoagulant.

Peppermint *(Mentha piperita)* strengthens the liver and glandular function.

Carrier Oil: Sesame seed oil.

Application:

Diffuse, directly inhale, or add 2-4 drops to bath water. Apply to ankle Vita Flex points, lower pelvis, or areas of concern. Use in hot compress. Dilute 1:15 with vegetable oil for body massage.

Motivation

Stimulates feelings of action and accomplishment, providing positive energy to help overcome feelings of fear and procrastination.

Ingredients:

Roman Chamomile *(Chamaemelum nobile)* combats restlessness, tension, insomnia. It purges toxins from liver where anger is stored.

Spruce *(Picea mariana)* helps to open and release emotional blocks, creating a feeling of balance and grounding.

Ylang Ylang *(Cananga odorata)* increases relaxation; balances male and female energies. It also restores confidence and equilibrium.

Lavender *(Lavandula angustifolia)* has been documented to improve concentration and mental acuity. Researchers at the University of Miami School of Medicine in Florida reported that patients felt less depressed, performing math computations faster and more accurately following inhalation of lavender oil (Diego et al., 1998).

Application:

Diffuse, directly inhale, or add 2-4 drops to bath water. Apply on feet (big toe), chest, nape of the neck, behind ears, wrists, or around navel. Put 4-8 drops on cotton ball and locate on vents.

PanAway

Reduces pain and inflammation, increases circulation, and accelerates healing. Relieves swelling and discomfort from arthritis, sprains, muscle spasms and cramps, bumps, and bruises.

Ingredients:

Helichrysum *(Helichrysum italicum)* is a powerful anaesthetic and analgesic. It quenches pain and inflammation and reduces muscle spasms.

Wintergreen *(Gaultheria procumbens)* is strongly anti-inflammatory and antispasmodic. It is analgesic and reduces pain.

Clove *(Syzygium aromaticum)* is used in the dental industry to numb gum and kill pain. It is one of the most antimicrobial and antiseptic of all essential oils.

Peppermint *(Mentha piperita)* has powerful pain-blocking, anti-inflammatory, and antispasmodic properties. A 1994 double-blind, placebo-controlled, randomized cross-over study at the University of Kiel in Germany found that peppermint oil had a significant analgesic effect (Gobel et al., 1994).

Application:

Dilute 1 part EO to 1 part vegetable oil. Possible skin sensitivity.

Diffuse/humidify, directly inhale, or add 2-4 drops to bath water. Apply on location or on temples, back of neck, forehead. Use as a compress or Raindrop style along spine.

Use Relieve It for deep tissue pain. Add helichrysum to enhance effect of PanAway. For bone pain use Wintergreen. All can be diluted with Ortho Ease Massage Oil.

Peace & Calming

Promotes relaxation and a deep sense of peace and emotional well-being, helping to dampen tensions and uplift spirits. When massaged on the bottom of the feet, it can be a wonderful prelude to a peaceful night's rest. It may calm overactive and hard-to-manage children. Reduces depression, anxiety, stress, and insomnia.

Ingredients:

Blue Tansy *(Tanacetum annuum)* is anti-inflammatory and helps cleanse the liver and lymphatic system. Emotionally, it combats anger and negative emotions.

Patchouli *(Pogostemon cablin)* is strongly grounding and centering. Very high sesquiterpenes that stimulate the limbic center of the brain. It reestablishes mental and emotional equilibrium and energizes the mind.

Tangerine *(Citrus nobilis)* contains esters and aldehydes that are sedating and calming, helping with anxiety and nervousness.

Orange *(Citrus sinensis)* is elevating to the mind and body and brings joy and peace. A 1995 Mie University study documented the ability of citrus fragrances to combat depression and boost immunity.

Ylang Ylang *(Cananga odorata)* increases relaxation; balances male and female energies. It also restores confidence and equilibrium.

Application:
Possible sun/skin sensitivity.

Diffuse, directly inhale, or add 2-4 drops to bath water. Apply to wrists, edge of ears, or foot Vitaflex points. Dilute 1:15 with vegetable oil for body massage. Put 4-8 drops on cotton ball and locate on vents.

Combine with Lavender (for insomnia) and German chamomile (for calming).

Present Time

An empowering fragrance that creates a feeling of being in the moment. Disease develops when we live in the past and with regret. Being in present time is key to progressing and moving forward.

Ingredients:

Neroli *(Citrus aurantium)* was used by the ancient Egyptians for healing the mind, body, and spirit. It is stabilizing and strengthening to the emotions, promoting peace, confidence, and awareness. It brings everything into focus.

Ylang Ylang *(Cananga odorata)* increases relaxation; balances male and female energies. It also restores confidence and equilibrium.

Spruce *(Picea mariana)* opens and releases emotional blocks, fostering a sense of balance and grounding.

Carrier Oil: Almond oil.

Application:
Diffuse, directly inhale, or add 2-4 drops to bath water. Apply to sternum and thymus area, neck and forehead.

Purification

Cleanses and disinfects the air and neutralizes mildew, cigarette smoke, and disagreeable odors. Disinfects and cleanses cuts, scrapes and bites from spiders, bees, hornet, and wasps.

Ingredients:

Citronella *(Cymbopogon nardus)* is antiseptic, antibacterial, antispasmodic, anti-inflammatory, insecticidal, and insect-repelling.

Lemongrass *(Cymbopogon flexuosus)* has strong antifungal properties.

Lavandin *(Lavandula* x *hybrida)* is antifungal, antibacterial, a strong antiseptic, and a tissue regenerator.

Rosemary *(Rosmarinus officinalis* CT cineol*)* is antiseptic and antimicrobial and may be beneficial for skin conditions and dandruff. It helps fight candida and is anti-infectious.

Melaleuca *(Melaleuca alternifolia)* is antibacterial, antifungal, antiparasitic, antiseptic, and anti-inflammatory.

Myrtle *(Myrtus communis)* is antibacterial and may support immune function in fighting colds, flus, and other infectious disease.

Application:
Dilute 1 part EO to 1 part vegetable oil.
Possible skin sensitivity.

Diffuse 15 to 30 minutes every 3 to 4 hours. Directly inhale, or add 2-4 drops to bath water. Apply on location to cuts, sores, bruise, or wound. Put 4-8 drops on cotton ball and locate on vents. Add 2 drops to a wet cloth and put in clothes dryer.

Raven

Treats respiratory disease and infections such as tuberculosis, influenza, and pneumonia. It is highly antiviral and antiseptic.

Ingredients:

Ravensara *(Ravensara aromatica)* is referred to by the people of Madagascar as the oil that heals. It is antiseptic, anti-infectious, antiviral, antibacterial, antifungal, and expectorant. It has been used to treat influenza, sinusitis, bronchitis, and herpes.

Eucalyptus *(Eucalyptus radiata)* may have a profound antiviral effect upon the respiratory system. It may also help reduce inflammation of the nasal mucous membrane.

Peppermint *(Mentha piperita)* is a powerful anti-inflammatory and antiseptic for the respiratory system. It is used to treat bronchitis and pneumonia. High in menthol and menthone, it helps suppress coughs and clears lung and nasal congestion.

Wintergreen *(Gaultheria procumbens)* is strongly anti-inflammatory and antispasmodic. It is analgesic and reduces pain.

Lemon *(Citrus limon)* increases micro-circulation and promotes immunity.

Application:

Dilute 1 part EO to 1 part vegetable oil. Possible sun/skin sensitivity.

Diffuse/humidify, directly inhale, or add 2-4 drops to bath water. Apply to throat and lung area and foot Vita Flex points. Use as hot compress over lungs or with Raindrop Technique. To use in suppository dilute with vegetable oil 1:10 and retain during the night.

R.C.

Gives relief from colds, bronchitis, sore throats, sinusitis, coughs and respiratory congestion. Decongests sinus passages, combats lung infections, and relieve allergy symptoms.

Ingredients:

Eucalyptus globulus has shown to be a powerful antimicrobial and germ-killer. It is expectorant, mucolytic, antibacterial, antifungal, antiviral, and antiseptic. It reduces infections in the throat and lungs, such as rhinopharyngitis, laryngitis, flu, sinusitis, bronchitis, pneumonia.

Eucalyptus radiata is anti-infectious, antibacterial, antiviral, an expectorant, and anti-inflammatory. It has strong action against bronchitis and sinusitis.

Eucalyptus australiana is antiviral, antibacterial, and antifungal.

Eucalyptus citriodora decongests and disinfects the sinuses and lungs. It is anti-inflammatory, anti-infectious, and antispasmodic.

Myrtle *(Myrtus communis)* supports the respiratory system and helps treat chronic coughs and tuberculosis. It is suitable to use for coughs and chest complaints with children.

Pine *(Pinus sylvestris)* opens and disinfects the respiratory system, particularly the bronchial tract. It has been used since the time of Hippocrates to support respiratory function and fight infection. According to Daniel Pénoël, M.D., pine is one of the best oils for bronchitis and pneumonia.

Spruce *(Picea mariana)* helps the respiratory and nervous systems. It is anti-infectious, antiseptic, and anti-inflammatory.

Marjoram *(Origanum majorana)* supports the respiratory system and reduces spasms. It is anti-infectious, antibacterial, and antiseptic.

Lavender *(Lavandula angustifolia)* is antispasmodic, hypotensive, anti-inflammatory, and antiseptic.

Cypress *(Cupressus sempervirens)* promotes blood circulation and lymph flow. It is anti-infectious, antibacterial, antimicrobial, mucolytic, antiseptic, refreshing, and relaxing.

Peppermint *(Mentha piperita)* is a powerful nasal and lung decongestant with antiseptic properties. It opens nasal passages, reduces cough, improves airflow to the lungs, and kills airborne bacteria, fungi and viruses. A 1994 double-blind, placebo-controlled, randomized cross-over study at the University of Kiel in

Germany found that peppermint oil exerted a significant analgesic effect (Gobel et al., 1994). Alan Hirsch, M.D., documented peppermint's ability to curb appetite when inhaled.

Application:
Dilute 1 part EO to 1 part vegetable oil. Possible skin sensitivity.

Diffuse/humidify, directly inhale, apply on chest, neck, throat, or over sinus area. Use as a hot compress or with Raindrop Technique. Dilute 1:15 with vegetable oil for body massage. Put 4-8 drops on cotton ball and locate on vents.

TO COMBAT SINUS/LUNG CONGESTION: Add R.C., Raven or Wintergreen to bowl of hot, steaming water. Place a towel over your head and water/oil mixture and inhale the steam. Combine with Raven (alternating morning and night) and Thieves to enhance effects.

Release

Helps release anger and memory trauma from the liver in order to create emotional well-being. Letting go of negative emotions and frustration enables one to progress in a positive way.

Ingredients:

Ylang Ylang *(Cananga odorata)* increases relaxation; balances male and female energies. It also restores confidence and equilibrium.

Lavandin *(Lavandula* x *hybrida)* is antifungal, antibacterial, a strong antiseptic, and a tissue regenerator.

Geranium *(Pelargonium graveolens)* stimulates nerves and assists in balancing hormones. Its aromatic influence helps release negative memories, thereby opening and elevating the mind.

Sandalwood *(Santalum album)* is high in sesquiterpene compounds which stimulate the pineal gland and the limbic region of the brain, the center of emotions and memory. Used traditionally in yoga and meditation.

Blue Tansy *(Tanacetum annuum)* is anti-inflammatory and helps cleanse the liver and lymphatic system. Emotionally, it combats anger and negative emotions and promotes a feeling of self-control.

Carrier Oil: Olive oil.

Application:
Diffuse, directly inhale, or add 2-4 drops to bath water. Apply over liver or as a compress. Massage on bottom of feet and behind ears. Dilute 1:15 with vegetable oil for body massage. Put 4-8 drops on cotton ball and locate on vents.

Relieve It

High in anti-inflammatory compounds that relieve deep tissue pain and muscle soreness.

Ingredients:

Spruce *(Picea mariana)* is anti-infectious, antiseptic, and anti-inflammatory.

Pepper, Black *(Piper nigrum)* is anti-inflammatory and combats deep tissue pain. It has been traditionally used to treat arthritis.

Peppermint *(Mentha piperita)* has powerful pain-blocking, anti-inflammatory, and antispasmodic properties. A 1994 double-blind, placebo-controlled, randomized cross-over study at the University of Kiel in Germany found that peppermint oil had a significant analgesic effect (Gobel et al., 1994).

Hyssop *(Hyssopus officinalis)* is anti-inflammatory and anti-infectious.

Application:
Dilute 1 part EO to 1 part vegetable oil. Possible skin sensitivity.

Apply on location to relieve pain. Use as cold or hot compress.

Sacred Mountain

Instills strength, empowerment, grounding, and protection with the sacred feeling of the mountains.

Ingredients:

Spruce *(Picea mariana)* opens and releases emotional blocks, fostering a sense of balance and grounding. Traditionally, it was believed to possess the frequency of prosperity.

Idaho Balsam Fir *(Abies balsamea)* has been researched for its ability to kill airborne germs and bacteria. As a conifer oil, it creates a feeling of grounding, anchoring, and empowerment.

Cedarwood *(Cedrus atlantica)* is high in sesquiterpenes, which stimulate the limbic part of the brain, the center of emotions and memory. It stimulates the pineal gland, which releases melatonin, thereby improving thoughts, cognition, and memory.

Ylang Ylang *(Cananga odorata)* increases relaxation; balances male and female energies. It also restores confidence and equilibrium.

Application:

Dilute 1 part EO to 1 part vegetable oil. Possible skin sensitivity.

Diffuse, directly inhale, or add 2-4 drops to bath water. Apply to crown of head, back of neck, behind ears, on thymus and wrists. Dilute 1:15 with vegetable oil for body massage. Put 4-8 drops on cotton ball and locate on vents. Add 2 drops to a wet cloth and put in clothes dryer.

SARA

Enables one to relax into a mental state to facilitate the release of the trauma of Sexual And/or Ritual Abuse. SARA also helps unlock other traumatic experiences such as physical and emotional abuse.

Ingredients:

Geranium *(Pelargonium graveolens)* helps release negative memories, thereby opening and elevating the mind.

Lavender *(Lavandula angustifolia)* is relaxant and grounding. University of Miami researchers found that inhalation of lavender oil increased beta waves in the brain, suggesting heightened relaxation. It also reduced depression and improved cognitive performance (Diego et al., 1998). A 2001 Osaka Kyoiku University study found that lavender reduced mental stress and increased alertness (Motomura et al., 2001). High in aldehydes and esters, it helps overcome insomnia, stress, and nervous tension.

Rose *(Rosa damascena)* possesses the highest frequency of all essential oils, creating balance, harmony, and well-being as it elevates the mind.

Blue Tansy *(Tanacetum annuum)* helps cleanse the liver and calm the lymphatic system, helping one to overcome anger and negative emotions, promoting a feeling of self-control. Its primary constituents are limonene and sesquiterpenes.

Orange *(Citrus sinensis)* is elevating to the mind and body and brings joy and peace. A 1995 Mie University study documented the ability of citrus fragrances to combat depression and boost immunity.

Cedarwood *(Cedrus atlantica)* is high in sesquiterpenes, which stimulate the limbic part of the brain, the center of emotions and memory. It stimulates the pineal gland, which releases melatonin, thereby improving thoughts, cognition, and memory.

Ylang Ylang *(Cananga odorata)* increases relaxation; balances male and female energies. It also restores confidence and equilibrium.

White Lotus *(Nymphaea lotus)* has been found to have anticancerous and strong immune supporting properties.

Carrier Oil: Almond oil.

Application:

Possible sun sensitivity.

Apply over energy centers and areas of abuse, on navel, lower abdomen, temples, nose, and foot Vitaflex points.

Sensation

Profoundly romantic, refreshing, and arousing. It amplifies excitement of experiencing new heights of self-expression and awareness.

Sensation is also nourishing and hydrating for the skin and is beneficial for many skin problems.

Ingredients:

Ylang Ylang *(Cananga odorata)* increases relaxation; balances male and female energies. It also restores confidence and equilibrium.

Rosewood *(Aniba rosaeodora)* is antiseptic, antifungal, and nourishing to the skin. It enhances skin elasticity.

Jasmine *(Jasminum officinale)* is beneficial for dry, oily, irritated, or sensitive skin. Combats muscle spasms, frigidity, depression.

Application:

Possible skin sensitivity.

Diffuse or add 2-4 drops to bath water. Apply on location, neck or wrists. Uses as a compress over abdomen. Dilute 1:15 with vegetable oil for body massage. Put 4-8 drops on cotton ball and locate on vents. Add 2 drops to a wet cloth and put in clothes dryer.

SclarEssence

Balances hormones naturally using essential oil phytoestrogens. Has been shown to increase estrogen levels. Combines the soothing effects of peppermint with the balancing power of fennel and clary sage and the calming action of sage lavender for an extraordinary dietary supplement.

Ingredients:

Clary Sage *(Salvia sclaria)* balances the hormones. It contains natural sclareol, a phytoestrogen that mimics estrogen function. It helps with menstrual cramps, PMS, and circulatory problems.

Peppermint *(Mentha piperita)* strengthens the liver and glandular function.

Sage Lavender *(Salvia avandulifolia)* is high in limonene which prevents DNA damage.

Fennel *(Foeniculum vulgare)* is antiseptic and stimulating to the gastrointenstinal system. It is antispasmodic so it may provide relieve from cramps.

Application:

Put 1-10 drops in a 00 capsule mixed with a pure vegetable oil (V6). Ingest 1 capsule daily as needed. Do not use in conjunction with any other hormone products.

Sensation

Leaves skin silky, youthful, and rejuvenated.

Vegetable Oils:

Fractionated Coconut Oil is distilled from pure coconut oil. It is colorless, odorless, never goes rancid, and is easily washed out from fabrics.

Grape Seed Oil is light-textured, odorless, and nourishing to the skin.

Almond Oil is high in vitamin E and phytonutrients. Highly nourishing to the skin, it protects cell membranes from oxidative damage.

Wheatgerm Oil is rich in lecithin, vitamin E, and B vitamins. Protects skin from free radical damage. Moisturizing and noncomedogenic.

Olive Oil is rich in cell-protecting phytonutrients and antioxidants like squalene.

Essential Oils:

Rosewood *(Aniba rosaeodora)*—is soothing and nourishing to the skin. Weber State University has documented its antibacterial action.

Ylang ylang *(Cananga odorata)* is calming and brings about a sense of relaxation.

Jasmine *(Jasminum officinale)* is beneficial for dry, oily, irritated, or sensitive skin. It can also be uplifting and stimulating.

Surrender

Helps one surrender aggression and a controlling attitude. Stress and tension are released quickly when we surrender our own will.

Ingredients:

Lavender *(Lavandula angustifolia)* has sedative and calming properties.

Roman Chamomile *(Chamaemelum nobile)* combats restlessness, tension, insomnia. It purges toxins from liver where anger is stored.

German Chamomile *(Matricaria recutita)* has an electrical frequency that promotes peace and harmony creating a feeling of security.

Angelica *(Angelica archangelica)* helps to calm emotions and brings memories back to the point of origin before trauma or anger was experienced, helping us to let go of negative feelings.

Mountain Savory *(Satureja montana)* it is stimulating and energizing.

Lemon *(Citrus limon)* is stimulating and invigorating, promoting a deep sense of well-being. A 1995 Mie University study found that citrus fragrances boosted immunity, induced relaxation, and reduced depression.

Spruce *(Picea mariana)* opens and releases emotional blocks, creating a feeling of balance and grounding. Traditionally, it was believed to possess the frequency of prosperity.

Application:
Possible sun/skin sensitivity.

Diffuse, directly inhale, or add 2-4 drops to bath water. Apply on location, or on forehead, solar plexus, along ear rim, chest and nape of neck. Dilute 1:15 with vegetable oil for body massage. Put 4-8 drops on cotton ball and locate on vents.

Thieves

A blend of highly antiviral, antiseptic, antibacterial, anti-infectious essential oils. Thieves was created from research of a group of 15th-century thieves who rubbed oils on themselves to avoid contracting the plague while they robbed the bodies of the dead and dying. When apprehended, these thieves disclosed the formula of herbs, spices, and oils they used to protect themselves in exchange for more lenient punishment.

Studies conducted at Weber State University (Ogden, UT) during 1997 demonstrating it's killing power against airborne microorganisms. One analysis showed a 90 percent reduction in the number of gram positive *Micrococcus luteus* organisms after diffusing for 12 minutes. After 20 minutes of diffusing, the kill-rate jumped to 99.3 percent. Another study against the gram negative *Pseudomonas aeruginosa* showed a kill rate of 99.96 percent after just 12 minutes of diffusion.

Ingredients:

Clove *(Syzygium aromaticum)* is one of the most antimicrobial and antiseptic of all essential oils. It is antifungal, antiviral, anti-infectious.

Lemon *(Citrus limon)* has antiseptic-like properties and contains compounds that amplify immunity. It promotes circulation, leukocyte formation, and lymphatic function.

Cinnamon Bark *(Cinnamomum verum)* is one of the most powerful antiseptics known. It is strongly antibacterial, antiviral, and antifungal.

Eucalyptus *(Eucalyptus radiata)* is anti-infectious, antibacterial, antiviral, and anti-inflammatory.

Rosemary *(Rosmarinus officinalis* CT cineol) is antiseptic and antimicrobial. It is high in cineol—a key ingredient in antiseptic drugs.

Application:
Dilute 1 part EO to 4 parts vegetable oil.
Possible sun/skin sensitivity.

Diffuse for 15 to 30 minutes every 3 to 4 hours. Apply to bottom of feet, throat, stomach, or abdomen. Dilute 1:15 in vegetable oil and massage over thymus. For headaches put 1 drop on tongue and push against roof of mouth. Dilute 1:15 with vegetable oil for body massage. Put 4-8 drops on cotton ball and locate on vents. Add 2 drops to a wet cloth and put in clothes dryer.

3 Wise Men

Opens the subconscious mind through pineal stimulation to release deep-seated trauma. Engenders a sense of grounding and uplifting through emotional releasing and elevated spiritual consciousness.

Ingredients:

Sandalwood *(Santalum album)* is high in sesquiterpene compounds which stimulate the pineal gland and the limbic region of the brain, the center of emotions and memory. Used traditionally in yoga and meditation.

Juniper *(Juniperus osteosperma* and *J. scopulorum)* elevates spiritual awareness creating feelings of love and peace.

Frankincense *(Boswellia carteri)* is considered a holy anointing oil in the Middle East and has been used in religious ceremonies for thousands of years. It stimulates the limbic part of the brain, which elevates the mind.

Myrrh *(Commiphora myrrha)* is referenced throughout the Bible, constituting a part of a holy anointing formula given to Moses (Exodus 30:22-27). It has one of the highest levels of sesquiterpenes, a class of compounds that stimulate the hypothalamus, pituitary, and amygdala, the control center for emotions and hormone release in the brain.

Spruce *(Picea mariana)* opens and releases emotional blocks, creating a feeling of balance and grounding. Traditionally, it was believed to possess the frequency of prosperity.

Carrier Oil: Almond oil.

Application:

Diffuse, directly inhale, or add 2-4 drops to bath water. Add 2 drops on crown of head, behind ears, over eyebrows, on chest, over thymus, and at back of neck. Dilute 1:15 with vegetable oil for body massage. Put 4-8 drops on cotton ball and locate on vents. Add 2 drops to a wet cloth and put in clothes dryer.

Transformation

Repressed trauma and tragedy from the past may be out of sight, but they are definitely not out of mind. Memories are imprinted in our cells for better or worse. Stored negative emotions need to be replaced with joy, hope and courage. Transformation blend radiates with the purifying oils of lemon and peppermint, along with the revitalizing power of sesquiterpenes from sandalwood and frankincense. Balsam fir anchors new mental programming.

Reaching into the deepest recesses of memory, Transformation empowers and upholds the changes you want to make in your belief system. Positive, uplifting beliefs are foundational for the transformation of behavior.

Ingredients:

Lemon *(Citrus limon)* is an antiseptic oil that is rich in limonene, which has been extensively studied for its ability to combat tumor growth in over 50 clinical studies. It increases microcirculation, which may improve vision.

Peppermint *(Mentha piperita)* Dr. William N. Dember of the University of Cincinnati found that inhaling peppermint oil increased mental accuracy by 28 percent.

Sandalwood *(Santalum album)* is high in sesquiterpenes, which stimulate the pineal gland and the limbic region of the brain, the center of our emotions. Used traditionally in yoga and meditation.

Clary Sage *(Salvia sclarea)* balances the hormones. It contains natural sclareol, a phytoestrogen that mimics estrogen function. It helps with menstrual cramps, PMS, and circulatory problems.

Frankincense *(Boswellia carteri)* stimulates the limbic part of the brain, which elevates the mind, helping to overcome stress and despair. It is used in European medicine to combat depression.

Idaho Balsam Fir *(Abies balsamea)* has been researched for its ability to kill airborne germs and bacteria. As a confer oil, it creates a feeling of grounding, anchoring and empowerment.

Rosemary *(Rosmarinus officinalis* CT cineol) helps overcome mental fatigue, stimulating memory and opens the conscious mind. University of Miami scientists found that inhaling rosemary boosted alertness, eased anxiety and amplified analytic and mental ability.

Cardamom *(Elettaria cardamomum)* is uplifting, refreshing and invigorating. It may be beneficial for clearing confusion. In a study done by Dember, et al., 1995, cardamom was found to enhance performance accuracy.

Application:

Diffuse for most effective use. May also be applied topically on appropriate Vita Flex points.

Trauma Life

Releases buried emotional trauma (ie., accidents, death of loved ones, assault, abuse). It combats stress and uproots traumas that cause insomnia, anger, restlessness, and a weakened immune response.

Ingredients:

Valerian *(Valeriana officinalis)* is calming, relaxing, grounding, and emotionally balancing. Clinically researched for its tranquilizing properties. German health authorities have pronounced valerian to be an effective treatment for restlessness and sleep disturbances resulting from nervous conditions. It helps minimize shock, anxiety, and the stress that accompanies traumatic situations.

Lavender *(Lavandula angustifolia)* is relaxant and helps overcome insomnia and anxiety.

Frankincense *(Boswellia carteri)* elevates the mind and helps overcome stress and despair. It stimulates the limbic region of the brain, the center of emotions. In ancient times, frankincense was known for its anointing and healing powers.

Sandalwood *(Santalum album)* is high in sesquiterpene compounds which stimulate the pineal gland and the limbic region of the brain, the center of emotions and memory. Used traditionally in yoga and meditation.

Rose *(Rosa damascena)* has the highest frequency among essential oils. It creates a sense of balance, harmony, and well-being and elevates the mind. It creates a magnetic energy that attracts love and brings joy to the heart.

Helichrysum *(Helichrysum italicum)* improves circulation and helps release feelings of anger promoting forgiveness.

Spruce *(Picea mariana)* opens and releases emotional blocks, fostering a sense of balance and grounding.

Geranium *(Pelargonium graveolens)* stimulates the nerves and helps release negative memories.

Davana *(Artemisia pallens)* is high in sesquiterpenes which help overcome anxiety.

Citrus hystrix *(Citrus hystrix)* has aldehydes and esters that are calming and sedating.

Application:

Possible sun/skin sensitivity.

Diffuse, directly inhale, or add 2-4 drops to bath water. Apply to bottom of feet, chest, forehead, nape of neck, behind ears, and along spine raindrop-style. Dilute 1:15 with vegetable oil for body massage. Put 4-8 drops on cotton ball and locate on vents. Add 2 drops to a wet cloth and put in clothes dryer.

Valor

Balances energies to instill courage, confidence, and self-esteem. It helps the body self-correct its balance and alignment.

Ingredients:

Rosewood *(Aniba rosaeodora)* is anti-infectious, antibacterial, antifungal, and antispasmodic.

Blue Tansy *(Tanacetum annuum)* helps cleanse the liver and lymphatic system helping one to overcome anger and negative emotions promoting a feeling of self-control.

Frankincense (Boswellia carteri) is considered a holy anointing oil in the Middle East and has been used in religious ceremonies for thousands of years. Stimulates the limbic part of the brain, elevating the mind and helping to overcome stress and despair. It is used in European medicine to combat depression.

Spruce *(Picea mariana)* opens and releases emotional blocks, fostering a sense of balance and grounding. Traditionally, it was believed to possess the frequency of prosperity.

Carrier Oil: Almond oil.

Application:

Diffuse, directly inhale, or add 2-4 drops to bath water. Apply 4 to 6 wrists, chest, and base of neck, bottom of feet, or along spine in raindrop technique. When using a series of oils, apply Valor first and wait 5 to 10 minutes before applying other oils. Dilute 1:15 with vegetable oil for body massage.

White Angelica

Increases the aura around the body to bring a delicate sense of strength and protection, creating a feeling of wholeness in the realm of one's own spirituality. Its frequency neutralizes negative energy and gives a feeling of protection and security.

Ingredients:

Ylang Ylang *(Cananga odorata)* increases relaxation; balances male and female energies. It also restores confidence and equilibrium.

Rose *(Rosa damascena)* has the highest frequency among essential oils. It creates a sense of balance, harmony, and well-being and elevates the mind. It creates a magnetic energy that attracts love and brings joy to the heart.

Melissa *(Melissa officinalis)* brings out gentleness. It is calming and balancing to the emotions, affecting the limbic part of the brain, the emotional center of memories.

Sandalwood *(Santalum album)* is high in sesquiterpene compounds which stimulate the pineal gland and the limbic region of the brain, the center of emotions and memory. Used traditionally in yoga and meditation.

Geranium *(Pelargonium graveolens)* stimulates the nerves and helps release negative memories thereby opening and elevating the mind.

Spruce *(Picea mariana)* opens and releases emotional blocks, fostering a sense of balance and grounding. Traditionally, it was believed to possess the frequency of prosperity.

Myrrh *(Commiphora myrrha)* is referenced throughout the Old and New Testaments, constituting a part of a holy anointing formula given to Moses (Exodus 30:22-27). It has one of the highest levels of sesquiterpenes, a class of compounds that stimulate the hypothalamus, pituitary, and amygdala, the control center for emotions and hormone release in the brain.

Hyssop *(Hyssopus officinalis)* is strongly balancing for emotions.

Bergamot *(Citrus bergamia)* is simultaneously uplifting and calming, with a unique ability to relieve anxiety, stress, and tension.

Rosewood *(Aniba rosaeodora)* is soothing and nourishing to the skin, enhancing elasticity. It is high in linalool, which has a relaxing, empowering effect.

Carrier Oil: Almond oil.

Application:
Diffuse, directly inhale, or add 2-4 drops to bath water. Apply to shoulders, along spine, on crown of head, on wrists, behind ears, base of neck, or foot Vitaflex points. Dilute 1:15 with vegetable oil for body massage. Put 4-8 drops on cotton ball and locate on vents. Add 2 drops to a wet cloth and put in clothes dryer.

9

Massage Oils

Massage and therapeutic touch have long been part of both physical and emotional healing. When essential oils are combined with massage, the benefits are numerous. Massage improves circulation, lymphatic drainage, and aids in the elimination of tissue wastes. The oils bring peace and tranquility as well as keen mental awareness. Massage opens and increases the flow of energy, balancing the entire nervous system and helping to release physical and emotional disharmony. The unrefined carrier vegetable oils are rich in fat-soluble nutrients and essential fatty acids.

Cel-Lite Magic

Cel-Lite Magic enhances circulation and helps to provide nutrients to reduce fat and cellulite.

Vegetable Oils:

Fractionated Coconut Oil is distilled from pure coconut oil. It is colorless, odorless, never goes rancid, and is easily washed out from fabrics.

Grape Seed Oil is light-textured, odorless, and nourishing to the skin.

Olive Oil is rich in cell-protecting phyto-nutrients and antioxidants like squalene.

Wheatgerm Oil is rich in lecithin, vitamin E, and B vitamins. Protects skin from free radical damage. Moisturizing and noncomedogenic.

Almond Oil is high in vitamin E and phytonutrients. Highly nourishing to the skin, it protects cell membranes from oxidative damage.

Essential Oils:

Cedarwood (*Cedrus atlantica*)—historically used for its calming, purifying properties; highly beneficial for skin.

Cypress (*Cupressus sempervirens*) increases circulation.

Juniper (*Juniperus osteosperma* and *J. scopulorum*) detoxifies and cleanses.

Grapefruit (*Citrus paradisi*) is a disinfectant. with unique fat-dissolving properties.

Clary Sage (*Salvia sclarea*) supports cells and hormones. It contains natural phytoestrogens.

Pepper (*Piper nigrum*) is anti-inflammatory and combats soreness and pain in deep muscles.

Directions: Apply on location. Can be used in massage or added to bathwater.

Dragon Time

Dragon Time combines essential oils that have been researched in Europe for their balancing effects on hormones.

Vegetable Oils:

Fractionated Coconut Oil is distilled from pure coconut oil. It is colorless, odorless, never goes rancid, and is easily washed out from fabrics.

Grape Seed Oil is light-textured, odorless, and nourishing to the skin.

Almond Oil is high in vitamin E and phytonutrients. Highly nourishing to the skin, it protects cell membranes from oxidative damage.

Olive Oil is rich in cell-protecting phyto-nutrients and antioxidants like squalene.

Wheatgerm Oil is rich in lecithin, vitamin E, and B vitamins. Protects skin from free radical damage. Moisturizing and noncomedogenic.

Essential Oils:

Clary Sage (*Salvia sclarea*) supports cells and hormones. It contains natural phytoestrogens.

Fennel (*Foeniculum vulgare*) has estrogren-like action; stimulating to circulatory system.

Lavender (*Lavandula angustifolia*)—is highly regarded for the skin. Excellent for burns and for cleansing cuts, bruises, and skin irritations. It is uniquely calming and relaxing.

Jasmine (*Jasminum officinale*) is beneficial for dry, oily, irritated, or sensitive skin. It can also be uplifting and stimulating.

Sage (*Salvia officinalis*) has estrogen-like activity and used for treating many types of skin condition. Strengthens the vital centers.

Ylang Ylang (*Cananga odorata*)—may be extremely effective in calming and bringing about a sense of relaxation.

Ortho Ease

An anti-inflammatory and pain-killing complex of vegetable and essential oils. Ideal for strained, swollen, or torn muscles and ligaments.. Also combats insect bites, dermatitis, and itching.

Vegetable Oils:

Fractionated Coconut Oil is distilled from pure coconut oil. It is colorless, odorless, never goes rancid, and is easily washed out from fabrics.

Wheatgerm Oil is rich in lecithin, vitamin E, and B vitamins. Protects skin from free radical damage. Moisturizing and noncomedogenic.

Grape Seed Oil is light-textured, odorless, and nourishing to the skin.

Almond Oil is high in vitamin E and phytonutrients. Highly nourishing to the skin, it protects cell membranes from oxidative damage.

Olive Oil is rich in cell-protecting phytonutrients and antioxidants like squalene.

Essential Oils:

Wintergreen (*Gaultheria procumbens*) contains a cortisone-like compound that combats pain from sore bones, muscles, and joints.

Juniper (*Juniperus osteosperma* and *J. scopulorum*) detoxifies and cleanses.

Marjoram (*Origanum majorana*) reduces pain and inflammation in sore muscles; antiseptic.

Red Thyme (*Thymus vulgaris*) is powerfully antiviral, antimicrobial, and antibacterial. It is also rubefacient or warming to the skin.

Vetiver (*Vetiveria zizanioides*) is an anti-inflammatory that soothes joint and muscle pain.

Peppermint (*Mentha piperita*)—cooling and invigorating, it blocks pain and itching. (Gobel et al., 1996). Antifungal and antibacterial.

Eucalyptus (*Eucalyptus ericifolia*)—is antibacterial and antifungal.

Lemongrass (*Cymbopogon flexuosus*)—has powerful antifungal properties that were documented in the journal *Phytotherapy Research*.

Ortho Sport

An anti-inflammatory and pain-killing complex of vegetable and essential oils. Ideal for strained, swollen, or torn muscles and ligaments. It has a higher phenol content than Ortho Ease and produces a greater warming sensation.

Vegetable Oils:

Fractionated Coconut Oil is distilled from pure coconut oil. It is colorless, odorless, never goes rancid, and is easily washed out from fabrics.

Wheatgerm Oil is rich in lecithin, vitamin E, and B vitamins. Protects skin from free radical damage. Moisturizing and noncomedogenic.

Grape Seed Oil is light-textured, odorless, and nourishing to the skin.

Olive Oil is rich in cell-protecting phytonutrients and antioxidants like squalene.

Almond Oil is high in vitamin E and phytonutrients. Highly nourishing to the skin, it protects cell membranes from oxidative damage.

Essential Oils:

Wintergreen (*Gaultheria procumbens*) contains a cortisone-like compound that combats pain from sore bones, muscles, and joints.

Oregano (*Origanum vulgare*) is high in carvacrol, a potent anti-inflammatory.

Marjoram (*Origanum majorana*) reduces pain and inflammation in sore muscles; antiseptic.

Red Thyme (*Thymus vulgaris)* is powerfully antiviral, antimicrobial, and antibacterial. It is also rubefacient or warming to the skin.

Peppermint (*Mentha piperita*)—cooling and invigorating, it blocks pain and itching. (Gobel et al., 1996). Antifungal and antibacterial.

Eucalyptus (*Eucalyptus globulus*)—is a powerful antimicrobial agent, rich in eucalyptol (a key ingredient in many antiseptic mouth rinses). It also repels insects.

Lemongrass (*Cymbopogon flexuosus*) has pain-killing and antifungal actions.

Vetiver (*Vetiveria zizanioides*) is an anti-inflammatory that soothes joint and muscle pain.

Elemi (*Canarium luzonicum*) used in Europe for hundreds of years in salves for skin and celebrated healing ointments. Elemi belongs to the same botanical family as frankincense and myrrh. Antiseptic and antimicrobial, it is widely regarded today for soothing sore muscles, protecting skin, and stimulating nerves.

Protec

Protec is designed to be used in a night-long retention enema or douche to support prostate and vaginal health. Suitable for both men and women. Use 1/2 to 1 ounce added to an enema or douche.

Vegetable Oils:

Olive Oil—a moisturizing agent in many organic cosmetics that will not clog pores.

Grapeseed Oil—makes an excellent carrier for essential oils.

Sweet Almond Oil—this nourishing oil is well suited for massage, aiding in a smooth application while reducing friction.

Wheatgerm Oil—a rich and lush oil high in lecithin, vitamin E, and B vitamins.

Vitamin E—protects skin and cell membranes against oxidative damage.

Essential Oils:

Frankincense (*Boswellia carteri*)—is considered a holy anointing oil in the Middle East and has been used in religious ceremonies for thousands of years. It is stimulating and elevating to the mind and helps overcome stress and despair as well as supporting the immune system.

Myrrh (*Commiphora myrrha*)—is an antimicrobial oil referenced throughout the Old and New Testaments (*A bundle of myrrh is my well-beloved unto me.* Song of Solomon 1:13). Antibacterial, it is widely used in oral hygiene products.

Sage (*Salvia officinalis*)—is used in Europe for numerous types of skin conditions.

Cumin (*Cuminum cyminum*)—studied for its anticancer properties in "The Anticarcinogenic Effects of the Essential Oils from Cumin, Poppy, and Basil" (Aruna et al., 1996), it is rarer and more expensive than the commonly used white cumin. Cumin is antiseptic, calming, and a powerful support to the immune system. Cumin seeds have been retrieved from the tombs of the pharoahs of Egypt.

Relaxation

Promotes relaxation and easing of tension.

Vegetable Oils:

Fractionated Coconut Oil is distilled from pure coconut oil. It is colorless, odorless, never goes rancid, and is easily washed out from fabrics.

Grape Seed Oil is light-textured, odorless, and nourishing to the skin.

Almond Oil is high in vitamin E and phytonutrients. Highly nourishing to the skin, it protects cell membranes from oxidative damage.

Wheatgerm Oil is rich in lecithin, vitamin E, and B vitamins. Protects skin from free radical damage. Moisturizing and noncomedogenic.

Olive Oil is rich in cell-protecting phytonutrients and antioxidants like squalene.

Essential Oils:

Tangerine (*Citrus nobilis*)—is soothing for anxiety and nervousness.

Rosewood (*Aniba rosaeodora*)—is soothing and nourishing to the skin. Weber State University has documented its antibacterial action.

Spearmint (*Mentha spicata*)—oil helps support the respiratory and nervous systems. Its hormone-like activity may help open and release emotional blocks and bring about a feeling of balance.

Peppermint (*Mentha piperita*)—cooling and invigorating, it blocks pain and itching. (Gobel et al., 1996). Antifungal and antibacterial.

Ylang ylang (*Cananga odorata*) is calming and brings about a sense of relaxation.

Lavender (*Lavandula angustifolia*)—is highly regarded for the skin. Excellent for burns and for cleansing cuts, bruises, and skin irritations, it is uniquely calming and relaxing.

V-6 Vegetable Oil Complex

A complex of nourishing, antioxidant vegetable oils that is colorless and odorless. It is the ideal carrier for essential oils.

Vegetable Oils:

Fractionated Coconut Oil is distilled from pure coconut oil. It is colorless, odorless, never goes rancid, and is easily washed out from fabrics.

Olive Oil is rich in cell-protecting phyto-nutrients and antioxidants like squalene.

Sesame Seed Oil—contains powerful phyto-nutrients and is nourishing to the skin.

Almond Oil is high in vitamin E and phytonutrients. Highly nourishing to the skin, it protects cell membranes from oxidative damage.

Sunflower Seed Oil is compatible with the skin's natural oils and sebum.

Wheatgerm Oil is rich in lecithin, vitamin E, and B vitamins. Protects skin from free radical damage. Moisturizing and noncomedogenic.

10

Dietary Supplements with Essential Oils

Many of these supplements contain herbs, nutrients and therapeutic-grade essential oils. These supplements are formulated using a unique process pioneered by D. Gary Young. The essential oils mixed in these supplements act as catalysts to help deliver nutrients through the cell membranes while assisting in the removal of cellular wastes.

It is important to remember that these supplements are usually dissolved and assimilated by the body within a couple of hours. Therefore, spacing them throughout the day will provide better assimilation and nutrient value than consuming a handful all at once.

When using supplements, a general guideline is to discontinue use for at least one or two days a week to allow the body to regain homeostasis and permit its natural recuperative powers to engage.

AD&E

The best source of natural vitamins A (mixed carotenoids), D, and E. These vitamins are essential for immune, cardiovascular, and eye health. To enhance it's effects use in conjunction with Longevity Essential Oil Capsules.

INGREDIENTS:

Beta Carotene (Vitamin A) is converted by the body to Vitamin A.

Vitamin A (Palmitate) is a fat-soluble vitamin that helps support the function of the eyes, liver, immune system. It acts as a superb antioxidant. It is needed for proper growth and development.

Vitamin D3 (Cholecalciferol) stimulates the absorption of calcium, thereby helping to prevent osteoporosis, estrogen and magnesium deficiency, and cancer.

Vitamin E (d-Alpha Tocopheryl Acetate) provides many health benefits including helping to prevent acne, AIDS, cancer, diabetes, cataracts, lupus, macular degeneration, myopathy, and works as a wonderful antioxidant.

In a base of grapeseed oil, and several tocopherols.

Directions: Take 5 drops once daily in 1/2 cup of distilled water.

Companion Products: Super C Chewable, Super B, Super Cal, Longevity Oil Blend.

AlkaLime

This specially designed alkaline mineral powder contains an array of high-alkaline salts and other yeast and fungus fighting elements, such as citric acid and essential oils. Its precisely balanced, acid-neutralizing mineral formulation helps preserve the body's proper pH balance—the cornerstone of health. By boosting blood alkalinity, yeast and fungus are deprived of the acidic terrain they require to flourish. The effectiveness of other essential oils is enhanced when the body's blood and tissues are alkaline.

AlkaLime may help reduce the following signs of acid-based yeast and fungus dominance:

- fatigue/low energy
- unexplained aches and pains
- overweight conditions
- low resistance to illness
- allergies
- headaches
- irritability/mood swings
- indigestion
- colitis/ulcers
- diarrhea/constipation
- urinary tract infections
- rectal/ vaginal itch.

INGREDIENTS:

Calcium carbonate provides calcium, which is needed for healthy bones.

Citric acid is added to help cleanse the digestive system.

Magnesium supports healthy intestinal flora, the first-line defense against fungus overgrowth.

Potassium bicarbonate added for electrolyte balance.

Sea salts have trace minerals that regulate pH.

Sodium bicarbonate used for electrolyte and pH balance.

ESSENTIAL OILS:

Lemon (*Citrus limon*) prevents cellular mutation and enhances DNA repair (Reddy et al., 1998).

Lime (*Citrus aurantiifolia*) decongests the lymphatic system.

Companion Products: Essentialzyme, Mineral Essence, Mint Condition, VitaGreen, Di-Tone, peppermint, Purification, spearmint, Thieves.

Directions: Stir one rounded teaspoon into six to eight oz. of distilled or purified water and drink immediately. To aid in alkalizing connective tissue, AlkaLime may be taken 1-3 times per day before meals or before eating. As an antacid, AlkaLime may be taken as needed. Otherwise, an ideal time to take AlkaLime would be prior to bedtime.

AminoTech

AminoTech is the ultimate energizing antioxidant nutrient complex for promoting strength, health and prime physical conditioning.

INGREDIENTS:

Creatine monohydrate is one of the best-documented muscle-builders and energy-enhancers.

L-Glutamine a key amino acid for supporting muscle growth.

L-Arginine is an amino acid that promotes circulation in the small capillaries of our tissues, allowing greater nutrient absorption and cellular metabolism.

L-Taurine occurs in large quantities in striated muscles. Taurine levels decline with increased physicial activity and need to be replenished.

MSM supports healthy hair, skin, liver, and immune function.

Magnesium is crucial for proper enzyme function, muscle contractions and heart rhythm. It reduces blood pressure, prevents arteriosclerosis, and improves insulin action.

Alpha lipoic acid is one of the most powerful known antioxidants. It is the only antioxidant that is both oil and water soluble. It has been used to treat dabetes, heart, and liver disease.

RNA (ribonucleic acid) is vital for energy production in the cells.

Zinc citrate is a trace mineral essential for normal immune function and good health. It is involved in numerous enzyme functions.

Chromium polynicotinate acts as a "spark plug" for supporting metabolism and carbohydrate burning. This essential mineral has been studied for its ability to increase lean body mass and decrease body fat.

L-Selenomethionine is a source of selenium, a powerful antioxidant mineral vital for the creation of superoxide dismutase. Studies at the University of Arizona have examined its ability to reduce the risk of cancer.

Fructooligosaccharides (FOS) are one of the best-documented natural nutrients for promoting the growth of the *lactobacilli* and bifidobacteri that are the linchpin of sound health. FOS has also been clinically studied for its ability to increase magnesium and calcium absorption, lower blood glucose, cholesterol, and LDL levels, and to inhibit production of the reductase enzymes that can contribute to cancer. Because FOS may increase magnesium absorption, it may also lead to lowered blood pressure and better cardiovascular health.

Wolfberry powder contains over 15 percent protein by weight. It is rich in immune-stimulating polysaccharides and is one of the highest antioxidant foods known.

ESSENTIAL OILS:

Lemon (*Citrus limon*) prevents cellular mutation and enhances DNA repair (Reddy et al., 1998).

Lime (*Citrus aurantiifolia*) decongests the lymphatic system.

Directions: Take 1 to 2 heaping scoops daily. Mix 1 serving (2 scoops) with water. For added flavor mix with rice, goat, or almond milk.

Companion Products: WheyFit, Power Meal, Be-FIt, Wolfberry Crisp.

Arthro Tune

An herbal complex that may help arthritis and rheumatoid conditions.

INGREDIENTS:

Alfalfa powder supports muscles and joints.

Butcher's broom has anti-inflammatory action.

Capsicum annuum is a powerful agent for improving blood circulation and blocking pain receptors.

Yucca improves blood circulation.

Uncaria tomentosa, known as Cat's Claw, is used as an immune system stimulant and possesses anti-inflammatory properties.

Magnesium relaxes muscles.

Alpha glutaric acid promotes joint repair.

ESSENTIAL OILS:

Basil (*Ocimum basilicum*) relaxes both striated and smooth muscles.

Wintergreen (*Gaultheria procumbens*) helps reduce bone, joint, and muscle pain.

Cypress (*Cupressus sempervirens*) can improve circulation.

Fir (*Abies alba*) is high in terpenes to soothe and tone the muscles.

Helichrysum (*Helichrysum italicum*) has been studied by European researchers for regenerating tissue and improving circulation.

Juniper (*Juniperus osteosperma* and *J. scopulorum*) has been used to stimulate nerve function.

Marjoram (*Origanum majorana*) is used extensively for soothing the muscles.

Pepper (*Piper nigrum*) has been used for soothing deep tissue muscle pain.

Spruce (*Picea mariana*) helps the respiratory and nervous systems.

Companion Products: BLM, Essentialzyme, Sulfurzyme (capsules or powder), Super Cal, Ortho Ease massage oil, Ortho Sport massage oil, PanAway, Relieve It

Directions: Take one capsule, twice daily. Best taken before meals. If you have sensitive digestion, take with meals.

Be-Fit

A high-powered formula for enhancing strength and endurance and promoting muscle formation.

INGREDIENTS:

Wolfberry powder contains over 15 percent protein by weight. It is rich in amino acids for supporting muscle integrity.

HMB (Betahydroxy beta-methylbutyrate) the best documented nutrient for increasing muscle mass.

Eleuthero root (formerly referred to as Siberian ginseng) strengthens the adrenal glands, enhances immune function, normalizes blood pressure, improves mental alertness, and promotes hormonal balance.

Ginkgo biloba extract improves energy, memory, and mood, due to its ability to enhance cerebral and peripheral circulation.

L-arginine is an amino acid that promotes circulation in the small capillaries of our tissues, allowing greater nutrient absorption and cellular metabolism.

L-lysine works to enhance the benefits of the amino acid L-leucine found in wolfberry powder.

Creatine monohydrate is a naturally occurring compound of three amino acids, providing high-energy fuel for muscles. It helps increase muscle mass as well as muscle contraction for improved intensity and endurance.

Cayenne dialates blood vessels to improve circulation, stamina, and energy.

ESSENTIAL OILS:

Wintergreen (*Gaultheria procumbens*) has a cortisone-like action for pain relief due to its high concentration of methyl salicylate.

Lemongrass (*Cymbopogon flexuosus*) is used for ligament support.

Nutmeg (*Myristica fragrans*) is used for its adrenal cortex-like activity, which helps support the adrenal glands for increased energy.

Rosemary (*Rosmarinus officinalis*) helps overcome mental fatigue.

Directions: Take 2 capsules in the morning and 2 capsules at night.

Companion Products: Master Formula HIS/HERS, Royal Essence, Power Meal, Ultra Young, Wolfberry Crisp

Berry Young Juice

This is the highest antioxidant liquid dietary supplement from whole food sources. Rich in ellagic acid, polyphenols, flavonoids, vitamins, and minerals.

INGREDIENTS:

Ningxia wolfberry (*Lycium barbarum*) juice is one of the highest known antioxidant nutrients. It is rich in polysaccharides that have been studied for their ability to combat cancer and strengthen the immune system. It is rich in polyphenols, carotenoids, magnesium, potassium, and vitamin C.

Blueberry Juice (from concentrate) is one of the highest antioxidant foods according to ORAC research developed by USDA researchers at Tufts University.. Animal studies at Tufts University have shown that blueberry extracts can reverse many of the signs of aging.

Raspberry Juice (from concentrate) is rich in ellagic acid, a vital anti-aging nutrient which provides powerful protection against cell mutation.

Pomegranate Juice (from concentrate) is an extremely high antioxidant nutrient that has been show to prevent heart disease in clincial studies.[1,2,3]

Apricot Juice (from concentrate) contains high concentrations of carotinoids, a class of high-powered antioxidants that includes beta carotene (provitamin A). Apricots are also rich in rutin, which strengthens blood vessels.

Organic Blue Agave Nectar is an extremely low-glycemic nutrient from the desert cactus *Agave tequilana*.

1. "Pomegranate juice consumption inhibits serum angiotensin converting enzyme and reduces systolic blood pressure" Pomegranate 2000 Israel Aviram, Dornfeld Atherosclerosis

2. "Pomegranate juice consumption reduces oxidative stress, atherogenic modifications to LDL, and platelet aggregation: Studies in humans and in atherosclerotic apolipoprotein E-deficient mice 1,2 Pomegranate, Free Radical, Heart Disease 1999 Israel Aviram, Dornfeld, Rosenblat, Volkova, Kaplan, Coleman, Hayek, Presser, Fuhrman *American Journal of Clinical Nutrition*

3. "Pomegranate juice supplementation to atherosclerotic mice reduces macrophage lipid peroxidation, cellular cholesterol accumulation and development of artherosclerosis" Pomegranate, 2001 Israel, Kaplan, Hayek, Raz, Coleman, Dornfeld, Vaya, Aviram, *Journal of Nutrition*

ESSENTIAL OILS:

Orange (*Citrus sinensis*) is very high in limonene, a supernutrient that has been studied extensively for its ability to prevent cellular mutations and reverse cancer. Over 50 peer-reviewed research papers have investigated limonene against a variety of cancers, including breast, lung, and colon.

Directions: Drink at least one ounce once a day. To maximize benefits, drink at least one hour before meals.

Companion Products: Wolfberry Crisp, Essential Omegas, Ultra Young, Essential Manna, Longevity.

Blue Agave Nectar, Organic

The ultimate low-glycemic sweetener, Blue Agave nectar is harvested from organic *Agave tequilana* plants. The hearts (heads) of the agaves are chopped, ground, and pressed for their juices. The result is a viscous, honey-like fluid that has a color and shelf stability similar to honey.

- A sugar alternative with a low glycemic index of 39 (it has minimal impact on blood sugar levels). This makes it a sweetener of choice for diabetics, hypoglycemics, or others who cannot tolerate sucrose or choose not use artificial sweeteners.

- Blue Agave is about 50 percent sweeter and has fewer calories per teaspoon than sucrose (table sugar).

- Records show that the ancient Meso-Americans used this plant as food as well as externally and internally for injuries and illnesses. Known as the Mexican Tree of Life and Abundance.

Directions: In recipes, substitute an amount of blue agave nectar equal to 3/4 of the amount of sugar called for in the recipe. You may also need to reduce the amount of liquid, just as you would for honey.

Companion Products: Stevia.

BLM (Bones, Ligaments and Muscles) Capsules

A high-powered arthritis treatment that includes essential oils and a special collagen complex for building bones, ligaments and muscles. The exclusive collagen and hyaluronic acid blend strengthens and rebuilds damaged joints and cartilage as it combats arthritis inflammation and pain.

INGREDIENTS:

Glucosamine Sulfate is a proteoglycan with over 30 years of double-blind placebo-controlled studies on its ability torebuild damaged cartilage and reduce arthritis symptoms. Derived from shellfish.

Collagen type II is the raw material from which joints are built. It contains the most proteoglycans of any cartilage source. Contains cartilage matrix glycoprotein which reduces oxidateive damage to joints. It also reduces inflammation by acting on lymphoid tissue in the digestive system. Derived from avian cartilage.

Rice flour

MSM—Methysulfonylmethane is an exceptionally bioavailable source of sulfur that restores flexibility to cell membranes and slows the breakdown of cartilage.

Manganese Citrate is a crucial cofactor in collagen creation.

ESSENTIAL OILS:

Idaho Balsam Fir (*Abies balsamea*) is a powerful inflammatory essential oil which reduces swelling and pain in joints

Wintergreen (*Gaultheria procumbens*) contains methyl salicylate, which has been used for decades for its anti-inflammatory and pain-relieving properties. Listed in the United States Pharmacopeia for combating muscle and joint pain.

Clove (*Syzygium aromaticum*) has been shown to have anti-inflammatory and antioxidant effects.

Directions: Take 1 capsule three times a day if you weigh less than 120 lbs, one hour after meals and/or before retiring.

Take 1 capsule four times a day if you weigh between 120 and 200 lbs, one hour after meals and/or before retiring.

Take 1 capsule five times a day if you weigh over 200 lbs.

Companion Products: BLM Powder, SuperCal, MegaCal, Sulfurzyme, Essential Omegas, Nutmeg, Clove, Idaho Balsam Fir, Wintergreen, Peppermint, PanAway, Aroma Siez

BLM (Bones, Ligaments and Muscles) Powder

Same powerful arthritis formula as found in BLM capsules with the addition of bacteria-fighting Xylitol as a bone strengthener.

INGREDIENTS:

Glucosamine Sulfate is a proteoglycan with over 30 years of double-blind placebo-controlled studies on its ability torebuild damaged cartilage and reduce arthritis symptoms. Derived from shellfish.

Collagen type II is the raw material from which joints are built. It contains the most proteoglycans of any cartilage source. Contains cartilage matrix glycoprotein which reduces oxidateive damage to joints. It also reduces inflammation by acting on lymphoid tissue in the digestive system. Derived from avian cartilage.

Xylitol a non-caloric, anti-bacterial sweetener

Rice bran

MSM—Methysulfonylmethane is an exceptionally bioavailable source of sulfur that restores flexibility to cell membranes and slows the breakdown of cartilage.

Manganese Citrate is a crucial cofactor in collagen creation.

ESSENTIAL OILS:

Clove (*Syzygium aromaticum*) has been shown to have anti-inflammatory and antioxidant effects.

Peppermint (*Mentha piperita*) known for its ability to relieve pain and inflammation

Idaho Balsam Fir (*Abies balsamea*) is a powerful inflammatory essential oil which reduces swelling and pain in joints

Wintergreen (*Gaultheria procumbens*) contains methyl salicylate, which has been used for decades for its anti-inflammatory and pain-relieving properties. Listed in the United States Pharmacopeia for combating muscle and joint pain.

Directions: Take 1 tablespoon daily with 8 oz. of water or juice, one hour after meals or medications and/or before retiring.

Companion Products: BLM Capsules, SuperCal, MegaCal, Sulfurzyme, Essential Omegas, Nutmeg, Clove, Idaho Balsam Fir, Wintergreen, Peppermint, PanAway, Aroma Siez

BodyGize

BodyGize is a milk and soy protein supplement fortified with vitamins, minerals, and essential oils. It helps balance the body at its ideal weight and promotes muscle formation. It contains soy solids that have been studied for their effects against breast and ovarian cancer.

INGREDIENTS:

Non-fat dry milk supplies organic calcium and high quality protein.

Ultrafiltered Microfiltered Whey is the best source of high quality protein, with the highest Protein Efficiency Ratio and Protein Digestability Corrected Amino Acid Score. It is rich in alpha-lactalbumin, beat lactoglobulin, immunoglobulins, lactoferrin, lactoperoxidase, calcium and magniesium. Ultrafiltered whey is far superior to the denatured protein found in ion exchange whey which is very high in sodium and low in calcium, potassium, and magnesium. Ion exchange whey is also devoid of glycomicropeptides, lactoperoxidase, and lactoferrin.

Fructose is a low-glycemic sweetener having minimal impact on blood sugar levels.

Potassium citrate prevents heart disease, strokes, and high blood pressure.

Vanilla Bean Extract from Madagascar vanilla beans.

Lecithin is a key phospholipid essential for cell membrane integrity and healthy liver function

Xanthan/Guar gum is a natural stabilizer.

Sodium chloride for electrolyte balance.

Magnesium is crucial for proper enzyme function, muscle contractions, and heart rhythm. It reduces blood pressure, prevents arteriosclerosis, and improves insulin action.

Vitamin C (ascorbic acid) helps the body manufacture collagen for connective tissue, cartilage, tendons, etc., and is used for proper immune function. It is also an antioxidant.

Vitamin E protects against cardiovascular disease and is beneficial for acne, allergies, and wound healing.

Vitamin A is an important antioxidant.

Calcium pantothenate is needed for the prevention of depression and tinnitus.

Niacinamide (vitamin B3) is essential for the production of energy, regulates blood sugar, and reduces cholesterol.

Zinc is crucial for proper immune function and is needed for proper action of many hormones, including insulin and growth hormone. It helps improve wound healing.

Copper is necessary for proper red blood cell formation and immune function.

Vitamin D helps with the absorption of calcium and has many anticancer properties.

Vitamin B6 supports immune function and protects the heart and blood vessels. It inhibits skin cancer growth and helps prevent kidney stones and PMS symptoms. Vitamin B6 requires folic acid and magnesium to maximize its effects.

Riboflavin (Vitamin B2) is crucial in the production of cellular energy, helps regenerate the liver, and prevents cellular mutations.

Thiamin (Vitamin B1) is essential for energy production, carbohydrate metabolism, and nerve cell function.

Vitamin B12 is critical for red blood cell formation and proper immune and nerve function. Works with vitamin B6 to prevent heart disease. Vegetarians often lack adequate B12.

Folic acid plays an important role in cardiovascular health.

Biotin helps convert fats and amino acids into energy. It promotes healthy nails and hair and combats yeast and fungus overgrowth.

ESSENTIAL OILS:

Lime (*Citrus aurantiifolia*) prevents cellular mutation and enhances DNA repair.

Tangerine (*Citrus nobilis*) is an anticoagulant that increases blood flow and circulation.

Orange (*Citrus sinensis*) prevents cellular mutation and enhances DNA repair (Reddy et al., 1998).

Lemon (*Citrus limon*) prevents cellular mutation and enhances DNA repair.

Cypress (*Cupressus sempervirens*) improves circulation and blood flow.

Grapefruit (*Citrus paradisi*) prevents DNA and cellular mutation.

Mandarin (*Citrus reticulata*) is antifungal, antispasmotic, and promotes digestion.

Directions: Add one measuring scoop to eight to ten oz. purified water, juice, or low-fat milk. Blend in blender for 30 seconds. Ice cubes may be added to thicken like a shake. BodyGize works with all juices. It is a predigested protein and may be taken anytime. For optimum results, take with Master Formula HIS or HERS and Thyromin.

Companion Products: Be-Fit, Power Meal, Wolfberry Crisp, Thyromin, Nutmeg, Longevity.

Tips for Getting the Most from BodyGize

1. **For fast weight reduction:** Enjoy BodyGize as an alternative for breakfast and dinner. Eat a sensible, low-fat, well-balanced lunch, which should include vegetables, fruits, and whole grains. As with any weight balancing program, fats, sugars, and high-caloric foods should be omitted from your diet. Raw organic vegetables and fruits are excellent snacks.

2. **For weight gain:** Enjoy BodyGize mixed with whole milk or apple juice. Add a banana or a pear and drink after each meal.

3. **For good health and weight maintenance:** After you have achieved your ideal weight, enjoy a BodyGize shake as a meal alternative daily, possibly for breakfast. BodyGize may also be used as a filling and nutritious snack. Drink plenty of distilled or purified water.

Note: Anyone who is pregnant or nursing, has health problems, or wants to lose more than 50 pounds or more than 20 percent of his/her body weight, should consult a physician before starting this or any other weight management program.

Carbozyme

Designed to relieve bloating, cramping, intestinal distress, and combat Candida and yeast overgrowth, Carbozyme is an advanced starch and sugar digesting vegetarian enzyme complex that contains pure amylase and therapeutic-grade essential oils. Clinical studies in 2002 using two capsules twice a day of Carbozyme eliminated the need for insulin in diabetic patients.

INGREDIENTS:

Amylase (alpha) is a powerful starch digesting enzyme prevents starch fermentation in the digestive system.

Bee pollen is rich in natural enzymes and coenzymes.

ESSENTIAL OILS:

Thieves is a powerful antiseptic and antifungal blend of therapeutic grade essential oils

Directions: Take 1 capsule three times daily or as needed just before meals containing carbohydrates.

Companion Products: Polyzyme, Lipozyme, Detoxzyme, Thieves

CardiaCare

Strengthens and supports the heart and cardio-vascular system.

INGREDIENTS:

Rhododendron caucasicum contains phenyl-propanoids that have been shown in clinical studies to increase the efficiency of the cardiovascular system.

Wolfberry powder contains the amino acids that are vital to supporting cardiovascular function.

Magnesium is crucial for proper enzyme function, muscle contractions and heart rhythm. It reduces blood pressure, prevents arteriosclerosis, and improves insulin action.

Hawthorn berry has been used for decades in European cardiac medicine. Active constituents in the berries dilate coronary blood vessels, thereby increasing blood circulation in the heart.

Coenzyme Q10 (CoQ10) is used by every cell in the body to convert food to energy. Heart cells require more CoQ10 than any other cell.

Vitamin E prevents oxidative damage to low-density lipoproteins (LDLs), a primary cause of clogged coronary arteries and heart disease.

ESSENTIAL OILS:

Helichrysum (*Helichrysum italicum*) helps regulate cholesterol, stimulates liver function, helps reduce blood stickiness.

Lemon (*Citrus limon*) decreases platelet stickiness and improves blood.

Marjoram (*Origanum majorana*) provides support for smooth muscles of the heart, relieves spasms, and may work as a diuretic.

Ylang Ylang (*Cananga odorata*) has been used traditionally to support heart functions.

Directions: Take three capsules two times daily.

Companion Products: AD&E, Longevity Capsules, HRT, Essential Omegas, Mineral Essence, Aroma Life.

Chelex

Chelex contains herbs that have been traditionally used to chelate and neutralize heavy metals and and disarm free radicals. Take 1 to three droppers three times a day.

INGREDIENTS:

Extracts:

Astragalus—used as a diuretic, a vasodilator, and respiratory infection treatment, this herb reputedly has immune-stimulating effects and increases energy.

Garlic—demonstrated by Louis Pasteur to have antibacterial properties in 1858. Albert Schweitzer used garlic to treat amoebic dysentery. Later, researchers found that garlic can protect against heart disease and cancer. Garlic juice halts the growth of more than 60 types of fungi and 20 types of bacteria.

Sarsaparilla—contains saponins, steroid-like molecules that neutralize endotoxins (poisons secreted by fungi and bacteria in the human body) that contribute to many kinds of disease.

Eleuthero root (formerly referred to as Siberian ginseng) strengthens the adrenal glands, enhances immune function, normalizes blood pressure, improves mental alertness, and promotes hormonal balance.

Red Clover—used to treat asthma, bronchitis, skin ailments, ulcers, and arthritis. Used in some cultures to prevent recurrence of cancer.

Royal jelly is the substance fed to queen bees that allows them to live thirty to forty times longer than worker bees. It is very rich in amino acids, minerals, and vitamins B5 and B6. It stimulates the adrenal glands to increase energy.

ESSENTIAL OILS:

Rosemary (*Rosmarinus officinalis*) is antiparasitic and balances the endocrine system.

Roman chamomile (*Chamaemelum nobile*) promotes bile flow and liver function.

Eucalyptus (*Eucalyptus globulus*) is a powerful antimicrobial agent, rich in eucalyptol (a key ingredient in many antiseptic mouth rinses).

Helichrysum (*Helichrysum italicum*) has been studied by European researchers for regenerating tissue and improving circulation. This oil has also been studied for its natural chelating action.

Directions: Take 3 ml three times daily or as needed.

Companion Products: JuvaCleanse, JuvaFlex, Detoxzyme, Essentialzyme, Polyzyme.

ComforTone

An herbal laxative complex of bentonite, apple pectin, and herbal extracts that may relieve constipation, enhance colon function, and dispel parasites and toxins.

ComforTone can help eliminate parasites from the body, break up encrustations along the colon wall, and relax intestinal spasms. If you experience nausea when using ComforTone, use Di-Tone or peppermint (diluted if necessary); if you experience constipation, increase your water intake and avoid using ICP. If you have a history of chronic constipation, do not start ICP and ComforTone at the same time. First use ComforTone until the system is open, and then follow with ICP. Drink ten glasses of water per day.

INGREDIENTS:

Licorice root cleanses the blood and supports the liver, the most important organ for cleansing.

Psyllium seed is a soft fiber that helps relieve abdominal pain, constipation, diarrhea, and protects against flatulence and nausea.

Apple pectin helps with enzyme production and supports proper digestive function.

Bentonite is an intestinal cleansing agent.

Fennel is antiparasitic, antimicrobial, antispasmotic, is a digestive aid, helps regulate intestinal flora, and increases gastric secretions.

Garlic is antifungal, antiparasitic, antiviral, an immune stimulant, works as a digestive aid, and is a catalyst for the oils.

German chamomile is antimicrobial, anti-inflammatory, limits the parasympathetic nervous system in its production of mucus, and relaxes spasms in the colon wall.

Echinacea is antimicrobial, antiparasitic, lowers bowel transit time, absorbs toxins in the colon, and stimulates the immune system.

Ginger root is anti-inflammatory, antispasmodic, helps lower cholesterol, and cleanses the colon.

Cascara sagrada works as an herbal laxative and as a liver cleanser.

Burdock root lowers bowel transit time, balances intestinal flora, and absorbs toxins from the bowels.

Diatomaceous earth is one of the best intestinal cleansers.

Cayenne pepper *(capsicum annuum)* is stimulating to circulation.

ESSENTIAL OILS:

Rosemary (*Rosmarinus officinalis*) is antiparasitic and balances the endocrine system.

German chamomile *(Matricaria recutita)* helps prevent acne, rashes, and eczema.

Tarragon (*Artemisia dracunculus*) has been used to reduce intestinal spasms, sluggish digestion, and fermentation.

Peppermint (*Mentha piperita*) reduces candida, nausea, and vomiting.

Ginger (*Zingiber officinale*) combats indigestion, diarrhea, loss of appetite, and congestion.

Anise (*Pimpinella anisum*) helps prevent flatulence, colon spasms, and indigestion.

Mugwort (*Artemisia vulgaris*) has been used traditionally to calm nerves.

Tangerine (*Citrus nobilis*) is cleansing and purifying to the digestive system.

Directions: Start with 2-5 capsules first thing in the morning, and 2-5 capsules just before bed. Drink eight to ten eight-ounce glasses of purified or distilled water per day for best results. If you get cramps, lower the dosage or skip one day and resume the following. After starting ComforTone do not stop completely. Take at least one in the morning and one in the evening. For maximum results, use with JuvaTone and Essentialzyme. ComforTone may be taken every day without becoming addictive.

Companion Products: Chelex, ICP, JuvaTone, Essentialzyme, ParaFree, Di-Tone, JuvaFlex, Juva Cleanse, Purification, Thieves

Safety Data: ComforTone may be taken during pregnancy, as long as you do not get diarrhea. Diarrhea might cause cramping, which could induce labor.

CortiStop - Women's

Designed to counter rising cortisol levels in women.

INGREDIENTS:

Pregnenolone is the precursor hormone from which all other hormones are created. It is an important precursor for the body's production of progesterone which blocks cortisol receptors.

Black Cohosh (root extract) has natural estrogen-like effects that counteract higher cortisol levels.

DHEA (Dioscorea villosa) is an important hormone precursor for progesterone.

ESSENTIAL OILS:

Conyza reduces cortisol levels and promotes hormone balance.

Peppermint hormone balancer.

Frankincense hormone balancer.

Fennel has estrogen-like activity that combats excess cortisol.

Clary Sage increases estrogen balance and blunts the effects of excess cortisol.

Directions: Take one capsule before retiring. If desired, for extra benefits take another capsule in the morning before breakfast.

Companion Products: Progessence, Prenolone, Prenolone+, Dragontime, Endoflex

If pregnant or under a doctor's care, consult a physician before using.

Detoxzyme

A vegetable enzyme complex designed to promote detoxification of the body. Combines essential oils with enzymes designed to digest starches, sugars, proteins, and fats. This formula is structured with trace minerals that help the body detoxify itself, reducing cholesterol and triglycerides. It helps in opening the gallbladder duct and cleansing the liver, preventing candida and yeast overgrowth, and promoting general detoxification.

The formula facilitates optimal absorption of nutrients from foods and supplements, delays the aging process, and maintains optimal energy levels. It also helps to regulate the pH level and reduce acidification and parasite colonization and infestation.

Detoxzyme also contains phytase, an enzyme essential for people eating vegetarian diets. Phytase is crucial for unlocking the mineral content of many grains, nuts, seeds, and other foods which contain high levels of essential minerals that are unavailable to the human body because they are bound up in insoluble indigestible phytate complexes. Up to 90% of the magnesium, potassium, and zinc in foods like barley, cashews, walnuts, and rice is irreversibly tied up by phytic acid and cannot be absorbed by the digestive system. Thus the phytase in Detoxzyme results in a a huge boost in mineral absorption from diets high in nuts, seeds, and whole grains.

The benefits of essential minerals to human health cannot be overemphasized. Magnesium is crucial for blood pressure regulation and antioxidant production, zinc is critical for normal immune function, and potassium is vital for blood pressure and water balance and is found inside of every cell in the body.

INGREDIENTS:

Amylase, glucoamylase, alpha-galactosidase, invertase, lactase, cellulase, protease, bromelain, lipase, phytase, cumin seed

ESSENTIAL OILS:

Cumin (*Cuminum Cyminum*) has been shown to be antiparasitic and antiviral. It supports immune function.

Anise (*Pimpinella anisum*) is antiparasitic and promotes digestion and protein breakdown.

Fennel (*Foeniculum vulgare*) is antiseptic and antiparasitic and improves digestive and pancreatic functions.

Directions: Take 2-3 capsules three times daily, between meals.

Companion Products: ComforTone, JuvaTone, Mint Condition, Di-Tone, JuvaFlex, JuvaCleanse.

Essential Manna - Carob, Apricot, Carob Mint, Spice

This is a nutritionally dense, fiber-rich superfood that is based on the diet of the Hunza people. The Hunza's longevity has been attributed to their consumption of a high potassium, high magnesium diet of dried fruits (especially apricots), nuts, and a variety of whole grains.

INGREDIENTS:

Apricots contain high concentrations of carotinoids, a class of high-powered antioxidants that includes beta carotene (provitamin A). Apricots are also rich in rutin, which strengthens blood vessels.

Ningxia wolfberry (*Lycium barbarum*) has been studied for its ability to combat cancer and strengthen the immune system.

Barley is exceptionally rich in soluble fiber and is an ideal food for type II diabetics.

Buckwheat is high in potassium, magnesium, and other essential minerals that improve cholesterol levels and glucose tolerance.

Amaranth is rich in lysine, an amino acid lacking in many traditional grains, such as wheat and corn.

Almonds contain high amounts of magnesium and vitamin E, which enhance immune support.

Millet is over 12 percent protein and a source of 12 essential minerals, including magnesium, potassium, zinc, and iodine.

Brown rice is rich in protein with high concentrations of the muscle-building amino acids, L-leucine, L-isoleucine, and L-valine. Brown rice is packed with a fiber content necessary for proper digestion.

Coconut is rich in potassium and low in sodium.

Rolled oats contain high amounts of manganese, selenium, and magnesium.

Pineapples are rich in potassium and contain bromelain, a protein-digesting enzyme.

Sesame seeds are rich in linoleic and oleic acid and contain unusual antioxidant compounds, used to prevent free-radical damage.

Stevia is an all-natural sweetening supplement. *(See Stevia).*

Also contains: pumpkin seeds, filberts, pecans, cashews, and papaya.

Directions: Eat throughout the day.

Companion Products: JuvaPower/Spice, Wolfberry Crisp, Berry Young Juice, Polyzyme, Power Meal, Longevity Capsules.

Essential Omegas

This is the only omega-3 fatty acid essential fat supplement to include essential oils such as clove, the highest known antioxidant that has the same anti-inflammatory blood thinning action as aspirin. Essential Omegas combines DNA and cell protecting essential oils with heart-protecting anti-inflammatory essential fatty acids such as alpha linolenic acid, a vital omega-3 fat that is essential for human health. This liquid supplement lowers the stickiness and viscosity of blood thereby preventing abnormal blood clot formation. Antioxidant essential oils prevent the creation of oxidized cholesterol (foam cells) that contributes to atherosclerosis and heart disease.

INGREDIENTS:

Flax Seed Oil (cold-pressed, organic) very high in Omega 3 (alpha linolenic acid) and rich in lignans, which combat cell mutation and cancer. Omega-3 fats reduce the risk of heart disease and decrease blood stickiness.

Black Current Oil rich in GLA, (gamma linoleic acid) which slows the creation of arachidonic acid (AA) and reduces inflammation in the body, a key contributing factor to many degenerative diseases.

GLA also supports nerve function and a deficiency in GLA and other essential fatty acids can lead to severe bone loss. Essential fatty acids may also enhance calcium absorption, boost bone growth, and slow calcium loss in urine. GLA has been shown to combat premenstrual syndrome (PMS) including mood swings, breast tenderness, irritability and swelling and bloating from fluid retention.

ESSENTIAL OILS:

Clove is more effective than aspirin for reducing platelet and blood stickiness and tendency to close. It also reduces the rate of rancidity and oxidation of essential fatty acids both outside and inside the body. It is also one of the most powerful antioxidants known.

Orange is rich in limonene with antioxidant activity and antimutagenic properties.

Directions: Take 1 tablespoon three times daily.

Companion Products: Longevity Capsules, Juva-Power/Spice, Wolfberry Crisp, Berry Young Juice, Longevity, Thyme, Clove.

Essentialzyme

A high-quality enzyme complex that may improve and aid digestion and the elimination of toxic waste from the body. Essentialzyme was formulated to help supply enzymes to those who have difficulty digesting or assimilating food. Essentialzyme helps reestablish proper enzyme balance in the digestive system and throughout the body and helps improve intestinal flora. It may also help retard the aging process.

Enzyme supplementation is particularly important for people suffering chronic pancreatitis, cystic fibrosis, or in any condition where the pancreas duct or common bile duct is blocked, thereby preventing enzymes from reaching the intestine.

INGREDIENTS:

Pancrelipase a powerful complex of fat, protein, and starch-dissolving enzymes derived from pork.

Trypsin is an animal product that has amino acid precursor action, carbohydrate conversion, and assimilation.

Carrot powder has the second highest concentration of natural enzymes in vegetables.

Alfalfa sprouts are a source of natural amylase.

Pancreatin 4X is a protein-digesting enzyme complex that has been used to treat cancer.

Papain is a vegetable enzyme and carbohydrate digester.

Bromelain is a natural enzyme and carbohydrate digester.

Betaine HCl helps with the digestion of protein.

Cumin seed has been used for centuries in the Middle East to help promote digestion and stimulate enzyme activity.

ESSENTIAL OILS:

Tarragon (*Artemisia dracunculus*) is antiviral, antibacterial, and anti-inflammatory.

Peppermint (*Mentha piperita*) improves digestion and intestinal health.

Anise (*Pimpinella anisum*) improves digestion and intestinal health

Fennel (*Foeniculum vulgare*) has been used for centuries for proper digestion.

Clove (*Syzygium aromaticum*) is beneficial for its antibacterial, antiviral, antifungal, anti-infectious, and antiparasitic properties.

Directions: Take 2 or 3 tablets three times daily or as needed. Take Essentialzyme with meals, especially high-protein meals, after 3 p.m., as it will help lessen the burden on the digestive system.

Companion Products: Polyzyme, Carbozyme Lipozyme, Mint Condition, Di-Tone

Exodus

Exodus is the ultimate supercharged antioxidant containing a biblical blend of essential oils and other nutritional herbs to provide important support for the immune system.

INGREDIENTS:

Uncaria tomentosa (Cat's Claw, Una de Gato) contains alkaloids including mitraphylline that substantially amplify immunity.

Amino acid complex of alanine, cystine, arginine, glycine, lycine, threonine, and thorine is used as the building block of the enzymes, proteins, and cells of our natural defenses.

Yucca cleanses the blood.

Echinacea is one of the best-studied immune boosters. It increases the number and activity of white blood cells, T-cells, and natural interferon.

Vitamin A is a powerful antioxidant is essential for proper immunity.

Grapeseed extract is one of the strongest known antioxidants.

Ionic minerals have proven immune stimulating properties.

Pantothenic acid boosts the formation of antibodies.

ESSENTIAL OILS:

Frankincense (*Boswellia carteri*) was historically used for its healing properties. It has antitumoral and immune-stimulating properties.

Hyssop (*Hyssopus officinalis*) has been recognized for thousands of years for its anti-inflammatory, anti-infectious, and antiparasitic properties. It helps discharge toxins and mucus.

Bay laurel (*Laurus nobilis*) has antiseptic and antimicrobial properties.

Spikenard (*Nardostachys jatamansi*) is highly regarded in India as a medicinal herb.

Myrrh (*Commiphora myrrha*) is anti-infectious and antitumoral, enhancing the immune system.

Directions: Take 3 capsules, 2 to 3 times daily.

Companion Products: ImmuPro, ImmuneTune, Super C Chewable, Exodus II, Thieves

HRT Tincture

HRT tincture combines concentrated extracts of some of the best-studied herbs for improving heart function, including hawthorn berry, garlic, and cayenne. Hawthorn berry's role in supporting the heart has been gaining increasing notice among both authors and physicians. According to Varro Tyler, Ph.D., one of the most highly esteemed herbalists in the U.S., "Studies are urgently needed for [an herb] as potentially valuable as this one."

EXTRACTS:

Hawthorn berries—used since the time of Dioscorides in the first century A.D., they are one of the best studied herbs to support the heart, protecting against heart muscle weakness, angina, and mild arrhythmia. J. L. Rodale published an entire book on the subject, *The Hawthorn Berry for the Heart.*

Garlic protects against heart disease and cancer. Garlic juice halts the growth of more than 60 types of fungi and 20 types of bacteria.

Lobelia protects and stimulates the heart muscle.

Cayenne possesses fibrinolytic activity (able to break down blood clots).

Royal jelly is a substance fed to queen bees that allows them to live thirty to forty times longer than worker bees. It is very rich in amino acids, minerals, and vitamins B5 and B6. It stimulates the adrenal glands to increase energy.

ESSENTIAL OILS:

Lemon (*Citrus limon*) decreases platelet stickiness and improves blood flow.

Rosewood (*Aniba rosaeodora*) has been researched at Weber State University for its antibacterial antimicrobial action.

Ylang ylang (*Cananga odorata*) is traditionally used to support heart function and circulation.

Cypress (*Cupressus sempervirens*) is an oil most used for the circulatory system.

Directions: Take 1 to 3 droppers three times daily in distilled water or as needed.

Companion Products: Cardiacare, Super Cal, Longevity Capsules

I.C.P.

ICP Multiple Fiber Beverage is a unique source of fiber and bulk for the diet, which helps speed the transit time of waste matter through the intestinal tract. Psyllium, oat bran, flax, and rice bran are specifically balanced in I.C.P. to eliminate allergy symptoms that many people experience when taking psyllium alone. Essential oils enhance I.C.P.'s flavor and may help dispel gas and pain. This formula is unsurpassed as an aid in enhancing normal bowel function.

INGREDIENTS:

Psyllium seed powder expands when mixed with water and is smooth and filling, not abrasive, to the intestinal walls.

Plant Cellulose is toxin-absorbing fiber.

Aloe vera extract is a natural laxative and lubricant that relaxes the colon.

Rice bran is an outstanding source of soluble and semisolid fiber.

Oat bran binds up fat so it does not enter the blood stream.

Guar gum has been used in expanding and cleansing the colon.

Flax seed is an excellent cleanser for intestinal walls and the digestive system. It is also a rich source of fiber, lignans, and omega-3 fats.

Yucca helps break up obstructions in the digestive system and contains enzymes for digestion.

Fennel seed stimulates the gastrointestinal mucous membrane, which in turn stimulates the pancreas to secrete digestive enzymes to dissolve undigested proteins. It is antiparasitic.

Pepsin is an enzyme to aid digestion.

ESSENTIAL OILS:

Fennel (*Foeniculum vulgare*) is antibacterial and antiparasitical.

Tarragon (*Artemisia dracunculus*) is anti-infectious, antispasmodic, and antiviral.

Ginger (*Zingiber officinale*) improves digestion and combats parasites.

Lemongrass (*Cymbopogon flexuosus*) is antifungal and promotes digestion.

Rosemary (*Rosmarinus officinalis*) reduces indigestion and helps regulate cholesterol.

Anise (*Pimpinella anisum*) helps colon spasms and indigestion.

Directions: Take five times a week for maintenance (1/2 cup water, 1/2 cup apple juice, and one heaping teaspoon of ICP). Take more often for cleansing (Start with one heaping teaspoon, 2 to three times a day with carrot or other vegetable juices. Increase to three teaspoons, three times a day.) ICP dilutes better in warm water. Drink immediately as this product tends to thicken quickly when added to liquid.

For best results, take ComforTone first, then ICP, morning and night. ICP absorbs toxins and can build and improve peristalsis, the wave-like movement of the intestinal walls.

Companion Products: ComforTone, JuvaTone, Essentialzyme, ParaFree (capsules or liquid), Di-Tone, JuvaFlex, Purification, Thieves

ImmuGel

ImmuGel is a unique blend of amino acids, trace minerals, herbal extracts, and essential oils. This blend creates one of nature's most powerful antioxidant and antimicrobial formulas. It destroys yeast, fungi and bacteria. This formula can be used for general maintenance, or it can be increased during times of fatigue, depression, or to help prevent illness.

INGREDIENTS:

Deionized water helps cleanse and purify the body's tissues and organs.

Hydrolyzed protein complex contains alanine, arginine, aspartic acid, glutamic acid, glycine, histidine, hydroxyproline, leucine and isoleucine, lycine, methionine, phenylalanine.

Methylcellulose has been used by parasitologists to inhibit single-cell parasites.

German chamomile extract is antibacterial and antifungal.

Trace minerals restore electrolyte balance in the cells, essential for normal immunity.

ESSENTIAL OILS:

Cinnamon bark (*Cinnamomum verum*) is antifungal, antibacterial, and antiviral.

Clove (*Syzygium aromaticum*) is anti-infectious, antiviral, antifungal, antiparasitic, and has been used in European hospitals for viral hepatitis, bronchitis, flu, sinusitis, and cholera.

Rosemary (*Rosmarinus officinalis*) is antiseptic.

Lemon (*Citrus limon*) promotes leukocyte formation and increases immune function.

Thyme (*Thymus vulgaris*) is one of the strongest antibacterial, antifungal, and antiviral oils.

Oregano (*Origanum compactum*) is antiviral and antibacterial.

Directions: Take 1/2 to 1 teaspoon, three times daily. May be taken with water.

Companion Products: Exodus, ImmuPro, ImmuneTune, Super C Chewable, Exodus II, ImmuPower, Thieves, Longevity Capsules

ImmuneTune

ImmuneTune is a super antioxidant complex that supports the immune system and fights free radicals. The curcuminoid blend in this product has been found to be 60 percent stronger in antioxidant activity than pine bark or grape seed extract. However, synergy is the key to obtaining maximum effect. Through combining curcuminoids with grapeseed extract, its antioxidant power is almost doubled.

INGREDIENTS:

Curcuminoids (from curcumin and turmeric) are potent antioxidants and immune supporters. They are also anti-inflammatory.

Grapeseed extract is one of the strongest natural antioxidants known.

Magnesium is essential for healthy immunity.

Potassium is critical for immune health.

Calcium pantothenate may serve as protection against high blood pressure and colon cancer.

Alpha lipoic acid is one of the most powerful known antioxidants. It is the only antioxidant that is both oil and water soluble. It has been used to treat dabetes, heart, and liver disease.

Chromium improves insulin sensitivity and blood sugar metabolism.

Selenium has been extensively researched for its anticancer and antioxidant properties.

Echinacea increases white blood cell count and stimulates the immune system.

Ginger extract has been used to treat indigestion, flatulence, diarrhea, and stomach ache.

Yucca is an excellent antioxidant that supports the liver and gall bladder.

ESSENTIAL OILS:

Orange (*Citrus sinensis*) contains limonene, a powerful antioxidant.

Pine (*Pinus sylvestris*) helps prevent respiratory infection and bronchitis.

Fir (*Abies alba*) has also been used for different types of respiratory infections and bronchitis.

Cistus (*Cistus ladanifer*) has been used to improve immune function.

Ravensara (*Ravensara aromatica*), known as the "oil that heals," may help support the immune system.

Lemon (*Citrus limon*) promotes leukocyte formation and increases immune function.

Directions: For slow metabolism, take 2 to 3 capsules daily. For fast metabolism, take 3 to 6 capsules daily. It is best taken on an empty stomach. For stomach sensitivity, take with meals.

Companion Products: Exodus, ImmuPro, ParaFree (capsules or liquid), Super C Chewable, Exodus II, ImmuPower, and Thieves.

ImmuPro

ImmuPro chewable is packed with some of the most powerful immune stimulants known, including wolfberry polysaccharide and beta glucan (a polysaccharide from reishi, maitake, and *Agaricus blazei* mushrooms). Numerous studies have documented the ability of these botanicals to reverse cancer and stimulate both cell-mediated and humoral immunity, dramatically boosting levels of macrophages, neutrophiles, phagocytes, B-cells, T-cells, natural killer cells, interleukins, and interferons. Contains a complex of the potent immune-boosting minerals zinc, copper, and selenium. Also contains melatonin, one of the most powerful immune stimulants known, shown to clinically reverse tumor growth. Melatonin levels steadily decrease with age and are a factor that contributes to accelerated aging.

INGREDIENTS:

Wolfberry polysaccharide used in China for centuries, has been shown to be one of the most powerful supporters of immune function.

Organic reishi, maitake, and *Agaricus blazei* mushrooms are the highest known sources of a rich variety of beta glucans, potent immune-stimulating polysaccharides which have been documented by numerous studies as having significant immune-boosting effects.

Orange oil (*Citrus sinensis*) contains over 90 percent d-limonene, one of the most powerful anticancer compounds studied in recent years. A potent antioxidant.

Zinc Citrate is a superb, bioavailable source of zinc, a mineral crucial to normal immune function.

Copper chelate (rice protein) an essential mineral which should always be combined with zinc at the correct ratio. This is due to the fact that copper and zinc compete for absorption in the intestines. Excess of either zinc or copper can create a mineral deficiency that can result in immune suppression instead of immune activation.

Selenomethionine is essential for normal immunity, activating T-lymphocytes, interleukins, interferons, and NK cells.

Melatonin is one the most powerful known immune stimulants, boosting both cell-mediated and humoral immunity. It has been documented as an immune treatment for tumors.

Directions: Take 1 tablet before retiring. If under stress take 2 to 4 tablets before retiring or as needed.

Companion Products: Exodus, ImmuneTune, ImmuGel, Thieves, Longevity.

JuvaPower/JuvaSpice

A whole food high antioxidant vegetable powder complex that is a rich source of acid-binding foods and high in liver-protecting nutrients like tocotrienols, xanthophylls, and tocopherols. It is also rich in antimutagenic sulphoraphane and squalene.

INGREDIENTS:

Rice Bran (*Oryza Sativa*): Stabilized, nonchemically treated. Contains gamma-oryzanol, tocotrienols, tocopherols, squalene, ferulic acid, IP6 (inositol hexaphosphate) and Gamma-oryzanol, a triterpene alcohol that is more effective than vitamin E in stopping oxidation of cholesterol. In studies at the Louisiana State University in Baton Rouge, researchers concluded that gamma-oryzanol "had activities higher than that of any of the 4 vitamin E components. Gamma-oryzanol may be a more important antioxidant of rice bran in the reduction of cholesterol oxidation than vitamin E."[4]

Rice bran is considered one of the best sources of squalene, an antimutagen and anti-cancer agent also found in olive oil and shark liver oil. [5,6]

Ferulic acid is also found in rice bran and acts as an antioxidative, hypotensive polyphenol that reduces blood pressure.[7]

---

4. Z. Xu et al., *J Agric Food Chem.* 2001.

5. TJ Smith, University of South Carolina (*Expert Opin Investig Drugs.* 2000)

6. HL Newmark, Rockefeller University, New York (*Ann N Y Acad Sci.* 1999)

7. Suzuki A et al., "Short- and long-term effects of ferulic acid on blood pressure in spontaneously hypertensive rats." *Am J Hypertens.* 2002 Apr;15(4 Pt 1):351-7.

Spinach Powder *(Spinacea oleracea)*: One of the highest known antioxidant foods (1,260 ORAC units/100g), rich in mixed carotenoids (ie., lutein, zeaxanthin), 9-cis-beta-carotene, flavonoids, and p-coumaric acid derivatives. "Neoxanthin from spinach significantly reduced cell viability to 10.9% for PC-3, 15% for DU 145 (prostate cell cancer lines)." E Kotake-Nara E, Hokkaido University.

Tomato Flake *(Lycospersicon esculentum)*: High in antimutagens lycopene, kaempferol, and chlorogenic acid.

Beet Root Powder *(Beta vulgaris)*: High-pigment red phenotypes have been shown to have the best liver-protecting properties, according to M. Wettasinghe, University of Wisconsin at Madison.

Flax Seed Bran *(Linum usitatissimum)*: high in lignans, which prevent cellular mutations according to over 50 peer-reviewed clinical studies. The lignans in flax seed also protect the liver against over burden of toxins, according to recent university research (Rakuno Gakuen University, Ebetsu, Japan).[8]

Oat Bran *(Avena sativa)*: high in immune-supporting beta glucans.

Peppermint Leaf *(Mentha piperita)*: studied for its ability to combat cellular mutation.

Broccoli Floret Powder *(Brassica oleracea ssp. cymosa)*: high in sulphoraphane, protective against cellular mutations; 890 TE/100g According to Cornell University scientists, "Broccoli possessed the highest total phenolic content, followed by spinach, yellow onion, red pepper, carrot, cabbage, potato." Y. Chu, Cornell University.

Cucumber Powder *(Cucumis sativus)*: 100 grams has 5,160 iu Vit. A, 312 mcg folate, 3,456 mg Vit. K

L-taurine: Essential for bile acid formation and liver protection.

Dill Leaf *(Anethum graveolens)*

Barley Sprout Powder *(Hordeum vulgare L.)*

Ginger Root Powder *(Zingiber officinale Rosc.)*

Aloe Vera Extract (Aloe barbadensis)

Slippery Elm, inner bark, (Ulmus fulva)

Psyllium Seed Husk (Plantago ovata), a key colon cleanser. A healthy liver requires a healthy colon.

Anise (Pimpinella anisum): seed and EO.

Fennel (Foeniculum vulgare): seed and EO.

Potassium Cloride (JuvaSpice)

Real Salt (Redmond Utah) (JuvaSpice)

Cayenne Pepper *(Capsium Annum)* (JuvaSpice only)

Directions: Sprinkle 1 tablespoon on food or add to purified drinking water.

Companion Products: JuvaTone, JuvaCleanse, Juvaflex

JuvaTone

JuvaTone is a special herbal complex designed to support the liver. The liver is one of the most important organs of the body. It purifies the blood and is a key to converting carbohydrates to energy. An overtaxed liver may affect our energy, digestion, and skin. Fats and bile within the liver can easily become oversaturated with oil-soluble toxins, synthetic chemicals, and heavy metals. As toxins build, the liver becomes taxed and stressed, resulting in aggravating skin conditions, rashes, fatigue, headaches, muscle pain, digestive disturbances, pallor, dizziness, irritability, mood swings, and mental confusion. The liver also plays a major role in helping the body detoxify. The final products of digestion are transported through the portal vein from the colon to the liver to be cleansed.

---

8. Endoh D et al., Rakuno Gakuen University, Ebetsu, Japan.

INGREDIENTS:

Choline bitartrate has been used in the treatment of many liver disorders, including elevated cholesterol levels, viral hepatitis, and cirrhosis.

Inositol helps the liver rid itself of fat and bile.

Beet root is a source of enzymes that protects the liver.

L-cysteine promotes the production of glutathione, one of the most powerful antioxidants and vital for protecting the liver.

Bee propolis supports liver detoxification.

Dl-methionine is one of the most powerful antioxidants in the body, and especially important to protect the liver.

Oregon grape root contains berberine, which has been studied as a liver protectant and for its effects against hepatitis.

Dandelion root is used for disturbances in bile flow and liver disorders.

Other INGREDIENTS: Alfalfa sprouts, echinacea root, parsley, sodium copper chlorophyllin in herbal extracts.

ESSENTIAL OILS:

Geranium (*Pelargonium graveolens*) has been used for centuries as a liver cleanser and to regenerate tissue and nerves.

German chamomile (*Matricaria recutita*) improves bile flow from the liver.

Rosemary (*Rosmarinus officinalis*) supports the liver and combats cirrhosis.

Lemon (*Citrus limon*) promotes leukocyte formation and increases immune function.

Blue tansy (*Tanacetum annuum*) is anti-inflammatory and is used for hypertension and arthritis.

Myrtle (*Myrtus communis*) helps break up mucus and stimulate the thyroid.

Directions: For slow metabolism, take 2 tablets, three times daily. Increase as needed up to 4 tablets, four times daily. For fast metabolism, take 3 tablets, three times daily and increase to 4 tablets, four times daily or as needed. Best taken between meals. Tablets may be chewed, broken, or swallowed whole. For optimum results, use with ComforTone.

Companion Products: ComforTone, ICP, Essentialzyme, ParaFree (capsules or liquid), Di-Tone, Forgiveness, JuvaFlex, Release, Surrender, JuvaCleanse

K & B Tincture

K & B tincture contains extracts of herbs that promote kidney and bladder health.

Extracts:

Juniper berries—long used by Greek, Arabic, and Native American peoples as a kidney stimulant to encourage cleansing and increased filtration.

Parsley is used to purify the urinary tract.

Uva Ursi a mild diuretic, astringent, and urinary tract infection remedy.

Dandelion root—traditionally used to treat edema and digestive, gallbladder, and liver disorders.

Roman chamomile increases bile flow and liver function.

Royal jelly is a substance fed to queen bees that allows them to live thirty to forty times longer than worker bees. It is very rich in amino acids, minerals, and vitamins B5 and B6. It stimulates the adrenal glands to increase energy.

ESSENTIAL OILS:

Clove (*Syzygium aromaticum*) is one of the most antimicrobial and antiseptic essential oils.

Juniper (*Juniperus osteosperma* and *J. scopulorum*) is a strong diuretic.

Sage (*Salvia officinalis*) strengthens the vital centers and supports metabolism.

Fennel (*Foeniculum vulgare*) is antiseptic to the digestive tract. Supports digestion.

Geranium (*Pelargonium graveolens*) opens the bile duct.

Roman chamomile (*Chamaemelum nobile*) promotes the flow of bile to and from the liver, a key aspect of cleansing and detoxification.

Directions: Take 1 to 3 droppers three times daily in distilled water or as needed.

Companion Products: Juniper, Essentialzyme, Detoxzyme, JuvaTone, JuvaCleanse, JuvaFlex

Lipozyme

A fat-digesting enzyme complex that promotes fat digestion and enhaces the absorption of fat-soluable vitamins such as vitmain A, vitamin D, and vitamin E.

INGREDIENTS:

Lipase a fat-digesting enzyme

Bee pollen is a natural source of amylase that is rich in natural enzymes and coenzymes.

Pancreatin 10X is a powerful natural full-spectrum enzyme complex of proteases, amylases, and lipases.

Trace minerals enhance enzyme activity.

ESSENTIAL OILS:

Di-Tone blend

Directions: Take 1 capsule three times daily or as needed just before meals.

Companion Products: Essentialzyme, Polyzyme, Detoxzyme

Longevity Capsules

Longevity essential oil capsules are the world's most powerful antioxidant supplement. With an ORAC antioxidant score of 150,000, this formula provides 700 times the antioxidant power of carrots. Packed with limonene, the subject of over 50 studies documenting its antimutagenic, antitumoral, anticancerous, and cellular DNA-protecting attributes. Contains thyme essential oil which preserves fats from degradation in the brain, heart, liver, and kidneys, while raising total antioxidant levels, including glutathione and superoxide dismutase. Orange essential oil is 90 percent limonene, a powerful antioxidant. Clove reduces the stickiness of blood cells, and decreases

joint pain and swelling. Dr. Nagashima of the Nihon University in Japan found eugenol (the active component of clove oil) inhibited the destruction of the fatty outer layer of human red blood cells.

ESSENTIAL OILS:

Thyme (*Thymus vulgaris*) is strongly antibacterial, antifungal, and antiviral.

Orange (*Citrus sinensis*) stops cellular mutation and DNA damage.

Clove (*Sygygium aromaticum*) has potent anti-parasitic, antibacterial, and antifungal properties.

Directions: Take 1 capsule once a day or as needed.

Companion Products: Berry Young Juice, Essential Omegas, Wolfberry Crisp, ImmuPro.

Master Formula HERS

The Master Formula Vitamin HERS is a unique complex of high potenacy vitamins and minerals. To enhance assimilation it contains the key amino acid L-phenylalanine.

INGREDIENTS:

Vitamin A and beta carotene are powerful antioxidants that support the eyes, hair, and skin.

Vitamin D is vital for calcium absorption and liver and kidney health.

Vitamin E protects the heart and blood and combats free-radical oxidative damage.

Vitamin C is vital for healthy immunity and blood vessel integrity. It fights free-radical damage and premature aging.

Folic acid prevents heart disease, breast cancer, birth defects. Requires Vitamin B6 and B12 to be assimilated.

Thiamine (vitamin B1) is essential for energy production, carbohydrate metabolism, and nerve cell function.

Riboflavin (vitamin B2) is crucial in the production of cellular energy, helps regenerate the liver, and prevents cellular mutations.

Niacin converts carbohydrates into energy. At least 4.4 mg is needed for every 1,000 calories consumed to avoid deficiency diseases.

Vitamin B6 protects the heart and blood vessels. Prevents cellular mutations. Requires folic acid. Vitamin B12, and magnesium to be assimilated.

Vitamin B12 is critical for red blood cell formation and proper immune and nerve function. Works with vitamin B6 to prevent heart disease. Vegetarians are often deficient in B12.

Biotin (Vitamin H) converts fats and amino acids into energy and promotes healthy hair while combating yeast and fungus overgrwoth.

Pantothenic acid is needed for the prevention of depression and tinnitus.

Choline bitartrate is a vital nutrient for liver health, used to combat hepatitis and cirrhosis.

Calcium is key for bone health and prevents high blood pressure.

Iodine (kelp) promotes thyroid hormone production, yielding faster metabolism, and higher energy.

Magnesium is crucial for proper enzyme function, insulin action, muscle contractions and heart rhythm. It reduces high blood pressure.

Copper is vital for red blood cell and immune function.

Zinc is crucial for healthy immunity, cell growth, wound healing, and proper action of many hormones, including insulin and growth hormone.

Potassium is vital for healthy muscle, nerve, heart, and adrenal function. It reduces high blood pressure and balances water distribution.

Manganese is needed for blood sugar control, energy metabolism, and proper thyroid function.

Chromium improves insulin sensitivity and blood sugar metabolism.

Selenium has been extensively researched for its anticancer and antioxidant properties.

Silicon is essential for formation of collagen in bone, cartilage, and other connective tissues.

In a base of betaine HCl, citrus bioflavonoids, L-cysteine, histidine, tyrosine, lysine, arginine, PABA (para amino benzoic acid), molybdenum, and amino acid complex.

Directions: For slow metabolism: take 3-6 tablets daily. For fast metabolism: take 4-8 tablets daily. Take 1/2 the amount before breakfast and 1/2 before dinner. Best taken before meals.

Companion Supplements: Super B, Super C Chewable, Super Cal, Essential Manna, Mineral Essence, Power Meal, Sulfurzyme, Wolfberry Crisp, Progessence.

Master Formula HIS

The Master Formula Vitamin HIS is a unique complex of high potenacy vitamins and minerals. To enhance assimilation it contains the key amino acid L-phenylalanine.

INGREDIENTS:

Vitamin A and beta carotene are powerful antioxidants that support the eyes, hair, and skin.

Vitamin D is vital for calcium absorption and liver and kidney health.

Vitamin E protects the heart and blood and combats free-radical oxidative damage.

Vitamin C is vital for healthy immunity, blood vessel integrity. It combats free-radical damage and premature aging.

Folic acid plays an important role in cardiovascular health.

Thiamin (vitamin B1) is essential for energy production, carbohydrate metabolism, and nerve cell function.

Riboflavin (vitamin B2) is crucial in the production of cellular energy, helps regenerate the liver, and prevents cellular mutations.

Niacin converts carbohydrates into energy. At least 4.4 mg is needed for every 1,000 calories consumed to avoid deficiency diseases.

Vitamin B6 protects the heart and blood vessels. Prevents cellular mutations. Requires folic acid. Vitamin B12, and magnesium to be assimilated.

Vitamin B12 is critical for red blood cell formation and proper immune and nerve function. Works with vitamin B6 to prevent heart disease. Vegetarians are often deficient in B12.

Biotin (Vitamin H) converts fats and amino acids into energy and promotes healthy hair while combating yeast and fungus overgrwoth.

Pantothenic acid is needed for the prevention of depression and tinnitus.

Choline bitartrate is a vital nutrient for liver health, using to combat hepatitis and cirrhosis.

Calcium is key for bone health and prevents high blood pressure.

Iodine (kelp) helps prevent goiters, stimulates the thyroid, and balances hormones.

Magnesium is crucial for proper enzyme function, insulin action, muscle contractions and heart rhythm. Reduces high blood pressure.

Copper is vital for red blood cell and immune function.

Zinc is crucial for healthy immunity, cell growth, wound healing, and proper action of many hormones, including insulin and growth hormone.

Potassium is vital for healthy muscle, nerve, heart, and adrenal function. It reduces high blood pressure and balances water distribution.

Manganese is needed for blood sugar control, energy metabolism, and proper thyroid function.

Chromium improves insulin sensitivity and blood sugar metabolism.

Selenium has been extensively researched for its anticancer and antioxidant properties.

Silicon is essential for formation of collagen in bone, cartilage, and other connective tissues.

In a base of betaine HCl, citrus bioflavonoids, L-cysteine, histidine, tyrosine, lysine, arginine, PABA (para amino benzoic acid), molybdenum, and amino acid complex.

Directions: Take 1-3 tablets with breakfast and 1-3 with lunch (take before meals).

Companion Supplements: Super B, Super C Chewable, Super Cal, Essential Manna, Mineral Essence, Power Meal, Sulfurzyme, and Wolfberry Crisp,

MegaCal

A high-powered calcium and essential mineral complex with a 1:1 calcium to magnesium ratio. Contains over 650 mg of elemental magnesium and calcium per serving along with key quantities of zinc, manganese, and copper, balanced to scientific ratios to avoid mineral interactions and competition. Calcium and magnesium are necessary not only for healthy bones and teeth, but also for proper heart and blood function and to keep nerve and muscles working properly.

INGREDIENTS:

Calcium: Calcium Lactate Pentahydrate, Calcium Glycerophosphate, Calcium Carbonate, Calcium Ascorbate

Magnesium: Magnesium Citrate, Magnesium Sulfate, Magnesium Carbonate

Zinc Gluconate

Copper Gluconate

Manganese Sulfate

Xylitol, as an anti-bacterial agent and bone strengthener

Lemon *(Citrus Limon)* essential oil, which prevents DNA mutation and enhances cellular repair.

Fractionated Coconut Oil, which is anti-fungal and can help prevent or eliminate candida infections.

Directions: Take 1 tablespoon daily, at least 1 hour after a meal.

Companion Products: Super Cal, BLM capsules and powder

Mineral Essence

A balanced organic, ionic mineral complex with more than 60 different minerals. Without minerals, vitamins cannot be properly assimilated or absorbed by the body. Mineral Essence has a natural electrolyte balance, helping to prevent disease and premature aging. Minerals are also necessary for proper immune and metabolism functions.

Mineral essence also includes essential oils to enhance bioavailability. To demonstrate this, a group of volunteers consumed a teaspoon of liquid trace minerals without essential oils. Each volunteer experienced diarrhea within 24 hours. Following a washout period of several days, the same volunteers were given double the dosage of the same liquid trace minerals blended with essential oils. None experienced diarrhea.

INGREDIENTS:

Purified water is needed to dilute the minerals for liquifying this blend.

Honey is an emulsifier and natural sweetener.

Royal Jelly is a very rich source of amino acids and natural enzymes.

Trace minerals include beryllium, bismuth, boron, bromine, calcium, carbon, cesium, chloride, chromium, copper, gallium, germanium, gold, hafnium, indium, iodine, iron, lithium, lutecium, manganese, magnesium, molybdenum, nickel, niobium, nitrogen, phosphorus, potassium, rubidium, scandium, selenium, silicon, silver, sodium, strontium, sulfur, tantalum, thallium, tin, titanium, tungsten, vanadium, yttrium, zinc, and zirconium.

ESSENTIAL OILS:

Lemon (*Citrus limon*) prevents cellular mutation and enhances DNA repair.

Cinnamon bark (*Cinnamomum verum*) is anti-infectious, antibacterial, antiviral, antifungal, antiparasitic and anticoagulant.

Peppermint (*Mentha piperita*) is promotes digestion and mineral absorption.

Directions: Take 5 droppers morning and evening or as needed for a mineral supplement.

Companion Products: Master Formula HIS/HERS and CHILDREN'S, Sulfurzyme, Super Cal, AD&E

ParaFree, Liquid/Soft Gels

An advanced blend of some of the strongest essential oils that have been studied for their antiparasitic properties.

BASE OILS:

Sesame seed oil and olive oil.

ESSENTIAL OILS:

Cumin (*Cuminum Cyminum*) has been shown to be antiparasitic and antiviral. It supports immune function.

Anise (*Pimpinella anisum*) is antiparasitic and promotes digestion and protein breakdown.

Fennel (*Foeniculum vulgare*) is antiseptic and antiparasitic and improves digestive and pancreatic functions.

Bay laurel (*Laurus nobilis*) is antiseptic, antibacterial, antiparasitic, and antiviral. It is also a diuretic, fungicidal, and digestive aid.

Vetiver (*Vetiveria officinalis*) is antiseptic, anti-inflammatory, and immune-supporting.

Nutmeg (*Myristica fragrans*) supports adrenal glands, is antibacterial and anti-inflammatory, and stimulates immune function. It has also been used to reduce diarrhea.

Tea Tree (*Melaleuca alternifolia*) is antifungal, antiparasitic, and antibacterial.

Clove (*Syzygium aromaticum*) has potent antiparasitic, antibacterial, and antifungal properties.

Idaho tansy (*Tanacetum vulgare*) is one of the most potent worm-expelling essential oils.

Thyme (*Thymus vulgaris*) is one of the strongest antibacterial, antifungal, and antiviral essential oils.

Companion Products: ComforTone, ICP, JuvaTone, JuvaCleanse, Thieves, ImmuPower, Detoxzyme, Polyzyme, Essentialzyme

Directions: Liquid: Take 2 to 4 droppers, three times daily for 21 consecutive days.

Gelcaps: Take 2 to 5 gelcaps, two to three times a day for 21 consecutive days out of each month.

Repeat for three cycles or as needed. Use ParaFree with ComforTone and ICP for cleansing. The ICP will help break up plaque along the intestinal walls.

Note: Use in moderation during pregnancy, possibly 2 capsules daily. If diarrhea occurs, discontinue. A good parasite cleanse is recommended before conception. Consult your health care provider before starting a cleansing program.

PD 80/20

PD 80/20 is a dietary supplement designed to provide natural hormone support for the body. As hormone levels decline with age, maintaining adequate hormone reserves becomes vital for sustaining health and preventing premature aging.

INGREDIENTS:

Pregnenolone (640 mg), DHEA (160 mg)

Companion Products: Essentialzyme, Sulfurzyme (capsules or powder), VitaGreen, Progessence, Prenolone, and Prenolone+

Companion Oils: Clary sage, fennel, Dragon Time.

Directions: Start with 1 capsule a day, then increase to 2 capsules a day as needed.

Polyzyme

The enzyme complexes in Polyzyme are used medically as powerful anti-inflammatories that combat arthritis, irritable bowel syndrome, fibromyalgia, ALS, and food allergies.

By promoting complete digestion of proteins, Polyzyme increases the production of key amino acids from food proteins. Amino acids are absolutely vital for healthy immunity and health and form the building blocks of hormone creation, tissue repair, and muscle formation. By promoting complete digestion, Polyzyme prevents putrifaction in the intestines that can lead to allergies, liver stress, and toxic blood.

Protease 3.0, 4.5, 6.0 are protein digesting enzymes designed to work in a broad range of pH conditions. Acid stable proteases are essential for amino acid creation in the acid environment of the stomach while alkaline proteases are more effective in the large intestine. This combination of proteases is scientifically formulated to maximize protein digestion and amino acid formation.

Phytase is an enzyme essential for people eating vegetarian diets. Phytase is crucial for unlocking the mineral content of many grains, nuts, seeds, and other foods which contain high levels of essential minerals that are unavailable to the human body because they are bound up in insoluble indigestible phytate complexes. Up to 90% of the magnesium, potassium, and zinc in foods like barley, cashews, walnuts, and rice is locked up by phytic acid and cannot be absorbed by the digestive system, unless phytase is present.

Lipase is a fat-dissolving enzyme vital for proper absorption of Vitamin D, E, and A.

Bromelain is a proteolytic enzyme from pineapple stems.

Papain is a plant enzyme from unripe papayas with a broad spectrum of digesting activity.

Peptidase promotes the creation and absorption of amino acids in the digestive system.

Rice bran is rich in ferulic acid and vitamin E.

ESSENTIAL OILS:

Anise (*Pimpinella anisum*) promotes digestion and helps eliminate parasites.

Peppermint (*Mentha piperita*) is a powerful promoter of digestion and peristalsis in the intestines. It is highly antifungal, combating candida, nausea, and vomiting.

Rosemary (*Rosmarinus officinalis* CT cineol) is highly antiseptic, with a broad-spectrum of antifungal activity that prevents fermentation and yeast/fungal overgrowth in the intestines.

Directions: Take 1 capsule three times daily or as needed just before meals with proteins.

Companion Products: Carbozyme, Lipozyme, Detoxzyme, Essentialzyme.

Power Meal

Power Meal is a complete vegetarian protein complex containing Ningxia wolfberry and rice protein with a large spectrum of antioxidant herbs, vitamins, enzymes, and minerals. Whether used as a meal alternative or snack, Power Meal can serve as an excellent weight management tool. Free of fats and synthetic ingredients, Power Meal provides the building blocks the body requires for regeneration and energy.

The protein-rich formula of Power Meal, when combined with exercise and proper nutrition, can help the body build lean muscle tissue, which is the foundation of a lean physique. Because muscle burns 22 times as many calories as fat, the addition of muscle tissue can significantly accelerate metabolism and contribute to a more slender body.

INGREDIENTS:

Ningxia wolfberry (*Lycium barbarum*) has 18 amino acids, 21 trace minerals, beta carotene, and vitamins B1, B2, B6, and E. It is an excellent whole food and has many functions in the body.

Rice protein concentrate is high in branched chain amino acids required for building muscles.

Eleuthero root (formerly referred to as Siberian ginseng) strengthens the adrenal glands, enhances immune function, normalizes blood pressure, improves mental alertness, and promotes hormonal balance.

Rice Bran (*Oryza Sativa*): Stabilized, nonchemically treated. Contains gamma-oryzanol, tocotrienols, tocopherols, squalene, ferulic acid, IP6 (inositol hexaphosphate) and Gamma-oryzanol, a triterpene alcohol that is more effective than vitamin E in stopping oxidation of cholesterol. In studies at the Louisiana State University in Baton Rouge, researchers concluded that gamma-oryzanol "had activities higher than that of any of the 4 vitamin E components. Gamma-oryzanol may be a more important antioxidant of rice bran in the reduction of cholesterol oxidation than vitamin E."

Rice bran is considered one of the best sources of squalene, an antimutagen and anti-cancer agent also found in olive oil and shark liver oil.

Ferulic acid is also found in rice bran and acts as an antioxidative, hypotensive polyphenol that reduces blood pressure. **Ginkgo biloba** extract increases energy, improves memory and is excellent for cerebral circulation, oxygenation, and blood flow.

Bee pollen is high in protein and low in fat and sodium. It contains many minerals and vitamins, including potassium, calcium, magnesium, zinc, manganese, copper, and B vitamins.

Guar gum promotes healthy colon function.

Calcium carbonate is needed for healthy bones, teeth, and joints.

Lecithin (food for the brain) is excellent for liver disorders and helps to balance cholesterol.

Choline bitartrate has been used in the treatment of many liver disorders (including elevated cholesterol levels), Alzheimer's disease, viral hepatitis, and cirrhosis.

Silicon is required for skin, ligaments, bones, and tendons.

Magnesium is crucial for proper enzyme function, muscle contractions and heart rhythm. It reduces blood pressure, prevents arteriosclerosis, and improves insulin action.

Potassium is important for proper muscle and nerve cell function.

MSM supports healthy hair, skin, liver, and immune function.

Inositol helps defat the liver and remove bile.

Betaine HCl promotes protein digestion.

Proteolytic Enzyme Blend containing lipase, protease, phytase and peptidase.

Kelp contains iodine, which is necessary to prevent goiters.

PABA (para amino benzoic acid) assists healthy bacteria in producing folic acid and helps form red blood cells.

L-carnitine helps convert fatty acids into energy.

Zinc is crucial for immunity, cell growth, wound healing, and proper action of many hormones, including insulin and growth hormone.

Boron promotes the absorption and utilization of calcium.

Betatene is a mixed-carotenoid complex containing lycopene, lutein, zeaxanthin, beta carotene and astaxanthin.

Copper is necessary for proper red blood cell and immune function.

Manganese citrate is an antioxidant that regulates blood sugar levels and increases cellular energy.

Vitamin C is vital for healthy immunity and blood vessel integrity. It fights free-radical damage and premature aging.

Vitamin E protects the heart and blood and combats free-radical oxidative damage.

Vitamin D3 stimulates the absorption of calcium and exerts many anticancerous properties, especially against breast and colon cancer.

Fructooligosaccharides (FOS) are one of the best-documented natural nutrients for promoting the growth of *lactobacilli* and bifidobacteria, the linchpin of sound health. FOS has also been clinically studied for its ability to increase magnesium and calcium absorption, lower blood glucose, cholesterol, and LDL levels, and to inhibit production of the reductase enzymes that can contribute to cancer. Because FOS may increase magnesium absorption, it may also lead to lowered blood pressure and better cardiovascular health.

In addition, FOS also has another benefit - It has a naturally sweet taste.

Alpha lipoic acid is one of the most powerful known antioxidants. It is the only antioxidant that is both oil and water soluble. It has been used to treat diabetes, heart disease, and liver disease.

Selenium has been extensively researched for its anticancer and antioxidant properties.

Riboflavin is important in the production of energy, regenerating glutathione and preventing cancer.

Thiamin (Vitamin B1) is essential for energy production, carbohydrate metabolism, and nerve cell function.

Chromium improves insulin sensitivity and blood sugar metabolism.

Vitamin B6 protects the heart and blood vessels. Prevents cellular mutations. Requires folic acid, Vitamin B12, and magnesium to be assimilated.

Folic acid plays an important role in cardiovascular health and helps prevent neural tube defects.

Niacin converts carbohydrates into energy. At least 4.4 mg is needed for every 1,000 calories consumed to avoid deficiency diseases.

Biotin helps convert fats and amino acids into energy. It promotes healthy nails and hair and combats yeast and fungus overgrowth.

Vitamin B12 is critical for red blood cell formation and proper immune and nerve function. Works with vitamin B6 to prevent heart disease. Vegetarians are often deficient in Vitamin B12.

Also includes: natural vanilla and fructose.

ESSENTIAL OILS:

Grapefruit (*Citrus paradisi*) prevents DNA and cellular mutation.

Orange (*Citrus sinensis)* contains the powerful antioxidant limonene, is anti-inflammatory, antispasmodic, and anticoagulant.

Lemon (*Citrus limon*) prevents cellular mutation and enhances DNA repair.

Cypress (*Cupressus sempervirens*) helps improve circulation and lymph flow.

Anise (*Pimpinella anisum*) promotes digestion and helps eliminate parasites.

Fennel (*Foeniculum vulgare*) is antiparasitic, antimicrobial, antispasmodic, helps regulate intestinal flora, is a digestive aid, and increases gastric secretions.

Nutmeg (*Myristica fragrans*) helps support the adrenal glands for increased energy.

Directions: Take 2 scoops in water or rice milk as a meal alternative or as needed for energy and endurance.

Companion Products: Essential Manna, Wolfberry Crisp, WheyFit, ThermaBurn.

ProGen

ProGen is an all-vegetable and herbal support for the prostate and male glandular system. Saw palmetto is one of the most widely used herbs to combat prostate enlargement, which affects most men over 45. *Pygeum africanum* prevents prostate atrophy and malfunction.

INGREDIENTS:

Serenoa serrulata (saw palmetto) reduces an enlarged prostate and relieves the inflammation and pain of benign prostatic hypertrophy.

Dioscorea villosa (wild yam) is antispasmodic and supports the reproductive organs.

Pygeum africanum is used to prevent prostate atrophy and malfunction.

L-glutathione is a sulfur-bearing liver antioxidant.

Di-methylglycine is excellent for heart muscle and tissue support.

L-carnitine supports prostate health.

Magnesium is vital for prostate health.

Eleuthero root (formerly referred to as Siberian ginseng) strengthens the adrenal glands, enhances immune function, normalizes blood pressure, improves mental alertness, and promotes hormonal balance.

Zinc is one of the most important minerals for prostate health. It helps restore sexual potency.

ESSENTIAL OILS:

Yarrow (*Achillea millefolium*) is supportive to the prostate and nerves.

Sage (*Salvia officinalis*) has estrogen-like properties and may help balance hormones.

Myrtle (*Myrtus communis*) helps prevent candida and helps prevent an inflamed prostate.

Myrrh (*Commiphora myrrha*) has hormone-like properties and is anti-inflammatory.

Peppermint (*Mentha piperita*) helps decongest the prostate and urinary tract.

Fennel (*Foeniculum vulgare*) has estrogen-like properties and helps balance the hormones.

Lavender (*Lavandula angustifolia*) is calming and balancing.

Directions: Take 2 capsules two times daily.

Companion Products: Be-Fit, Master Formula HIS, Protec, Power Meal

Rehemogen

Rehemogen tincture contains herbs that were used by Chief Sundance and other Native Americans to cleanse, purify, disinfect and build the blood.

Extracts:

Red clover blossom prevents cellular mutations and builds blood.

Chaparral—used by Native American healers as an internal disinfectant and to treat tuberculosis.

Licorice root—traditionally used to to combat circulatory dysfunction and liver disorders.

Oregon grape root—contains berberine, a powerful liver protectant.

Sarsaparilla—contains saponins, steroid-like molecules that neutralize endotoxins (poisons secreted by fungi and bacteria in the human body), that contribute to many kinds of disease.

Cascara sagrada—used to support the liver, pancreas, gallbladder, and stomach.

Burdock root—eaten as a vegetable in Japan to cleanse the blood.

Royal jelly is the substance fed to queen bees that allows them to live thirty to forty times longer than worker bees. It is very rich in amino acids, minerals, and vitamins B5 and B6. It stimulates the adrenal glands to increase energy.

ESSENTIAL OILS:

Rosemary (*Rosmarinus officinalis*) combats fatigue.

Thyme (*Thymus vulgaris*) is highly antimicrobial and antiseptic.

Melaleuca (*Melaleuca alternifolia*) is antimicrobial and antiseptic.

Roman chamomile (*Chamaemelum nobile*)—promotes the flow of bile to and from the liver, a key part of cleansing and detoxification.

Also contains: Buckthorn bark, stillingia, and prickly ash bark.

Directions: Mix 1 to 3 droppers, three times daily in distilled water or as needed.

Companion Products: Essentialzyme, Polyzyme, Detoxzyme, Di-Tone

Stevia Extract

Stevia extract is a super-sweet, low-calorie dietary supplement that helps regulate blood sugar and supports the pancreas. It is valuable for anyone with diabetes and hypoglycemia.

It is a first-rate aid to weight loss and weight management because it contains no calories. In addition, research indicates that it significantly increases glucose tolerance and inhibits glucose absorption. People who ingest stevia daily often report a decrease in their desire for sweets and fatty foods. It may also improve digestion and gastrointestinal function, soothe upset stomachs, and help speed recovery from minor illnesses.

Stevia also inhibits the growth of some bacteria and infectious organisms, including those that cause tooth decay and gum disease. Many individuals using stevia have reported a lower incidence of colds and flu. Many who have used stevia as a mouthwash have experienced a significant decrease in gum disease.

When topically applied, stevia softens the skin and smooths out wrinkles while healing various skin blemishes, acne, seborrhea, dermatitis, and eczema. When used on cuts and wounds, stevia promotes rapid healing without scarring.

INGREDIENTS:

Stevia leaf extract—intensely sweet with a mild, licorice-like aftertaste.

Directions: Use as a supplemental sweetener.

Companion Products: Blue Agave Nectar.

Sulfurzyme Powder and Capsules

Sulfurzyme is a unique combination of methyl-sulfonylmethane (MSM), the protein-building compound found in breast milk, fresh fruits and vegetables, and Ningxia wolfberry (*Lycium barbarum*). Together, they create a new concept in balancing the immune system and supporting almost every major function of the body. Of particular importance is the ability of MSM to equalize water pressure inside of the cells—a considerable benefit for those plagued with bursitis, arthritis, and tendonitis.

Ningxia wolfberry supplies nutrients to enhance the proper assimilation and metabolism of sulfur.

INGREDIENTS:

MSM is a special organic sulfur that combats autoimmune diseases including arthritis, asthma, lupus, and scleroderma. MSM is critical to proper skin, hair, and liver health. MSM is the subject of a bestselling book, *The Miracle of MSM, The Natural Solution for Pain*, authored by UCLA neuropsychiatrist Ronald Lawrence M.D., Ph.D., and Stanley Jacob, M.D.

Ningxia wolfberry (*Lycium barbarum*) contains minerals and coenzymes to support sulfur metabolism.

Directions:

CAPS: Take 2 capsules two times daily one hour before or after meals.

POWDER: Take 1/2 teaspoon with distilled water two times daily one hour before or after meals

Companion Products: BLM, Super Cal, ArthroTune, Essentialzyme, Ortho Ease, PanAway, Mega Cal

Super B

Super B is a comprehensive source of the B vitamins essential for good health, including, thiamine (vitamin B1), riboflavin (vitamin B2), niacin (vitamin B3), pyridoxine (vitamin B6), vitamin B12, biotin, folic acid, and PABA. It also includes minerals that aid the assimilation and metabolism of B vitamins.

B vitamins are particularly important during times of stress when reserves are depleted. Although research has shown that megadoses of B vitamins are not healthy, it has been known that the diets of many Americans do not provide the recommended amount of B vitamins essential for normal functions of immune response.

When many B vitamins are combined at once in the stomach, it can cause a fermentation resulting in stomach upset. To avoid this, Super B uses a synergistic suspension isolation process to isolate the various vitamins so they are released at different times.

INGREDIENTS:

Folic acid protects heart and blood vessels.

Thiamin (vitamin B1) required for carbohydrate metabolism, and nerve cell function.

Riboflavin (vitamin B2) is crucial in the production of cellular energy, helps regenerate the liver, and prevents cellular mutations.

Niacin is essential for turning carbohydrates into energy. It lowers cholesterol and helps regulate blood sugar. At least 4.4 mg are needed for every 1,000 calories consumed to avoid pellagra.

Vitamin B6 supports immune function and protects the heart and blood vessels. It inhibits skin cancer growth and helps prevent kidney stones and PMS symptoms. Vitamin B6 requires folic acid and magnesium to maximize its effects.

Vitamin B12 is critical for red blood cell formation and proper immune and nerve function. Works with vitamin B6 to prevent heart disease. Vegetarians often lack adequate B12.

Biotin helps convert fats and amino acids into energy. It promotes healthy nails and hair and combats yeast and fungus overgrowth.

Magnesium is crucial for proper enzyme function, insulin action, muscle contractions and heart rhythm. It reduces high blood pressure.

PABA (para amino benzoic acid) assists healthy bacteria in producing folic acid. It also helps the bones form red blood cells.

Zinc is crucial for immunity, cell growth, wound healing, and proper action of many hormones, including insulin and growth hormone.

Selenium has been extensively researched for its anticancer and antioxidant properties.

Directions: Take 1/2 to 1 tablet daily, preferably with meals. If taken on an empty stomach, one may experience a niacin flush, a normal reaction which may last up to an hour.

Companion Products: Super C Chewable, Super Cal, AD&E, Longevity Capsules

Super C

Physical stress, alcohol, smoking, and using certain medications may lower the blood levels of this essential vitamin. When citrus fruits are not readily available, diets may not contain enough vitamin C. Super C is properly balanced with rutin, biotin, bioflavonoids, and trace minerals to work synergistically, balancing the electrolytes and increasing the absorption rate of vitamin C. Without bioflavonoids, vitamin C has a hard time getting inside cells; and without proper electrolyte balance and trace minerals, it will not stay there for long.

INGREDIENTS:

Vitamin C is an antioxidant essential for the creation of collagen, connective tissue, cartilage, tendons, and vital for immunity.

Citrus bioflavonoids dramatically enhance vitamin C activity and act as potent antioxidants.

Rutin helps prevent capillary fragility, preventing easy bruising, swelling, and nosebleeds.

Calcium is needed for healthy bones, teeth, and joints.

Cayenne is excellent as a general stimulant and stamina booster.

Zinc is crucial for immunity, cell growth, wound healing, and proper action of many hormones, including insulin and growth hormone.

Potassium is required for proper electrolyte balance and to prevent high blood pressure.

ESSENTIAL OILS:

Orange (*Citrus sinensis*) contains the powerful antioxidant limonene.

Tangerine (*Citrus nobilis)* is an anticoagulant and helps decongest the lymphatic system.

Lemon (*Citrus limon*) promotes leukocyte formation and increases lymphatic function.

Grapefruit (*Citrus paradisi*) prevents DNA and cellular mutation.

Lemongrass (*Cymbopogon flexuosus*) is antiparasitic, antifungal, and promotes digestion.

Directions: For reinforcing immune strength, 2 tablets daily. For maintenance, one tablet daily. Best taken before meals.

Companion Products: Exodus, ImmuPro, ImmuneTune, VitaGreen, Citrus Fresh, Exodus II, ImmuPower

Super C Chewable

The only vitamin C chewable vitamin in the world to combine citrus essential oils, citrus bioflavonoids, and whole-food natural vitamin C in one tablet.

According to Dr. Victor Herbert, professor of medicine at the Mount Sinai School of Medicine in New York, synthetic vitamin C as a supplement "is not an antioxidant. It'a redox agent--an antioxidant in some circumstances and a pro-oxidant in others." In other words, synthetic ascorbic acid can actually be a free-radical in some cases. Only natural vitamin C that occurs naturally in foods has no oxidizing effects.

Scientists are also discovering that Vitamin C needs be combined with citrus bioflavonoids to fully unlock its therapeutic effects. Bioflavonoids are known to have a vitamin P-type action that improves microcirculatory and blood vessel integrity.

INGREDIENTS:

Acerola cherry *(Malphighia glabra)* is one of the highest natural sources of vitamin C.

Citrus bioflavonoid *(Citrus limon)* enhances vitamin C activity. It is extremely high in antioxidants and flavonoids.

Calcium Carbonate is a source of dietary calcium to enhance vitamin C activity and absorption into the cell.

ESSENTIAL OIL:

Orange *(Citrus sinensis)* is rich in limonene, which prevents DNA and cellular mutation.

Directions: Take 2 to 4 tablets between meals. If under stress take 4 to 8 tablets during the day..

Companion Products: Exodus, ImmuPro, ImmuneTune, VitaGreen, Citrus Fresh, Exodus II, ImmuPower, Berry Young Juice.

Super Cal

A high-powered calcium, potassium, and magnesium complex. Restores proper electrolyte and hormonal balance, and improves muscle and bone development.

INGREDIENTS:

Calcium is essential for healthy bones and teeth. Calcium citrate is one of the best absorbed calciums available.

Magnesium works with calcium to build bones.

Potassium is vital for improving bone density.

Boron increase calcium utilization.

Zinc enhances calcium absorption and is crucial for proper hormone activity and growth hormone production

ESSENTIAL OILS:

Wintergreen (*Gaultheria procumbens*) relieves bone, joint, and muscle pain.

Marjoram (*Origanum majorana*) supports muscles and nerves.

Lemongrass (*Cymbopogon flexuosus*) is used for ligament support.

Myrtle (*Myrtus communis*) supports muscles.

Directions: Take 1 to 2 capsules before meals.

Companion Products: ArthroTune, BLM, Ortho Sport, Ortho Ease, Sulfurzyme, Idaho Balsam Fir, Peppermint, Mega Cal

COMPARISON OF YOUNG LIVING'S CALCIUM SUPPLEMENTS

	MegaCal	SuperCal
Calcium per Serving	618 mg	242 mg
Percent of RDI of Calcium	61%	24%
Type of calcium	Lactate, Carbonate, Glycerophosphate Ascorbate	Citrate
Source of Calcium	High purity precipitated	High purity precipitated
Calcium:Magnesium Ratio	1:1	3:1
Other minerals	Potassium, Zinc, Copper, Manganese	Potassium Zinc, Boron
Additional nutrients	Xylitol, vitamin C	
Benefits	Fights osteoporosis, alleviates muscle cramps; supports normal thyroid function	Fights osteoporosis, Jointsupport, improves metabolism; supports normal thyroid function
Designed for	Diets high in dairy products	Vegetarians, diets restricted in calories or high in carbonated beverages
Directions	Take 1 tbsp. 1 hour after meals	Take 1-2 capsules between meals
Other info	Time-released mineral complex	

ThermaBurn

A revolutionary appetite-suppressing, weight-control herbal complex with thermogenic essential oils. It is the only herbal, fat-reducing supplement to contain liver cleansers and defatters to increase metabolism and prevent oxidative damage from excess fat-burning.

INGREDIENTS:

Chromium polynicotinate acts as a "spark plug" for revving metabolism and carbohydrate burning.

Boron promotes calcium utilization.

Inositol hexaniacinate improves circulation and insulin action.

Di-methionine protects the liver cells from oxidative damage due to increased metabolism.

Theobromine is a natural energizer that increases red blood cells. When combined with niacin, it boosts blood flow.

L-carnitine is an amino acid so powerful that an entire book was written discussing its fat-burning and energizing effects (*The Carnitine Miracle* by R. Crayhon, M.S.).

Garcinia cambogia increases metabolism and fat burning on a cellular level. It speeds the oxidation/burning of carbohydrates while suppressing fat synthesis (*Lowenstein, 1971; Sullivan et al., 1974; Rao et al., 1988*).

Guarana extract is high in xanthines, which provide energizing and appetite-suppressing effects (Engels et al., *1999*).

Licorice root extract increases fat utilization and glycogen production in the liver.

Yerba mate extract contains matein, which exerts a safe, energizing effect that combats fatigue. This herb has been used for centuries to increase endurance and promote health.

ESSENTIAL OILS:

Nutmeg (*Myristica fragrans*) helps support the adrenal glands for increased energy.

Spearmint (*Mentha spicata*) improves digestion.

Peppermint (*Mentha piperita*) has the ability to directly affect the brain's satiety center, triggering a sense of fullness after meals.

Myrtle (*Myrtus communis*) may help increase thyroid function.

Frankincense (*Boswellia carteri*) is a thermogenic antioxidant.

Canadian fleabane (*Conyza candensis*) increases growth hormone production.

Directions: Take 1 to 2 capsules two hours before or after meals.

Companion Products: Thyromin, Power Meal, En-R-Gee, BodyGize

ThermaMist Oral Spray

A revolutionary appetite-suppressing, weight-control herbal complex with thermogenic essential oils. It has a very high nutrient absorption rate due to its oral absorption method of delivery. It affords unmatched appetite and metabolism control.

INGREDIENTS:

Vitamin B3 (Niacin) is a critical coenzyme used in cellular reactions involved with energy metabolism.

Guarana leaf extract is high in xanthines, which provide energizing and appetite-suppressing effects (Engels et al., *1999*).

Yerba mate extract contains matein, which exerts a safe, energizing action that helps combat fatigue (Weiner, 1994) and enhance metabolism.

Yohimbe extract is an energizing herb grown in Africa.

Schizandra supports normal liver function and the breakdown of fats in the liver. It is also a superb antioxidant (Naggai et al., 1988; Zhao et.al., *1990*)

Garcinia cambogia increases metabolism and fat burning on a cellular level. It speeds the oxidation/burning of carbohydrates while suppressing fat synthesis (*Lowenstein, 1971; Sullivan et al., 1974; Rao et al., 1988*).

5-HTP (5-hydroxytryptophan) is known to help suppress the appetite and reduce hunger.

Stevia increases insulin efficiency.

Chromium nicotinate helps burn fats, and enhances insulin utilization.

ESSENTIAL OILS:

Peppermint (*Mentha piperita*) has the ability to directly affect the brain's satiety center, triggering a sense of fullness after meals.

Spearmint (*Mentha spicata*) has hormone-like properties that support the thyroid.

Grapefruit (*Citrus paradisi*) stimulates fat-burning and cellulite elimination.

Directions: Spray 3 sprays into buccal cavity of the mouth 3 times a day or whenever "cravings" occur. Individual needs may vary.

Companion Products: ThermaBurn, Be-Fit, Thyromin

Thyromin

This product was developed to nourish the thyroid, balance metabolism, and reduce fatigue. It contains a combination of specially selected glandular nutrients, herbs, amino acids, minerals, and essential oils. All of the oils are therapeutic-grade quality and are perfectly balanced to bring about the most beneficial and nutritional support to the thyroid.

INGREDIENTS:

Adrenal/pituitary extracts from bovine sources (Argentina) provide the building blocks to thyroid hormone synthesis.

Vitamin E is a potent antioxidant.

Iodine (kelp) is a key component of the T3 and T4 thyroid hormones that are pivotal for increasing energy levels and metabolism.

Potassium supports healthy thyroid function.

CoQ10 is used by cells in the body to convert food to energy.

L-cysteine is an amino acid for thyroid health.

ESSENTIAL OILS:

Peppermint (*Mentha piperita*) supports digestion and pancreatic function.

Spearmint (*Mentha spicata*) has hormone-like properties that support the thyroid.

Myrtle (*Myrtus communis*) may help increase thyroid function.

Myrrh (*Commiphora myrrha*) is also a thyroid supporter.

Directions: Take 1 to 2 capsules daily, immediately before going to sleep.

Companion Products: VitaGreen, ThermaBurn, ThermaMist, En-R-Gee, EndoFlex

Ultra Young

Ultra Young is a revolutionary spray supplement that supports healthy pituitary and growth hormone secretion. It contains *Vicia faba*, which contains L-dopa. In 1976 a National Institute of Aging study found that administration of L-dopa to patients over 60 years of age resulted in a dramatic increase in growth hormone levels. A study conducted by Dr. George Cotzias showed that mice, fed small doses of L-dopa, lived twice as long as the control group not receiving L-dopa.

INGREDIENTS:

Vicia faba major contains L-dopa, an amino acid shown to restore the sensitivity of the hypothalamus and increase growth hormone production.

Ningxia wolfberry (*Lycium barbarum*) is rich in polysaccharides, which have potent immune-stimulating effects, raising levels of immunoglobulin A (IgA), an immune protein that steadily declines with age.

L-arginine is an amino acid that helps increase natural growth hormone production.

L-glutamine is an amino acid that boost growth hormone levels.

Zinc complex plays a pivotal part in maintaining optimal pituitary function.

GABA (Gamma-aminobutyric acid) is a nutrient that can amplify growth hormone production.

Vitamin B3 provides nutritional support for the hypothalamus and pituitary.

Vitamin B6 supports glandular function.

Vitamin E protects the heart and blood and combats free-radical oxidative damage.

Selenium has been extensively researched for its anticancer and antioxidant properties.

Stevia is a super-sweet supplement.

ESSENTIAL OILS:

Sandalwood (*Santalum album*) stimulates the hypothalamus and pituitary glands and boosts natural growth hormone production.

Fleabane (*Conyza canadensis*) stimulates growth hormone secretion from the pituitary.

Directions: Spray Ultra Young directly inside cheeks and on the roof of the mouth. Avoid swallowing for 1 to 2 minutes. Spray upon waking, between meals, and just before retiring. Avoid spraying on the tongue because this reduces its effectiveness. It is best used 1 to 2 hours before or after meals, with no snacking in-between because high blood sugar levels also reduce its effectiveness.

Companion Products: Essential Manna, Wolfberry Crisp, Berry Young Juice, Longevity Capsules, ImmuPro, JuvaPower/Spice

Ultra Young +

Contains the same ingredients as Ultra Young but with the addition of DHEA, a precursor to many important hormones.

VitaGreen

This supplement is a high protein, high-energy chlorophyll formula that invigorates and revitalizes the cells. It supports the immune, thyroid, and digestive health.

Clinical experience has shown that before putting oils in VitaGreen, there was 42 percent blood absorption in 24 hours. After adding essential oils to VitaGreen, blood absorption increased to 64 percent in 30 minutes and 86 percent in an hour. The conclusion was that the cells were now receiving nutrients that they had previously not been able to assimilate.

INGREDIENTS:

Spirulina is a source of chlorophyll, a magnesium-rich pigment that has been linked to improved energy and metabolism. Spirulina has been used as a tonic, purifier, and detoxifier. It targets the immune system, liver, kidneys, blood, intestinal flora, and cardiovascular systems.

Barley grass juice concentrate is an antioxidant that is rich in minerals.

Bee pollen is high in protein and low in fat and sodium. It is loaded with vitamins and minerals, including potassium, calcium, magnesium, zinc, manganese, copper, and B vitamins.

Panax ginseng boosts energy and reduces stress. It also has the unique ability to stimulate lymphocyte formation (an essential part of the immune system).

L-arginine is an amino acid that promotes circulation in the small capillaries of our tissues, improving nutrient delivery and cellular metabolism.

L-cystine is an amino acid that supports healthy liver function and hair.

L-tyrosine supports the formation of neurotransmitters, such as dopamine and serotonin.

Choline bitartrate has been used in the treatment of Alzheimer's disease. It is essential for liver health.

Kelp contains nutrients to prevent thyroid hormone deficiency and estrogen imbalance.

ESSENTIAL OILS:

Melissa (*Melissa officinalis*) is anti-inflammatory and energizing.

Lemon (*Citrus limon*) prevents cellular mutation and enhances DNA repair.

Lemongrass (*Cymbopogon flexuosus*) is antiparasitic, antifungal, and boosts digestion.

Rosemary (*Rosmarinus officinalis*) fights candida and balances the endocrine system.

Directions: Take 3 capsules, three times daily.

Companion Products: Power Meal, Thyromin, Wolfberry Crisp, En-R-Gee

WheyFit

The only high-protein nutrient complex to include powerful whole-food antioxidants, thermogenic essential oils, and liver protectors to enhance fat burning. When used conscienciously, WheyFit reduces body fat as it helps build muscles and increase endurance. It contains antioxidant ingredients promoting insulin action and protecting the body from oxidative stress.

INGREDIENTS:

Protein (from whey, egg whites, and soy)

Whey is proven to be one of the most complete proteins and the most easily digested, it helps build and tone muscle tissue when used with any fitness or exercise program.

Ultrafiltered Microfiltered Whey is the best source of high quality protein, with the highest Protein Efficiency Ratio and Protein Digestability Corrected Amino Acid Score. It is rich in alpha-lactalbumin, beat lactoglobulin, immunoglobulins, lactoferrin, lactoperoxidase, calcium and magnesium. Ultrafiltered whey is far superior to the denatured protein found in ion exchange whey which is very high in sodium and low in calcium, potassium, and magnesium, Ion exchange whey is also devoid of glycomicropeptides, lactoperoxidase, and lactoferrin.

Lecithin is rich in phosphatidylcholine an essential nutrient for liver health. A healthy liver is essential for keeping metabolic systems at peak potential and vital for increasing fat oxidation.

Protein-Digesting Enzyme Complex contains an array of proteases designed to work in different acid/alkaline environments, amplifying protein digestion. As the human body ages, enzyme production drops dramatically, which increases protein underabsorption and malabsorption. This creates an amino acid deficiency and triggers allergic reactions from putrifying proteins in the intestinal tract.

FOS (Fructooligosaccharides) is one of the best-documented natural fibers for improving the healthy balance of bacteria in the digestive system. Technically a fiber, rather than sugar, FOS triggers no spikes in blood sugar levels the way sucrose and glucose do. It has been shown to balance blood sugar levels, help support liver function, and improve calcium and magnesium absorption (Cambell et al., 1997; Alles et al., Morohashi et al., 1998).

Blueberry powder has been documented to be one of the most powerful antioxidants known, rich in flavonoids that quench free radicals and protect against cellular DNA damage (Cao et al., 1999; Edenharder et al., *1994*).

Strawberry powder is high in ellagic acid, a powerful antioxidant that protects against cellular mutation and liver damage. (Narayanan et al., 1999; Singh et al., 1999).

Zinc is crucial for immunity, cell growth, wound healing, and proper action of many hormones, including insulin and growth hormone.

L-selenomethionine is a source of selenium, a powerful antioxidant mineral vital for the creation of superoxide dismutase. Studies at the University of Arizona have examined its ability to reduce the risk of cancer.

ESSENTIAL OILS:

Lemon (*Citrus limon*) prevents cellular mutation and enhances DNA repair (Reddy et al., 1998).

Directions: Mix 1 level scoop with 1 cup of distilled water, rice milk or goat milk.

Companion Products: AminoTech, ThermaBurn, Be-Fit, Royal Essence, Vitagreen, PowerMeal, BodyGize

Wolfberry Crisp

A whole food, low-glycemic super-nutrient complex containing over 14 grams of protein per serving. It is rich in antioxidants and phytonutrients and does not significantly raise blood sugar levels. Can be used as a meal replacement.

INGREDIENTS:

Soy & Whey Protein Complex is an ideal source of balanced, quality protein

Organic blue agave (*Agave tequilana*) **nectar** is a very low glycemic index (39) organic cactus extract that is sweeter than sucrose.

Raw almond butter is high in monounsaturated fats, minerals (magnesium and potassium) and fiber.

Ningxia wolfberry fruit is the highest antioxidant food known, rich in alpha carotene, beta carotene, lutein and zeaxanthin.

Raw pumpkin (*Curcubita pepo*) **seeds** are high in zinc, magnesium, calcium and phytosterols and sterolins. They also contain fatty acids that neutralize parasites. Pumpkin seeds must be eaten raw, since roasted or cooked seeds harbor altered fat that creates arterial plaque.

Raw cashews (*anacardium occidentale*) have high levels of monounsaturated fatty acids and selenium, magnesium, and potassium.

Raw walnuts (*Juglans regia*) are very high in ALA (Alpha lipoic acid), an important Omega-3 fat crucial for human health. Of all the nuts, it has the second-best omega 3 to omega 6 ratio. According to a recent study at the Thomas Jefferson University in Philadelphia, PA, "walnuts, when consumed as part of a low fat, low-cholesterol diet, have a beneficial effect on serum cardiovascular risk factors."

Unsweetened carob chips

Pure vanilla bean (*Vanilla planifolia*) **extract** is a pure extract of Madagascar vanilla beans.

Natural banana flavoring is a natural flavoring that is completely free of propylene glycol.

Directions: Eat 1 bar a day, or as a meal alternative.

Companion Products: JuvaPower, JuvaSpice, Berry Young Juice, Longevity capsules, Berrgyize Bar

11

Topical Hormone Therapy

Declining Hormones Signal Old Age

As we age, critical hormone imbalances can contribute to accelerated aging and heighten risk of cancers and other chronic diseases. Hormone replacement therapy using natural hormones (not synthetic analogues or look-alikes) in a cream application for transdermal absorption may be the best solution for reducing risk of cancer and alleviating other chronic diseases such as osteoporosis, disturbed sleep, depression, and obesity. In the specific case of progesterone, Harvard University researcher, John R. Lee, MD, found that natural progesterone is "very well absorbed through the skin, 40 to 70 times more efficiently than if you take it by mouth."

Research also indicates that essential oils enhance the penetration of topical hormone into the blood. This means that topical hormone creams with essential oils are more effective than other creams without penetration enhancers.

Hormones that decline with age include, DHEA, melatonin, testosterone, and progesterone. Estrogens (estradiol) can also drop with age, although not as quickly as progesterone, which creates an estrogen dominant condition common in women over 40. Cortisol, sometimes referred to as the death hormone, increases with age, contributing to a number of age-related problems.

Insomnia, Immunity, and Cancer

Declines in melatonin are directly linked with lowered immunity, disturbed sleep cycles, and heightened cancer risk. Declines in DHEA are correlated with lower energy and central obesity.

CAUTION: Before commencing any regimen of natural progesterone, pregnenolone, or DHEA supplementation, you should have your hormone levels tested and evaluated by a health care professional or a reliable laboratory which specializes in saliva hormone tests. In an arena as complex as hormone therapy, it is critical that any deficiencies be correctly identified BEFORE supplementation is initiated.

ZRT Laboratories offers affordable, accurate at-home testing of the following hormones:

Progesterone	DHEA
Estradiol	Estrone
Estriol	Testosterone
Melatonin	

ZRT Labs can be contacted at:
PHONE: (503) 466-2445
WEBSITE: www.salivatest.com/index.html

Cortisol: The Death Hormone

Hormones that increase with age, such as cortisol can also contribute to many age-related chronic diseases such as high blood pressure, abdominal obesity and blood sugar imbalances. Lowering cortisol levels not only increases immunity but also increases insulin sensitivity and enhances fat metabolism.

Dangers of Synthetic Hormones

Recent research has discredited many of the supposed benefits of synthetic hormones such as conjugated (horse urine) estrogens and medroxyprogesterone acetate and other synthetic progestins.

These patented synthetic imposters of human hormones are very different biochemically than the natural hormones found in plants and in the human body, and their effects can be hazardous to health. Long term use of these synthetic hormones has been linked with dramatically higher risks of heart disease, ovarian cancer, breast cancer, and osteoporosis. (Natural hormones cannot be patented.)

In contrast, the natural hormones found in the human body are some of the safest natural compounds to prevent heart disease and cancer. A good example of natural hormone safety is illustrated by progesterone. When a woman reaches the late stage of pregnancy, her levels of progesterone rise to over 300 times that of normal, and both mother and child thrive on this.

Osteoporosis and Prostate Cancer

Natural progesterone has been used to successfully treat osteoporosis, heart disease, and breast cancer in women. Research by Dr. John R. Lee, MD has shown that progesterone can be to used to effectively treat prostate cancer and Benign Prostate Hyperplasia (BPH) in men.

Lowering Cancer Risk Naturally

As women grow older and approach menopause (between age 35 and 45), they become increasingly susceptible to estrogen dominance, due to an increased frequency of ovulation and dramatically lowered production of progesterone. This shortage of progesterone can lead to osteoporosis, mood swings, depression, weight gain, and increased risk of breast, endometrial, cervical, and uterine cancers.

Premenopausal women can also suffer from an estrogen deficiency, which can markedly raise their risk of heart disease (which is one reason why women's risk of heart disease reaches the equivalents of men's after age 40). A simultaneous estrogen and progesterone deficiency is one of the most common and insidious conditions afflicting women over age 40 and can result in significant deleterious effects on both physical and mental health.

Transdermal hormone creams have revolutionized the way women can manage hormone control. Because natural progesterone, pregnenolone, and DHEA are readily absorbed through the skin and into the tissues, they are rapidly becoming the standard for convenient and economical hormone replacement therapy in the United States.

Usage Guide for Progessence, Prenolone, and Prenolone+

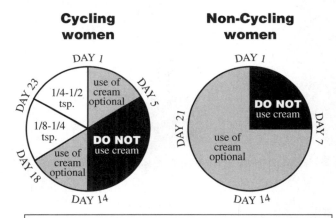

Hormone Content in mg (per ounce)			
	Pregnenolone	Progesterone	DHEA
Progessence	0	400	
Regenolone	1000	5	
NeuroGen	1000	5	100
Prenolone	1000	5	
Prenolone+	1000	5	250
PD80/20	640		160

A variety of transdermal hormone creams are available to target both progesterone, estrogen, and DHEA deficiencies among women. Women who are primarily progesterone deficient and estrogen dominant, primarily need progesterone supplementation. Women who are both estrogen and progesterone deficient, need both pregnenolone and progesterone hormones (the body converts pregnenolone into the needed amounts of estrogen).

Andropause: Menopause in Men

Declining testosterone and DHEA occurs in men over 40 and has the following symptoms

Loss of sexual desire
Lower strength (shrinking muscles)
Reduced energy
Depression
Increased anxiety
Thinning hair
Wrinkles
Prostate Problems (restricted urine flow, sexual performance etc.)

To combat these symptoms, a cream containing DHEA and pregnenolone is a first line of defense treatment.

Essential Oils: Hormone Skin Penetration Enhancers

A number of clinical studies have shown that essential oils enhance by many times the ability of hormones and other medicines to penetrate the skin and enter the blood stream.

Studies conducted at Pisa University in 2002 found that essential oils (ie., cajeput, cardamom, melissa, myrtle, niaouli, orange oil) and essential oil components (1,8 cineole, alpha-pinene, alpha-terpineol, d-limonene) dramatically boosted estradiol hormone penetration through the skin and into the blood and tissues. Studies at the University of Bradford in the UK also found that essential oil compounds enhanced drug penetration by 13 times. A 1996 study at the China Pharmaceutical University in Nanjing similarly found a dramatic increase in drug absorption following eucalyptus and peppermint essential oils. [1,2,3]

Products

ImmuPro

Boosts MELATONIN and T-lymphocyte immune cells. Designed for people who have interrupted or shortened sleep cycles, low immunity, or high risk of cancer.

ACTIVE INDREDIENTS:

4 mg/oz melatonin

Directions: Take 2-4 tablets before bed.

(See Chapter 10 for more information on this product)

NeuroGen

NERVE REGENERATION cream. Designed for people who suffer nerve degeneration (diabetics) or pain.

A topically applied pregnenolone cream that contains essential oils, hormones, and nutrients designed to stimulate nerve regeneration.

For more information on pregnenolone's ability to regenerate nerves, please consult: *Pregnenolone: A Radical New Approach to Health, Long Life, and Emotional Well-Being* by D. Gary Young.

ACTIVE INDREDIENTS:

1,000 mg/oz pregnenolone from soybeans
5 mg/oz natural progesterone from soybeans
100 mg/oz natural DHEA from wild yam

INGREDIENTS: Moisture cream base, lecithin, pregnenolone, trace minerals, wheat germ oil, wild yam, eluethero, black cohosh, blue cohosh.

Essential Oils: Helichrysum, juniper, peppermint, lemongrass, frankincense, and spearmint.

Directions: Apply 1/8 to 1/4 tsp. on location 3 x day or as needed for nerve regeneration.

Companion Products: Sulfurzyme, BLM, PanAway.

Prenolone

Boosts ESTROGEN & PROGESTERONE levels. Designed for people who either have insufficient results with **Progessence** or have deficient levels of both estrogen and progesterone.

A topically applied pregnenolone cream that is designed as a broad-spectrum hormone supplement for men and women.

A powerful natural hormone cream that treats osteoporosis, depression, bloating, mood swings, weight gain, PMS, menstrual irregularity, cramps.

Pregnenolone is the precursor hormone from which the body creates all other sex and adrenal hormones, including progesterone, estradiol, estrone, estriol, testosterone, DHEA, and aldosterone.

ACTIVE INDREDIENTS:

1000 mg/oz pregnenolone from soybeans
5 mg/oz natural progesterone from soybeans

INGREDIENTS: Moisture cream base, lecithin, pregnenolone, trace minerals, wheat germ oil, wild yam, eluethero, black cohosh, blue cohosh.

1. Abdullah D, Ping QN, Liu GJ. "Enhancing effect of essential oils on the penetration of 5-fluorouracil through rat skin." *Yao Xue Xue Bao.* 1996;31(3):214-21.

2. Monti D, et al., "Effect of different terpene-containing essential oils on permeation of estradiol through hairless mouse skin." *Int J Pharm.* 2002 Apr 26;237(1-2):209-14.

3. Cornwell PA, Barry BW. "Sesquiterpene components of volatile oils as skin penetration enhancers for the hydrophilic permeant 5-fluorouracil." *J Pharm Pharmacol.* 1994 Apr;46(4):261-9.

Essential Oils: Clary sage, conyza, geranium, fennel, sage and blue yarrow.

Directions: Massage 1/4 to 1/2 tsp. thoroughly into soft tissue areas of the body (arms, thighs, abdomen, neck etc.) until absorbed. Rotate sites of application daily. Individual needs may vary. Apply for three weeks out of the month (See chart on page 168).

Companion Products: Prenolone+, Progessence, Sulfurzyme, PD80/20.

Prenolone +

Boosts ESTROGEN, PROGESTERONE, & DHEA levels. Designed for people who either have inadequate results with **Progessence** or **Prenolone**, or have deficient levels of estrogen, progesterone, and DHEA or testosterone.

Contains pure pregnenolone derived from soy. Also contains DHEA derived from wild yam. This triple hormone cream is designed for those who require a more rounded hormone balance or who have insufficient levels of testosterone or DHEA. For usage, instructions, and ingredients, see Prenolone.

ACTIVE INDREDIENTS:

1000 mg/oz pregnenolone from soybeans
5 mg/oz natural progesterone from soybeans
250 mg/oz natural DHEA from wild yam

Progessence Cream

To combat ESTROGEN DOMINANCE and amplify progesterone levels. The first treatment of choice for women over 40.

Increased progesterone is very powerful anti-aging therapy for women over 40, and has been shown effective to reverse osteoporosis, depression, bloating, weight gain, PMS menstrual problems, and heightened risk of breast, cervical, ovarian, and uterine cancer and heart disease. For those who are deficient in both progesterone and estrogen, use **Prenolone**.

Progessence contains high levels of natural, soy-derived progesterone identical to that produced in the human body. It combats estrogen dominance, a condition common in women over 40 years of age.

Symptoms of estrogen dominance include hot flashes, depression, bloating, weight gain, excessive bone loss, and increased risk of breast and endometrial cancer and heart disease.

John Lee, MD, discusses in detail the benefits of topically applied progesterone in his book, "What Your Doctor May Not Tell You About Menopause." According to Dr. Lee, progesterone can actually reverse bone loss in older women as well as reduce the need for hormone replacement in women lacking ovaries or not ovulating.

Studies have shown the skin application of progesterone creams results in far better absorption than hormones taken orally. Further studies have shown that combining hormones with essential oils further amplifies skin absorption into the blood stream.

ACTIVE INDREDIENTS:

400 mg/oz pure progesterone from soybeans.

INGREDIENTS: Moisture cream base, lecithin, pregnenolone, trace minerals, wheat germ oil, wild yam, eluethero, black cohosh, blue cohosh.

Essential Oils: Clary sage, conyza, geranium, fennel, sage and blue yarrow.

Directions: Massage 1/4 to 1/2 tsp. thoroughly into soft tissue areas of the body (arms, thighs, abdomen, neck etc.) until absorbed. Rotate sites of application daily. Individual needs may vary. Apply for three weeks out of the month (See chart on page 168).

Companion Products: PD 80/20, Dragon Time

Regenolone

MUSCLE AND JOINT PAIN cream. Designed for people who suffer severe pain, inflammation, and stiffness from arthritis, rheumatism, or other muscle and joint conditions.

Contains pure pregnenolone derived from soy. Also includes MSM and essential oils to provide unmatched relief from arthritis pain, back pain, and other muscle and skeletal inflammation and pain..

ACTIVE INDREDIENTS:

1,000 mg/oz pregnenolone from soy beans
5 mg/oz natural progesterone from soybeans

INGREDIENTS: Moisture cream base, lecithin, pregnenolone, trace minerals, wheat germ oil, wild yam, eluethero, black cohosh, blue cohosh.

Essential Oils: Wintergreen, peppermint, douglas fir, oregano and spearmint.

Directions: Apply 1/8 to 1/4 tsp. on location 3 x day or as needed to combat pain associated with arthritis, sciatica, back pain, and carpal tunnel syndrome.

Companion Products: Sulfurzyme, Essential Omegas, BLM, OrthoEase, Lemon-Sandalwood Bar Soap, Peppermint-Cedarwood Bar Soap, AromaSiez, PanAway

OTHER HORMONE SOLUTIONS FOR WOMEN (See Chapter 10 for more detailed information on these products.)

CortiStop WOMEN

Contains progesterone and hormone precursors which slow cortisol production in women.

PD 80/20

Contains pregnenolone and DHEA in a capsule for ingestion. It is designed for people who do not benefit from hormone creams such as Progessence, Prenolone, or Prenolone+.

Each capsule contains 640 mg of pure pregnenolone from soy and 160 mg of pure DHEA from wild yam.

Essential Oils

Many women ages 40-plus have found that essential oils effectively combat PMS and menopause problems. Oils with estrogen-like activity include fennel, anise, clary sage, and sage.

Fennel, anise, and clary sage can be combined in equal proportions in a double 00 capsule and ingested 2 to 8 capsules per day to raise estrogen levels. Find an endocrinologist who will monitor your estrogen levels through blood testing every 30 days until you have

reached the levels you want. Research at the Young Life Research Clinic has shown that ingestion of these oils in capsules up to 8 per day **does not** cause side effects or toxicity to the human body or liver.

The blends of Dragon Time, SclarEssence, Lady Sclareol and Transformation have been used with excellent results by many women to balance and normalize hormone levels.

HORMONE SOLUTIONS FOR MEN
(See Chapter 10 for more detailed information on these products.)

ProGen

Contains high-powered herbal extracts (i.e., saw palmetto, Pygeum africanum) that improve prostate function. It slows the body's production of DHT, a hormone that creates abnormal cell proliferation in the prostate. BPH (benign prostate hyperplasia), common in men over age 40, can eventually lead to prostate cancer, one of the most common forms of cancer in the United States. BPH symptoms include incontinence, restricted urine flow, and impotence.

Maintenance: Take 2-3 capsules, 2 times daily

Aggressive deterioration: 6 capsules, 3 times daily.

Mister

An essential oil blend that supports the male reproductive system. May be taken as a dietary supplement: 3-10 drops under tongue, 2-3 times daily. Take 10-20 drops in water or in a capsule, 2 times daily. Use no more than 7 days and then rest 4 days. Massage on Vita Flex points between scrotum and rectum.

12

Water Treatment

According to Environmental Protection Agency (EPA) reports, 40 million Americans are exposed to levels of lead in water that exceed the EPA-proposed maximum contaminant allowances. Even at low levels, lead in water causes reduced birth weight, premature births, delayed mental development, and impaired mental abilities.

Scientists at the U.S. Public Health Service report that trihalomethanes (dangerous toxins made from chlorine) found in tap water have been linked to higher-than-normal rates of miscarriage and birth defects.[1]

Using information gathered from the EPA, the National Resources Defense Council (NRDC) reports that more than 45 million Americans drink tap water polluted with fecal matter, pesticides, toxic chemicals, radiation, and lead.

The inhalation of trihalomethanes (in a vapor form that occurs with hot water) while showering is more toxic than drinking chlorinated water. Buying drinking water does not protect consumers from inhaling vapors.

Reports from the EPA indicate that entities such as mining companies and electrical power plants release 7.8 billion pounds of toxic substances per year onto the land, into the water, and into the air, and the amount is increasing.

The NRDC reports that over 940,000 Americans are sickened by contaminated tap water annually. In addition, the council reports that contaminated tap water kills 900 people each year. For more information on water pollution, see Appendix M

H₂Oils - Lemon, Lemon/Grapefruit, Lemon/Orange, Peppermint

H2Oils are special packets of essential oils that allow passive and gradual diffusion of essential oils into water or ambient air. Each packet contains up to 10 ml of essential oil.

Directions: Place one or more individual oil packets in sealed water dispenser. Allow them to steep for several hours or overnight. Packets can be left in water dispenser for up to four days.

RainSpa Shower Head

The RainSpa Shower Head is a refreshing alternative to the necessity of drawing a bath to enjoy bath salts. Simply pour your bath salts (or mix your own using essential oils and Epsom salts) into the showerhead, attach to your current plumbing and enjoy a shower as invigorating as a walk in the spring rain.

How to use: Attach to shower outlet. Detach bath salt container, fill half-full with bath salts, and reattach container. Make sure the on/off button of the shower head is in the off position. Begin flow of shower water, and switch the on/off button to the on position and enjoy your fragrant shower.

Shower Mate Filter

The Shower Mate Filter is a revolutionary portable water filter using a patented metal-alloy filtering system. The metal-alloy attracts organic particles, bacteria, and viruses and then binds them to a metal membrane where they are subjected to a

---

1. Magnus, P., et al. "Water Chlorination and Birth Defects." *Epidemiology,* 10:513-517 (1999)

small electrical charge that inactivates them. The key to the filter's effectiveness is a patented, copper-zinc membrane that generates an electrostatic charge when wet. This charge literally captures toxic metals found in ordinary tap water so that they are filtered out, providing cleaner, purer water. It filters out 99% of the chemicals in municipal water.

How to use: First remove the RainSpa (or other) Shower Head from the overhead pipe, remove any existing filter, insert the Shower Mate Filter coupling mate into the overhead shower pipe.

Whole House Water Filtration System

This commercial-quality filter is able to purify 150,000 gallons of water before a cartridge change is necessary (about once a year). Not only does this unit last five times longer than most other similar filters, but a manufactuer five-year guarantee against defects. Lifetime warranty on casing. This filter removes hazards that include:

- Giardia
- Cryptosporidium
- Trihalomethanes
- Chlorine
- Pesticides
- Lead

Water is filtered through two state-of-the art cartridges.

CARTRIDGE 1: DUAL GRADIENT FILTER

The first contains a dual-gradient filter that has one layer wrapped around the other to provide finer filtration than is found in most other filters. In the second, water flows through a high-powered carbon briquette filter system not available through retail channels.

The dual-gradient cartridge has three times the dirt-holding capacity of similarly sized cartridges. It removes sediment (dirt, sand, grit, rust, etc.) from the water to extend the life of the charcoal filters. In addition, the inner layers reduce the levels of fine particles.

CARTRIDGE 2: CARBON BRIQUETTE

The superior carbon filter system contains a carbon-briquette cartridge of bonded powdered charcoal. The powdered consistency of the briquette allows for increased surface contact that results in maximum absorption of chlorine.

The 0.5 micron post filter greatly reduces bacteria, including giardia and cryptosporidium.

The carbon filter removes trihalomethanes, which might otherwise be consumed, absorbed through the skin, or inhaled during a shower. It also reduces lead, and removes pesticides, odors, and objectionable tastes.

CARTRIDGE 3 (optional): UV FILTER

A third UV filtration unit is available separately. It will kill all types of viruses, bacteria, and fungi.

13

Skin Care

Human skin is like a large sponge. It absorbs traces of almost everything that comes into contact with it—both harmful and beneficial. The skin is especially susceptible to exposure to organic solvents and petroleum-based chemicals. When some of these come into contact with the skin, they can be absorbed in far higher volumes than other types of substances.

This means that many questionable petrochemicals commonly found in personal care products, such as Soldium Laurel Sulphate (SLS), Triethanol amine (DEA), PEGs, and quarterniums can be absorbed into the skin. Over time, some of these chemicals may accumulate in the organs and tissues and result in mounting brain, nerve, and liver damage (Matthew et al., 1995).

A Troubling Trend

The most troubling indication that the synthetic chemicals in cosmetics and shampoos may be leaching into our bodies was provided by the government-funded Human Adipose Tissue Survey (Bock, 1996). According to this study, almost every person tested showed measurable levels of petroleum-based, carcinogenic chemicals, such as toluene, benzene, and styrene, in their fatty tissues.

This is why increasing numbers of health professionals are recommending personal care formulas that are completely natural and free of synthetic or petroleum-based ingredients. "To stay healthy, people have do more than just exercise and eat healthy," states Denver physician Terry Friedmann, M.D. "Consumer should also avoid personal care products that contain toxic synthetic ingredients that can penetrate the skin and accumulate in their tissues. In some cases, these products can have a greater impact on health than either diet or exercise." AromaSilk skin care products contain wolfberry seed oil, a costly and unusual ingredient that makes important contributions to healthy skin (see box). Along with wolfberry seed oil, AromaSilk products contains MSM, an essential nutrient that has an unsurpassed ability to strengthen the skin. "MSM is absolutely dynamite for the skin," says international fashion model Teri Williams, who was a cover model for Vogue Magazine. "In my experience, it is the single most important nutrient to support healthy skin and hair."

Ronald Lawrence, M.D., Ph.D. agrees. "The importance of MSM for healthy skin and hair cannot be overemphasized. In my clinical practice, I have seen the difference that MSM makes. It is outstanding whether applied topically or taken as dietary supplement."

In addition to wolfberry seed oil and MSM, the AromaSilk skin products also contain therapeutic-grade essential oils that have a long history of use in skin care. Pure myrrh, sandalwood, geranium, rosewood, frankincense, and Roman chamomile essential oils have been used to preserve the health of the skin throughout recorded history.

AromaSilk also includes a proprietary blend of antioxidant herbal extracts, such as Ginkgo biloba, orange blossom, witch hazel, cucumber, horse chestnut, and aloe vera gel, as well as special blends of pure vegetable oils such as almond, jojoba, avocado, and rose hip seeds oils.

"They feel fabulous on my skin," raves Kay Cansler, a former Director of Educational Diagnostics. "Without question, these are products for the new millennium. I've been using them for six months, and I can feel and see a huge difference. I am very, very impressed."

A.R.T. Day Activator

Age Refining Technology (A.R.T.) Day Activator cream combines the skin revitalizing power of essential oils with a proprietary anti-aging peptide complex that reduces the look of fine lines and wrinkles, diminishes age spots, evens skin tone and increases the elasticity and density of your skin. A.R.T. Day Activator delivers a noticeable difference—more youthful-looking skin.

Ingredients (all plant-derived):

Base: Deionized Water, Pentylene glycol, Glycerine, Glycerol stearate, Cetearyl alcohol, Caprylic triglycerides

Plant Extracts: Plankton,Meadowfoam Seed Oil, Shea Butter, Aloe *(Aloe barbadensis),* Dipotassium Glycyrrhizate, Green Tea *(Camellia oleifera), Chlorella vulgaris,* Lecithin, Grape Seed *(Vitis vinifera),* Algae, Mugwort *(Artemisia vulgaris)*

Preservatives: Phenoxyethanol, Chloraphenecin, Benzoic Acid

Stabilizers: Xanthan gum, Sodium stearoyl lactylate, Carbomer, Polysorbate 20, Dimethicone

Nutrients: Tetrahexyldecyl ascorbate, Tocopheryl acetate, Squalane, Sodium hyaluronate, Retinyl palmitate, Sodium PCA,

Active Ingredients: Wolfberry oil *(Lycium barbarum),* Chamomile, German EO *(Matricaria recutita),* Micrococcus lysate, Palmityl oligopeptide, Palmitoyl tetrapeptide-3, Sandalwood EO *(Santalum album),* Frankincense EO *(Boswellia carteri)*

Directions: Apply in the morning after cleansing. Using fingertips, massage a generouis amount (usually 2 to 4 pumps) of Day Activator over face and neck regions as needed. Suitable for all skin types. For maximum benefit, Day Activator should be used with A.R.T. Gentle Foaming Cleanser and A.R.T. Night Reconstructor Cream.

A.R.T. Gentle Foaming Cleanser

This unique foaming cleanser was designed to clean the skin by gently removing oil, dirt and makeup. Gentle Foaming Cleanser is formulated from naturally occurring sugars and contains ingredients that penetrate the epidermis to remove unwanted oils and impurities. This cleanser also includes a quarter of pure therapeutic-grade essential oils that were specifically selected for their skin-enhancing benefits.

Ingredients (all plant derived):

Base:, Deionized Water, Sodium cocoyl glutamate, Sodium methyl cocoyl taurate, Sodium lauroamphoacetate, Decyl glucoside, Glycerine

Plant Extracts:, Aloe *(Aloe barbadensis),* Melissa leaf *(Melissa officinalis),* Gingko leaf *(Gingko biloba),* Camellia Oleifera Leaf *(Camellia oleifera),* Lavender leaf *(Lavandula angustifolia)*

Preservatives: Chlorphenesin, Benzoic Acid

Stabilizers: Sorbic Acid, NaOH, Cetyl hydroxyethylcellulose

Nutrients: Tocopheryl acetate, Retinyl palmitate,

Active Ingredients: Sandalwood EO *(Santalum album),* Frankincense EO *(Boswellia carteri),* Lemon EO *(Citrus Medica Limonum)*

Directions: Splash face with warm water. Dispense and lather a small amount of cleanser from pump. With wet hands, massage gently over face. Rise thoroughly. To be used twice daily for a refreshing cleanse in the morning and a thorough cleansing at night. Suitable for all skin types. For maximum benefit, immediately apply A.R.T. Day Activator after morning cleansing and A.R.T. Night Reconstructor after the evening cleansing.

A.R.T. Night Reconstructor

While you rest, your body is hard at work replacing and repairing cells. A.R.T. Night Reconstructor facial cream will also be working to keep your skin hydrated and nourished. This full-bodied cream uses an amazing endonuclease enzyme to support cell revitalization all through the night. This formula is also inreiched with three skin-soothing essential oils, German chamomile, sandalwood and frankincense.

Ingredients (all plant derived):

Base: Deionized Water, Pentylene glycol, Glycerine, Glycerol stearate, Cetearyl alcohol

Plant Extracts: Meadowfoam Seed Oil, Shea Butter, Aloe *(Aloe barbadensis),* Dipotassium Glycyrrhizate, Green Tea *(Camellia oleifera), Chlorella vulgaris,* Lecithin, Grape Seed *(Vitis vinifera),* Algae, Mugwort *(Artemisia vulgaris)*

Preservatives: Phenoxyethanol, Chlora-phenecin, Benzoic Acid

Stabilizers: Xanthan gum, Sodium stearoyl lactylate, Carbomer, Polysorbate 20, Dimethicone

Nutrients: Tetrahexyldecyl ascorbate, Tocopheryl acetate, Squalane, Sodium hyaluronate, Retinyl palmitate, Sodium PCA,

Active Ingredients:, Wolfberry oil *(Lycium barbarum),* Chamomile, German EO *(Matricaria recutita),* Micrococcus lysate, Palmityl oligopeptide, Palmitoyl tetrapeptide-3, Sandalwood EO *(Santalum album),* Frankincense EO *(Boswellia carteri)*

Directions: Apply in the evening after cleansing. Using fingertips, massage in a generous amount (usually 2 to 4 pumps) of Night Reconstructor cream over face and neck regions as needed. For maximum results, Night Reconstructor should be used with A.R.T. Gentle Foaming Cleanser and A.R.T. Day Activator cream.

Boswellia Wrinkle Creme

Ingredients: Calendula extract, chamomile extract, rosebud extract, orange blossom extract, St. John's wort extract, aloe vera gel, kelp extract, *Ginkgo biloba* extract, grapeseed extract, ASC 111, goat's cream, glyceryl stearate, caprylic/capric triglyceride, shea butter, wolfberry seed oil, stearic acid, stearyl alcohol, sodium PCA, sodium hyaluronate, allantoin, panthenol, retinyl palmitate (vitamin A), tocopheryl acetate (vitamin E)

Essential Oils: Frankincense, sandalwood, myrrh, geranium, ylang ylang

Directions: Boswellia Wrinkle Creme is a collagen builder. Used daily, it will help minimize and prevent wrinkles. Put small amount in hand, emulsify, and apply to face and neck using upward strokes.

Clara Derm (spray)

Helps relieve a variety of skin irritations, burning and itching, particularly in sensitive female areas. Its gentle spray helps control rashes, candida, etc. Especially suited for the vaginal area before and after childbirth.

Ingredients:

Fractionated coconut oil base

Myrrh *(Commiphora myrrha)* has been used in the Middle East for many skin conditions, including rashes and chapped or cracked skin. It contains sesquiterpenes which stimulate the limbic system of the brain and the hypothalamus. The hypothalamus is the master gland of the human body, producing many vital hormones including thyroid and growth hormone.

Tea Tree *(Melaloeuca alternifolia)* is a powerful anti-bacterial, antifungal and anti-inflammatory essential oil that has been successful used to heal many skin conditions, including acne and sores. It is an excellent topical cleanser that promotes healing.

Lavender *(Lavandula angustifolia)* relieves muscles spasm/spsrains/pains, headaches, inflammation, anxiety. It is excellent for skin problems such as psoriasis, and is known for its ability to heal burns and other injuries without scarring. Has been used to reduce stretch marks. It is hypotensive, anti-infectious, anticoagulant.

Frankincense *(Boswellia carteri)* is considered a holy anointing oil in the Middle East. It stimulates the hypothalamus to amplify immunity. Research at Ponce University in Puerto Rico shows that it inhibits breast cancer and enhances DNA repair. In ancient times, it was well-known for its healing powers, and was reportedly used to treat every conceivable ill.

Roman chamomile *(Chamaemelum nobile)* is calming and relaxing and has been historically used to calm crying children. It is used in Europe for skin conditions including acne, dermatitis and eczema). Its calmative effects can help with restlessness, anxiety, depression and insomnia.

Helichrysum (*Helichrysum italicum*) iimproves circulation and reduces blood viscosity. It is anticoagulant, regulates cholesterol, stimulates liver cell function and reduces plaque deposits from veins and arteries.

Directions: Spray on affected area 1-3 times daily as needed.

Cinnamint Lip Balm

Is a natural lip balm enriched with essential oils and vitamins to soothe and prevent chapping.

Ingredients: Sweet almond oil, beeswax, MSM, hemp seed oil, sesame oil, orange wax, orange oil, tocopherol palmitate (vitamin E), ascorbyl palmitate (vitamin A), ascorbic acid (vitamin C), citric acid, wolfberry seed oil

Essential Oils: Peppermint, spearmint, cinnamon bark

Directions: To soften and moisturize lips, apply Cinnamint Lip Balm as often as needed.

Genesis Hand and Body Lotion

Ingredients: MSM, glyceryl stearate, stearic acid, glycerin, grape seed extract, sodium hyaluronate, sorbitol, rose hip seed oil, shea butter, mango butter, wheat germ oil, kukui nut oil, lecithin, safflower oil (*Carthamus tinctorius*), apricot oil, almond oil (*Prunus dulcis*), tocopheryl acetate (vitamin E), retinyl palmitate (vitamin A), jojoba oil (*Simmondsia chinensis*), sesame oil (*Sesamum indicum*), calendula extract (*Calendula officinalis*), chamomile extract, orange blossom extract, St. John's wort extract, algae extract, aloe vera gel, ascorbic acid (vitamin C), gingko biloba extract

Essential Oils: Rosewood, palmarosa, geranium, jasmine, lemon, roman chamomile, bergamot, ylang ylang

LavaDerm Cooling Mist

The essential oil of lavender has been highly regarded as a burn treatment since cosmetic chemist René Gattefossé used the oil to heal severe burns suffered in a laboratory explosion. Lavender oil has both antiseptic properties and an ability to reduce to the formation of scar tissue.

This cooling mist assists the healing of most topical burns, ranging from sunburn to second-degree thermal burns. It contains a highly purified concentrate of aloe vera gel, freshly processed from the leaves of aloe barbadiensis.

Ingredients: Re-structured water, aloe vera,

Essential Oil: lavender

Directions: Mist as often as needed to keep the skin cool and promote tissue regeneration.

Orange Blossom Facial Wash

Ingredients: MSM, wolfberry oil, decyl polyglucose, mixed fruit acid complex, hydrolysed wheat protein, citric acid, calendula extract, chamomile extract, rosebud extract, prange blossom extract, St. John's wort, algae extract, aloe vera gel, kelp extract, ginkgo biloba extract, grapeseed extract, dimethyl lauramine oleate.

Essential Oils: Lavender, patchouli, lemon, rosemary verbenon

Directions: Use either morning or night to cleanse and exfoliate the skin.

Rose Ointment

Is a skin ointment that protects and nourishes the skin and is outstanding when applied over essential oils to lock in their benefits. Note: Not recommended for burns initially, but is very helpful to maintain, protect, and keep the the scab soft.

Ingredients: Lecithin, lanolin, beeswax, mink oil, sesame seed oil, wheat germ oil, rose hip seed oil, carrot seed oil.

Essential Oils: Melaleuca alternifolia, myrrh, palmarosa, patchouli, rose, and rosewood.

Directions: Apply directly to skin or over open wound following essential oil application.

Sandalwood Moisture Creme

Ingredients: Deionized water, calendula extract, chamomile extract, rosebud extract, orange blossom extract, St. John's wort extract, aloe vera gel, kelp, *Ginkgo biloba* extract, grapeseed extract, caprylic/capric triglyceride, sorbitol, shea butter, goat's cream, glyceryl stearate, wolfberry seed oil, rosehip seed oil, sodium PCA, algae extract, stearic acid, allantoin, lecithin, retinyl palmitate (vitamin A), tocopheryl acetate (vitamin E), ascorbic acid (vitamin C), locust bean gum, hydrolyzed wheat protein, sodium hyaluronate, tocopheryl linoleate.

Essential Oils: Myrrh, sandalwood, rosewood, lavender, rosemary verbenon

Directions: For best results, use after cleansing and toning the face and neck to promote younger, healthier skin. Put small amount in hand, emulsify, and apply to face and neck using upward strokes.

Sandalwood Toner

Ingredients: Deionized water, MSM, glycerin, sorbitol, sodium PCA, allantoin, aloe vera gel, cucumber extract, chamomile extract, rosemary extract, echinacea extract, gotu kola extract, sodium hyaluronate, arnica extract, witch hazel extract, horse chestnut extract, wolfberry seed oil.

Essential oils: sandalwood, Roman chamomile, rosewood, myrrh

Directions: Lightly mist face and neck. For best results follow with Sandalwood Moisture Creme.

Satin Facial Scrub - Juniper

An exfoliating scrub designed for oily skin. It gently eliminates layers of dead skin cells with a revolutionary combination of fruit acids and jojoba beads.

This scrub can be used as a drying face mask to draw impurities from the skin.

Ingredients: Glycerin, caprylic/ capric triglyceride, MSM, sorbitol, glyceryl stearate, carnuba wax, beeswax, jojoba sax beads, aloe vera gel, stearic acid, algae extract, rosemary extract, chamomile extract, tocopheryl acetate (vitamin E), retinyl palmitate (Vitamin A), sodium PCA, shea butter, grape seed extract, titanium dioxide, mango butter, L-ascorbic acid (vitamin C), sodium hyaluronate, tocopheryl linoleate, allantoin, hydrolyzed wheat protein, hydrolyzed soy protein, malic acid, lactic acid, citric acid, and green tea extract.

Essential Oil: Juniper.

Directions: Apply warm water to the face to moisten skin. Apply scrub directly to the face and gently massage in a gentle circular motion, creating a lather. Rinse thoroughly and gently pat dry. Use four or five times weekly, depending on need.

Satin Facial Scrub - Mint

A gentle exfoliating scrub designed for normal skin. It gently eliminates layers of dead skin cells with a revolutionary formula of jojoba beads and other natural ingredients.

This scrub can be used as a drying face mask to draw impurities from the skin.

Ingredients: Glycerin, caprylic/capric triglyceride, MSM, sorbitol, glyceryl stearate, carnuba wax, beeswax, jojoba sax beads, aloe vera gel, stearic acid, algae extract, rosemary extract, chamomile extract, tocopheryl acetate (vitamin E), retinyl palmitate (Vitamin A), sodium PCA, shea butter, grape seed extract, titanium dioxide, mango butter, L-ascorbic acid (vitamin C), sodium hyaluronate, tocopheryl linoleate, allantoin, hydrolyzed wheat protein, and hydrolyzed soy protein.

Essential Oil: Peppermint.

Directions: Apply warm water to the face to moisten skin. Apply scrub directly to the face and gently massage in a gentle circular motion, creating a lather. Rinse thoroughly and gently pat dry. Use four or five times weekly, depending on need.

Satin Hand and Body Lotion

Nourishes and moisturizes skin. Also good for scars, burns, rashes, itching, and sunburns. Contains herbal extracts, essential oils, and vitamin C.

Ingredients: MSM, glyceryl stearate, stearic acid, glycerin, goat's cream, sorbitol, wolfberry seed oil, grapeseed, sodium hyaluronate, rosehip seed oil, shea butter, mango butter, wheat germ oil, kukui nut oil, lecithin, safflower oil, apricot oil, almond oil, jojoba oil, sesame oil, calendula extract, chamomile extract, orange blossom extract, St. John's wort extract, algae extract, aloe vera gel, *Ginkgo biloba* extract, grape seed extract, tocopheryl acetate (vitamin E), retinyl palmitate (vitamin A), ascorbic acid (vitamin C), sodium hyaluronate.

Essential oils: Geranium, rosewood, ylang ylang, jasmine, sandalwood, peppermint, Roman chamomile, melaleuca alternifolia

Directions: To moisturize the skin, promote healing, and leave the skin feeling soft, silky and smooth, apply to hands, body, and feet.

Sensation Hand and Body Lotion

Leaves the skin soft and moist as it protects from harsh weather, chemicals, and dry air.

Ingredients: Includes dionized water, MSM, grape seed extract, rose hip seed oil, mango butter, wheat germ oil, kukui nut oil, lecithin, safflower oil, apricot oil, almond oil, tocopheryl acetate (vitamin E), retinyl palmitate (vitamin A), jojoba oil, sesame oil, calendula extract, chamomile extract, orange blossom extract, St. John's wort extract, rosewood

Essential Oils: ylang ylang, jasmine

Directions: Apply directly to skin.

Chinese Secret to Youthful Skin

For centuries, the Chinese living in Inner Mongolia have been using a very unusual vegetable oil with exceptional benefits for the skin: Wolfberry seed oil. This rare and expensive oil from Inner Mongolia is painstakingly extracted from the seeds of the Ningxia variety of the Lycium berry. Not only is the oil rich in vitamin E, linoleic, and linolenic acids, but it also has an unusual chemistry that makes it ideal for nourishing and hydrating the skin. "The wolfberry seed oil is one of the best oils for the skin," according to researcher Sue Chao. "It is sought-after throughout Asia and has some very unusual regenerative properties, such as protecting aging skin and adding luster to skin."

Wolfberry Eye Creme

Eases eye puffiness and dark circles, and promotes skin tightening. Can be used before bed and in the morning.

Ingredients: Aloe vera gel, caprylic/capric triglyceride, MSM, sorbitol, glycerin, glyceryl stearate, goat's cream, avocado oil, shea butter, kukui nut oil, rose hip seed oil, wolfberry seed oil, hydrocotyl extract, coneflower extract, sodium PCA, lecithin, dipalmitoyl hydroxyproline, phenoxyethanol, beta-sitosterol, linoleic acid, tocopherol, sodium ascorbate, mannitol, almond oil, jojoba oil, mango butter, sodium hyaluronate, cucumber extract, green tea extract, tocopherol acetate, tocopherol palmitate (vitamin E), ascorbyl palmitate (vitamin A), ascorbic acid (vitamin C), citric acid, soy protein, wheat protein, allantoin, witch hazel extract, horse chestnut extract.

Essential oils: Lavender, rosewood, Roman chamomile, frankincense, geranium

Directions: Apply a tiny amount under eye area and on the eyelid before bed. Repeat in morning if needed.

14

Hair Care

Three Secrets to Great Hair

1. Use the right product for the right hair type.

No hair care product—regardless of its quality—works for all types of hair at all times. Hair that is naturally curly requires different hair treatments than those that are permed. Similarly, Asian hair (which tends to consist of thicker and rounder hair follicles) needs different hair care than does African hair (which tends to be very fine and frizzy).

This why the AromaSilk line of hair products is segmented into three different lines:

- The Lavender Volumizing line adds volume and fullness to hair. This collection includes a Scalp Wash, Nourishing Rinse, and Sealer that is specifically designed for long, flat, or dull hair.

- The Rosewood Moisturizing line moisturizes dry or damaged hair. This trio of scalp washes, nourishing rinses, and sealers contains essential oils and herbal extracts that helps defrizz and protect damaged, dry, or overprocessed hair. Naturally curly, thin, or oily hairs will benefit the most from this line.

- The Lemon-Sage Clarifying line prepares hair for perms or coloring. It contains essential oils and special herbal extracts that help remove buildup from chemicals, pollutants, and chlorine. Designed for all types of hair.

2. Use the right scalp washes and rinses.

First, the hair and scalp is cleansed with the Hair and Scalp Wash to open up the hair follicle and remove buildup, grease, and chemicals. After the hair follicle is cleansed and opened up, it is then nourished with the Nourishing Rinse. This allows nutrients to penetrate into the hair. It also protects the hair follicle from dirt and pollution, imparting shine, bounce, and vigor. It also locks in the nutrients.

3. Keeping hair free of petrochemical residues

Avoid synthetic hair treatments and styling aids. These can damage hair over time, breaking the sulfur bonds that make hair lustrous and alive.

Lavender Volume Shampoo

Contains all natural ingredients for gently cleansing and volumizing fine hair. MSM provides sulfur to help build and strengthen hair. Fortified with vitamin complex, including panthenol, and vitamins A, C, and E. Contains essential oils for a beautiful fragrance.

Ingredients: Coconut oil; olive oil; decyl polyglucose; MSM (methylsulfonalmethane); deionized water, meadow seed oil (dimethicone copolyol meadowfoamate); vegetable soya protein; vegetable wheat protein; vegetable oat protein; lemon *(Citrus medica limonum)* extract; sugar maple *(Acer sacchrinum)* extract; orange *(Citrus aurantium dulcis)* extract; aloe vera *(Aloe barbadersis)* gel; almond *(Prunus amygdalus dulcis)* glyceride; soapwort *(Saponaria officinalis)* extract; dimethyl lauranine cleate; cetyl triethylmonium dimethicone copolyol phthalate; acetamide MEA; dimethlcanol panthenol; keratin; linoleic acid; hyaluronic acid; sorbitol; wheat germ oil; dimethiconol cysteine; jojoba *(Simmondsia chinensis)* oil; inositol; and niacin.

Essential Oils: Lavender, Clary Sage, Lemon, Jasmine

Instructions: Wet hair thoroughly. Apply small amount of Lavender Volume Hair & Scalp Wash. Massage thoroughly into hair and scalp. Rinse well. Repeat if desired.

Lavender Volume Conditioner

Conditions and volumizes fine hair with MSM, amino acids, and a multi-vitamin complex. Essential oils enhance and provide vital components for healthy hair.

Ingredients: Unsaporified Oils of Coconut and Olive, Shea Butter, Phytantriol, MSM, Guar Gum, Mineral Water, Glycerine, Panthenol, Sodium PCA, Aloe Vera Gel 10X, Silk protein, MICA, Natural Vitamin E, Blue Agave Nectar, Avocado, Keratin, Evening Primrose, Hawaiian White Ginger, Horsetail, Plankton (Bladderwrack), Spirulina, Sunflower, BOIS II, Hyaluronic Acid, Jojoba Oil, Mineral Complex, Lecithin, Benzyl Alcohol, Allantoin, Inositol, Vitamin B3, Vitamin A,

Essential Oils: Lavender, Geranium, Rosewood, Palmarosa, Roman Chamomile, Ylang Ylang, Rose, Lemon, Bergamot, Jasmine, Sandalwood, Cedarwood.

Instructions: Apply Lavender Volume Nourishing Rinse through the hair. Leave on hair for just a few seconds for light conditioning or for several minutes for deep conditioning. Rinse well.

Lemon Sage Clarifying Shampoo

Removes buildup of styling products, leaving hair feeling naturally clean and healthy. Contains herbal extracts, vitamins, and essential oils to enhance the hair.

Ingredients: Saponified Oils of Coconut and Olive, Decylpolyglucose, MSM, Mineral Water, Decylpolyglucose-Extra Glycerine, Soapwort, Guar Gum, MICA, Polysorbate, Silk protein, Aloe Vera Gel 10X, MSM-Extra, Sodium PCA, Blue Agave, Panthenol, Whole Egg, Hyaluronic Acid, BOIS II, Avocado, Bee Balm, Hawaiian White Ginger, Jaborandi, Plankton (Bladderwrack), Quince, Rosemary, Spirulina, Sunflower Extract, Vitamin E, Jojoba Oil, Mineral Complex, Benzyl Alcohol, Retinyl Palmitate, Allantoin, Inositol, Vitamin B3, Glycerin.

Essential Oils: Peppermint, Lemon, Cedarwood

Instructions: Wet hair thoroughly. Apply small amount of Lemon-Sage Clarifying Hair & Scalp Wash. Massage thoroughly into hair and scalp. Rinse well. Repeat if desired.

Lemon Sage Conditioner

Conditions hair of all types without building up on hair. Herbal extracts, vitamins, and essential oils work together to improve hair condition.

Ingredients: Unsaponified base of Shea Butter, Phytantriol, MSM, Guar Gum, Glycerine, Mineral Water, Sodium PCA, Aloe Vera Gel 10X, Silk protein, MICA, Lecithin, Natural Vitamin E, Blue Agave Nectar, Whole Egg, Avocado, Hawaiian White Ginger, Jaborandi, Peony, Rosemary, Spirulina, Sunflower, Hyaluronic Acid, Panthenol, BOIS II, Mineral Complex, Benzyl Alcohol, Allantoin, Inositol, Vitamin B3, Vitamin A.

Essential Oils: Peppermint, Lemon, Cedarwood

Instructions: Apply Lemon-Sage Clarifying Nourishing Rinse to hair from roots to ends. Leave on hair for just a few seconds for light conditioning or for several minutes for deep conditioning. Rinse well.

Rosewood Moisturizing Shampoo

Contains natural ingredients to moisturize dry hair while gently cleansing. Contains herbal extracts, vitamins, and essential oils for nourishing the hair.

Ingredients: Saponified Oils of Coconut and Olive, Decylpolyglucose, Guar Gum, MSM, Mineral Water, Decylpolyglucose Extra, Guar Gum Extra, Glycerine, Blue Agave Nectar, MSM Extra, Sodium PCA, Silk protein, Polysorbate, MICA, Whole Egg, Natural Vitamin E, Aloe Vera Gel, Hyaluronic Acid, Phantenol, Jojoba Oil, Avocado, Evening Primrose, Irish Moss, Peony, Plankton (Bladderwrack), Quince, Slippery Elm, Spirulina, Sunflower, Yucca, Wheat Germ Oil, Mineral Complex, Benzyl Alcohol, Retinyl Palmitate, Allantoin, Inositol, Vitamin B3.

Essential Oils: Rosewood, Cedarwood, Orange

Instructions: Wet hair thoroughly. Apply small amount of Rosewood Moisturizing Hair & Scalp Wash. Massage thoroughly into hair and scalp. Rinse well. Repeat if desired.

Rosewood Moisturizing Conditioner

Conditions and moisturizes dry hair with natural vegetable fatty acids, MSM, milk protein, vitamins, and essential oils.

Ingredients: Unsaponified Oils of Coconut and Olive, Shea Butter, Phytantriol, MSM, Guar Gum, Glycerine, Blue Agave Nextrar, Fractionated Coconut Oil, Sodium PCA, Aloe Vera Gel 10X, Silk protein, MICA, Mineral Water, Natural Vitamin E, Avocado, Evening Primrose, Irish Moss, Peony, Slippery Elm, Spirulina, Sunflower, Yugga, Vitamin E, Whole Egg, Hyaluronic Acid, Jojoba Oil, Panthenol, BOIS II, Mineral Complex, Benzyl Alcohol, Allantoin, Retinyl Palmitate, Inositol, Vitamin A.

Essential Oils: Rosewood, Cedarwood, Orange

Instructions: Apply Rosewood Moisturizing Nourishing Rinse to hair from roots to ends. Leave on hair for a few seconds for light conditioning or for several minutes for deep conditioning. Rinse well.

15

Body Care

Aqua Essence Essential Oil Packs

Aqua Essence Essential Oil packs use a special inert material to slowly diffuse essential oils into the air or water. Once the impermeable outer packet is opened, the inner packet then gradually releases a measured amount of essential oils for purification, odor control, or mood enhancement.

Each packet contains 4 individual inner packs of 10 ml of essential oil blend.

Directions: These packs can be placed in your central ventilation system, or left opened in the room to passively diffuse. The also can be used in bath or drinking water

Joy

Essential Oils: Bergamot, ylang ylang, geranium, rosewood, lemon, mandarin, jasmine , Roman chamomile, palmarosa, rose

Peace & Calming

Essential Oils: Tangerine, orange, ylang ylang, patchouli, blue tansy

Sacred Mountain

Essential Oils: Spruce, ylang ylang, balsam fir, cedarwood

Valor

Essential Oils: Spruce, rosewood, blue tansy, frankincense,

Shower Gels

Bath & Shower Gel Base

Bath Gel Base is a dispersing agent to help unlock the full effects of your aromatherapy bath. Contains natural botanical ingredients for cleansing the pores. You may add single essential oils or blends to create your own fragrance or specific therapeutic action.

How to use: Add 5-10 drops of an essential oil or blend (depending on the strength of the oil) to 3 Tbsp. Bath Gel Base. Mix well before using.

Ingredients: Saponified oils of coconut and olive, vegetable gum, aloe vera, rosemary extract, glycerin

Dragon Time Bath & Shower Gel

This bath and shower gel was blended for women's stressful time of the month. This custom-formulated blend of essential oils and vegetable oils is exceptionally balancing and uplifting, both physically and emotionally.

Ingredients: Saponified oils of coconut and olive, vegetable gum, aloe vera, rosemary extract, glycerin

Essential Oils: Bergamot, clary sage, geranium, jasmine, lemon, palmarosa, Roman chamomile, rosewood, lavender, blue tansy, mandarin, sage, fennel, marjoram, and ylang ylang.

Evening Peace Bath and Shower Gel

Evening Peace blends natural botanical ingredients with therapeutic-grade essential oils to relax tired, fatigued muscles and help dampen stress and tension.

Ingredients: Saponified oils of coconut and olive, vegetable gum, aloe vera, rosemary extract, glycerin.

Essential Oils: Bergamot, Roman chamomile, clary sage, geranium, jasmine, lemon, palmarosa, rosewood, Blue tansy, sandalwood, and ylang ylang.

Morning Start Bath & Shower Gel

Morning Start is an invigorating gel that combines uplifting, energizing essential oils to jumpstart your vigor and energy.

Ingredients: Saponified oils of coconut and olive, vegetable gum, aloe vera, rosemary extract, glycerin

Essential Oils: Lemongrass, rosemary, juniper and peppermint.

Sensation Bath & Shower Gel

Sensation contains an enchantingly fragrant mix of oils used by Cleopatra to enhance love and increase desire to be close to someone special.

Ingredients: Saponified oils of coconut and olive, vegetable gum, aloe vera, rosemary extract, glycerin

Essential Oils: Rosewood, ylang ylang, and jasmine.

Bar Soaps

The Body's Largest Organ: The Skin

With skin covering the approximately 20 square foot outside surface of the human body, it is the largest human organ and the first line of defense against harmful substances, infection, and dehydration. For adults, the skin is between 15 and 20 percent of total body weight.

Because of its large surface area, the skin can soak in many types of toxins and petrochemicals. This can result in cancer-causing compounds leaching into the body and accumulating in the fat.

Many people complain that commercial soaps make their skin feel dry and itchy, or worse. Trapped free alkali is the most common irritant in soap. Soap is made from oils (an acid) mixed with water and alkali (a base). Acids and bases neutralize each other to form a salt, in this case soap, with glycerine as a by-product. Oils that did not combine with the alkali are "free" which creates a "superfatted" soap. These mild soaps are exceptionally good for the skin, even though they have a reduced lather and shelf life. Alkali that is not neutralized by essential oils is "free alkali", which makes soap harsh and drying. The handcrafting process for natural soap removes the excess alkali that other soaps leave in.

Benefits of Handmade Natural Soaps

Handcrafted in small batches, natural bar soaps are not only pure, natural, and nontoxic; they are also good for the skin. Handmade soaps have a "hand-lotion-in-the-soap" effect created by the natural vegetable oils and waxes in the soap as well as an emulsion of water and glycerin formed when the soap was made. While the "hand-lotion-in-the-soap" effect may reduce lathering, this is what makes handmade soap extraordinarily mild and moisturizing for dry and sensitive skin.

Secret to Creating the Best Handmade Soap

The best handmade soaps are made exclusively with natural ingredients that are blended in small batches and poured into wooden block molds. The soap is then wire cut into bars, dried on oak frames, and aged for over four weeks in a humidity and temperature-controlled curing room. The extended curing process is usually time-consuming and expensive, but it effectively eliminates most of the free alkali from the bar soap, a major cause of dryness and irritation.

Handmade natural soap can be made from a number of vegetable ingredients, such as saponified oils of palm, coconut, and olive, as well as therapeutic-grade essential oils. Rosemary extract can also be used as a natural preservative.

The result is a soap that does more than just cleanse the skin. It can also act as a therapeutic skin treatment with powerful antioxidant and skin-protecting properties that can be used to treat eczema, prsoriasis, dermatitis, pigmentation, inflammation, and more.

"Natural" Can be Unnatural

Unfortunately, the term "natural" can be used in very deceptive ways. If an ingredient is a five generation derivative of coconut meat, some will claim it to be natural, even if you can't pronounce the name of the ingredient.

The main ingredients in many mass-produced bar soaps are substances known as "sodium tallowate" and "potassium tallowate." These are the fatty remains of slaughtered cows, sheeps, and horses. Brains, fatty tissues, other unwanted parts of dead and sometimes diseased animals are collected into large vats and used to create "tallow." This tallow is shipped off to commercial soapmakers where it is processed into bar soaps.

Unfortunately, the U.S. Food & Drug Administration does not regulate the ingredients in soap. Some ingredients in mass-marketed soap including isopropyl alcohol, fragrances, DEA, FD&C colors, propylene glycol and triclosan have been proven harmful to human health. Isopropyl alcohol's drying effects can also remove protective oils and create microscopic cracks in the skin, which can trap and harbor bacteria and other pathogens. DEA (diethanolamine) is a hormone disrupting chemical known to form cancer-causing nitrates and nitrosamines. Dr. Samuel Epstein of the University of Illinois has found that repeated skin applications of DEA-based detergents resulted in a major increase in the incidence of liver and kidney cancers.

Regarding coal-tar derived FD&C colors, A Consumer's Dictionary of Cosmetic Ingredients states "many pigments cause skin sensitivity and irritation…and absorption (of certain colors) can cause depletion of oxygen in the body and death."

Instead of synthetic colors, German chamomile can be used. Rich in chamazuline, an intense blue pigment, chamomile actually has anti-inflammatory properties that accelerate skin healing. Moreover, other compounds in chamomile and other essential oils combine therapeutic action with delightful aromas. Peppermint oil imparts a delightful fresh fragrance to a soap while containing compounds such as menthol that act as pain-relievers and anti-inflammatory agents.

Sadly, many of the compounds in the commercial fragrances used in bath and body products are carcinogenic or otherwise toxic. The word "fragrance" on a soap label refer to over 4,000 ingredients, most of which are synthetic. Not only are fragrances potentially carcinogenic, according to Home Safe Home author Debra Lynn Ladd. "Clinical observation by medical doctors has shown that exposure to synthetic fragrances can affect the central nervous system, causing depression, hyperactivity, irritability, inability to cope and other behavioral changes." A surprising number of people experience a dry-skin reaction from many common synthetic fragrances.

AromaSilk Bar Soaps

Aromasilk soaps are created through a proprietary soap-making process derived from a sixteenth century Spanish recipe which was combined with modern technology and a propriety blend of ultrapure ingredients.

Hand-poured and cured for almost a month. AromaSilk bar soaps are unlike any other soaps on earth. Mild and longlasting, the soaps are made with therapeutic-grade essential oils that are redefining natural skin therapy.

AromaSilk Bar Soaps—

- Contain less than 1% free alkali. The proprietary soap-making process used in AromaSilk bar soaps minimizes the presence of irritating skin-drying alkali salts.

- Use a moisturizing vegetable base that contains over 50% moisturizers.

- Include therapeutic-grade essential oils, many of which have been studied for their antiseptic, anti-inflammatory, and antifungal properties. These oils are added at the optimum moment of the soap-making process to preserve their beneficial compounds.

- Contain only the finest organic ingredients, including:

  - Saponified oils of palm, coconut, and olive
  - Organic oatmeal
  - Therapeutic-grade essential oils
  - Liquid aloe vera extract
  - Rosemary extract (as an antioxidant)

Lavender Rosewood Moisturizing Soap

Excellent for toning and nourishing the skin.

Essential Oils: Lavender, rosewood

Lemon Sandalwood Bar Soap

Very cleansing and purifying to the skin. Lemon oil is highly antifungal, combating ringworm, athlete's foot and other fungal infections. Sandalwood has been show to protect the skin against viruses, such as the human papilloma virus, which is related to herpes.

Essential Oils: Lemon, sandalwood

Melaleuca Geranium Bar Soap

Designed specifically to combat acne, this soap contains highly antiseptic essential oils designed to dissolve away excess sebum and disinfect the skin.

Essential Oils: Tea tree, *Melaleuca ericifolia*, geranium, vetiver

Morning Start Bar Soap

An invigorating blend of energizing and antifungal essential oils. It contains lemongrass which has been documented as a powerful anti-fungal agent in clinical studies. Ideal for combating ringworm, athlete's foot, and other fungal skin conditions.

Essential Oils: lemongrass, rosemary, peppermint, juniper

Peppermint Bar Soap

Offers an anti-inflammatory blend of essential oils to combat pain and itching. It is analgesic and pain-relieving and combats tendon, ligament, bone, and muscle pain.

Essential Oils: Peppermint, cedarwood

Sacred Mountain Soap

This soap is for oily skin. Dissolves away excess sebum and gently exfoliates.

Essential Oils: Spruce, fir, cedarwood

Thieves Cleansing Soap

A disinfecting soap that contains a powerful blend of highly antibacterial and antiseptic essential oils.

Essential Oils: Clove, lemon, cinnamon bark, eucalyptus, rosemary

Valor Bar Soap

A highly moisturing soap made with pure frankincense essential oil.

Essential Oils: spruce, rosewood, blue tansy, frankincense

Deodorants

Most deodorants today are loaded with toxic chemicals ranging from aluminum to antifreeze. As these chemical leach through the skin into the blood and tissues, these can create a toxic buildup in the body that can lead to cancer, liver damage, and neurological diseases.

Perils of Aluminum

Glen Scott, MD, of Cincinnati and Patricia Saunders, a government microbiologist, warned of aluminum neurotoxicity, causing the FDA to require aluminum-bearing antiperspirants to carry a renal dysfunction warning (June 9, 2003).

According the Antiperspirant Products Final Monograph, the FDA is "concerned that people with renal dysfunction may not be aware that the daily use of antiperspirant drug products containing aluminum may put them at higher risk because of exposure to aluminum in the product."Young children are "at higher risk resulting from exposure to aluminum." Parents and others "must keep these products away from children, and to seek professional assistance if accidental ingestion occurs."

Sources of Aluminum Exposure

Over the Counter: Deodorants, antiperspirants, baby wipes, skin creams, suntan lotions, toothpaste, buffered asprin.

Medical: Vaccinations, intervenous solutions, wound and antacid irrigation, ulcer treatment, blood oxygenization, bone or joint replacement and burn treatments.

Foods: Aluminum cans, foils, containers, baking powder, cake mixes, frozen dough, pancake mixes, self-rising flour, grains, processed cheese.

Studies of Aluminum Toxicity

UNIVERSITY OF WESTERN ONTARIO

"Regardless of the host, the route of administration, or the speciation, aluminum is a potent neurotoxicant."

— MJ Strong, Department of Clinical Neurological Sciences, University of Western Ontario, Canada

UNIVERSITY OF STIRLING

"Aluminium is acutely toxic to fish in acid waters. The gill is the principal target organ and death is due to a combination of ionoregulatory, osmoregulatory and respiratory dysfunction. The mechanism of epithelial cell death is proposed as a general mechanism of aluminium-induced accelerated cell death."

— C Exley, University of Stirling, Scotland

BIOFACTORS

"Experimental evidence is summarized to support the hypothesis that chronic exposure to low levels of aluminum may lead to neurological disorders."

— JG Joshi, Aluminum, a neurotoxin which affects diverse metabolic reactions. Biofactors (1990 Jul)

THOMAS JEFFERSON UNIVERSITY

"This data defines a new model in which aluminum kills liver cells by mechanisms distinct from previously recognized pathways of lethal cell injury. It is hypothesized that aluminum binds to cytoskeletal proteins intimately associated with the plasma membrane. This interaction eventually disrupts the permeability barrier function of the cell membrane, an event that heralds the death of the hepatocyte."

— JW Snyder et al., Department of Pathology, Thomas Jefferson University, Philadelphia, Pennsylvania (Arch Biochem Biophys 1995)

STATE UNIVERSITY AT GENT, BELGIUM

"Epidemiological studies from Norway and England suggest a relation between the frequency of Alzheimer's disease and the concentration of aluminum in the drinking water. Estimates, made in this study, show that the role of aluminum from tooth pastes may be even more important than that from the drinking water. For that reason we determined in samples of tooth pastes taken from the BENELUX market which brands contained aluminum. This appeared to be the case for about 22% of the brands which according to the manufacturers cover about 60% of the market."

— RM Verbeeck, Laboratory for Analytical Chemistry, State University, Gent, Belgium (Acta Stomatol Belg 1990 Jun)

UNIVERSITY OF VIRGINIA

"Attention was first drawn to the potential role of aluminum as a toxic metal over 50 years ago… the accumulation of aluminum is associated with the development of toxic phenomena; dialysis encephalopathy, osteomalacic dialysis osteodystrophy, and an anemia. Aluminum has also been implicated as a toxic agent in the etiology of Alzheimer's disease, Guamiam amyotrophic lateral sclerosis, and parkinsonism-dementia."

— CD Hewitt et al., University of Virginia Health Sciences Center, Charlottesville

Aromaguard - Meadow Mist

The first deodorant stick in the world to use an aluminum-free, petrochemical-free essential oil formula made from edible ingredients and therapeutic-grade essential oils.

Ingredients: Fractionated coconut oil (Cocos nucifera), pure beeswax (Cera alba), pure vegetable esters, zinc oxide, Vitamin E

Essential Oils: Lemon, geranium, rosemary, rosewood, lavender, tea tree, niaouli, clove

Aromguard - Mountain Mint

The first deodorant stick in the world to use an aluminum-free, petrochemical-free essential oil formula made from edible ingredients.

Ingredients: Fractionated coconut oil (Cocos nucifera), pure beeswax (Cera alba), pure vegetable esters, zinc oxide, Vitamin E

Essential Oils: Clove, lemon, peppermint, rosemary, *Eucalyptus radiata*, white fir

16

Oral Health Care

Toothpastes

The Dirtiest Place on the Body

It is common medical knowledge the dirtiest part of the body is not the colon or bowels but the mouth. The back of the tongue is literally teeming with pathogenic microorganisms. According to Dr. John Richter founder of the Richter Center for the Diagnosis and Treatment of Breath Disorders, "more bacteria per square inch live [on the back of the tongue] than on any other part of the body."

The problem is that few people use a toothbrush to remove these bacteria. And even if the tongue were to receive a thorough scrubbing, many would remain and quickly repopulate the mouth.

The Heart Disease Link

At the 2001 annual session of the American College of Cardiology, researchers were stunned by new research that showed that gingivitis is actually linked to heart disease. "There is sufficient evidence to conclude that oral lesions, especially advanced periodontopathies, place certain patients at risk for cardiovascular disease and stroke," stated Louis F. Rose, DDS, MD, of the University of Pennsylvania.

The same oral pathogen *Porphyromonas gingivalis* that causes gum disease, also contributes to the inflammation along arteries and arterial damage that leads to heart and vascular disease.

Brushing Is Not Enough

Most toothpastes work to prevent cavities by merely hardening the tooth enamel with fluoride or using abrasive salts to mechanically scrub away microorganisms from teeth and gums.

The problem is that brushing is not enough to eliminate bacterial, fungal, and viral presence in the mouth. Such microorganisms typically hide between teeth and under the tongue. While brushing mechanically removes some of the plaque and pathogens, it still leaves 40 to 70% of microorganisms behind unscathed to later repopulate the mouth. Oral hygiene could be vastly improved by adding proven and potent antiseptics to the toothpaste matrix, rather than relying on either fluoride or scrubbing.

Antibacterial and Antiseptic

Essential oils are ideal for use in oral care products because they are both antiseptic and non-toxic—a rare combination. Jean Valnet, M.D., who used essential oils for decades in his clinical practice emphasized this: "Essential oils are especially valuable as antiseptics because their aggression toward microbial germs is matched by their total harmlessness toward tissue."

Dentarome, Dentarome Plus, Fresh Essence Mouthwash and Fresh Essence Plus Mouthwash use therapeutic-grade essential oils at the heart of their formulas. These oils include peppermint, wintergreen, eucalyptus, thyme, and a proprietary blend of therapeutic-grade essential oils, including clove, lemon, cinnamon, and rosemary. This blend was tested at Weber State University in Ogden, Utah, and found to dramatically inhibit the growth of many types of bacteria (both gram negative and gram positive), including *Micrococcus luteus* and *Staphylococcus aureus*. Even more remarkably, this blend exhibited a 99.96 percent kill rate against tough gram negative bacteria, like *Pseudomonas aeruginosa*. These bacteria, because of their thicker cell walls, tend to be far more resistant to antiseptics.

The essential oils of thyme, clove and cinnamon possess significant inhibitory affects against 23 different genera of bacteria.

—*International Journal of Food Microbiology*

Essential oils constituents, such as thymol, menthol and eucalyptol, have been used in mouth rinses for over 100 years [and] have been documented to be antibacterial in laboratory tests. With the association of microorganisms and plaque formation, and [their] suspected involvement with carious lesions (tooth decay) and gingivitis, the effect of essential oils takes on new interest.

—*Journal of the Soc. of Cosmetic Chemists*

The Truth about Thyme

A comprehensive 2002 survey of medical literature has shown that thyme oil is one of the strongest natural antiseptics known. Researchers found that thyme oil kills over 60 different strains of bacteria (both gram negative and gram positive) and 16 different strains of fungi. A 1995 study by Nicole Didry at the College of Pharmaceutical and Biological Sciences in Lille, France, found that

thyme oil at even very small concentrations (500 parts per million or less), killed the pathogenic organisms responsible for the tooth decay, gingivitis, and bad breath, *Streptococcus mutans*, *Streptococcus sanguis*, *Streptococcus milleri*, *Streptococcus mitis*, *Peptostreptococcus anaerobius*, *Prevotella buccae*, *Prevotella oris*, and *Prevotella intermedia*.

Clinical Research on Essential Oils in Dental Hygiene

Over 100 studies have documented how essential oils kill the microbes that cause tooth decay and gingivitis. According to Christine Charles and colleagues in a study published by the *Journal of the American Dental Association*, "The efficacy of an essential-oil-containing antiseptic mouthrinse has been demonstrated in numerous double-blind clincial studies."[1,2,3,4,5]

Researchers at the University of Maryland have also stated in the *Journal of Clinical Periodontology* that "Antiseptic mouthrinses are well known for their antibacterial effectiveness and are widely used for the prevention and treatment of periodontitis and to prevent the formation of supragingival plaque."[6]

Bacteria	Cinnam Aldehyde from cassia/cinnamon EO	Thymol from thyme EO	Carvacrol from oregano EO	Eugenol from clove EO
Streptococcus mutans	250	250	250	500
Streptococcus sanguis	250	125	125	250
Streptococcus milleri	31	125	125	125
Streptococcus mitis	125	125	125	250
Peptostreptococcus anaerobius	500	500	500	1000
Prevotella buccae	125	250	250	500
Prevotella oris	63	250	250	500
Prevotella intermedia	125	125	125	250

MIC µg/ml (PPM or parts per million)

Didry et al., 1995

1. CH Charles et al., "Comparative efficacy of an antiseptic mouthrinse and an antiplaque/ antigingivitis dentifrice. A six-month clinical trial." *J Am Dent Assoc.* 2001 May;132(5):670-5.

2. IG DePaola et al., "Chemotherapeutic inhibition of supragingival dental plaque and gingivitis development." *J Clin Periodontol.* 1989 May;16 (5):311-5.

3. CD Overholser et al., "Comparative effects of 2 chemotherapeutic mouthrinses on the development of supragingival dental plaque and gingivitis." *J Clin Periodontol.* 1990 Sep;17 (8):575-9.

4. KR Eldridge et al., "Efficacy of an alcohol-free chlorhexidine mouthrinse as an antimicrobial agent." *J Prosthet Dent.* 1998 Dec;80(6):685-90.

5. BG Riep et al., "Comparative antiplaque effectiveness of an essential oil and an amine fluoride/ stannous fluoride mouthrinse." *J Clin Periodontol.* 1999 Mar;26(3):164-8.

6. AA Baqui et al., "In vitro effect of oral antiseptics on human immunodeficiency virus-1 and herpes simplex virus type 1." *J Clin Periodontol.* 2001 Jul;28(7):610-6.

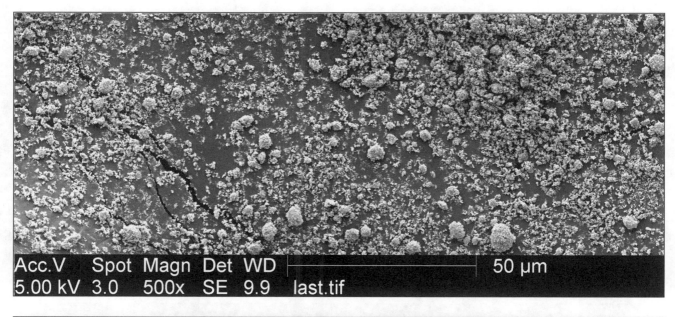

Acc.V Spot Magn Det WD ⊢————————— 50 µm
5.00 kV 3.0 500x SE 9.9 last.tif

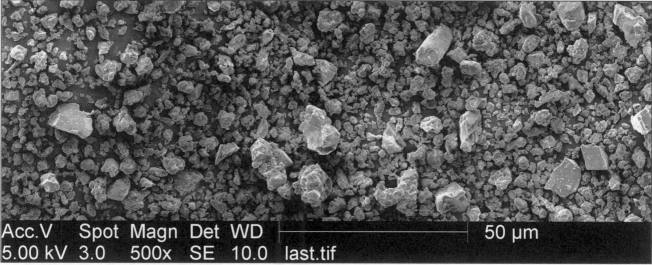

Acc.V Spot Magn Det WD ⊢————————— 50 µm
5.00 kV 3.0 500x SE 10.0 last.tif

ABOVE: Shown at 500 times magnification are scanning electron microscope photos of ultrafine particle zinc oxide (top) and calcium carbonate (bottom) which form the base of the most advanced toothpastes in the world. These ultrafine particle sizes allow for gentle removal of dental plaque with minimal erosion of tooth enamel.

NEXT PAGE: Shown at 500 times magnification are scanning electron microscope photos of three common brand toothpastes. The top photo shows a popular toothpaste which has article sizes so large that a single grain nearly fills up the entire image area. Such huge particles are extremely corrosive to teeth, cleaning teeth while at the same time accelerating the erosion of enamel. The middle photo shows the large angular structure of a leading whitening toothpaste, whose sharp oversized structure whitens teeth by stripping away enamel with a sandpaper-like action. The lower photo shows a popular household toothpaste with less anguler but large particle sizes with a rough, coarse, abrasive texture that can be highly damaging to dental structure. Long term use of such dentrifices can hasten the loss of enamel and eventually increase the risk of tooth loss.

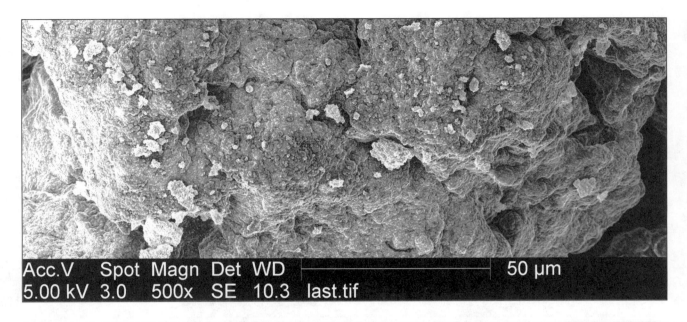

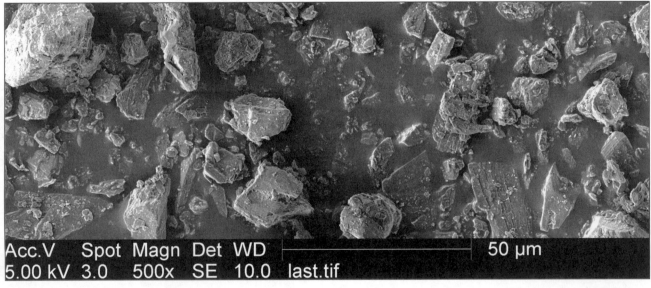

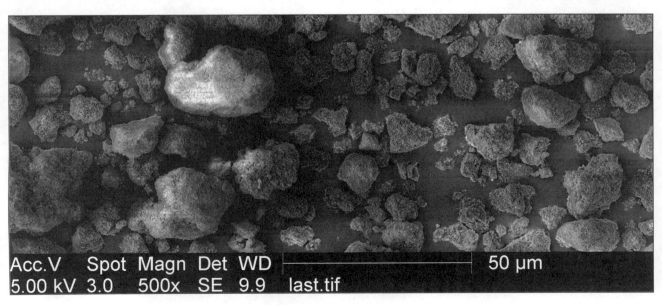

Excess Abrasion Destroys Tooth Enamel

The problem with many common brand toothpastes is that they contain very large-sized abrasive particles that can quickly wear away tooth enamel. Because tooth enamel is not regenerated by the body, its loss is permanent. It is never replaced. As tooth enamel is lost, the softer dentin material underneath is exposed and thereby greatly enhances the risk of dental decay and tooth loss.

To preserve dental enamel, a toothpaste (dentifrice) should have extremely fine particle size: Particles fine enough to not damage or abrade irreplaceable enamel, but yet sufficiently strong to remove the biofilm of dental plaque (caused by *Streptococcus mutans* bacterial) that can cause tooth decay, gingivitis and dental disease.

Removing Tarter Naturally

Most toothpastes use questionable chemicals such as pentasodium triphosphate and tetrasodium pyrophosphate to control tartar, the scale that builds up on teeth and irritates gums, leading to gingivitis, tooth loss, and periodontal disease. However, recent studies published in the *American Journal of Dentistry* have documented the significant tartar-reducing effects of zinc citrate. Among these clinical studies was a randomized, double-blind six-month trial which showed that a zinc-citrate containing toothpaste could reduce tartar by 26%.[7]

Essential Oils as Effective Antiseptic Mouthrinses

Essential oils have proved to be even more effective as antiseptic mouthrinses than even FDA-recognized plaque-control antiseptic drugs such as stannous fluoride. A 1999 study published in the Journal of Clinical Periodontology found that an essential oil mouthrinse containing thymol, methyl salycilate (wintergreen), menthol (peppermint), and eucalyptol (Eucalyptus globulus) was far more effective than a stannous fluoride antiseptic.

Comparing Toothpastes

	Dentarome Ultra	Common Brand
Active Ingredients	Thieves* blend Eucalyptus Oil Peppermint Oil Thyme Oil Wintergreen Oil	Sodium Fluoride Sodium Monofluorophosphate
Foaming Agent	None	Sodium Laurel Sulfate (SLS) **
Tartar Control	Zinc Citrate	Pentasodium triphosphate
Tooth Health Agent	Wintergreen Oil	Tetrasodium pyrophosphate
Moisturizer	Vegetable Glycerine	Glycerine, sorbitol
Sweetener	Xylitol	Sodium saccharin
Coloring	None	Titanium Dioxide FD&C Blue #1
Cleansing Agent	Ultrafine Calcium Carbonate	Abrasive Silica Synthetic Glycerine
Flavoring	Therapeutic-grade Essential Oils	Artificial Sources Natural Sources
Thickener	Xanthum Gum	Xanthum Gum, Cellulose Gum

* A proprietary blend of clove, lemon, cinnamon, *Eucalyptus radiata*, rosemary.
* Also known as sodium laureth sulfate.

Dentarome Toothpaste

Dentarome is formulated with pure, natural edible ingredients, such as vegetable glycerine, sodium bicarbonate, ionic minerals, and steviocide (a natural, intensely-sweet extract from a tropical plant native to South America). In addition, Dentarome uses an exclusive formula of uniquely antiseptic and antimicrobial therapeutic-grade essential oils to combat plaque-causing microorganisms. Dentarome leaves the mouth fresh, fragrant, and clean.

Dentarome was tested at Weber State University and found to have potent antimicrobial properties against a wide range of oral microbes, including *Streptococcus oralis, Streptococcus pneumoniae,* and *Candida albicans.*

---

7. SL Santos et al. Anticalculus effect of two zinc citrate/essential oil-containing dentifrices. Am J Dent. 2000 Sep;13(Spec No):11C-13C.

Dentarome Plus Toothpaste

Includes a higher concentration of thymol and eugenol for extra antiseptic action. Thymol is derived from thyme oil *(Thymus vulgaris)* and eugenol is derived from clove oil *(Syzygium aromaticum)*.

Dentarome Ultra Toothpaste

This high-powered essential oil toothpaste has a special two-part essential oil system that has:

- Anti-stain whitening enzymes
- Time-released essential oil mouthwash
- Therapeutic-grade essential oils of Thieves (EO of clove, cinnamon, rosemary cineol, and lemon)

- Low abrasion formula contains the smallest particle-size commercially available calcium carbonate and zinc oxide
- Special tartar-control agents
- All food-grade edible ingredients

Patented Liposome Technology

- Uses only water and lecithin
- Emulsifies and protects essential oils from oxidation
- Binds essential oils to the mucus membranes in the mouth for unmatched breath-freshening and oral hygiene

Mouthwash and Lozenges

Essential Oil Mouthrinses Reduce Plaque and Fight Tooth Decay

A number of clinical studies over the past 20 years have documented the ability of essential oil mouthrinses to control plaque and fight gingivitis. Typical of these is 1999 study at Humboldt University in Berlin, Germany. Researchers using an observer-blind, randomized, cross-over design found that median plaque reductions generated by twice-daily essential oil mouthrinses were 23% greater than a placebo. The essential oils used were thyme, peppermint, wintergreen, and eucalyptus. (Riep et al., 1999).

A six-month, double blind controlled clinical study at the University of Maryland similarly found that the essential oils of thyme, peppermint, wintergreen, and eucalyptus dramatically improved oral hygiene, killing the bacteria that cause plaque, tooth decay, and gingivitis. In this case, 20 ml of mouthrinse used twice daily produced a 34% inhibition of both plaque and gingivitis compared with a control.

Comparing Mouthwashes		
	Fresh Essence Mouthwash	Common Brand
Active Ingredients		
Thieves*		
Thyme oil	Thymol	
Eucalyptus oil	1,8 cineol	
Wintergreen oil	Methyl Salicylate	
Peppermint oil	Menthol	
Base	Water	Alcohol, SD Alcohol
Sweetener	Steviocide Sorbitol	Sodium saccharin
Coloring	None	D&C Yellow #10 FD&C Green #3 FD&C Blue #1 FD&C Yellow #5
Flavoring	Peppermint	Artificial Sources
Preservatives	None	Benzoic Acid Polysorbate 80
Dispersant	Natural Lecithin	Poloxamer 403 Sodium Hydroxide
(Lye)		Synthetic Glycerine

* A proprietary blend of clove, lemon, cinnamon, *Eucalyptus radiata*, rosemary.

Critical Kill Time Against Representative Oral Pathogens			
	TYPES of MOUTHRINSES		
	Essential Oil	Stannous Fl	Sterile Water Control
Fusobacterium nucleatum	<0.5 min	<0.5 min	>5 min
Streptococcus mutans	<0.5 min	<1 min	>5 min
Prevotella intermedia	<0.5 min	<2 min	>5 min
Lactobacillus casei	<0.5 min	>2 min	>5 min
Candida albicans ATCC 28366	<0.5 min	>5 min	>5 min
Candida albicans ATCC 18804	<0.5 min	>5 min	>5 min
Pan et al., 1999			

Controlled Release
Retention of thymol in the mouth

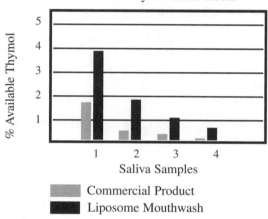

Commercial Product
Liposome Mouthwash

Figure 3. The retention of thymol was measured over a period of five minutes in various saliva samples. The level of thymol remaining in the saliva dropped off rapidly following usage of the commercial product. However, following usage of the liposome-based mouthwash, there was a significantly higher level of thymol in each saliva sample analyzed.

Liposomal Binding to Teeth

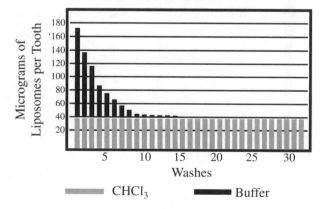

CHCl₃   Buffer

Figure 1. A saliva-coated human tooth was dipped in a solution of dental liposomes and rinsed repeatedly with 1.0 ml of water.

Comparison of Coolness
Retention of menthol flavor in the mouth

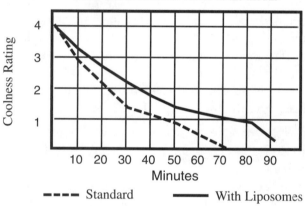

---- Standard   ——— With Liposomes

Figure 2. Lozenges made with mucin-binding system to release menthol flavor slowly are compared to control menthol lozenges. Timing began when the lozenge was completely dissolved in the mouth.

Benefits of Liposomes in Fresh Essence

Controlled-release liposomes are a key ingredient in Fresh Essence Mouthwash. These liposomes adhere to either tooth enamel or mucus membranes in the mouth. The two primary benefits of using liposome technology are:

1. **Controlled release of active ingredients**

2. **Ingredient protection**

The controlled-release aspect of liposome technology is enhanced through the use of a patented "liposome anchoring" system. Liposomes that adhere to dental enamel can be used to improve dental health, because they contain active materials to prevent plaque formation, treat periodontal disease, and prevent dental caries. These active materials can be released slowly, enhancing their benefits.

The ability of dental liposomes to slowly release their therapeutic cargo is demonstrated in Fig. 1. A saliva-coated tooth is dipped into a solution containing dental liposomes. The liposomes contain a test material. The tooth is sequentially washed with 1.0 ml of buffer 30 times. The test material is removed slowly with the washes. Even after 30 washes, some active material is retained on the tooth.

Slow Release Systems for Oral Soft Tissues

Liposomal systems that adhere to mucus membranes are designed to slowly release beneficial chemical compounds in the mucus membranes of the mouth and nose. This is useful in the slow release of flavors. For example, a breath lozenge containing menthol that is contained in a mucin-binding system can provide extended oral freshness longer than a standard menthol lozenge (Fig. 2).

In another experiment, two thymol-based mouthwashes were compared side by side. The first was a standard commercial product with no liposome-based delivery; the second used a liposomal delivery system. The results of the experiment are illustrated in Fig. 3. The level of thymol measured in saliva over a period of five minutes was measured. With the commercial product, thymol levels dropped off quickly, whereas with the liposome-based mouthwash, there was a significantly higher level of thymol in each saliva sample.

Fresh Essence Plus Mouthwash

Fresh Essence Plus is formulated with dionized water, mouthwash liposome-concentrate, essential oils of peppermint, Thieves, spearmint, and vetiver; melissa floral water, and peppermint floral water.

By utilizing a patented liposome technology (using soy-derived lecithin) that binds the essential oils to the mucus membrane inside the mouth, the essential oils remain in the mouth longer, providing long-lasting, germ-killing and breath-freshening effects.

Free from dyes, alcohol, preservatives, and other synthetic ingredients, Fresh Essence uses food-grade medicinal essential oils such as thyme, eucalyptus, wintergreen, peppermint, manuka, and the blend Thieves. These oils contain natural compounds clinically proven to kill the bacteria that can cause bad breath, plaque, and gum diseases, such as gingivitis. **By using the entire essential oil rather than isolated active ingredients, Fresh Essence gains significant advantages in safety and antiseptic power.** The complete oils of eucalyptus and thyme exhibit far stronger anti-microbial power than their active constituents alone. These whole oils are also safer because they contain a natural balance of elements that makes them nondamaging to human tissue.

Thieves Lozenges

A special throat lozenge that contains the essential oil blend of Thieves, university tested for it's ability to kill 99.6% of bacteria tested.

INGREDIENTS:

Xylitol is important for maintaining good oral hygiene.

Sorbitol is a noncarcinogenic flavoring agent.

ESSENTIAL OILS:

Clove EO has been shown to inhibit over 60 strains of gram negative and positive bacteria and 13 types of fungi according to over two dozen clinical studies.

Lemon EO inhibits the growth of fungi and yeasts.

Cinnamon EO is one of the strongest known antimicrobial, antiviral, and antifungal essential oils.

Eucalyptus radiata has been used to purify the air for centuries.

Rosemary is a special chemotype of rosemary in rich in eucalyptol, on the key ingredients in antiseptic mouthwashes.

Orange EO is fungicidal.

Peppermint EO is antibacterial.

17

Personal Care Products for Children

KidScents Bath Gel

A shower gel with a neutral pH, perfect for young skin. pH neutral and noncomedogenic.

Ingredients: deionized water, decylpolyglucose, glycerin, sorbitol, MSM, aloe vera gel, panthenol, tocopheryl acetate, chamomile extract, comfrey extract, PG-hydroxyethycellulose cocodimonium chloride, coneflower extract, kiwi nut oil, jojoba oil, citrus seed extract, babassu oil, grape seed extract, dimethicone copolyol meadowfoamate, soap bark extract, soapwort extract, hyaluronic acid, wheat germ oil, keratin, linoleic acid, linolenic acid

Essential Oils: Cedarwood and geranium.

Companion Products: KidScents Shampoo, Kidscents Moisturizing Lotion

KidScents Moisturizing Lotion

An extraordinarily gentle lotion with the ideal pH for young skin. pH neutral and noncomedogenic.

Ingredients: Dionized water, MSM, glyceryl stearate, stearic acid, glycerin, grape seed extract, sodium hyaluronate, sorbitol, rose hip seed oil, shea butter, mango butter, wheat germ oil, kukui nut oil, lecithin, safflower oil, apricot oil, almond oil, tocopheryl acetate (vitamin E), retinyl palmitate (vitamin A), jojoba oil, sesame oil, calendula extract, chamomile extract, orange blossom extract, St. John's wort extract, algae extract, aloe vera gel, ascorbic acid (vitamin C), ginkgo biloba extract

Essential Oils: Cedarwood, rosewood, Canadian red cedar, and geranium.

Companion Products: KidScents Tender Tush Ointment

KidScents Shampoo

Contains the finest and most nontoxic natural ingredients for gently cleansing young, delicate hair. Perfectly pH-balanced formula.

Ingredients: Deionized water, decylpolyglucose, MSM, aloe vera gel, panthenol, tocopheryl acetate, chamomile extract, coneflower extract, kiwi nut oil, jojoba oil, citrus seed extract, babassu oil, grape seed extract, dimethicone copolyol meadowfoamate, hyaluronic acid, wheat germ oil, keratin, linoleic acid, linolenic acid

Essential Oils: Tangerine, lemon, and blue tansy.

Companion Products: KidScents Bath Gel, Kidscents Moisturizing Lotion

KidScents Tender Tush Ointment

An ointment designed to protect and nourish young skin and promote healing. pH neutral and noncomedogenic.

Ingredients: Coconut oil, cocoa butter, bees wax, wheat germ oil, olive oil, almond oil

Essential Oils: Sandalwood, rosewood, Roman chamomile, lavender, cistus, blue tansy, and frankincense.

Directions: Apply as needed to areas with diaper rash, redness, or irritation.

Companion Products: Rose Ointment, German chamomile, Roman chamomile.

KidScents Toothpaste

KidScents Toothpaste is a revolutionary all-natural, vegetarian formula with edible ingredients. Ultra-fine calcium carbonate, a natural tooth-health agent, gently scrubs plaque and debris from teeth without damaging enamel. Contains xylitol which has been proven to reduce tooth decay. Also contains an antiseptic, antimicrobial complex of essential oils which kill the oral bacteria responsible for gingivitis, periodontal disease, and tooth decay.

Ingredients: Calcium carbonate, natural strawberry Flavor, vegetable glycerine, zinc oxide, xanthum gum, trace minerals, xylitol, steviocide

Essential Oils: Peppermint, Thieves, Spearmint, Orange, Lemon

Companion Products: Fresh Essence Plus Mouthwash, Thieves Lozenges

KidScents MightyMist

A special spray multivitamin with wolfberry polysaccharide and therapeutic-grade essential oils.

Ingredients: Wolfberry (*Lycium barbarum*) polysaccharide, vitamin A, vitamin D3, vitamin E, vitamin C, folic acid, vitamin B-1, vitamin B-2, niacin-niacinamide, vitamin B-6, vitamin B-12, biotin, pantothenic acid, calcium, iodine, magnesium, copper, zinc, manganese, chromium, selenium, potassium, fructose, sorbitol, Bee pollen, inositol, stevia (*Stevia rebaudiana*)

Essential Oils: Lime, mandarin, orange

Directions: Spray inside mouth three times between meals.

Companion Products: MightyVites, Mightyzymes

KidScents MightyVites

A special chewable multivitamin formulated for children in the early growth years and for adult maintenance in late years. It is made with Chinese wolfberry (*Lycium barbarum*) and grain proteins for added immune support, with beta carotene, vitamin C, amino acids, and stevia.

Essential Oils: Lime, mandarin, orange

Directions: Chew three tablets daily with breakfast as a dietary supplement.

Companion Products: Body Balance, Essential Manna, Power Meal, Essential Omegas, Mightyzyme, Mightymist, Wolfberry Crisp.

18

Household Care

Thieves Household Cleaner

A nontoxic, biodegradable, cleansing solution that uses therapeutic-grade essential oils as emulsifiers and germ-killers. It contains Thieves Essential Oil Blend, which is docmented to kill over 99.96% of bacteria it comes into contact with (ie., *Pseudonomas aeroginosa*).

Ingredients:

Cleansing solution base: Nontoxic, biodegradable

Soy Lecithen is used as a natural emulsifier

Thieves Essential Oil Blend:

Clove (Syzygium aromaticum)
Lemon (Citrus limon)
Cinnamon Bark (Cinnamomum verum)
Eucalyptus Radiata (Eucalyptus radiata)
Rosemary (Rosmarinus officinalis)

Thieves Antiseptic Spray

An all-natural petro-chemical-free antiseptic spray that uses therapeutic-grade essential oils. It contains Thieves Essential Oil Blend, which is docmented to kill over 99.96% of bacteria it comes into contact with (ie., *Pseudonomas aeroginosa*).

Ingredients:

Pure Grain Alcohol is denatured with pure cinnamon essential oil; no toxic, harmful or synthetic denaturants used.

Soy Lecithen is used as a natural emulsifier

Thieves Essential Oil Blend:

Clove (Syzygium aromaticum)
Lemon (Citrus limon)
Cinnamon Bark (Cinnamomum verum)
Eucalyptus Radiata (Eucalyptus radiata)
Rosemary (Rosmarinus officinalis)

Thieves Antiseptic Wipes

A pack of 30 essential-oil-impregnated wipes using Thieves Essential Oil. Docmented to kill over 99.96% of bacteria it comes into contact with (ie., *Pseudonomas aeroginosa*).

Ingredients:

Pure Grain Alcohol is denatured with pure cinnamon essential oil; no toxic, harmful or synthetic denaturants used.

Soy Lecithen is used as a natural emulsifier

Thieves Essential Oil Blend:

Clove (Syzygium aromaticum)
Lemon (Citrus limon)
Cinnamon Bark (Cinnamomum verum)
Eucalyptus Radiata (Eucalyptus radiata)
Rosemary (Rosmarinus officinalis)

19

Animal Care and Horses

Products

Animal Scents Shampoo

This shampoo is designed to clean all types of animal fur and hair. It has insect-repelling and killing properties, and is designed to rid hair of lice, ticks, and other insects.

Ingredients: Saponified coconut oil and olive oil, glycerin, guar gum (*Cyamopsis tetragonoloba*), aloe vera (*Aloe barbadensis*), rosemary extract (*Rosmarinus officinalis*)

Essential Oils: Citronella, lavandin, lemon, geranium, spikenard

Animal Scents Ointment

This ointment has been tested in the field for many years. It is designed cover and seal infected wounds and seal in essential oils.

Ingredients: Mink oil, lecithin, bees wax, lanolin, sesame seed oil, Wheat germ oil, carrot seed oil (*Daucus carota*), rose hip seed oil

Essential Oils: Palmarosa, geranium, patchouli, Idaho balsam fir, myrrh, tea tree, rosewood

Veterinary Medicine

Essential oils have been used very successfully on many different kinds of animals from kittens to 2,000-pound draft horses. Animals generally respond to essential oils in much the same way as humans do.

How Much Should I Use?

Most animals are even more sensitive to the effects of the oils than humans. They often seem to have a natural affinity to the healing influence of the oils. Adjust dosage proportionately, based on body weight. If the protocol for a human being (at about 160 lbs) calls for 3-5 drops, then a horse (at 1600 lbs or more) could use as much as 10 times that amount, while a dog (at 16 lbs) would use as little as one tenth that amount. Generally speaking, if you have never put oils on an animal before, you should start carefully, applying them only to the feet, paws, or hooves (on the frog and cornet bands) at first.

In the case of cats and small dogs, essential oils should ALWAYS be diluted before applying, because they are actually MORE sensitive to the

---

Use Special Caution with Cats

Cats metabolize things very differently from dogs and other animals. Certain oils are potentially toxic to cats and could result in injury or even death, if applied incorrectly. For example, cats generally have adverse reactions to citrus products, and citrus oils are sometimes used to deter cats from frequenting an area. Also, cats are very sensitive to strong odors. A safe alternative, when in doubt, would be to mist them lightly with floral water. Consulting with a veterinarian is a good policy before applying oils to cats for the first time.

---

biochemicals in the oils than humans. Be careful to avoid high phenol oils, such as oregano and thyme, on cats because they can be extremely sensitive to these stronger oils. They should only be used in high rates of dilution (90%) and the diluted oil should only be applied to the paws.

General Guidelines:

For small animals: (cats and small dogs) Apply 3-5 drops DILUTED (80-90%) oil mixture per application.

For larger animals: (large dogs) Apply 3-5 drops NEAT per application.

For large animals: (cattle and horses) Apply 20-30 drops NEAT per application.

How to Administer EOs Internally

For internal use (ingestion), essential oils can be put into a capsule and mixed with the feed.

On large animals, the animal's bottom lip can be pulled out and (for example, in the case of a horse) 10 or 15 drops of oil put in. The animal will feel the effect quickly because capillaries in the lip will carry the oil into bloodstream immediately. For a large dog, 1 to 3 drops is sufficient.

When treating animals with essential oils internally, make certain the oils used are pure and free of chemicals, solvents, and adulterants. Always seek the advice of a qualified veterinarian before allowing the animals to ingest essential oils.

Other Helpful Tips:

- When treating large animals for viral or bacterial infection, arthritis, or bone injury, generally use the same oils and protocol recommended for humans.
- For applying to large open wounds or hard-to-reach areas, it helps to put the oils in a spray bottle and spray them directly on location.
- After an oil application to an open wound, cover the wound with Animal Scents Ointment to seal it and protect it from further infection. The ointment will also prevent the essential oils from evaporating into the air.
- There is no right or wrong way to apply essential oils. Every animal is a little different. Use common sense and good judgment as you experiment with different methods. Observe carefully how the animal responds to the treatment.

- Take special care not to get essential oils in the animal's eyes.
- Make sure the animal is drinking pure water. **Chlorinated water will suppress thyroid and immune function** in animals even quicker than in humans, and when that happens, you will suppress the healing process of that animal whether it is a dog, a horse or a cat. (see CHAPTER 12: WATER TREATMENT).

- Quality protein is vitally important to promote healing, which makes the use of organic feed essential. Unfortunately many commercial feeds contain bovine byproducts that have high risk for BSE disease and make them unfit for animal care. Avoid these at all costs. Enzymes are also essential to maximize digestion and protein assimilation.

Where to Apply Essential Oils to Animals:

For non-ungulate animals (not having hooves) such as dogs or cats, oils (neat or diluted) can be applied to paws for faster absorption.

For hoofed animals, sprinkle a few drops on the spine or flanks and massage them in. Also apply on the gums, tongue or underneath the top lip; also apply on the frog and cornet bands of hooves. These are all good locations for oils to be applied to cows, horses, etc., all animals with hooves. Oils can also be applied to auricular points of the ears.

When the Animal is Jittery and Resists:

If you have a high-spirited, jittery animal that won't be still to receive the application, apply Peace & Calming and/or Valor on yourself first. As you approach the animal, it will react it perceives the aroma. Kneel down or squat beside the animal and remain still for several minutes, so that it can become accustomed to the smell. As the animal breathes in the fragrances, it will become calmer and easier to manage.

Essential Oils First Aid Kit for Animals

- **Animal Scents Ointment** to seal and disinfect open wounds.

- **Exodus II** for infection, inflammation; to promote tissue regeneration.

- **Helichrysum** as a topical anesthetic.

- **Idaho Tansy** is one of the most versatile oils for animals. It is purifying, cleansing, tissue-regenerating, anti-inflammatory, and anesthetic, and is used for bruised bones, cuts, wounds, and colic. It repels flies.

- **Laurel** for bruising and soreness.

- **Lavender** for tissue regeneration, desensitizing wound.

- **Melrose** for disinfecting and cleaning wounds.

- **Mountain savory** for reducing inflammation.

- **Myrrh** for infection, inflammation; to promote tissue regeneration.

- **Ortho Ease** to dilute essential oils and act as a pain-reliever and anti-inflammatory.

- **PanAway:** If the pain originates from a broken bone rather than an open wound, use PanAway to kill pain in points where there is no open, raw tissue. NOTE: Do not apply PanAway to open wounds because it will sting and traumatize the animal. Instead use helichrysum and balsam fir to reduce bleeding and pain.

- **Purification** is more effective than using iodine or hydrogen peroxide for washing and cleansing wounds. It repels ticks and mites.

- **Roman chamomile** for tissue regeneration, desensitizing wound.

- **Thieves** for inflammation, infection and bacteria; for proudflesh (where new tissue continues to rebuild itself causing excessive granulation) to promote tissue regeneration.

- **Valerian** can be used internally and externally for controlling pain.

- **Vetiver** can be used internally and externally for controlling pain.

Animal Treatment A to Z

ARTHRITIS:

(common in older animals and purebreeds). Ortho Ease or PanAway (massage on location or put several drops in animal feed).

Use Raindrop-like application of PanAway, wintergreen, pine, or spruce and massage the location. For larger animals use at least 2 times more oil than a normal Raindrop Technique would call for on humans.

For prevention: Put Power Meal and Sulfurzyme in feed or fodder. Small animals: 1/8 to 1/4 serving per day. Large animals: 2-4 servings per day.

BIRTHING:

Gentle Baby.

BLEEDING:

Geranium, helichrysum (Shave the hair over the area being treated.)

BONES: (pain, spurs—all animals):

R.C., PanAway, wintergreen, lemongrass, and spruce. All conifers are very powerful in the action for bones and in promoting bone health. For more effective absorption, it is helpful to shave the fur/hair away from the area being treated. BLM is an excellent supplement for building animal bones.

BONES: (fractured or broken):

Mix PanAway with 20-30 drops of wintergreen and spruce. Cover the area. After 15 minutes rub in 10-15 more drops of wintergreen and spruce. Cover with Ortho Sport Massage Oil. BLM can be used as a supplement to help speed bone healing.

CALMING:

Peace & Calming, Trauma Life, lavender (domestic animals respond very quickly to the smell).

COLDS AND FLU:

For small animals put 1-3 drops Exodus II, ImmuPower, or Di-Tone in feed or fodder. For large animals, use 10-20 drops.

COLIC:

For large animals (cows) put 10-20 drops of Di-Tone in feed or fodder. For small animals, use 1-3 drops.

FLEAS AND OTHER PARASITES:

Single oils: Lemongrass, tea tree, eucalyptus (all types), citronella, and peppermint.

Blends: Di-Tone. Also add 1-2 drops of lemongrass to Animal Scents shampoo, and use to shampoo the animal.

Oils repel fleas and other external parasites. Wash blankets with oils added to the wash during the rinse cycle. Also, place 1-2 drops of lemongrass on collar to help eliminate fleas.

For internal parasites, daily rub Di-Tone on the pads (bottom) of the feet. Many people have reported that they have seen the parasites eliminated from the animal within days after starting this procedure.

INFLAMMATION:

Apply Ortho Ease, PanAway, pine, wintergreen, or spruce on location. Put Sulfurzyme in feed. Mineral Essence may also be good.

INSECT REPELLENT:

Put 10 drops each of citronella, Purification, *Eucalyptus globulus,* and peppermint in 8 ounce spray bottle with water. Alternate formula: Put 2 drops pine, 2 drops Eucalyptus globulus, and 5-10 drops citronella in a spray bottle of water. Shake vigorously and spray over area. Floral waters, such as peppermint and Idaho tansy, can also be used.

LIGAMENTS/TENDONS (torn or sprained):

Apply lemongrass and lavender (equal parts) on location and cover area. For small animals or birds, dilute essential oils with V-6 Mixing Oil (2 parts mixing oil to 1 part essential oil).

MINERAL DEFICIENCIES:

Mineral Essence. (In one case, an animal stopped chewing on furniture once his mineral deficiency was met).

MITES (ear mites):

Apply Purification and peppermint to a Q-Tip and swab just the inside of the ear.

NERVOUS ANXIETY:

Valor, Trauma Life, Roman or German chamomile,geranium, lavender, and valerian.

PAIN:

Helichrysum, PanAway, Relieve It, clove, or peppermint diluted 50-50 with V6 Oil Complex.

SHINY COATS:

Rosemary and sandalwood. Essential Omegas, sulfurzyme, or AD&E, will be beneficial as well.

SINUS PROBLEMS:

Diffuse Raven, R.C., pine, myrtle, and *Eucalyptus radiata* in animal's sleeping quarters or sprinkle their on bedding. Thieves, Super C, Exodus, Exodus II, and ImmuneTune have been reported as being extremely beneficial for sinus and (lung also) congestion.

SKIN CANCER:

Frankincense, lavender, clove, and myrrh. Apply neat.

TICKS:

To remove ticks, apply 1 drop cinnamon or peppermint on cotton swab and swab on tick. Then wait for it to release the head before removing from animal's skin.

TRAUMA:

Trauma Life, Valor, Peace & Calming, melissa, rosewood, Gentle Baby, lavender, valerian, and chamomile.

TUMORS OR CANCERS:

Mix frankincense with ledum, lavender or clove and apply on area of tumor.

WORMS AND PARASITES:

ParaFree and Di-Tone.

WOUNDS (open or abrasions):

Melrose, helichrysum, and Animal Scents Ointment.

Further Helps for Equine Care

BRUISED ANKLE (ie., from hobble injury):

Apply bay laurel, Melrose, and mountain savory to reduce tenderness, bruising, and inflammation.

CANCER:

Shave area near the tumor and inject with a hypodermic needle. Keep saturated with frankincense. If the area is open, put a plug in the opening to hold the oil in the tumor cavity. Alternate with clove oil every four days. Continue for six months.

COLIC: (The leading cause of death in horses.)

Symptoms:
- Pawing the ground with head down
- Trotting in circles
- Lying down and looking bloated
- No churning or rumbling in the stomach. Quiet is a sign of colic.

Causes:
- Eating off the ground and mineral imbalance (getting too much dirt in the gut). The accumulated dirt can cause the gut to twist, abscess, and spasm.
- Parasites
- Eating too much alfalfa and not enough feed. Alfalfa can stress kidneys and liver in horses. In general, grass hay is best for horses of all kinds. As a rule of thumb, the more a horse works, the more alfalfa he needs and can tolerate.
- Getting too hot.

Treatment Protocol:
Keep the horse standing or walking. If the horse lies down, keep the animal's head tied up to prevent him from rolling.

1st hour:
Internal Use:
8 to 10 Detoxzyme capsules
15 drops of DiTone

Put into animal's feed grain or drop inside lip. You can open the capsules and make an enzyme/oil paste to put inside the horse's lip)

Massage
- Rub 10 drops DiTone up each flank and massage out towards umbilical area.
- Rub 10 drops DiTone around the coronet band.
- Rub DiTone on auricular points of ears.

Enema
Mix 30 drops of Di-Tone in 6 ounces olive oil or V-6 oil and insert in the horse's rectum as enema. Do not use castor oil-it dehydrates the colon.

2nd hour:
Put 10 to 20 drops Di-Tone in the mouth and on the flanks and coronet band.

4th hour:
Repeat 1st hour protocol except for enema.

6th hour:
Repeat 1st hour protocol, adding 5 drops of peppermint to the 15 drops of Di-Tone.

8th hour:
Repeat 1st hour except for enema and add 1 scoop of Power Meal (add to water if the animal is drinking).

10th hour:
Continue administering 6-8 Detoxzyme capsules every 2 hours until the horse's bowels are moving well.

DISTEMPER, WHOOPING COUGH OR ASTHMA

Daily Regimen:
- Mix 30 drops each of R.C. and Raven in 4 ounces of V-6 Oil Complex and insert into the rectum.
- Put 15 drops each of R.C. and Raven in the bottom lip.
- Massage oils on the chest between the front legs and auricular points of ears.
- Raindrop Technique down the spine and neck hair.
- 4 Longevity capsules.

FRACTURES/BONE CHIPS

Shave area around affected bone
Apply mixture of
5 drops wintergreen
5 drops balsam fir
2 drops oregano

Add to feed: 2 tablespoons Sulfurzyme
Continue the above daily for 3 months

Case History:

In 1997 a horse's back hock was fractured, with two 50-cent-sized pieces splintered off. The animal was diagnosed at stage 5 lameness and the vet urged euthanizing the animal. After wintergreen essential oil was applied for several months, the bone regenerated and the break healed. Today the horse (Goliath) is ridden in jousting tournaments. (Note: Other oils that may be effective for this condition include helichrysum, spruce and Idaho balsam fir. Sulfurzyme can be used internally.)

HIDE INJURIES

Case History:

A 4-month-old colt had the hide on one side of its body stripped off. The wound was sprayed with Melrose to disinfect and helichrysum to control pain. The wound was then sealed with the formula now known as Animal Scents Ointment. Within several months the hair and skin had completely grown in and the animal had made a full recovery.

HOOF INFECTIONS

Case History:

In 2000, a show horse received some kind of severe bit on the pastern. Although the vet diagnosed a rattlesnake bite, it may have been caused by something else. Two weeks later, the entire pastern and coronet band were inflamed (the size of a cantaloupe) and the rotting, decaying flesh revealed a large hole where the bone was visible and had separated from the hoof. The vet suggested amputating the foot. Instead the following protocol was initiated:

Day 1: Wound was cleaned and disinfected with Thieves and helichrysum and the foot was bandaged. This treatment decreased pain enough to allow the mare to put weight on the foot.

Day 2: Swelling dropped by 50 percent. Wound was again cleaned with Thieves and helichrysum and then packed with Animal Scents Ointment

Day 3 to 14: Wound was washed morning and night with Thieves, melrose and helichrysum and packed with Animal Scents Ointment.

RESULT: The animal today walks with no discomfort. A brand new hoof has appeared with only a small scar where the wound was. Although there was minor swelling in the pastern for a while, it faded 8 months later.

IMPRINTING ON NEW FOALS

Recommended Essential Oils:

Valor, Highest Potential, Sacred Mountain, Joy, Surrender, Acceptance

As soon as a colt is born, pick up the foal, hold it in your arms. Massage 5-6 drops of oil along the spine and a drop on each ear; then rub oils all over colt's body, a few drops at a time. Lay the colt in your lap. Lay its head back, stroke its neck, and pass over its nose (avoid putting any oils on the nose; it is very sensitive). Repeat every day for 21 days.

JITTERINESS:

To calm a horse, apply a few drops of oil on the hands; then put one hand on the base of the tail and the other on the withers. The animal should relax. Relaxation is the first step to healing.

Put several drops of Trauma Life, Surrender or Peace & Calming in your hand and briefly hold it up to the animal's muzzle or nostrils. If the horse pulls away and returns to it several times--perhaps out of curiosity or perhaps thinking that food may appear--feed him some grain as a reward and then put your hand with oil on his muzzle and gently rub it in. As he relaxes, work your hand around the side of his jaw and up along the neckline to the ears. Then rub his ears and top of head/crop. As he further relaxes, you can add more oil to the palm of your hand (Peace & Calming or valerian) and continue rubbing his ears, head and crop.

KIDNEY FAILURE:

- Administer 10 drops (about 1/2 dropper) K & B tincture morning and night
- Raindrop-type application on the spine: 5 drops each of cypress and juniper daily for 10 days

LAXATIVE FOR FOALS:

Put 4 drops of Di-Tone in bottom lip daily until bowels are moving.

OPEN WOUNDS

Case History:

A large thoroughbred gelding was attacked by a cougar who clawed a chunk of flesh out of the horse's buttocks half the size of a soccer ball. The horse bled terribly, blood squirting from ruptured blood vessels. The vet said the prognosis was grim because there was too much torn, damaged, and removed tissue. Even if the horse didn't die, the wound would leave a size scar and indentation.

TREATMENT PROTOCOL:

DAY 1:

To reduce pain and stop bleeding, a 5cc hypodermic syringe was filled with helichrysum and sprayed into the wound. The horse became less jittery and the bleeding stopped.
Several minutes later a larger 10cc syringe of Purification was sprayed into the open wound It took over 15 ml of Purification to spray down and cover the entire wound.

After several hours, the wound was sprayed with Melrose to disinfect it and packed with the formula now known as Animal Scents Ointment. To keep hair out of the wound and reduce the possibility of infection, the tail was wrapped and tied up. Because there was no way to cover or close the wound, the horse was kept in the stable to prevent him from moving around. The animal was closely monitored to reduce the possibility of reinfection caused by the animal lying down, rolling around, and scratching the wound.

DAY 2-7

The horse's grain was supplemented with enzymes (crushed up Essentialzyme--Polyzyme is also helpful--and four scoops of Power Meal, which is dense in the nutrients required for healing and tissue rebuilding. Three times daily the open wound was irrigated with Purification and helichrysum. The vet came regularly to monitor the horse's progress. He remarked that he had never seen muscle tissue regenerate to such a degree.

WEEKS 2 to 4

Two times a day the open wound was irrigated with Purification and helichrysum

WEEKS 4 to 8

Once a week the wound was irrigated with Purification and helichrysum until it was closed.

RESULTS:

Today no indentation or concavity is visible, only a small circular two-inch scar.

PUNCTURE WOUNDS

Put 1cc of Thieves in a hypodermic syringe, insert the needle deeply into the wound, and irrigate thoroughly. Repeat 1 to 2 times a day for 2 to 3 days if still infected or swollen continue for up to 10 days.

SADDLE SORES and RAW SPOTS

(ie., where packs rub against flesh):

Use Melrose and Animal Scents ointment for at least 3 days.

SCOURS (diarrhea caused by bacteria):

- Put 5 drops Di-Tone in the horse's lower lip and rub 5-8 drops up in flank,
- Put I.C.P. in water or pouring it down the throat.
  Continue for four days.

SCREW WORM

There is a round worm called a bore or screw worm that bores into the spine of a horse (especially wild horses). It will cause a huge boil-like abscess on the spine. When lanced a larva worm will come out of that abscess. Sometimes the abscess will actually break open and ooze. Pour Thieves into the hole to flush out the larva worm and then fill the hole with a mixture of 12 drops Melrose and 5 drops mountain savory.

STRANGLES (*Streptococcus equi* infection):

- Perform Raindrop Technique with Thieves.
- 4 drops of Thieves on the inside of the bottom lip (for a large horse, 8 drops).
- 1 teaspoon of ImmuGel for a small horse, 1 tablespoon for a big horse.

- After 2 hours repeat RT with oregano and thyme; Put 2 drops of oregano and 2 drops of thyme on the inside of the bottom lip (for a large horse, 4 drops each).
- 1 teaspoon of ImmuGel for a small horse, 1 tablespoon for a big horse.

Repeat the last two steps every 2 hours until the horse begins to improve. As the horse continues to improve, alternate treatments every four hours, every 6 hours, and then morning and night.

SWOLLEN SHEATH

Geldings and stallions occasionally suffer swollen sheath, with an abscess and infection. It can be caused by

1. Eating hay too rich in protein (ideal levels of protein should be 12 to 15%; alfalfa hay can have protein as high as 26%).

2. Not extracting the penis and letting it clean off.

TREATMENT:

1. Put on rubber gloves.
2. Clean inside the sheath and remove debris with soap and water. (Use half a cap of Thieves household cleanser diluted in a half gallon of water).
3. Clean outside of the sheath, apply myrrh oil and rosemary with bay laurel. The ratio is 15 drops of myrrh, 15 drops of rosemary, and 10 drops of laurel.
4. Perform cleaning and disinfecting morning and night until infection and swelling subsides.
5. Maintenance: The sheath should be cleaned out once a month Make sure the horse is fed adequate water and grass hay and gets sufficient exercise to increase circulation.
6. Perform Raindrop Technique with oregano, thyme and mountain savory every three to six months.

UMBILICAL CORDS OF NEWBORN FOALS:

Instead of iodine, put myrrh oil on the umbilical cord of newborn foals. Myrrh will dry the umbilical cord and facilitate a good separation. Exodus II can also be used to treat infections in a foals umbilical cord.

Tips on Performing Raindrop Technique on Horses

Although many veterinarians have developed their own variations on this technique, the simplicity of this procedure is what makes it effective. RT for horses is similar to that for humans except that there must be practical modifications because of the difference in size and shape of the patient. Trying to exactly duplicate the human-version of Raindrop Technique on animals is not advised.

STARTING POINT:

Apply 6 drops of Valor to the tailbone (the base of the tail where it connects with the spine). Then place one hand on the withers and the other on the tailbone and hold for 5 minutes. There is no difference energetically, whether you use your right or left hand in these spots. Once the horse relaxes (i.e., drops its head and eyelids droop) the procedure can start.

DON'TS:

- Do not spend too much time stroking the horse's spine. Usually three repetitions is sufficient
- Avoid dripping oils on the hair of the horse's spine and stroking them in. You will be stroking against the grain of the hair and oil will be flicked off the spine rather than rubbed in. (This is not so important with animals with fine hair).
- Once you make contact with the animal you are applying oils, never break it.
- Don't work on the animal with multiple partners. RT is more effective when only one pair of hands makes continuous contact with the animal because:
1) The energy stays the same.
2) Animals get skittish when two or more people touch them at the same time.

HOW TO APPLY OILS:

- Where feasible, shave the spine area for direct application of the oil (you will use less oil).
- If shaving is not feasible, stand the hair up and part it; then drip the oil down through the hair so the oil contacts the spine. Hold the oil six inches above the spine as you drop it in.
- For coarse-haired animals stroke in the oils using small, circular motions, working from the base of the tail to the shoulders of the spine.

- For fine-haired animals, stroke in oils using regular Raindrop Technique straight-strokes
- Spend enough time massaging to get oils down into the skin and not sitting on top of the hair

When dripping the oils on spine, use
- 12 drops on a draft horse
- 6 drops on a saddle horse
- 3-4 drops on a miniature horse, Shetland or Welch pony

ADDITIONAL TIPS:

Carefully use your fingertips and thumb tips to perform Vita Flex along the auricular points of the ear. Be gentle. If you inflict a little discomfort, the horse will distrust you and pull away.

Stretching the spine is problematic in horses, so instead place one hand over the tail, the other hand on the withers and focus moving the energy along the spine.

Rubbing oils around the coronet band will allow them to reach the bloodstream and travel through the nerves in the legs to the spine.

Drip Marjoram and Aroma Siez into the hair of the outside muscles away from the spine and rub in with a larger circular motion massages. (Idaho tansy, Bay Laurel or Melrose--which are anti-inflammatory, anaesthetic, insect-repelling, relaxing and healing--

can also be used). This is important because horses used for packing, riding, or working have extra stress to the spine and muscles in the back.

Avoid having two people working on opposite sides of the horse at the same time. No two people's energy are the same and this produces an energetic imbalance.

Use a stool (mounting block) to reach both sides of the spine without having to break contact, potentially creating tension in the animal.

Some people mistakenly believe that if they don't have all the oils in the Raindrop kit, they can't do a raindrop. One does not need to apply every single oil to have an effective treatment. You can perform an excellent, beneficial Raindrop procedure with one oil, if that's all you have. Using just oregano and thyme or even Idaho tansy can produce excellent results. Similarly, Melrose, tea tree, mountain savory, or bay laurel can also be used.

Is it OK to stroke oils down off the hips and down the legs? Yes

Is it OK to put a hot towel on the spine? Yes, it is recommended.

Following a raindrop, you can apply a saddle blanket then a horse blanket and leave the animal standing in the stall. Usually after about 10 minutes they will lie down and go to sleep.

EO Testimonials from Animal Owners

The following is a small selection of the dozens of testimonials received from animal owners:

"My cat developed a pink bald spot, near his tail, which was losing hair by the day. The veterinarian didn't know what it was, so she tested for a virus and sold me antibiotics to give him just in case. She mentioned that it had the appearance of a burn.

"When I got home, I decided to re-think the antibiotic idea: if it might be a burn, why not simply put on lavender, I asked myself? So I applied less than a drop on that spot, by just barely touching it. In the morning it was clearly improved. I applied lavender again the same way, a second time only. His fur grew back in so fast I didn't worry about it again.

"Later I learned that this is a common spot where a cat will scratch another when it runs away from a standoff. In hindsight, I believe the bald spot was just that: a cat scratch infection."

— *Barbara J. Ullrich, Tacoma, WA*

"My cat Nigel has to be rushed to three different animal hospitals one night due to a ruptured urethra. He was in severe pain and had been anesthetized twice over the course of about 6 hours.

"By 11:00 pm we were wearily on our way to the third hospital, which was over an hour away, when I thankfully found my Young Living lavender oil in my coat pocket. After applying several drops to my forehead, temples and neck to help calm me down, I simply held the open bottle next to Nigel's carrier where he was loudly despairing and restlessly trying to stand despite his dizziness from the anesthesia.

"Within seconds of introducing the oil to him, he became silent. I was so amazed that I had to check to make sure he was still alive! I left the bottle open for the duration of the trip. He remained calm for the remainder of the drive, meowing only occasionally, and made it through his final surgery beautifully. Thanks to the lavender oil, Nigel and I got through the final hours of that very long, traumatic night with comfort and ease."

— *Sarah George, Newburyport, MA*

"Three years ago, my corgi, Dickens, ruptured a disc in his back. As a result, his back legs were paralyzed. He was 5 years old at the time. He underwent surgery and recovered very well, but he was left with an odd gait, with swinging hips. He was able to run and play, go on long walks and, most importantly, was pain free.

"But a year and a half ago, while laying on the sofa, he rolled over on his back and immediately began yelping in pain. We had no idea what was wrong. Since it was 8 pm on a Friday night, we took him to an emergency animal clinic. He was examined and x-rayed. Nothing showed up on the x-ray, but Dickens continued to howl and shake, so the vet thought that maybe he had a pinched nerve in his neck. She gave him a shot for pain and a cortisone shot, and prescribed both pain and cortisone pills. We took him to our regular vet the following Monday, who agreed the problem was most likely a pinched nerve, and gave us enough pills to last 2 weeks. Dickens did fine for two weeks, and after a final check up, the vet released him. He recommended that we use a harness, not a leash, to relieve any neck stress.

"Things went along well for about 10 days. Then all at once, Dickens started howling in pain. This time I decided to try my own therapy. I got out a 15 ml bottle and made up a "Raindrop concoction" consisting of 5 ml Valor, 2 ml Aroma Siez and 1 ml each of oregano, thyme, basil, wintergreen, cypress, marjoram, and peppermint.

"I applied 5-7 drops of this mixture along his spine, starting at the atlas and moving down to his tail bone. I massaged it in, and then applied a little V6 Oil Complex to "seal" it. I repeated this treatment 3-4 times daily. On the second day, Dickens was running and playing again. I continued the treatment for about 3 weeks. Several times since then, Dickens has come over to me and stared expectantly until I got out the "Raindrop concoction" and applied it to his back.

"Now over 8 years old, he has remained healthy and happy, and I know what to do if the condition flares up again."

— *Linda Chandler, Carmel, CA*

"Early one morning I received a call from Marie, one of my massage clients I had seen the day before. Her 14 year old dog, Precious, had been to the groomer--whom she doesn't like--and fell off the table while the groomer wasn't watching. The dog could not walk or squat. Marie took her to the vet, who examined and x-rayed Precious and found no broken bones. Precious received a shot and an anti-inflammatory, but she still could not walk. Marie wanted me to come help with her dog. Although Marie had complete faith in my abilities, I was hesitant to go. I suggested other things that might help, but Marie was insistent. I told her I would be there within the hour.

"On the way I was sorting out what I could do for the dog. I had the essential oil blend, PanAway, with me, but I wasn't sure the dog would like the aroma, and I wondered if an animal in pain would allow me to work on it. I know Precious, so that was a help. She was glad to see me. She was on Marie's bed and that was a good place to work.

"I tried gentle massage to the back and spinal area. It was soon evident she liked what I was doing and seemed to know I was trying to help her. After about 10 or 15 minutes, we encouraged her to get up. She stood, but her hind legs were rubbery and she could not walk. As she lay down I noticed her left back leg was stuck, out straight. I massaged the left leg, hip, and knee with PanAway, especially the tendons in the knee, and we then took Precious outside. She emptied her bladder, came inside under her own power, drank a whole bowl of water and ate a little food. (She had not been drinking or eating.) Marie called me the next day to say Precious was walking and feeling fine. 'It's a miracle!' she said."

— *Kathy Smith, CMS, NMT, Atlanta GA*

"My horse Katie, is a beautiful Shire draft horse, of the type used in jousting. Katie had a serious abscess on the bottom of her foot. Fixing this involves digging a huge hole into the foot to get the abscess out, and is a painful situation for the horse--which is very rarely anaesthetized. My vet was trying to get to the abscess and of course Katie was skittish. The farrier was helping him, but Katie weighs a ton (yes, a ton--as I said, she is a jousting-type horse), and it was very slow going. She was upset, scared, and I knew she was in pain. It's hard because you can't tell an animal it's "going to be all right" when the doctor is done. I didn't know what to do.

"So I had my friend go to my car to get some Peace & Calming, as I figured anything could help. She mistakenly brought back PanAway, and before realizing it was a different blend, I put it up to Katie's nose. At that moment, I realized it was not the oil I had intended to use and had my friend go back to the car to get the Peace & Calming. The thing was, as soon as I had put the PanAway to Katie's face, she had gotten "interested" in the small; her ears had pricked forward and she had stopped moving around as much. Then when I put the P & C up to her nostrils, it calmed her down *immediately.* The vet was able to 'doctor' her up and an unpleasant task became manageable. In fact, the farrier didn't even have to continue to help the vet. Katie relaxed so much that you could see her shoulder go down and she stopped trying to pull her foot away from the vet. There was blood all over her hoof from the vet trying to dig out that abscess! My friend and I were honestly amazed that 'suddenly' she just relaxed and even dropped her head down. Now, mind you, I used almost the entire bottle of the P & C, because the work on the abscess took a long time. But from the moment I put it up to her nostrils until the vet packed her foot up and wrapped it with an enormous bandage. her shoulders were relaxed, and her head was down (a good sign with horses that they are not stressed). The vet didn't even give me a 'butte' (horse painkiller); he just said "whatever you were doing, keep doing that."

— *Sandra Shepard, CMT, JD, Petaluma, CA*

"I recently used the oils in a case with a mare that had colic, and they seemed to work just like the drug, Banamine. I had on hand three oils that were suggested for use on smooth muscles (intestines) in the Desk Reference--marjoram, clary sage and lavender. For each application, I used 5 drops of the same oils on each flank with a warm compress. Each application took effect in about 30 minutes and kept the mare calm and comfortable for 2.5-3 hours. I alternated oils throughout the night with each application. Marjoram and clary sage seemed to work better than lavender. By 7:30 the next morning, the mare showed marked improvement and went for water."

— *Janis Early, Tallahassee, FL*

20

Vita Flex Technique

Vita Flex Technique means "vitality through the reflexes." It is a specialized form of hand and foot massage that is exceptionally effective in delivering the benefits of essential oils throughout the body. It is said to have originated in Tibet thousands of years ago, and was perfected in the 1960s by Stanley Burroughs long before acupuncture was popular in Western medicine.

It is based on a complete network of reflex points that stimulate all the internal body systems. Essential oils are applied to contact points, and energy is released through electrical impulses created by contact between the fingertips and reflex points. This electrical charge follows the nerve pathways to a break or clog in the electrical circuit usually caused by toxins, damaged tissues, or loss of oxygen. As

Vita Flex Foot Chart

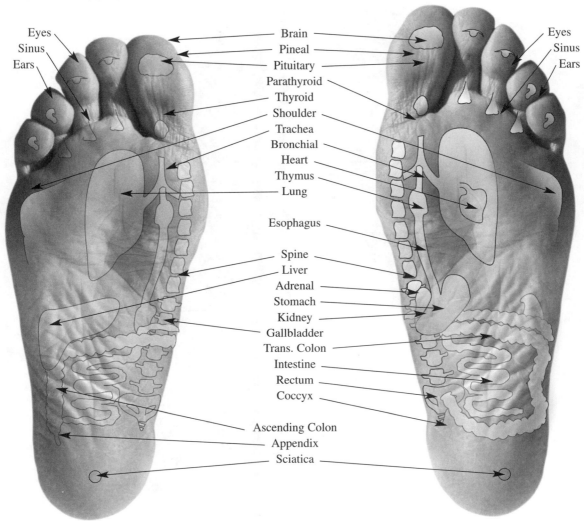

Eyes
Sinus
Ears

Brain
Pineal
Pituitary
Parathyroid
Thyroid
Shoulder
Trachea
Bronchial
Heart
Thymus
Lung

Esophagus

Spine
Liver
Adrenal
Stomach
Kidney
Gallbladder
Trans. Colon
Intestine
Rectum
Coccyx

Ascending Colon
Appendix
Sciatica

Eyes
Sinus
Ears

with acupressure there are hundreds of Vita Flex reflex points throughout the human body, encompassing the entire realm of body and mind, that are capable of releasing many kinds of tension, congestion, and imbalances.

In contrast to the steady stimulation of Reflexology, Vita Flex uses a rolling and releasing motion that involves placing fingers flat on the skin, rolling onto the fingertips, and continuing over onto the fingernail using medium pressure. Then moving forward about half the width of the finger, this rolling and releasing technique is continually repeated until the Vita Flex point, or area, is covered. This movement is repeated over the area three times.

Combine this technique with 1-3 drops of essential oil applied to those areas of the feet that correspond to the system of the body you wish to support (see the diagram on previous page). Rapid and extraordinary results are experienced when combining essential oils with Vita Flex stimulation, as it increases the effect of both.

The diagram below shows the nervous system connection to the spine for the electrical points throughout the body.

Nervous System Connection Points

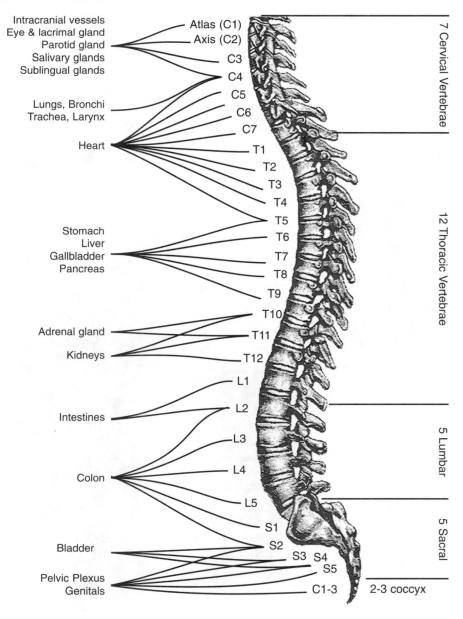

21

Raindrop Technique®

D. Gary Young developed the Raindrop Technique® (RT) during the 1980s based on his research with essential oils as antimicrobial agents, and prompted by some fascinating information he learned from an elder among the Lakota Indian Nation in South Dakota. This Lakota elder related that several generations ago, his ancestors regularly migrated north across the Canadian border into the northern regions of Saskatchewan and Manitoba, where they often witnessed the Aurora Borealis, or Northern Lights. When the Aurora Borealis was on display, those who were ill or had complicated health problems would stand facing the dancing lights and hold their hands out toward the lights and inhale deeply. Their belief was that the air was charged with healing energy from the Aurora Borealis. Mentally, they would "inhale" this energy into their spine and then out through nerve pathways to afflicted areas of the body.

This process stimulated an incredible healing effect for many of his ancestors. Effleurage (feathered finger stroking) became associated with this tradition after the borders were closed and the Lakota could no longer migrate north. Restricted to their reservations, they began practicing this energy process mentally, coupled with light stroking to facilitate the spreading of energy through the body.

It was this tradition that provided the promptings and began the process that gave birth to the development of Raindrop Technique (RT). Since 1989, RT has received an enormous amount of praise from users around the world for its ability to help ameliorate spinal abnormalities such as scoliosis and kyphosis, and facilitate tissue cleansing.

RT is based on the idea—now being explored in a number of scientific studies—that many types of scoliosis and spinal misalignments are caused by viruses or bacteria that lie dormant along the spine. These pathogens create inflammation, which, in turn, contorts and disfigures the spinal column.

RT is a powerful, non-invasive tool for assisting the body in correcting defects in the curvature of the spine by utilizing the antiviral, antibacterial, and anti-inflammatory action of several key essential oils. During the years that it has been practiced, it has resolved numerous cases of scoliosis, kyphosis, and chronic back pain. Further, it has eliminated the need for back surgery for hundreds of people. By integrating Vita Flex and massage, the power of essential oils brings the body into structural and electrical alignment.

Consistent with the French Model

The use of undiluted essential oils in RT is consistent with the French model for aromatherapy—which is the most extensively practiced and studied model in the world. With over 40 years of experience using essential oils clinically, the French have consistently recommended neat (undiluted) use of essential oils. An illustrious roster of 20th century French physicians provides convincing evidence that undiluted essential oils have a valuable place in the therapeutic arsenal of clinical professionals. René Gattefossé, PhD; Jean Valnet, MD; Jean-Claude Lapraz, MD; Daniel Pénoël, MD; and many others have long attested to the safe and effective use of undiluted essential oils and the dramatic and powerful benefits they can impart. According to Dr. Pénoël, "What happens when we use [essential oils] without diluting them? With many current essential oils, nothing dangerous or serious can happen."

In the case of Raindrop Technique®, the use of certain undiluted essential oils typically causes minor reddening and "heat" in the tissues. Normally, this is perfectly safe and not something to be overly concerned about. Blondes, redheads, and persons whose systems are toxic are more susceptible to this temporary reddening. Should the reddening or heat become excessive, it can be remedied within a minute or two by the immediate application of several drops of pure, quality vegetable oil to the affected area. This effectively dilutes the oils and the warming effect. Temporary mild warming is normal for RT. Typically it is even milder than that of many capsicum creams or sports ointments. Indeed, rather than being a cause of concern, this warming indicates that positive benefits are being imparted. In cases where the warmth or heat exceeds the comfort zone of the recipient, as mentioned before, the facilitator can apply any pure vegetable oil to the area until the comfort level is regained and reddening dissipates (usually within 2 minutes).

NOTE: If a rash should appear, it is an indication of a chemical reaction between the oils and synthetic compounds in the skin cells and interstitial fluid of the body (usually from conventional personal care products). Some misconstrue this as an allergic reaction, when in fact the problem is not caused by an allergy but rather by foreign chemicals already imbedded in the tissues.

A number of medical professionals throughout the United States have adopted RT in their clinical practice and have found it to be an outstanding resource for aiding sciatica, scoliosis, kyphosis, and chronic back pain. Ken Krieger, DC, a chiropractor practicing in Scottsdale, Arizona, states, "As a chiropractor, I believe that the dramatic results of RT are enough for me to rewrite the books on scoliosis." Similarly, Terry Friedmann, MD, of Westminster, Colorado, states that "these essential oils truly represent a new frontier of medicine; they have resolved cases that many professionals had regarded as hopeless."

Do Infections Cause Scoliosis and Sciatica?

A growing amount of scientific research shows that certain microorganisms lodge near the spinal cord and contribute to deformities. Studies at Western General Hospital in Edinburgh, Scotland, linked virus-like particles to idiopathic scoliosis.[1,2] Researchers at the University of Bonn have also found the varicella zoster virus can lodge in the spinal ganglia throughout life.[3]

Research in 2001 further corroborated the existence of infectious microorganisms as a cause of spine pain and inflammation. Alistair Stirling and his colleagues at the Royal Orthopedic Hospital in Birmingham, England, found that 53 percent of patients with severe sciatica tested positive for chronic, low-grade infection by gram-negative bacteria (particularly Propionibacterium acnes) which triggered inflammation near the spine. Stirling suggested that the reason these bacteria had not been identified earlier was because of the extended time required to incubate disc material (7 days).[4]

The tuberculosis mycobacterium has also been shown to contribute to spinal disease and possibly deformations. Research at the Pasteur Institute in France, published in The New England Journal of Medicine, documented increasing numbers of patients showing evidence of spinal disease (Pott's disease) caused by tuberculosis.[5, 6, 7, 8]

In addition, vaccines made from live viruses have been linked to spinal problems. A 1982 study by Pincott and Taff found a connection between oral poliomyelitis vaccines and scoliosis.[9]

1. Green RJ, Webb JN, Maxwell MH. The nature of virus-like particles in the paraxial muscles of idiopathic scoliosis. J Pathol. 1979 Sep;129(1):9-12.

2. Webb JN, Gillespie WJ. Virus-like particles in paraspinal muscle in scoliosis. Br Med J. 1976 Oct 16;2(6041):912-3.

3. Wolff MH, Buchel F, Gullotta F, Helpap B, Schneweiss KE. Investigations to demonstrate latent viral infection of varicella-Zoster virus in human spine ganglia. Verh Dtsch Ges Pathol. 1981;65:203-7.

4. Stirling AL, et al., Association between sciatica and Propionibacterium acnes. Lancet 2001:V357.

5. Nagrath SP, Hazra DK, Pant PC, Seth HC. Tuberculosis spine—a diagnostic conundrum. Case report. J Assoc Physicians India. 1974 May;22(5):405-7.

6. Jenks PJ, Stewart B. Images in clinical medicine. Vertebral tuberculosis. N Engl J Med. 1998 June 4;338(23):1677.

7. Monaghan D, Gupta A, Barrington NA. Case report: Tuberculosis of the spine—an unusual presentation. Clin Radiol. 1991 May;43(5):360-2.

8. Petersen CK, Craw M, Radiological differentiation of tuberculosis and pyogenic osteomyelitis: a case report. J Manipulative Physiol Ther. 1986 Mar;9(1):39-42.

9. Pinott JR, Taffs LF. Experimental scoliosis in primates: a neurological cause. J Bone Joint Surg Br. 1982;64(4):503-7.

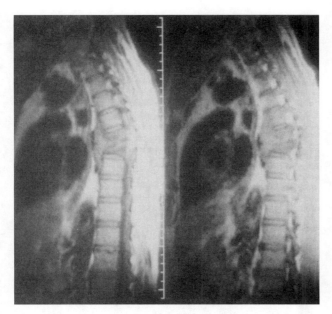

Example of kyphosis (hunchback) caused by an infectious microorganism (tuberculosis) in the spine. The above X-rays show two views of the spine of a 62 year-old man with a 3-month history of increasing back pain and inflammation due to kyphosis. The problem had become so severe that he could no longer walk unaided; however, there was no history of tuberculosis. The X-rays show the collapse of the seventh thoracic vertebra. He subsequently underwent back surgery to help correct the problem. Specimens taken during the surgery did not immediately show a bacterial infection, but after 12 weeks of incubation, the presence of Mycobacterium tuberculosis was detected, confirming the original diagnosis of spinal tuberculosis.

Source: Jenks, Peter J. and Stewart, Bruce. Images in Clinical Medicine. Vertebral Tuberculosis. New England Journal of Medicine, 1998 June 4, 338 (23);1677.

Powerful Infection-Fighters

Essential oils are some of the most powerful inhibitors of microbes known, and as such are an important new weapon in combating many types of tissue infections. A 1999 study by Marilena Marino and colleagues found that thyme oil exhibited strong action against stubborn gram-negative bacteria.[10] Similarly, basil essential oil also demonstrated strong bactericidal action against microorganisms Aeromonas hydrophila and Pseudomonas fluorescens.[11] A study at the Central Food Technological Institute in Mysore, India, found that a large number of essential oil components had tremendous germ-killing effects, inhibiting the growth of Staphylococcus, Micrococcus, Bacillus, and Enterobacter strains of bacteria. These compounds included menthol (found in peppermint), eucalyptol (found in rosemary, eucalyptus, and geranium), linalool (found in marjoram), and citral (found in lemongrass).[12] A 2001 study conducted by D. Gary Young, Diane Horne, Sue Chao, and colleagues at Weber State University in Ogden, Utah, found that oregano, thyme, peppermint, and basil exhibited very strong antimicrobial effects against pathogens such as Streptococcus pneumoniae, a major cause of illness in young children and death in elderly, and immune-weakened patients.[13] Many other studies confirm these findings.[14]

The ability of essential oils to penetrate the skin quickly and pass into bodily tissues to produce therapeutic effects has also been studied. Hoshi University researchers in Japan found that cyclic monoterpenes (including menthol, which is found in peppermint) are so effective in penetrating the skin that they can actually enhance the absorption of water-soluble drugs.[15] North Dakota State University researchers have similarly found that cyclic monoterpenes such as limonene and other terpenoids such as menthone and eugenol easily pass through the dermis, magnifying the penetration of pharmaceutical drugs such as tamoxifen.[16]

It is interesting to note that many essential oils used in RT—in addition to being highly anti-microbial—are also among those classified as GRAS (Generally Regarded As Safe) for internal use by the U.S. Food and Drug Administration. These include basil, marjoram, peppermint, oregano, and thyme. These and many other GRAS essential oils have a decades-long history of being consumed as foods or flavorings with virtually no adverse reactions.

In sum, RT is one of the safest, noninvasive techniques available for spinal health. It is also an invaluable tool to promote healing from within using topically applied essential oils.

10. Marino M, Bersani C, Comi G. Antimicrobial activity of the essential oils of Thymus vulgaris L. measured using a bioimpedometric method. Journal of Food Protection, Vol. 62, No. 9, 1999 pp. 1017-1023.

11. Wan J, Wilcock A, Coventry MJ. The effect of essential oils of basil on the growth of Aeromonas fluorescens. Journal of Applied Microbiology, 1998, 84, 152-158.

12. Beuchat LR. Antimicrobial properties of spices and their essential oils. Center for Food Safety and Quality Enhancement, Department of Food Science and Technology, University of Georgia, Griffin, Georgia.

13. Horne D, et al., Antimicrobial effects of essential oils on Streptococcus pneumoniae. Journal of Essential Oil Research, (September/October 2001). 13, 387-392.

14. Moleyar V, Narasimham P. Antibacterial activity of essential oil components. International Journal of Food Microbiology, Vol. 16 (1992) 337-32.

15. Obata Y, et al. Effect of pretreatment of skin with cyclic monoterpenes on permeation of diclofenac in hairless rat. Biol Pharm Bull. 1993 Mar;16(3)312-4.

16. Zhao K, Singh J. Mechanisms of percutaneous absorption of tamoxifen by terpenes: eugenol, d-limonene and menthone. Control Release. 1998. Nov 13;55(2-3)253-60.

Introduction to the Technique

Raindrop Technique® uses a sequence of highly antimicrobial essential oils synergistically combined to simultaneously kill the responsible viral agents and reduce inflammation. The principle single oils used include:

- oregano *(Origanum compactum)*
- thyme *(Thymus vulgaris)*
- basil or balsam fir *(Ocimum basilicum or Abies balsamea)*
- cypress *(Cupressus sempervirens)*
- wintergreen *(Gaultheria procumbens)*
- marjoram *(Origanum majorana)*
- peppermint *(Mentha piperita)*

The oils are dispensed like little drops of rain from a height of about six inches above the back and very lightly massaged along the vertebrae and back muscles. Although the entire process takes about 45 minutes to complete, the oils will continue to work in the body for up to one week following treatment, with continued re-alignment taking place during this time.

One caution: RT is not a cure-all or a magic bullet. A healthy balanced body is the result of a well-rounded program of exercise and proper diet. Health is everything we do, say, hear, see, and eat. RT is only one tool to help restore balance in the body. Healthy eating habits and a positive, open mind will also help prepare the body and skin to accept the oils better and more rapidly.

Although this technique is explained as simply as possible, you may want to contact Essential Science Publishing to purchase a demonstration video. Every step of the technique is carefully demonstrated in an actual hands-on presentation. You can order the video by visiting the ESP website at www.essentialscience.net or by calling toll-free 800-336-6308. Viewing this video and following the outline presented here will make this revolutionary technique easy to understand and easy to put into practice.

If you intend to offer the Raindrop Technique® as a service, please be advised that some states require that you be a licensed massage therapist, aesthetician or chiropractor prior to offering any service where physical touch is involved. Please check the regulations for your jurisdiction.

The Raindrop Technique®

It is recommended that RT be performed in a quiet, semi-darkened area free of distractions. Soft and relaxing music will make the recipient more comfortable. The temperature should be cool enough to prevent sweating, but warm enough to be comfortable as the recipient's back and legs will be exposed. In describing the technique, "facilitator" refers to the person giving the Raindrop Technique; "recipient" refers to the person receiving it.

For This Technique, You Will Need:

1. Massage table (ideally) or a comfortable, flat surface for the recipient to lie on. The surface should be high enough that the facilitator can perform the technique without back strain. It is best to cover the surface with sheets or towels that are expendable as several of the oils may stain certain fabrics. Also, some of the oils can react with the vinyls used to cover massage tables so be sure vinyl surfaces are covered well.

2. Two medium-sized towels and a twin-sized bed sheet. The towels will be used to make a warm compress; the sheet to protect the modesty of the recipient.

3. Easy access to hot water.

4. Timer, clock, or watch.

5. A stable tray on which to place oils (and instructions, if needed) near the receiver.

6. Each of the 10 oils listed throughout this chapter. (Seven single oils, two blends and a vegetable or massage oil.)

Preparation

- Both the facilitator and the recipient should remove all jewelry. This includes watches, pendants, chains, rings, bracelets, belts, earrings, etc.

- The facilitator should wear clothing that is loose and comfortable, and may wish to remove their shoes.

- The recipient should be draped in a bed sheet or towel, or dressed in hospital gown-attire so the facilitator can apply essential oils to the shoulders, neck, back, legs, and feet of the recipient.

- The facilitator should make sure their fingernails are clipped and filed down as short as possible to prevent unintentionally scratching the recipient's skin, particularly when doing the Vita Flex Technique.

- The facilitator should make sure fingernails are free of fingernail polish. Essential oils remove many polishes and lacquers.

- Only perform RT if you are feeling healthy, energized, and emotionally/ mentally clear and focused.

- For optimum results, the recipient should drink extra purified or distilled water for the first few days following RT. This will aid the body in flushing toxins from the tissues.

NOTE: Facilitators may choose to apply frankincense to themselves (on wrists, shoulders, neck, and top of the head) to help counter any negative energies coming from the recipient.

To begin:

- The recipient should lie on their back, face up on the massage table with the head resting in the face cradle.

- The recipient should lie as straight as possible with the hips flat on the table. The arms should rest alongside the body.

- The facilitator should keep constant physical contact with the recipient to prevent feelings of insecurity, anxiousness, or abandonment.

- Check for evenness of feet and in the length of the legs. Hold recipient's ankles just below the shin bone (with the right hand on the left ankle and the left hand on the right ankle) with the index finger of each hand touching the center of the outside ankle bone. While holding the ankles in this position, the thumbs of the facilitator should be even with one another. Unevenness could indicate a pelvic rotation or structural misalignment.

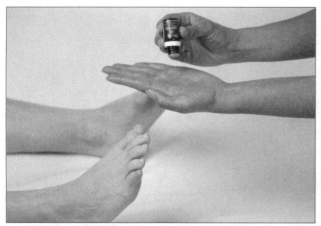

Fig. A — Putting Energy Balance Blend in the hand

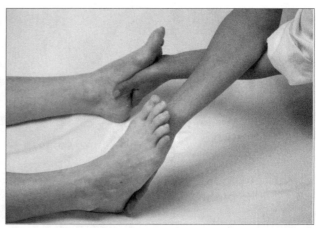

Fig. B — Placing hands on the recipient's feet

STEP 1 – Apply Valor blend to feet and shoulders

Oregano, thyme, and the Valor blend are the foundation oils for all Raindrop Technique work. The technique always begins with the application of Valor to the feet and shoulders. This is one of the most important steps for a successful RT because it works on the physical, electrical, spiritual, and emotional levels, supporting the physical and energy alignment of the body. The key to using this oil blend is patience. Once the frequencies begin to balance, a structural alignment will much more likely begin to occur.

This first step forms the foundation for everything that follows.

- According to energy medicine principles, female energy relates to the left side of the body, male energy to the right side. So this application begins differently for males and females.

- Put 6 drops of Valor into your left hand and apply to the left foot first if the recipient is a woman (See Fig. A); put the oil in the right hand and apply to the right foot first if the recipient is a man. Then apply the oil on the other foot.

STEP 2 – Place hands on recipient's feet and shoulders

Step 2 works best if there are two facilitators: one to hold the feet, the other to make contact at the shoulders. However, if you are working by yourself, the application works well just holding the feet, which is the most important. You may kneel or sit

while holding the feet or shoulders of the recipient. You should be in a comfortable position to maintain contact for several minutes.

- Cross your hands and place your palms as flat as possible against the soles of the receiver's feet. This hand crossing enables the facilitator to place the right palm on the right foot and the left palm on the left foot. The facilitator should hold this position for at least 5 minutes. (See Fig. B)

- If two facilitators are available, the second should sit or stand at the recipient's head and apply three drops of Valor to each shoulder. The right palm is placed on the recipient's right shoulder and left palm is placed on the left shoulder at the same time (without crossing arms). There must be as much palm-to-shoulder contact as possible.

- Let your mind be free and peaceful. Encourage the recipient to take deep breaths, inhaling and exhaling deeply and slowly, so they engage in their own healing. The recipient may feel a little heat or tingling on the feet, or an energy working up through the legs to the back, even moving as high as the head. Some facilitators may feel their hands become warm or tingly. Sometimes the facilitator may feel a pulsating effect. The facilitator should try to feel the energy coming through the recipient's feet. Look for:

  - Temperature change
  - A "pulsing" feeling
  - Subtle vibration

Once you feel energy and it is equal in both feet, you can release.

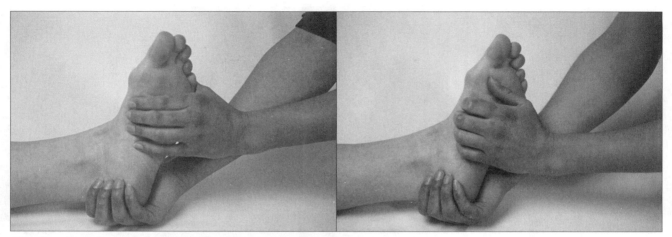

Fig. C — Applying thyme to the Vita Flex points of the foot

The vertebrae can achieve some realignment with this initial application alone. However, if there are people present with hidden negative attitudes, the results may be less than optimal. Only perform the RT if you are feeling healthy, energized, and emotionally/mentally clear and focused.

CAUTION: If there is a fold in the skin on the back of the neck or elsewhere, please note that essential oils can accumulate there. Be aware of this as you proceed, and if the recipient notices a burning sensation in a skin fold, be prepared to add V6 Oil Complex or massage oil there.

STEP 3 – Apply seven essential oils to the feet

In this step we will apply the seven single oils in a specific order to the spinal Vita Flex area of the soles of the feet (see chart on pages 204-205) using the Vita Flex Technique. The seven oils in their application sequence are:

- Oregano has potent antimicrobial and anti-inflammatory properties.

- Thyme is highly antimicrobial, inhibiting the growth of infectious microorganisms. It easily penetrates the skin and travels throughout the body.

- Basil or Balsam Fir: Basil has antispasmodic properties that relax muscles. It is also anti-inflammatory and antimicrobial. Balsam fir is an excellent substitute for basil and is less irritating to sensitive skin.

- Cypress oil improves circulation, relieves spasms and swelling, and helps heal damaged tissue.

- Wintergreen is anti-inflammatory and analgesic (pain-relieving) due to it's high methyl salicylate content. It is excellent for bones and joints.

NOTE: Be careful of your sources in obtaining wintergreen. Much of the wintergreen sold today has been chemically extended and adulterated with synthetic methyl salicylate.

- Marjoram oil is antispasmodic and muscle-relaxing.

- Peppermint enhances the effects of all the preceding essential oils. It also has pain-killing and antimicrobial properties, stimulating circulation and cooling inflamed tissue.

The procedure for this portion of RT involves a series of substeps as follows:

A. Place 2-3 drops of oregano (small feet require only 1-2 drops of essential oil) in the palm of the left hand. Dip the fingertips of the right hand in the oil, stir clockwise three times and apply along the spine Vita Flex points of the right foot (see chart on pages 204-205). This is the area along the bottom inside edge of the foot from the heel to the tip of the big toe. Massage with Vita Flex Technique the full length of this area three times. Remember to use the right hand for both oil application and Vita Flex massage on the right foot. (See Fig. C)

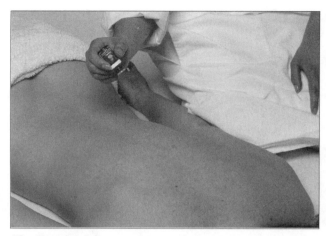

Fig. D — Applying oregano and thyme to the spine

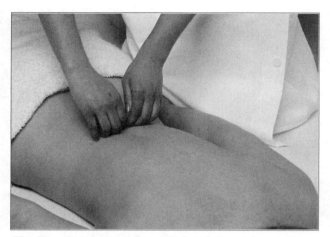

Fig. E — Brush strokes up the spine

B. Place 2-3 drops of thyme essential oil in the palm of the left hand. Dip two fingertips of the right hand in the oil, stir clockwise three times and apply—just as above with oregano oil—along the spinal Vita Flex area of the right foot. Massage along the full length of this spinal area using the Vita Flex Technique once to apply the oil, then two more times.

C. Place 2-3 drops of basil or balsam fir in the same manner as above on the right foot.

D. Place 2-3 drops of cypress in the same manner as above on the right foot.

E. Place 2-3 drops of wintergreen in the same manner as above on the right foot.

F. Place 2-3 drops of marjoram in the same manner as above on the right foot.

G. Place 2-3 drops of peppermint in the same manner as above on the right foot.

Repeat steps A-G, on the left foot, placing the oils in the palm of the right hand and applying them and doing Vita Flex on the left foot with the left hand.

STEP 4 – Apply oregano and thyme to spine

• Have the recipient turn over on their stomach to expose the back. Do this carefully to protect the recipient's modesty.

• Hold the bottle six inches above the skin and evenly space **2-4 drops** of oregano oil along the center of the spine from bottom to top (sacrum to atlas). (See Fig. D)

• Immediately after applying oregano, with 6-inch brush-like strokes, brush the backs of your fingertips along the spine as you "feather up" the back from the sacrum (base of spine) to the atlas (hair line on back of neck). Repeat this feathering process two more times. (See Fig. E)

• In the same way as above, evenly space 3-5 drops of thyme oil along the center of the spine from bottom to top. Feather in the thyme just as you did for oregano.

CAUTION: More is not better. If there is a slight warming or burning sensation along the spine or on the neck, apply a pure vegetable or massage oil. The high phenol content of oregano and thyme essential oils can produce excess warming or reddening to the skin, particularly with fair-skinned people. Following the application of thyme and oregano, if the recipient becomes uncomfortable with burning sensations, apply 5-10 drops of vegetable or massage oil over affected areas.

NOTE: For more information about each of the Raindrop Technique oils, refer to the single oils and oil blend chapters of this book.

STEP 5 – Apply basil or balsam fir; massage spinal muscles using circular motions

• Evenly drop **6-10 drops** of basil or balsam fir evenly along the center of the spine.

• Spread the oil over the back by using the feathering technique described in step 4.

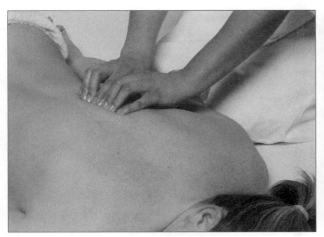

Fig. F — Easing muscles away from spine

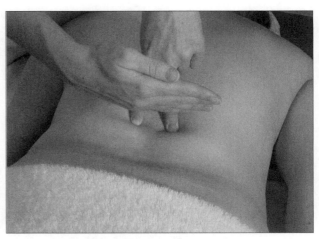

Fig. G — Two fingers straddling spine

- In small circular clockwise motions (using the pads of the fingertips of both hands placed side by side) massage the muscles on each side of the spine. Start at the sacrum and work up to the atlas, using the fingertips to gently push or pull the tissue away from the spine. After finishing one side of the spine, start on the other side. Do not work directly on the spine, but on the muscles on either side of the spine. Do not apply direct pressure to the vertebrae. Repeat this step two more times. (See Fig. F)

STEP 6 – Apply cypress and do a finger straddle/hand "saw" massage

- Evenly drop **6-10 drops** of cypress along the center of the spine.

- Spread the oil over the spine and spinal muscles using the feathering technique described in Step 4.

- Stand on the recipient's left side (right side if the facilitator is left handed) near the shoulder area, facing the recipient's feet. Straddle the spine at the sacrum (base) with the index and middle fingers of the non-dominant hand. Place the bottom edge of the dominant hand (ulnar or pinky side down) just below the middle joints of the two straddling fingers. (See Fig. G)

Simultaneously perform the following two motions:

1. Apply moderate downward pressure with the straddling fingers while pulling them slowly to the atlas (top) of the spine.

2. Using an equal downward pressure, "saw" the dominant hand back and forth, using short, rapid 1-inch strokes, moving the two straddling fingers back and forth as you slide them up the spine all the way to the hairline.

Repeat this step two more times.

STEP 7 – Apply wintergreen and thumb-roll up the spine

- Evenly drop **6-10 drops** of wintergreen along the center of the spine.

- Spread the oil over the spine and spinal muscles using the feathering technique described in Step 4.

- With your thumbs one inch apart on either side of the spine, use the Vita Flex method of thumb-rolling to work up the spine a thumbwidth at a time, from the sacrum to the atlas. Apply mild pressure. You may want to offset your thumbs by one inch to avoid bumping thumbs on the inward roll. Continue to roll your thumbs lightly over onto the nails and then release. Repeat this step two more times. (See Figs. H and I)

STEP 8 – Apply marjoram and peppermint to spinal muscles using flared feather strokes

In this step we apply the last two single essential oils—in the sequence listed—to the muscles along either side of the spine and feather them to the rib and shoulders areas of the back. The two oils are marjoram and peppermint.

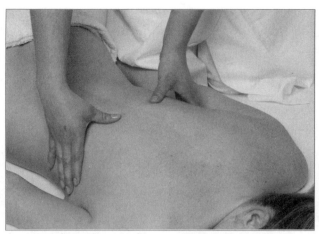

Fig. H — Thumb-rolling up spine (Down position)

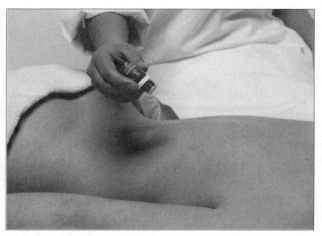

Fig. J — Applying basil, wintergreen, cypress, marjoram, and peppermint to muscles on each side of spine

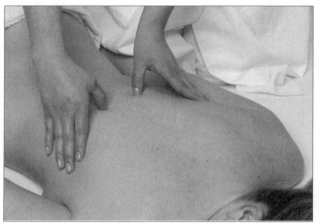

Fig. I — Thumb-rolling up spine (Up position)

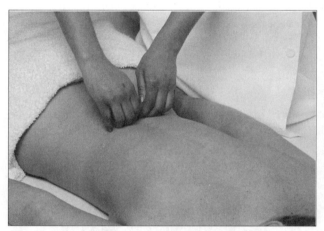

Fig. K — Brush strokes up the back muscles

- Evenly drop (Raindrop-style) **6-10 drops** (depending on the length of the recipient's spine) of marjoram onto the muscles along each side of the spine (12-20 drops total). (See Fig. J)

- After applying marjoram, with the nail side of your fingertips, use 6-inch brush-like strokes to feather the oil up the spine from the sacrum to the atlas. Repeat this step two more times. (See Fig. K)

- Then, extending the feather strokes (about 8 inches), lightly flare the fingertips out towards the sides of the back as you feather up the spine. Flare right hand to the right side of the back, and the left hand to the left side of the back, moving all the way to the side of the rib cage. Repeat this step two more times. This light stroking, or feathering, is called "effleurage." (See Fig. L)

- Starting at the sacrum, do a second set of flared feather strokes moving up the full length of the

spine to the atlas (the hairline on the back of the neck). Flare your fingertips out over the shoulders and neck when you reach the atlas. Repeat this two more more times, for a total of three times.

- Apply and feather a total of **6-10 drops** of peppermint essential oil using the same process.

STEP 9 – Apply Aroma Siez to the back

The Aroma Siez blend contains several highly antispasmodic essential oils that help relax sore, tense, or inflamed muscles.

- Apply at least **6-8 drops** of Aroma Siez over the entire length of each side of the spine (**12-16 drops** total). Feather in the blend as in Step 8, then, using circular motions with the flat of the hands, gently massage into the back muscles.

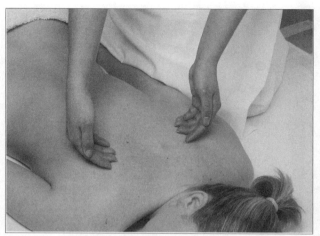

Fig. L — "Feathering up" the back over muscles next to the spine

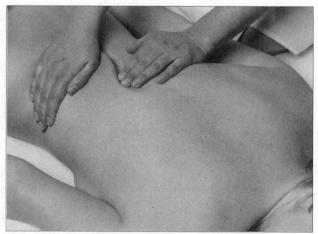

Fig. M — Palm rub massage on the back

Include the areas along the outer edges of the rib cage and shoulders that have not been previously worked.

STEP 10 – Massage entire back and neck with a quality vegetable or massage oil, finishing with palm rub

This application helps to seal in the essential oils, enhancing penetration.

- Put **12-20 drops** (depending on the size of the back) of V6 Oil Complex or massage oil, in your palm to warm the oil before spreading onto the muscles of the entire back and back of the neck. Use a gentle massage to evenly spread the massage oil.

- Place both hands on the receiver's back, palms down, near the base of the spine, one hand close to you, one hand on the far side of the back. Then slide the palms, with mild downward pressure, in opposite directions from the far side of the back to the near side, working slowly up the back toward the neck. Continue this alternating back and forth massage up to the nape of the neck. (See Fig. M) Do this massage up and down the back three times.

STEP 11 – Apply Valor to the spine

Apply **6-10 drops** of Valor, raindrop-style, along the center of the spine, from the sacrum to the atlas. Feather in the blend as in Step 8. Gently massage into the spine and spinal muscles using circular motions with the flats of your hands, moving from the sacrum to the atlas. Repeat two more times.

STEP 12 – Apply moist warm towel; perform back press

CAUTION: Special care must be taken with this step because the back can become hot! The heat will usually build slowly and peak in about 3-8 minutes, before cooling down to the point where it feels quite pleasant. The greater the inflammation and viral infection along the spine, the hotter the area along the spine will become.

If the heat becomes uncomfortable, place a dry, folded towel between the back and the damp towel (see first point below). If the warming sensation continues to be uncomfortable, remove all towels and massage the area with 10-15 drops of vegetable or massage oil.

- Soak one of the towels in warm water, wring it out, fold it in thirds, and lay it along the entire length of the spine.

- Place the other dry towel (folded in half) over the wet towel.

- Allow the heat from the wet towel to penetrate, usually about 8–10 minutes. If the heat fades before 8 minutes are up, it may be helpful to apply the warm moist towel a second time.

- Pay very close attention to the recipient's comfort. Ask questions.

- After the warmth of the oils has subsided (from 8–15 minutes), with the towels still in place, perform the back press by crossing the hands and placing them 1-2 inches apart at the base of

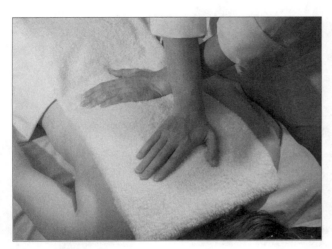

Fig. N — Back Press

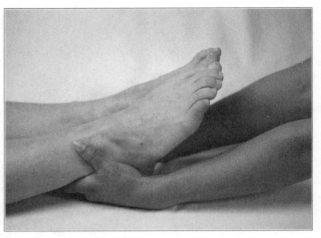

Fig. O — Stretching the spine

the back. Gently press the hands down and away from each other, vibrating the hands and spreading them slightly. Repeat this process of pressing, vibrating and spreading the hands 3-5 times, each time starting further up the spine, until reaching the top of the spine (See Fig. N). Repeat this step two more times.

STEP 13 – Remove towels and inspect spine

- Remove the towels. Make sure the person is lying with their head snug in the head cradle of the massage table and with their spine straight (hips aligned with shoulders).

- Check the spine. Corrections may or may not be visible. Results may take several days to take full effect. You may need to perform another technique at a later time.

STEP 14 – Gently stretch the back and neck

- Have the recipient turn over onto their back. Be careful to keep the receiver covered to protect modesty.

- If you are working alone, hold the ankles firmly and apply light pressure to stretch the back as shown (See Fig. O). If there is a second facilitator, they should hold the ankles while you cradle the individual's head in your hands (see cranial hold on next page), place your thumbs around the chin, and gently lift and ease back to

create slight tension. Hold for 3 seconds, then release for 3 seconds. Repeat three times.

Best results are achieved when two people perform this stretching step: one gently tensioning the neck while the other holds the legs. If there is only one facilitator, this step can be done in two sequential steps—ankles first, then neck.

STEP 14A – Finger placement for cranial hold

- Place both hands under the recipient's neck, with the fingers touching each other and the thumbs just below the jaw. (See Fig. P)

STEP 14B – Basic cranial hold

- Gently pull the recipient's head back from the torso using the cranial hold. Pull back gently for 3 seconds, then release for 3 seconds. Repeat this cycle slowly and gently three times. Check with the recipient during this process to verify that they are not experiencing any pain. If there is pain, immediately discontinue the stretch. (See Fig. Q)

STEP 14C – Modified cranial hold

This is an alternate version of the cranial hold, which differs in the hand placement on the receiver's head.

- Hold the recipient's head with one hand under the neck, palm up, and the other hand cradling the receiver's chin. Gently create tension in the neck by slowly pulling the head away from the

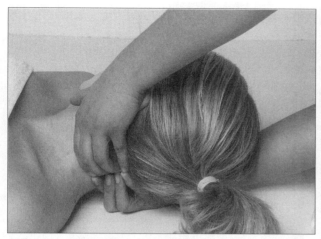

Fig. P — Finger placement for cranial hold stretch

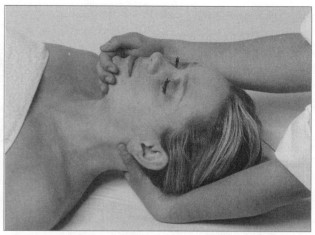

Fig. R — Holding chin during modified cranial hold

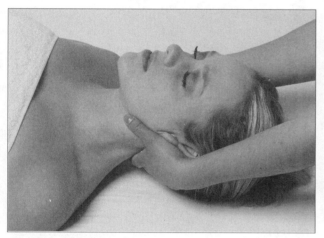

Fig. Q — Cranial hold

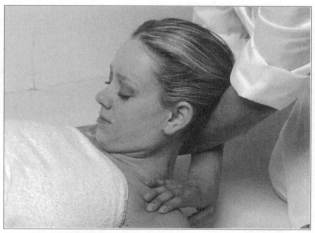

Fig. S — Neck Flex

torso. Hold for 5 seconds, then release for 5 seconds. Repeat two more times. (See Fig. R)

- Do not pull too hard. An assistant, if available, can anchor the feet while you gently tension the neck.

STEP 15 – Neck Flex

- Kneel or sit so that your shoulders are parallel to the recipient's shoulders.

- Cross your arms and place your hands (palm side down) on the recipient's shoulders (left hand on the right shoulder and visa versa).

- Make sure the recipient's tongue is not between their teeth.

- Raise your elbows in order to gently lift and stretch the recipient's neck until their chin touches the chest.

- Repeat this step two more times. (See Fig. S)

- For optimum results, the recipient should drink extra purified or distilled water for the first few days following RT. This will aid the body in flushing toxins from the tissues.

Customizing Raindrop Technique® to Address Specific Health Issues

Raindrop Technique can be customized to address different health issues that are not directly related to back problems. Lung infections, digestive complaints, hormonal problems, liver insufficiencies, and other problems can all be dealt with by substituting standard RT essential oils with other oils that are specifically targeted for that body system.

As a rule, when customizing RT, you will generally want to start with the Valor, oregano, and thyme. These three oils form the basis or "hub" of all Raindrop applications. (For extra antiviral effect, add mountain savory.) The other essential oils such as basil, wintergreen, marjoram, thyme, or cypress can be omitted or replaced by essential oils specific for the condition being treated.

For example, if a lung infection is present, basil and wintergreen should be replaced with ravensara, cypress replaced with Eucalyptus radiata, and marjoram replaced with mountain savory. (See diagram on next page)

There are several variations to the basic Raindrop Technique. These variations are not easy to explain and require class instruction and demonstration.

SUMMARY:

Raindrop Technique (RT) is a powerful tool that assists both professionals and lay people to achieve true balance in the body. Out of the thousands of RT sessions that have been performed, there have been hundreds of instances where the results were amazingly profound and immediate. Here are just a few examples:

A young man from Denver, Colorado who suffered from chronic scoliosis was able—for the first time in eight years—to fully bend over after the application of RT. With an overhead camera televising an image of his spine as he bent over, an audience of over 400 watched the vertebrae in his spine literally move into place. When he stood up, he was measured and had gained an inch in height.

Another case involved a professional model in her early 40s, who had developed early adult-onset scoliosis. She had to alter clothing so it would fit properly for modeling sessions. She wasn't able to sit still for any length of time. After receiving RT, her spine straightened to such a degree that she, too, gained an inch in height. She followed up with more RT in the next few months and reported that all discomfort was gone. She now dances and rides horses pain-free.

It is quite common that individuals with scoliosis who receive RT will gain 1/2 an inch or more in stature from a single application. Many others have reported pain relief, congestion relief, and cold and flu relief as a result of RT. This is why RT has captured so much interest among those involved in the healing arts.

Older children can benefit from RT, but it is critical to adjust the amount of oil used in proportion to their body size. Amounts should be adjusted to reflect the difference in body size relative to an adult.

Every person is biochemically different, and what works for one may not work for another. Different body types respond to the applications in ways you may not expect. Learn to be sensitive to the person on whom you are working so that you can respond to their needs.

The question is often asked, "How long do the effects of this application last?" Again, each person responds differently. Generally speaking, a high level of health and proper diet are key factors, as are exercise and attitude. The effects of one application may last several months for one person, but for another it may be necessary to have repeated applications weekly until the body begins to respond. The goal is to retrain the tissues of the body. This may take a few weeks or even a full year.

Spinal alignment may have a completely different look when the individual is lying down, rather than sitting. There is more torque on the spine in a sitting or standing position, so these are the positions in which X-rays are usually taken. The spine may appear to be totally corrected when the receiver is lying down, but then appear to be crooked when they are in a sitting position. This variance is normal and may be apparent until a total retraining of the muscles occurs. The object is to achieve proper alignment in all positions.

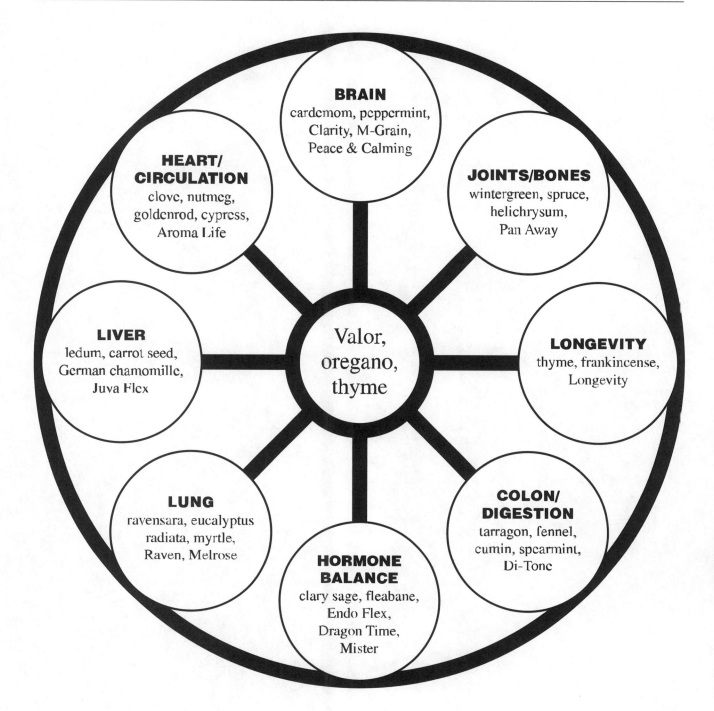

BRAIN
cardemom, peppermint,
Clarity, M-Grain,
Peace & Calming

**HEART/
CIRCULATION**
clove, nutmeg,
goldenrod, cypress,
Aroma Life

JOINTS/BONES
wintergreen, spruce,
helichrysum,
Pan Away

LIVER
ledum, carrot seed,
German chamomille,
Juva Flex

Valor,
oregano,
thyme

LONGEVITY
thyme, frankincense,
Longevity

LUNG
ravensara, eucalyptus
radiata, myrtle,
Raven, Melrose

**COLON/
DIGESTION**
tarragon, fennel,
cumin, spearmint,
Di-Tone

**HORMONE
BALANCE**
clary sage, fleabane,
Endo Flex,
Dragon Time,
Mister

22

Lymphatic Pump

Maintaining lymph circulation is one of the keys to keeping the immune system adequately functioning. This technique is designed to promote lymph circulation. It is an excellent tool for those who are sedentary or bedridden.

1. With the recipient lying on their back, hold one leg with one hand just above ankles with your palm on the underside of the leg (covering the Achille's tendon).

2. Place the other hand on the bottom of the recipient's foot with your palm over the ball of their feet and your fingers curled around their toes.

3. Push the top of the recipient's foot away from you. (See Fig. A)

4. Then, pull the recipient's foot toward you by the toes until the ball of the foot is as close to the table as possible. (See Fig. B)

5. Check with the recipient during the pump to verify that the muscles in their feet are not being overextended. This should be an active process, but not a painful one.

6. Pull and push their foot using this "pumping motion" at least 10 times on each leg for maximum benefit. Note that their entire body should move during each step of the Lymphatic Pump.

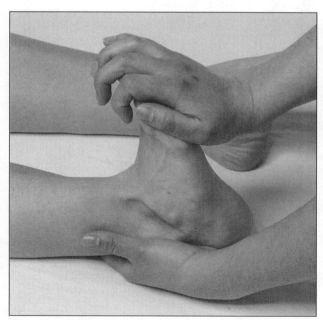

Fig. A — Pushing the foot

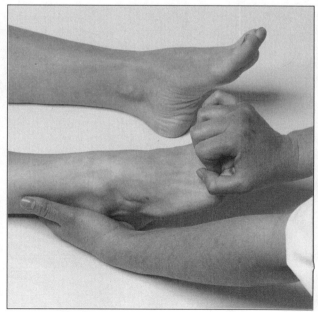

Fig. B — Pulling the foot

233

23

Auricular Aroma Technique

D. Gary Young developed auricular aroma technique, the integration of essential oils with standard auricular technique, after using essential oils in acupuncture applications in his clinic. He found that using essential oils in conjunction with acupuncture was extremely beneficial. He also found that acupuncture stimulation with essential oils was noticeably greater than either acupuncture or essential oil applications by themselves.

Emotional Ear Chart

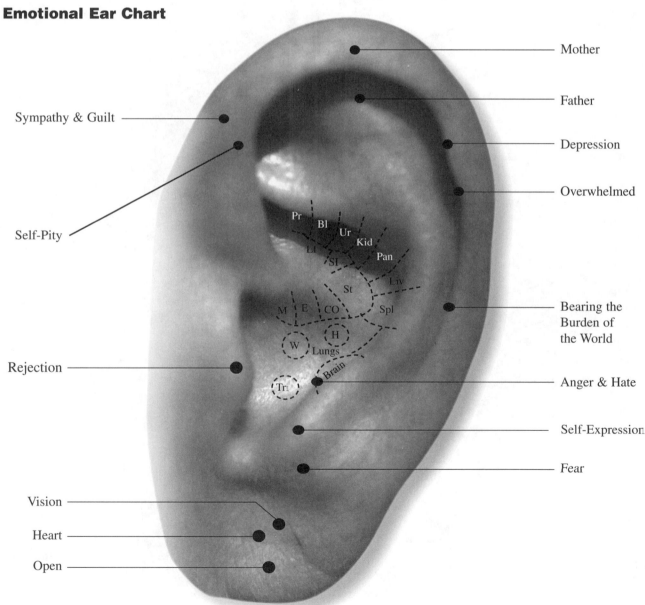

Mother

Father

Depression

Overwhelmed

Sympathy & Guilt

Self-Pity

Bearing the
Burden of
the World

Rejection

Anger & Hate

Self-Expression

Fear

Vision

Heart

Open

Pr
Bl
Ur
Kid
LI
SI
Pan
St
Liv
M E CO
Spl
W
H
Lungs
Tri
Brain

Acupuncture with essential oils seems to enhance benefits substantially. As Gary left his first clinical practice and began researching, farming, and teaching, he knew he could not continue the practice of acupuncture, so he started developing a simplified technique that everyone could use. That technique is called auricular probe technique, using a small, pen-shaped instrument with a rounded end to apply the oils to the acupuncture meridians or Vita Flex points on the ears. This concept can be used in both the emotional and physical realm.

For working the spine and dealing with neurological problems that exist because of spinal cord injury, auricular probe technique was found to be extremely beneficial to deliver the oils to the exact location of the neurological damage.

Auricular probe technique is a program that Gary continues to research and develop, and teach to doctors. It has shown tremendous potential and will grow to be a well-known modality in the future.

Physical Ear Chart

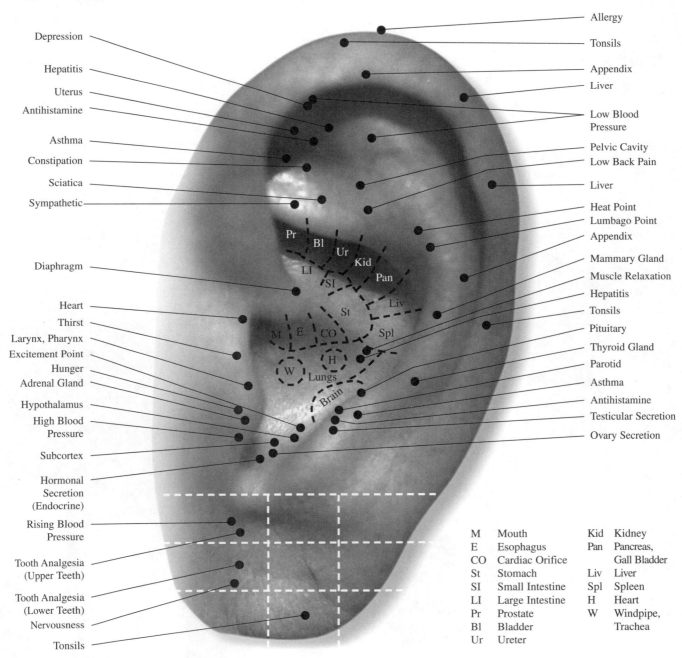

M	Mouth	Kid	Kidney
E	Esophagus	Pan	Pancreas,
CO	Cardiac Orifice		Gall Bladder
St	Stomach	Liv	Liver
SI	Small Intestine	Spl	Spleen
LI	Large Intestine	H	Heart
Pr	Prostate	W	Windpipe,
Bl	Bladder		Trachea
Ur	Ureter		

24

Emotional Response with Essential Oils

Today, we live in a society of emotional turmoil. There is more focus on emotional behavior and psychological conditions of the body now than at any time in our history. Many doctors are recognizing the possibility that a number of diseases are caused by emotional problems that link back to infancy and perhaps even to the womb. These emotional problems may have compromised our immune system or genetic structuring, causing children to become allergic to something that the mother ingested while pregnant.

Essential oils play an important role in assisting people to move beyond these emotional barriers. The aldehydes and esters of certain essential oils are very calming and sedating to the central nervous system (including both the sympathetic and parasympathetic systems). These substances allow us to relax instead of letting anxiety build up in our body. Anxiety creates an acidic condition that activates the transcript enzyme which then transcribes that anxiety on the RNA template and stores it in the DNA. That emotion then becomes a predominant factor in our lives from that moment on.

When we encounter an emotionally charged situation, instead of being overwhelmed by it, we can diffuse essential oils, put them in our bath, or wear them as cologne. The aromatic molecules will absorb into the bloodstream from the nasal cavity to the limbic system. They will activate the amygdala (the memory center for fear and trauma) and sedate and relax the sympathetic/parasympathetic system. The oils help support the body in minimizing the acid that is created so that it does not initiate a reaction with the transcript enzyme.

Because essential oils affect the amygdala and pineal gland in the brain, they can help the mind and body by releasing emotional trauma and sharpening focus.

People have many distractions in today's fast-paced world. Essential oils may assist people to stay centered in their goals. Those who are struggling to retain or remember information can breathe the essential oils of peppermint, cardamom, or rosemary to stimulate the brain and memory functions for better concentration. Those who find it difficult to stay focused can breathe the essential oils of galbanum, frankincense, sandalwood, and melissa. These oils are extremely beneficial for clarifying one's purpose. The blend Gathering will also bring focus to people's minds. For emotional clearing and release, the combination of essential oils called Trauma Life is especially helpful.

Oils For Emotional Application

ABUSE

Single Oils: Geranium, ylang ylang, sandalwood.

Blends: SARA, Hope, Joy, Peace & Calming, Inner Child, Grounding, Trauma Life, Valor, Forgiveness, White Angelica

AGITATION

Single Oils: Bergamot, cedarwood, clary sage, frankincense, geranium, juniper, lavender, myrrh, marjoram, rosewood, rose, ylang ylang, sandalwood.

Blends: Peace & Calming, Joy, Valor, Harmony, Forgiveness, Chivalry

ANGER

Single Oils: Bergamot, cedarwood, Roman chamomile, frankincense, lavender, lemon, marjoram, myrrh, orange, rose, sandalwood, ylang ylang.

Blends: Release, Valor, Sacred Mountain, Joy, Harmony, Hope, Forgiveness, Present Time, Trauma Life, Surrender, Christmas Spirit, White Angelica

ANXIETY

Single Oils: Orange, Roman chamomile, ylang ylang, lavender.

Blends: Valor, Hope, Peace & Calming, Present Time, Joy, Citrus Fresh, Surrender, Believe

APATHY

Single Oils: Frankincense, geranium, marjoram, jasmine, orange, peppermint, rosewood, rose, sandalwood, thyme, ylang ylang.

Blends: Joy, Harmony, Valor, 3 Wise Men, Hope, White Angelica, Motivation, Passion, Highest Potential

ARGUMENTATIVE

Single Oils: Cedarwood, Roman chamomile, eucalyptus, frankincense, jasmine, orange, thyme, ylang ylang.

Blends: Peace & Calming, Joy, Harmony, Hope, Valor, Acceptance, Humility, Surrender, Release, Chivalry

BOREDOM

Single Oils: Cedarwood, spruce, Roman chamomile, cypress, frankincense, juniper, lavender, rosemary, sandalwood, thyme, ylang ylang, black pepper.

Blends: Dream Catcher, Motivation, Valor, Awaken, Passion, Gathering, En-R-Gee

CONCENTRATION

Single Oils: Cedarwood, cypress, juniper, lavender, lemon, basil, helichrysum, myrrh, orange, peppermint, rosemary, sandalwood, ylang ylang.

Blends: Clarity, Awaken, Gathering, Dream Catcher, Magnify Your Purpose, Brain Power

CONFUSION

Single Oils: Cedarwood, spruce, cypress, peppermint, frankincense, geranium, ginger, juniper, marjoram, jasmine, rose, rosewood, rosemary, basil, sandalwood, thyme, ylang ylang.

Blends: Clarity, Harmony, Valor, Present Time, Awaken, Brain Power, Gathering, Grounding

DAY-DREAMING

Single Oils: Ginger, spruce, lavender, helichrysum, lemon, myrrh, peppermint, rosewood, rose, rosemary, sandalwood, thyme, ylang ylang.

Blends: Sacred Mountain, Gathering, Valor, Harmony, Present Time, Dream Catcher, 3 Wise Men, Magnify Your Purpose, Envision, Brain Power, Highest Potential

DEPRESSION

Single Oils: Frankincense, lemon, sandalwood, geranium, lavender, angelica, orange, grapefruit, ylang ylang.

Blends: Valor, Motivation, Passion, Hope, Joy, Brain Power, Present Time, Envision, Sacred Mountain, Harmony, Highest Potential

DESPAIR

Single Oils: Cedarwood, spruce, clary sage, frankincense, lavender, geranium, lemon, orange, lemongrass, peppermint, spearmint, rosemary, sandalwood, thyme, ylang ylang.

Blends: Joy, Valor, Harmony, Hope, Gathering, Grounding, Forgiveness, Motivation

DESPONDENCY

Single Oils: Bergamot, clary sage, cypress, geranium, ginger, orange, rose, rosewood, sandalwood, ylang ylang.

Blends: Peace & Calming, Inspiration, Harmony, Valor, Hope, Joy, Present Time, Gathering, Inner Child, Trauma Life, Envision, Chivalry

DISAPPOINTMENT

Single Oils: Clary sage, frankincense, geranium, ginger, juniper, lavender, spruce, orange, thyme, ylang ylang.

Blends: Hope, Joy, Valor, Present Time, Harmony, Dream Catcher, Gathering, Legacy, Magnify Your Purpose, Passion, Motivation

DISCOURAGEMENT

Single Oils: Bergamot, cedarwood, frankincense, geranium, juniper, lavender, lemon, orange, spruce, rosewood, sandalwood.

Blends: Valor, Sacred Mountain, Hope, Joy, Dream Catcher, Into the Future, Legacy, Magnify Your Purpose, Envision, Believe

FEAR

Single Oils: Bergamot, clary sage, Roman chamomile, cypress, geranium, juniper, marjoram, myrrh, spruce, orange, sandalwood, rose, ylang ylang.

Blends: Valor, Present Time, Hope, white Angelica, Trauma Life, Gratitude, Highest Potential

FORGETFULNESS

Single Oils: Cedarwood, Roman chamomile, frankincense, rosemary, basil, sandalwood, peppermint, thyme, ylang ylang.

Blends: Clarity, Valor, Present Time, Gathering, 3 Wise Men, Dream Catcher, Acceptance, Brain Power, Highest Potential

FRUSTRATION

Single Oils: Roman chamomile, clary sage, frankincense, ginger, juniper, lavender, lemon, orange, peppermint, thyme, ylang ylang, spruce.

Blends: Valor, Hope, Present Time, Sacred Mountain, 3 Wise Men, Humility, Peace Y Calming, Surrender, Live With Passion, Gratitude

GRIEF/SORROW

Single Oils: Bergamot, Roman chamomile, clary sage, *Eucalyptus globulus*, juniper, lavender.

Blends: Valor, Release, Inspiration, Inner Child, Gathering, Harmony, Present Time, Magnify Your Purpose

GUILT

Single Oils: Roman chamomile, cypress, juniper, lemon, marjoram, geranium, frankincense, sandalwood, spruce, rose, thyme.

Blends: Valor, Release, Inspiration, Inner Child, Gathering, Harmony, Present Time, Magnify Your Purpose, Gratitude

IRRITABILITY

Single Oils: All oils except eucalyptus, peppermint, black pepper.

Blends: Valor, Hope, Peace & Calming, Surrender, Forgiveness, Present Time, Inspiration

JEALOUSY

Single Oils: Bergamot, *Eucalyptus globulus*, frankincense, lemon, marjoram, orange, rose, rosemary, thyme.

Blends: Valor, Sacred Mountain, White Angelica, Joy, Harmony, Humility, Forgiveness, Surrender, Release, Gratitude

MOOD SWINGS

Single Oils: Bergamot, clary sage, sage, geranium, juniper, fennel, lavender, peppermint, rose, jasmine, rosemary, lemon, sandalwood, spruce, yarrow, ylang ylang.

Blends: Peace & Calming, Gathering, Valor, Dragon Time, Mister, Harmony, Joy, Present Time, Envision, Magnify Your Purpose, Brain Power

OBSESSIVENESS

Single Oils: Clary sage, cypress, geranium, lavender, marjoram, rose, sandalwood, ylang ylang, helichrysum.

Blends: Sacred Mountain, Valor, Forgiveness, Acceptance, Humility, Inner Child, Present Time, Awaken, Motivation, Surrender, Live With Passion

PANIC

Single Oils: Bergamot, Roman chamomile, frankincense, lavender, marjoram, wintergreen, myrrh, rosemary, sandalwood, thyme, ylang ylang, spruce.

Blends: Harmony, Valor, Gathering, White Angelica, Peace & Calming, Trauma Life, Awaken, Grounding, Believe

RESENTMENT

Single Oils: Jasmine, rose, tansy.

Blends: Forgiveness, Harmony, Humility, White Angelica, Surrender, Joy

RESTLESSNESS

Single Oils: Angelica, bergamot, cedarwood, basil, frankincense, geranium, lavender, orange, rose, rosewood, ylang ylang, spruce, valerian

Blends: Peace & Calming, Sacred Mountain, Gathering, Valor, Harmony, Inspiration, Acceptance, Surrender

SHOCK

Single Oils: Helichrysum, basil, Roman chamomile, myrrh, ylang ylang, rosemary CT cineol.

Blends: Clarity, Valor, Inspiration, Joy, Grounding, Trauma Life, Brain Power, Highest Potential, Australian Blue

25

Cleansing and Diets

Using Essential Oils and Supplements

The Risks of Internal Pollution

As the human body ages there is a risk of greater and greater buildup of chemical contamination in our tissues. As toxins accumulate, the body is more likely to suffer the energy-robbing effects of poor health and degenerative diseases.

This is why cleansing the body is so important. When the body is purged of heavy metal contamination, undigested foods, and internal pollution, it relieves enormous stress on the organs and tissues. Immune function is enhanced and particularly the stress on the liver is reduced.

Cleansing becomes especially important whenever animal products are consumed, such as meats and dairy products. These foods are loaded with naturally-occurring, disease-related microbes. According to Robert O. Young, Ph.D., D.Sc., meats contain an average of 300,000 to 3 million microorganisms per gram, or roughly 336 million per serving. Cheese contains from 300,000 to 1 million microorganisms per gram; milk, 20,000. These animal products can be a major source of internal pollution. Clean plant food, on the other hand, contains only 10 microbes per gram.

Humans were built to be primarily plant-eaters, not meat-eaters. Our long intestinal tracts are similar to many plant-eating species and are specifically designed by nature to digest a high-fiber, high-roughage, plant-based diet. Its long length allows enzymes a chance to unlock the nutrient value of the food. This contrasts markedly with the short intestines of flesh-eating animals, which are designed to quickly digest and pass through meats, without allowing them to putrefy, feed fungi, and create illness.

What happens when meats and dairy products are consumed by humans without adequate fiber? Lacking fiber, these proteins move through our lengthy intestines very slowly and easily become trapped in the intestine's many nooks and crannies. Acting like toxic time bombs, putrefying pockets of maldigested food gradually release their payload of heavy metals, chemicals, hormones, and toxins directly into the blood and tissues. Even worse, this undigested debris is fermented by our body's naturally-occurring yeast and fungi, polluting us with toxic by-products called mycotoxins. These mycotoxins have been linked to many diseases.

Who Needs Cleansing?

Everyone needs cleansing. All of us are stressed, to a lesser or greater degree, by an ever-mounting buildup of toxins, chemicals, bacteria, and parasites. A distinguished medical researcher, Kenneth Bock, M.D., states that humans are "walking toxic dumps." Why? Because of the industrial wastes, herbicides, pesticides, additives, and heavy metals we unknowingly absorb from our food, cosmetics, air, and water—even the mercury fillings in our teeth. Moreover, humans are at the top of the food chain meaning we are subjected to concentrated doses of potentially harmful chemicals from the meats and dairy products we consume.

According to a large 1990 survey by the Environmental Protection Agency, every single person tested showed some evidence of petrochemical pollution in their tissues and fats. Some of the chemicals found included styrene (used in plastics), xylene (a solvent in paint and gasoline), benzene (a chemical found in gasoline), and toluene (another carcinogenic solvent).

Inflamation is one of the main factors contributing to disease in the human body today—heart disease being a prime example. Many people do not understand how someone relatively healthy, with low cholesterol levels, normal arterial function, and healthy arterial walls can unexpectedly suffer a heart attack, yet it happens all too often. The explanation is inflammation.

What causes this inflammation and how does it occur in the body? Inflammation has various causes: bacterial infection (such as clamydia pneumoniae), poor diet, chemicals, hormonal imbalance, or physical injury.

A protein called "C-reactive" is released by the liver when inflammation is present. The level of this protein indicates the degree of inflammation in places like the linings of the arteries of the heart. Accumulation of C-reactive protein and an excess of blood protein plasma can change pH in the blood and cellular function and hasten the onset of tumors and a predisposition for heart disease. In fact, C-reactive protein testing may help doctors predict heart attack or stroke risk.

Cleansing allows the body to work towards fighting off the disease and not be encumbered or overloaded with the accumulation of toxins, mucous, and parasites that have built up over the years.

Understanding a Complete Cleansing

The ideal cleansing program should combine high water consumption with high-potency herbs, digestive enzymes, and therapeutic-grade essential oils. Essential oils have a special lipid-soluble makeup, which gives them a remarkable ability to penetrate cell membranes, break up undigested food, and oppose toxins. Essential oils also deliver oxygen, which has an unparalleled ability to inhibit the growth of many types of microbes. In fact, many essential oils have been studied for their unique antimicrobial, antifungal, and antiparasitic properties. Some oils, like rosemary, have demonstrated significant antiseptic activity, with documented research appearing in many scientific journals.

Consult your physician

Anyone cleansing or fasting for more than three days should do so under the supervision of a health care professional. Never begin a shut-down fast unless you have been fasting regularly for at least two years. This type of a fast should always be done under supervision.

A cleansing program should target many different parts of the body (colon, intestine, stomach, liver, pancreas) and cover many different types of internal pollution, including waste buildup, heavy metals, parasites, fungi, and yeast.

When Should You Cleanse?

Cleansing your system should not be just a once- or twice-a-year event. It should be continuous.

Cleansing is especially important for anyone over 40. With age comes a greater buildup of debris in our bodies caused by decreased production of the stomach acids and enzymes. Without proper enzyme production, we lack the ability to properly break down undigested proteins and other fermenting debris that obstruct our digestive system and impede the assimilation of nutrients.

To get the most out of any cleansing regimen, one must drink plenty of distilled or purified water (never chlorinated tap water) throughout the day. A good rule of thumb is to divide your body weight (in pounds) by half, then drink that number of ounces of water. For example, a 150 pound person should drink 75 ounces (about 7-8 glasses) of water daily.

The Stanley Burroughs Master Cleanse

The Master Cleanse is not a fast, but a cleansing program. A true fast consists only of water, while the original Master Cleanse incorporates a mixture of lemon juice, maple syrup, and cayenne pepper that is consumed throughout the day and is a source of calories, vitamins, and minerals.

NOTE: Clinical experience has shown that people do better when the Grade B Maple Syrup is replaced with Blue Agave nectar, as shown in the program below. Stanley Burroughs never had the opportunity to test this during his lifetime, so his recipe remains with the maple syrup.

The Master Cleanse is ideal for anyone who is not diabetic and can safely cleanse for at least three to seven days. The ideal duration of a cleanse is one to three weeks. As with any program of caloric restriction, however, it is *strongly* recommended that you consult with your health care professional before undertaking any extended fast or cleanse.

Program:

Take juice of 1/2 fresh lemon (preferably organic)

Mix juice into 8 oz. of distilled water

Add 1-2 tablespoons of blue agave nectar (in place of Grade B maple syrup)

Add up to 1/10th tsp. cayenne pepper (red)

Start with a pinch or two of cayenne and gradually increase to 1/10 tsp. Do not put cayenne pepper (capsicum) in capsules and take separate from the lemonade drink. It changes the action of the formula, and if sent directly to the stomach can cause inflammation and excessive mucous secretion. This may lead to sinusitis or to bowel mucous, and can even contribute to inflammatory bowel syndrome.

Drink as many 10 oz. glasses as required according to your body weight per day. If you weigh 100 pounds then you would drink half your weight in ounces which would be 50 ounces or 5 glasses.

Blue Agave nectar and Grade B maple syrup are two of the most balanced of all sugars, containing a balance of positive and negative ions. Neither enters the bloodstream as rapidly as honey or sugar which is better for people who react adversely to sugars, (becoming restless, sleepless, and energetic after consuming sugar), or may be borderline or pre-diabetic. Diabetics should definitely substitute blue agave for the maple syrup, using up to 1/4 tablespoon. (If you have difficulties locating Grade B Maple Syrup in your area, it is available through Creer Labs in Utah (801-465-5423).

Contrary to popular belief, lemon is not acidic in the body. It turns alkaline in the mouth. If an acid-like reaction is observed when using lemon with water, it is because of the minerals in the water. Distilled water will not react in this manner.

Tips

To aid the transition to vegetarianism and help re-program the system, take Body Gize three or four times per week. Also, for two weeks, take VitaGreen, then follow the master cleanse for another 30 days.

Cayenne pepper is a blood vessel dilator, a thermal warmer, and provides vitamin A. People who have type O blood tend to have poor circulation. As a result, their body temperature may drop during a cleanse. Because cayenne is an herb known for its ability to warm and restore circulation, it may be taken internally and used topically (especially on the feet, but in small amounts).

Cayenne pepper is also thermogenic. When used in a dietary program, it can facilitate an increase in the body's ability to burn fat.

For the deepest cleanse, it is recommended that you cleanse for at least two weeks. Exercise enhances the cleansing action of the program.

During the middle and later phases of the cleanse, the body chemistry changes, and energy levels may begin to increase. One may experience minor discomforts, such as headaches, upset stomach, or low energy, as toxins and parasites are released from the body. These symptoms will be short-lived.

It is important to have a positive attitude during cleansing or fasting. If you are unaccustomed to the process, you can prepare yourself by fasting one day a week. Sunday, or your Sabbath day, is a wonderful day for this purpose. The biggest obstacle to successful cleansing is fear of failure and not knowing what to expect.

To fast for 24 hours, it is easiest if you begin at noon and finish at noon on the following day or from one dinner to the next.

Again, drink plenty of water.

As you begin to fast, you may experience some unpleasant side effects of cleansing, such as headache, nausea, bloating, or irritability. These symptoms are part of the cleansing response and are often a result of toxins and waste matter being purged from the body which usually takes place within 12 to 36 hours.

If you experience these symptoms, you can cut back on your fluid intake, and turn to vegetable juices: carrot juice, carrot and celery—and 50/50 mixes, carrot with celery, spinach, and broccoli is really good. Carrot with a little apple juice or carrot, apple, and a little lemon juice is good to facilitate the continuation of the cleansing. Six ounces of of carrot juice, one ounce of apple, and 1/2 ounce of lemon juice will help keep the pH steady, slow the diarrhea, and keep the cleansing action going.

If you are feeling nauseated and bloated, it is an indication of two possibilities: (1) poisons are being released at a very rapid rate and may be backing up into the liver. Keeping the liver cleansed and flushed is extremely important. So it would be good to take ledum essential oil in a capsule at night or early morning. Ledum has a very strong effect on the liver and kidneys as a diuretic and a bile duct dilator.

The second reason for feeling ill is that the colon may not be eliminating as well because of spastic colon, loss of peristalsis (the wavelike motion of the intestines that moves waste matter out of the body), and/or from prolapsing with restrictions from kinks, loops, or twists in the colon. Hydro Colon therapy is a powerful treatment for cleansing the body and assisting in restoring peristalsis. You can call a colon hydrotherapist or buy a colima board. Portable colon hydrotherapy units that are available for use in the home are available from the Young Life Research Clinic (801) 489-8650.

Colon Hydrotherapy Mixture

Mix:
- 5 drops rosemary
- 5 drops basil
- 4 drops fennel

Add to colonic water and mix well.

In any case, you may also want to consult your health care professional.

During cleansing you may have an unexpected emotional clearing. There are various essential oil blends designed to help control your emotions, and modulate and facilitate the emotional release. Herbs, such as St. John's wort, kava, and hops extract, are excellent for managing stress and negative emotions. The essential oils of valerian, Roman and German chamomile, and lavender, are exceptionally beneficial. Essential oil blends, with tangerine, lavender, Roman chamomile, blue tansy, are calming and relaxing. Lemon oil is also calming. Most citrus oils containing aldehydes can be very calming in these situations. Vitamin B12 and folic acid are also important for emotional stability.

Ideally, these herbs or oils should be taken using oral infusion therapy (sprayed into the inside of the mouth where they can be most efficiently delivered into the blood).

The first 2 to 4 days of the fast are often the most difficult, since you will be overcoming the powerful psychological need to eat. As your body is cleansed of parasites and putrefying toxins, you will experience a sudden surge in energy and well being. Tapeworms, pinworms, and roundworms often start to appear in your stools after 4 to 6 days. Physical hunger will fade away. As the cleansing progresses, your mind will become sharper, your memory will improve, and your spirit will become more buoyant.

Remember: It is crucial to drink plenty of distilled water throughout the day, at least 8 to 10 eight ounce glasses. Water is crucial for not only flushing out toxins, but maintaining the metabolic machinery of your cells and tissues in proper working condition.

The Complete Cleanse

It is difficult to control internal pollution with a simple one-time fix or a single magic-bullet type solution. Complete cleansing requires a battery of different solutions all targeted at specific systems of the body. Cleansing the liver needs different herbs, oils and minerals than cleansing the colon which requires a different cleansing solution than the intestines.

Complete cleansing also requires a broad array of products that are effective against a wide variety of contaminants and microorganisms—not just one or two. Contaminants, like heavy metals, need a different set of tools to deactivate and purge them from the body than parasites do.

An important part of a complete cleansing program is essential oils. Highly antibacterial, antifungal, antiviral, and anti-inflammatory, essential oils help dissolve and chelate toxic chemicals and poisons in the body. They also promote digestive function by promoting the secretion and production of natural enzymes that enhance colon peristalsis that is the cornerstone of waste elimination.

The Herbal Colon Cleanse: ComforTone

Some of the best natural laxatives include cascara sagrada, diatomaceous earth, buckthorn bark, licorice root, apple pectin, bentonite, and black current extract. These herbs are particularly effective in cleansing the colon (large intestine) and can help counteract bloating and constipation. Purging the colon of toxins and impurities is just as important as cleaning the small intestine. Waste products and gases that are held in the colon have a far higher concentration of toxic byproducts than those in the small intestine. When these leach into the organs and tissues, they can wreak havoc in our bodies.

The essential oils of *Melaleuca alternifolia, rosemary officinalis cineol,* tarragon artemisa, bergamot, fennel, St. John's wort, German chamomile, and melissa along with basil eugenol, promote peristalsis and increase digestive secretions in the intestinal tract in helping to promote more and better digestion. Peppermint oil also promotes peristalsis.

Program:

Take two capsules every morning and two every night for two days.

Bowel movements should increase to 3-4 daily.

If elimination does not improve, then increase capsules to 3 each night and morning.

Do not exceed 8 capsules per day without advice from your physician.

If you feel cramping without results, you may have a dehydrated colon, spastic colon, loss of peristalsis, or a prolapsed colon.

Hydro colon therapy may be helpful. You can also drink 8 ounces of aloe vera and/or prune juice daily, which will work as a lubricant.

You should drink half your body weight of water in fluid ounces daily. When cleansing, you need 20 percent more water. However, water is not a lubricant. It works to soften and flush. Clay-like and hard stools and spastic colon indicate dehydration caused by not drinking enough fluids.

When bowel movements occur 3 to 4 times per day, ComforTone has done its job. If you retain this regularity, after stopping ComforTone, you have taken enough. An ideal bowel movement is 1 movement for each meal consumed per day; i.e.: 3 meals per day equal 3 bowel movements per day. When the movement slows to 1 or 2 per day or you begin to feel sluggish, begin again with ComforTone. You may be able to completely reduce your ComforTone dosage to zero or you may find that you need 1-2 capsules daily for a few weeks until you feel you do not need it any more.

Anyone, including pregnant women, should stop ComforTone if diarrhea occurs for more than 1 or 2 days. Restart again with a smaller amount. Other than this, it is safe to take the supplement through the entire pregnancy.

ComforTone and JuvaTone should not be taken together as they might cause a release of too many toxins at the same time, creating nausea, vomiting, dizziness or real discomfort. They are best taken at least one hour apart to allow them to work separately within the body.

The Intestinal Fiber Cleanse: ICP

Coarsely ground grains rich in soluble and semi-soluble fiber are some of the best intestinal cleansers known. Psyllium powder and husks, rice bran, oat bran, flax seed, and fennel seed all help loosen and expel undigested and fermenting materials from the intestines that may block nutrient absorption and poison the body's internal environment.

Fibers act as a biochemical sponge for the body, absorbing impurities, gases, and toxins. They also speed up the flow of waste matter through the intestines, helping to minimize the exposure to harmful substances. The slower the "transit time," or movement of waste matter through the gastro-intestinal tract, the higher the incidence of disease.

Fiber satisfies the appetite by giving people a feeling of fullness without adding excessive calories. Fiber may also help balance blood sugar levels. It also helps maintain regularity as we grow older, preventing and overcoming constipation, diarrhea, and gas. Essential oils, such as fennel, tarragon, ginger, lemongrass, rosemary, basil, St. John's wort, bergamot, German chamomile, lemon verbena, and melissa, not only help dissolve and chelate toxins, but they also combat pathological microorganisms that reside in the intestines.

Program:

Take 1 tbs. ICP, mixed in a glass of water, morning and night for two or three days.

After 2-3 days, increase dosage to 2 tbs. morning and night while you cleanse and drink plenty of water.

Maintenance dosage: 2 tbs., 3-4 time per week.

Mint Condition can be taken with ComforTone to soothe, help digestion, and relieve upset stomach.

Beta carotene, found in carrot juice and beet juice, also helps elimination.

Carrot seed oil detoxifies the liver, and in combination with geranium and lemongrass essential oils, may help in eliminating gallstones, cleaning the bowel, and relieving flatulence. For kidney stones, ledum, juniper, and geranium are best. To relieve flatulence, use fennel oil, St. John's wort, tarragon, and peppermint.

To maintain a healthy colon, it is best to stay away from processed and pasteurized dairy products, including all cheeses except goat cheese. Other items to avoid are refined white sugar, white flour, processed salt, starchy processed foods and fried foods. These are deadly to the intestinal tract. Also avoid bread made from hybrid wheats and grains that are damaging to the digestive tract. White bread is converted into sugar by the body and the sugar will turn to fat.

If ComforTone or ICP produce heartburn, this indicates that the digestive system is not working properly. If the cleansing process reduces the intestinal flora, add the following to the program:

- Essentialzyme: 1-3 tablets per meal and up to 6 with heavy meat meals late in the day or at night. Oils that can accelerate digestion are tarragon, fennel, St. John's wort, anise seed, and German chamomile. Take 3 or 4 drops of each of the above in a double 00 capsule taken before or after a meal to enhance digestion.

- Yogurt: Take 1/2 hour before meals on an empty stomach.

These supplements provide the stomach with the friendly bacteria and enzymes necessary for good digestion, conversion, and assimilation. Master Formula HERS/HIS and CHILDREN'S, Royal Essence, and Mineral Essence provide trace minerals that the body requires to make enzymes.

When taken together, ComforTone and Essentialzyme have synergistic effects, so less of each is required to achieve similar benefits.

The Enzyme Cleanse: Essentialzyme

Enzymes help break down foods and proteins that might otherwise ferment and putrefy in the gastrointestinal tract. Undigested foods tax our bodies, sap our energy, and spur the overgrowth of yeast, fungi, parasites, bacteria, and microorganisms that contribute to viral conditions, gastritis, Crohn's disease, and inflammatory diverticulitis. Inadequate digestive enzyme activity has also been linked to chronic inflammations elsewhere in the body, such as fibromyalgia, herpes, inability to gain or lose weight, bad breath, body odor, skin rashes, and migraines. Enzymes like pancreatin, pancrelipase, chymotrypsin, and trypsin are very efficient in breaking down proteins.

However, if the body is acidic, the chymotrypsin, trypsin, and enzymes will not effectively activate in the body. Vegetable enzymes from the unripe papaya and pineapple (papain and bromelain) provide enzyme support.

Digestive enzymes promote complete digestion and help those who have difficulty digesting and assimilating food. The older we get and the more food we consume, the more enzymes we need for complete digestion. Enzymes are essential in unlocking and metabolizing the vitamins, minerals, and amino acids in food.

Enzymes help digest cooked and processed foods that lack the natural enzymes of fresh foods.

Program:

For maintenance: 2-3 Essentialzyme or Polyzyme tablets 3 times daily. Best taken before meals.

Eating out: Carry tablets with you or take them when you return home. After a heavy meal at night and before going to bed, make sure to take tablets to help prevent fermenting.

A, B, and AB blood types: 2-4 tablets

O blood types: 3-6 or more tablets if you feel it necessary.

Cancer or other degenerative diseases

Use the following Ramping Enzymes Program

Ramping Enzymes Program:

Phase 1: Take 3 tablets 3 times daily. Increase by one tablet every day until you become nauseated. Then discontinue Essentialzyme for 24 to 36 hours.

Phase 2: Take 4 tablets 3 times daily. Increase daily by one tablet until you become nauseated. Rest (discontinue) again for 24-36 hours.

Phase 3: Take 5 tablets 3 times daily. Increase daily by one tablet until you become nauseated. Rest again for 24-36 hours.

Phase 4: Start again with the amount that was being taken before nausea occurred the third time. For example: If you were taking 30 tablets when you became nauseated, you would then start Phase 4 with 29 tablets spread out over each day. Continue with this amount for 6 weeks.

Phase 5: In the 7th week, start the enzyme ramping program all over again. This means that you begin Phase 1 and increase the amount by one each day until nausea or vomiting starts again. Repeat and continue for 6 weeks as previously described.

If your doctor determines that you are in remission, you can maintain with 20-30 tablets daily for one year, 6 days a week.

Maintenance: 6 Essentialzyme tablets, 2 times daily.

Caution: This is a very rigorous program so you should consult with your doctor before starting and have your doctor monitor your progress during the program.

The Liver Cleanse: JuvaTone, JuvaFlex, Juva Cleanse and Lipozyme

The liver is one of the most important organs in the body. It is pivotal for purifying the blood and plays a key role in converting carbohydrates to energy, as well as storing energy in the form of glycogen and fats. An overburdened liver can affect our energy, digestion, skin and blood.

Fats and bile within the liver can easily become saturated with toxic chemicals and heavy metals. As these toxins accumulate, the liver becomes taxed and becomes unable to properly detoxify the blood. Symptoms of a stressed and poorly functioning liver include skin conditions (ie., rashes, eczema, dermatitis), fatigue, headaches, pallor, dizziness, irritability, and poor digestion.

Several nutrients are essential for cleansing the liver. Choline, inositol, milk thistle, schizandra, and dl-methionine, have been researched for their ability to protect, defat and purge toxins from the liver. Oregon grape root is a source of berberine, a compound researched for its ability to slow the liver damage and scarring (cirrhosis) associated with alcohol consumption and hepatitis B and C.

Some essential oils can also be valuable in increasing the flow of bile from the liver. These oils include ledum, German chamomile, carrot seed, helichrysum, and geranium. Carrot seed oil is well-regarded by herbalists for its role in liver cleansing.

Mercury Toxicity

Mercury is present in harmful amounts in almost every person in the Unites States, due to consumption of seafood (methyl mercury levels in canned tuna are especially problematic) and amalgam dental fillings (which are about 50% mercury). It is estimated that every year, 22 million pounds of mercury are put in peoples mouths in the form of fillings. It is estimated that a person who consumes a 6 oz can of one of the top 5 brands of tuna fish will (with over 0.64 ppm methyl mercury levels) have consumed over 20 times the mercury considered safe by the Environmental Protection Agency.

According to the Centers for Disease Control, statistics show that one in eight women of childbearing age in the United States suffers from tissue levels of mercury that can be dangerous to a developing fetus.

Heavy metals are some of the most toxic poisons on earth and can slowly accumulate in human tissues and cause neurological diseases, cardiovascular problems and some types of cancers. [1]

---

1. Grandjean P, et al., "Cardiac autonomic activity in methylmercury neurotoxicity: 14-year follow-up of a Faroese birth cohort." *J Pediatr.* 2004 Feb;144(2):169-76.

The problem is that heavy metals such as mercury and lead form insoluble metallic salts that become trapped in the fat and in the kidneys and cannot be quickly excreted by the liver. Because liver plays a major role in trapping and stabilizing mercury, liver cleansing using essential oils can be an outstanding treatment in purging the body of heavy metal contamination that can contribute to many chronic neurological diseases.[2,3,4,5,6]

Clincial Studies Using Helichrysum, Ledum, Celery Seed Essential Oils (JuvaCleanse)

Clinical studies show that an essential oil blend of helichrysum, ledum, and celery seed (JuvaCleanse) dramatically amplified the elimination from the body of heavy metals, especially mercury, one of the most toxic of all non-radioactive metals. Mercury is particularly damaging to the brain and nervous system because it can pass through blood-brain barrier and accumulate indefinitely in motor neurons.

A 2003 clinical study involving a group of four patients tested the effect of three essential oils on the urinary output of mercury.

Four healthy individuals (ages 27 to 69) took two capsules per day (approximately 1,500 mg) of a blend of helichrysum, ledum, and celery seed (JuvaCleanse). The first urine collection occurred prior to essential oil therapy, with the second and third urine collections occurring two and four days after essential oil therapy had begun. The results showed that all four participants more than doubled their urinary elimination of mercury over the four days of evaluation.

Liver Cleanse Regimen:

Week 1: Take 3 JuvaTone tablets, 3 times daily for one week.

Week 2: Increase to 4 tablets, 3 times daily for one week.

Week 3: Increase to 5 tablets, 3 times daily for one week.

Week 4: Increase to 6 tablets, 3 times daily for 1 week.

Then decrease in the reverse order.

Rest for two weeks after completing the 8 week cycle.

The above regimen can be significantly enhanced with the addition of 10 drops daily of Juva Cleanse (taken in a capsule, in the morning upon rising, with 12 oz of pure water) and 1-3 tsp daily of Juva Power, added as a seasoning to foods.

JuvaFlex Essential Oil Blend may be massaged over the liver once daily and may also be applied in a hot compress application (see Compress method in Applications Methods at beginning of Chapter 30). A combination compress can be made with JuvaFlex and a castor oil poultice. Compresses may be applied several times a day. JuvaFlex may also be applied on the bottom of the feet through the Vita Flex technique over the liver points. It may also be taken as a dietary supplement, 4 drops twice daily mixed in soy/rice milk.

Nausea or vomiting indicates a toxic liver. Stop and rest 2-3 days and then start again with 1-2 tablets per day. Gradually increase amount.

JuvaTone and ComforTone should not be taken together as they might cause a release of too many toxins at the same time creating nausea, vomiting, dizziness or discomfort. They are best taken an hour apart to allow them to work individually as the body needs.

For more information on liver cleansing and a detailed daily protocol, consult "Re-JUVA-nate Your Health," a book on liver cleansing by D. Gary Young.

For more information on JuvaTone and Lipozyme, see Chapter 10 - DIETARY SUPPLEMENTS. For more information on JuvaFlex and Juva Cleanse, see Chapter 3 - BLENDS.

2. Stankovic RK, et al., "The expression and significance of metallothioneins in murine organs and tissues following mercury vapour exposure." *Toxicol Pathol.* 2003 Sep-Oct;31(5):514-23.

3. Kennedy CJ. "Uptake and accumulation of mercury from dental amalgam in the common goldfish, Carassius auratus." *Environ Pollut.* 2003;121(3):321-6.

4. Song KB, et al., "Mercury distribution and concentration in rats fed powdered dental amalgam." *Arch Oral Biol.* 2002 Apr;47(4):307-13.

5. Zalups RK, Lash LH. "Depletion of glutathione in the kidney and the renal disposition of administered inorganic mercury." *Drug Metab Dispos.* 1997 Apr;25(4):516-23.

6. Stoltenberg M et al., "Autometallographic tracing of mercury in pilot whale tissues in the Faroe Islands." *Int J Circumpolar Health.* 2003 May;62(2):182-9.

The Parasite Cleanse: ParaFree

Almost everyone has parasites in one form or another. For the most part, they go entirely unnoticed until they begin to cause fatigue and unwellness.

Pure essential oils have some of the strongest antiparasitic properties known. Some of these oils include thyme, clove, anise, nutmeg, fennel, vetiver, Idaho tansy, cumin, *Melaleuca alternifolia*, ledum, melissa, bergamot, and bay laurel.

Select three or four of the oils. Mix in equal proportions and fill a double 00 capsule. Take 3 to 6 a day for 7 days, resting for 7 days and repeating for 7 days. repeat this 3 week cycle seven times.

Oils that may be helpful for natural chelation would be helichrysum, orange or lime, cypress, and ledum.

Program:

The duration of this program depends on the individual.

Take 3-6 ParaFree gelcaps, 2 times daily for one week. Rest for one week to allow the parasite eggs to hatch and become active.

Resume dosage for a minimum of 3 weeks and then rest for 3 weeks. Repeat this cycle three times.

The Heavy Metal Cleanse: Chelex Tincture

Heavy metals such as lead, mercury and cadmium in microscopic amounts can cause severe damage to our bodies. They disrupt normal functions and can cause allergic reactions, fatigue, headache, muscle pains, digestive disturbance, dizziness, depression and mental confusion.

Of even graver concern is their tendency to accumulate in the brain, kidneys, nerves, immune system, and fatty tissues. Some highly poisonous heavy metals, such as cadmium, can remain in the body for up to 30 years. As a result, they can lead to degenerative diseases including Alzheimer's, multiple sclerosis, and even cancer.

Herbs such as astragalus, garlic, sarsaparilla, and red clover have the ability to bind heavy metals so they can be expelled from the body. Essential oils also have a natural ability to dissolve insoluble heavy metal salts so that they can be eliminated.

Program:

Put 3-4 droppers of Chelex Tincture in distilled water and drink 3-4 times daily for up to 120 days. Depending on the type of mineral or chemical toxicity, it may be necessary to follow this regimen for as long as 18 months.

Maintenance: 1-2 droppers, 2 times daily, 5 days a week. The duration of this program depends on one's own knowledge of exposure and contamination.

Hair analysis may help in determining the proper duration of this program.

Blood Cleanse: Rehemogen Tincture

This tincture contains herbs that were traditionally used by Chief Sundance and Native Americans for cleansing and purifying the blood. It builds red blood cells and is recommended for any blood disorder. It works as a strong companion with Chelex.

Program:

Chelation (use with above Chelex program): 2 droppers Rehmogen (50 drops) in water 2-3 times daily.

Blood disorders: Put 2-3 droppers Rehmogen (50-75 drops) in distilled water every 2-3 hours.

JuvaTone with Rehemogen is invaluable.

Maintenance Cleansing

Our lifestyles should incorporate cleansing at all times. The intensity of the cleansing depends on the individual. ComforTone, Essentialzyme and ICP taken at the same time, provide a powerful, synergistic cleansing force.

Program:

ComforTone: 3-5 capsules AM and PM.

Essentialzyme: 3 tablets, 3 times daily to continue the digestion of toxic waste in your body from everyday metabolism.

ICP: 1 tbsp. in a glass of water, A.M. and P.M.

JuvaPower: 1 Tbsp 2 x daily

Babies and Children

Babies and children respond very well to oils and supplements. The only difference from adult use is smaller dosage.

Babies: Put 1-2 drops of oil in your hand and rub them together until the hands are practically dry. Then hold them over any particular area of the baby. This works very well without direct application.

Direct application: Mix 1-2 drops of an essential oil in V-6 Mixing oil or Massage Oil Base and apply to bottom of feet.

Children: Put 1-2 drops on bottom of feet or anywhere else on the body as long as the oil is diluted in V-6 Mixing oil, Massage Oil Base, or any vegetable or massage oil. The dilution is always the important factor in comfortability.

Balancing Body Frequency

Much of the cause of imbalance is in the endocrine glands, which create the electrical balance throughout the physical body.

Where the imbalance is due to allergy in sinuses, throat, or pituitary insufficiency, apply the complementary oil to the crown of the head, the forehead, and the thymus.

The blend Release stimulates harmony and balance by releasing memory trauma from liver cells, which store emotions of anger, hate, and frustration. Apply neat over liver, apply compress over liver, or massage Vita Flex points on feet and hands.

Sandalwood oxygenates the pineal/pituitary gland, thus improving attitude and body balance. Rose has a frequency of 320 MHz, the highest of all oils. Its beautiful fragrance is aphrodisiac-like and almost intoxicating. The frequency of every cell is enhanced, bringing balance and harmony to the body. Rose is stimulating and elevating to the mind, creating a sense of well being.

Lavender is very good unless it is an oil that is disliked. Harmony will probably work in most situations. Inner Child is also excellent.

For overall body electrical imbalance, put a couple of drops of the complementary oil in each palm, have the person hold the right palm over the navel and the left palm over the thymus and take three slow, deep breaths. Place the dominant hand over the navel and the other hand over the thymus and rub clockwise three times. This works through the body's electrical field by pulling the frequency in through the umbilicus, the thymus, and the olfactory to the limbic system in the brain to create electrical balance.

Apply Thieves on the bottom of the feet. Sage is good for balancing frequencies when disease lowers body frequency.

Harmony on the energy centers (or chakras) helps balance the body, enhancing the healing process and facilitating the release of stored emotions.

The energy points corresponding to the endocrine glands are:

- The crown (top) of the head (pineal)
- Forehead (pituitary)
- Neck (thyroid)
- Thymus
- Solar plexus (adrenal)
- Navel (pancreas)
- Groin (ovaries/gonads)

Other oils that can be used are frankincense, myrtle, Valor, 3 Wise Men, and Joy.

Blood Types and Food Supplements

In 1996, Dr. Peter J. D'Adamo's book, *Eat Right 4 Your Type*, presented the concept of separate diets for each of the four blood types.

People with blood type A and AB are natural vegetarians and have the easiest time converting to a vegetarian diet. However, these people also have a tendency for thyroid problems and tend to be overweight. For them, exercise that increases heart rate is necessary to have weight reduction.

People with type B blood are probably the most balanced in nutritional needs and can more easily be either vegetarians or meat-eaters.

People with type O blood need additional protein, possibly through meat consumption. They have a more difficult time converting to vegetarianism. These people can get all the protein they need if they consume the correct portions of seeds, nuts and grains. VitaGreen should be a mainstay for this group. These people often have digestive deficiencies. They eat more but assimilate less, have excess gas, get full quickly but are hungry sooner, and tend to weigh less.

People who have type O blood tend to have poor circulation and as a result tend to be cold when fasting. Cayenne pepper improves this situation. One can also put some cayenne in one's shoes and socks when they are worn. Cayenne becomes damp from foot perspiration creating warmth to the feet.

During fasting, O blood types may require more protein. During the first two weeks these people should take Body Gize twice a day and should also take VitaGreen three times per day. These supplements will provide the necessary proteins. After two weeks, the supplements should be ceased, because protein intake must be zero in order to effect DNA memory change. The body will convert its minimal protein requirements as needed.

Blood type is one of many variables to be considered in selecting what you eat and the supplements you take.

Building the Body

Nutritional supplements enhanced with essential oils can help support and balance body systems. The following products will nourish, strengthen and build your body.

Program:

Power Meal—The all-vegetarian protein drink with Chinese wolfberries.

> Use 2 scoops (4 tbs.) in liquid 2-3 times per day. Mix in water, rice or soy milk. It can be mixed in orange or apple juice, but this may make it too sweet and lower the pH. It also may be mixed with cereal, fruits, desserts, and other foods.

> Combine equal parts Power Meal and Body Gize for a high-powered protein blend.

> Drink as needed.

Master Formula HERS/HIS—Premium multi-vitamin, mineral, and amino acid supplements.

> O Blood Type: 8-10 tablets daily.

> B Blood Type 6-8 tablets daily.

> A Blood Type 4-6 tablets daily.

Essentialzyme—Enzyme function for mental clarity and physical activity.

> O Blood Type: 4-8 tablets daily (depending on type of food eaten and time of day).

> B Blood Type: 8-10 tablets daily.

> A Blood Type: 10-12 tablets daily (A types tend to have more digestive needs).

Note: When eating heavy protein foods after 3:00 p.m., it is very helpful to additionally take Polyzyme before going to bed.

Exodus—Supercharged antioxidant formula for immune supporting.

> O Blood Type: 6-8 capsules daily.

> B Blood Type: 6-7 capsules daily.

> A Blood Type: 4-6 capsules daily.

VitaGreen—Protein-rich chlorophyll formula.

> O Blood Type: 8-10 capsules daily.

> B Blood Type: 6-8 capsules daily.

> A Blood Type: 4-6 capsules daily.

Ultra Young—Supports healthy pituitary and growth hormone secretion.

> Apply 3 sprays on the inside of the cheeks to maximize absorption. Avoid swallowing as long as possible to promote more buccal cavity absorption.

> Age 15-30: 3 sprays, 2 times daily (for immune support).

> Age 30-45: 3 sprays, 2-3 times daily.

> Age 45-65: 3 sprays, 4-6 times daily.

> Juvenile Pituitary Retardation: 3 sprays, 3-6 times daily.

> Spray 6 days a week for 3 weeks and rest for one week and then repeat.

ImmuneTune

> O Blood Type: 6-8 capsules daily.

> B Blood Type: 6 plus capsules daily.

> A Blood Type: 4 plus capsules daily.

Super C

> 1 tablet daily for maintenance.

> 2 tablets daily for reinforcing immune strength.

251

Super Cal

2-6 capsules daily or as needed.

Mineral Essence

3-6 droppers (75 to 150 drops) in water 1-2 times daily.

Sulfurzyme

Start: 1-2 tsp daily for 1-2 days

Increase: 1-2 tbs 2 times daily for maximum results.

The Clock Diet

The Clock Diet was originated by Dr. Charlotte Holms who maintained a private practice even at 100 years of age in 1989. This diet was based on the fact that stomach acid and enzyme production (pepsin and hydrochloric acid) begins in the morning (about 6 a.m.) and tapers off during the afternoon (between 1:00 and 3:00 p.m.).

This diet mandates that we should schedule our consumption of animal and plant protein to coincide with the highest output of stomach acid and enzymes. Unless our body produces the enzymes to break down protein, high-protein foods will merely ferment in the stomach and lead to fungal and bacterial overgrowth, laying the groundwork, not only for indigestion, but also for disease.

Ideally, we should consume all of our high-protein foods once a day during the morning meal. These foods include grains, such as oats, cornmeal, millet, soy milk, and brown rice, and animal products, such as cheese, milk, and meats.

When the stomach's production of acid and enzymes drops during midafternoon, the best foods to eat consist of simple and complex carbohydrates such as fresh fruits and cooked and raw vegetables. Avoid mixing protein and carbohydrates in the same afternoon or night meal.

Daily Maintenance

The human body has a daily need for nutrients to keep it in peak condition. The nutritional products listed below contain essential oils to help support normal digestive function and nutrient absorption.

Power Meal or Body Gize—Complete protein foods.

Combine or use individually: 1-2 scoops in water, rice milk, oat milk, or other liquid.

VitaGreen—Protein-rich chlorophyll formula very beneficial for vegetarians and O blood types.

O Blood Type: 8-10 capsules daily.

B Blood Type: 6-8 capsules daily.

A Blood Type: 4-6 capsules daily.

Master HIS/HERS—Gender-specific vitamin, mineral, and amino acid complexes.

O Blood Type: 8-10 tablets daily.

B Blood Type: 6-8 tablets daily.

A Blood Type: 4-6 tablets daily.

ComforTone—All natural colon cleanser.

Essential Manna—Whole food complex, a fiber- and mineral-rich snack.

Fasting

Fasting has been called nature's single-greatest healing therapy. Fasting is the avoidance of solid food with liquid intake varying from no liquids to just water to fresh juices. A fast can last 24 hours or several weeks. Fasting has long been a tradition in Judaism, Christianity and the Eastern religions. Religious fasting can involve purification, penitence or preparation for approaching God. An increasing number of doctors are recognizing that fasting can be physically healing while allowing us to focus our energy inward, bringing clarity and change.

Gabriel Cousens, M. D. writes that "fasting in a larger context, means to abstain from that which is toxic to mind, body and soul. A way to understand this is that fasting is the elimination of physical, emotional and mental toxins from our organs, rather than simply cutting down on or stopping food intake. Fasting for spiritual purposes usually involves some degree of removal of oneself from worldly responsibilities. It can mean complete silence and isolation during the fast which can be a great revival to those of us who have been putting our energy outward.

Fasting is generally safe but those with medical conditions should check with their health care professional.

Elson M. Haas, M. D. notes that fasting is a catalyst for change and an integral part of transformational medicine. He writes, "Fasting clearly improves motivation and creative energy; it also enhances health and vitality and lets many of the body systems rest."

An extremely important benefit of fasting is the elimination of toxins. By minimizing the work our digestive system must do, we allow it to repair itself and clean up stored toxins. In the beginning of a fast, the liver will convert stored glycogen to energy. As the fast continues, some proteins will be broken down unless juices provide calories.

The best way to convert to vegetarianism is by fasting. To be healthy, have energy, be free of sickness and disease, you must learn to discipline yourself and listen to the needs of your body.

Our bodies do not need meat to maintain good health, even though many of us have programmed ourselves through years of meat consumption to have the desire to eat meat. Our bodies can get all the protein required from a diet containing a wide variety of non-meat foods: beans, lentils, vegetables, whole grains, seeds, some cheeses, dairy products (preferably unpasteurized and natural colored), and occasionally eggs. However, you must be sure to eat enough protein to maintain a balanced, healthy body.

Exercise makes fasting work better, particularly if one is trying to lose weight.

NOTE: Pregnant or lactating mothers should seek medical supervision before beginning a fast.

Fitness

Power Meal—2 scoops, 4-6 times daily in water or rice milk or as needed.

Be-Fit—Women, 2 capsules before workout and 2 capsules after workout. For men to increase muscle mass, 6 capsules before and six capsules after workout.

> Capsules may be increased or decreased as needed according to body weight and blood type.

VitaGreen—As desired, anywhere from 4-10 capsules daily.

Master HIS/HERS—As desired, anywhere from 4-8 capsules daily.

Fortifying the Immune System

The immune system is the most important body system. It must be strong and responsive in order to combat infectious diseases and counteract toxins. Some 40 percent of immune system function is found in the intestinal tract and is called *pirus patchet*. Another 40 percent is accounted for by the thymus gland, which produces immune-stimulating cells.

Dietary supplements containing essential oils can boost immune system function.

ImmuPro—a complex of polysaccharides, beta glucans, minerals and essential oils that is regarded as the strongest immune stimulant known.

> **Maintenance:** 1 chewable once a day before retiring.

> **Deficiencies:** 2-4 chewables before retiring; 1-2 morning and afternoon.

> **Therapeutic Dosages:** 4-8 chewable before retiring; 2-3 morning and afternoon.

Exodus II—blended with oils referenced in the Old and New Testaments.

> Massage 3-6 drops on bottom of feet, thymus, throat, or wherever desired.

Exodus—a strong immune builder.

> **Maintenance:** 2-4 capsules daily; O blood types may increase amount.

> **For weaker system:** Take 6-10 capsules, 3 times daily for 10 days and then reduce. Type A's may want to use less.

Sulfurzyme—contains MSM and Chinese Wolfberry.

> **Maintenance:** 1-2 tsp. daily in water or juice. May increase as needed.

> **Deficiencies:** Begin 1-2 tsp. daily and work up to 3-4 tbs. daily or more if desired.

ImmuPower—a blend to strengthen, build, and protect the body.

> **Maintenance:** 1 capsule a day 3 or 4 times a week.

> **Deficiencies:** For pneumonia, flu or colds, 4 capsules a day for 10 days, resting 4 days, and then 1 capsule a day for another 10 days.

ImmuneTune—has strong antioxidant, anti-inflammatory, and anti-tumoral properties. Helps maintain electrolyte and pH balance.

Maintenance: 2-4 capsules daily.

Radex—contains herbs and essential oils that have been researched for their antioxidant properties and their effects on DNA-damaging free radicals. This blend also contains Super Oxide Dismutase, widely reported to be another powerful free-radical scavenger.

Super C—a special formula of ascorbic acid, scientifically balanced with rutin, bioflavonids, and trace minerals to balance electroytes and assist in the absorption of vitamin C. The essential oils of grapefruit, tangerine, lemon, and mandarin may increase the oxygen and bioflavonoid activity.

Thyromin—a special blend of glandular extracts, herbs, amino acids, minerals, and essential oils to support the thyroid. This gland regulates body metabolism and temperature and is important for immune function.

Protec—a blend of essential and vegetable oils designed for a night-long retention enema. Studies by Terry Friedmann, MD showed reversal of prostate cancer in a number of patients.

Mineral Essence—a precisely balanced complex of essential oils and more than 60 trace minerals that are essential to a healthy immune system. It includes well-known antioxidants and immune-supporters such as zinc, selenium and magnesium.

Other Products for Supporting the Immune System

Single oils:

- Frankincense with ravensara, thyme, helichrysum, oregano, rosemary, chamomile, Idaho tansy, mountain savory, melissa, lavender, grapefruit, lemon, cinnamon, clove, cumin, cistus, melaleuca, myrrh, myrtle, rose, vetiver, or lemongrass.

Blends:

- Frankincense with Thieves, ImmuPower, Abundance, Acceptance, Humility, R.C., or 3 Wise Men.

Supplements:

Super B, Royal Essence, VitaGreen, Power Meal, ArthroTune, Rehemogen, AlkaLime, Ultra Young, Cleansing Trio, JuvaTone, and Wolfberry Bar.

Other Steps for Maintaining a Healthy Immune System

1. Cleanse the colon and liver of toxins and accumulated waste that can sap energy and down-regulate immune response.

   —The Cleansing Trio is a complete cleansing solution.

2. Avoid excess fear, anxiety, and depression, which can undermine and compromise immune function. Continual daily use of essential oils is optimal to overcome stress (see STRESS).

3. Avoid physical and mental overexertion which can down regulate immune response. Essential oils, such as lavender, can have powerful relaxant effect on the mind and body, and thus stimulate immune function.

4. Maintain a healthy, balanced diet. A diet high in minerals, such as magnesium, potassium, selenium, zinc, and folic acid play a crucial role in optimizing immune response.

   —Berry Young Juice is rich in essential minerals, documented to double macrophage activity in studies at Weber State University.

   —Essential Manna is rich in potassium, magnesium, selenium, zinc and numerous other nutrients.

   —Berry Bars are loaded with essential minerals, phytonutrients, and FOS (to enhance mineral absorption).

5. Avoid contaminated or chlorinated water.

   Chlorine inhibits thyroid function interfering with its uptake of iodine and the amino acid tyrosine and therefore slows down metabolism, circulation, and immune function. Chlorine has also been linked to birth defects in children (see Chlorine, Appendix R).

— Add 1 drop of lemon, peppermint, or spearmint to drinking water.

— Use chlorine-free water for showering and bathing. The RainSpa shower head is specially designed to accept bath salts loaded with essential oils.

6. Stimulate the immune system using selected essential oils and supplements.

— Grapefruit, lemon, lemongrass, and R.C. promote leukocyte (white blood cell) formation.

— ImmuneTune, ImmuPro (polysaccharide complex) and Exodus (herbal complex) build and support the immune system. Exodus II (essential oil blend) is a companion to both supplements.

— VitaGreen encourages healthy blood and boosts immune function.

7. Diffuse essential oils to reduce airborne pathogens and viruses that can overwhelm the immune system.

— ImmuPower and Thieves.

NOTE: Do not diffuse Thieves more than 15 to 30 minutes at a time as the cinnamon may irritate the nasal passages. Also be sure that the room is well ventilated.

8. Inhalation of essential oils can increase immune function through their ability to stimulate the hypothalamus. According to studies conducted by Dr. Asawa of Japan and Dr. Richardson of England, inhalation of unadulterated essential oils increase blood flow to the brain by 15 percent and brain blood oxygen levels by 25 percent.

9. Eliminate parasites which compromise immune function by overloading the system (see PARASITES).

10. Use essential oils in massage applications or take as dietary supplements. Research from the Universities of Cairo, Geneva, and Paris indicate that essential oils are one of the highest known sources of antioxidants.

— Thieves, Exodus II, mountain savory, abundance, ImmuPower.

Dilute 1 or 2 drops in massage oil or V-6 Mixing Oil and massage on the thymus, bottom of feet, and throat. These oils can also be used as dietary supplements: Use 3 drops, four to six times daily for seven days. Repeat the cycle again, if needed, after four day rest.

11. Support the thyroid gland. The thyroid is crucial to regulating body metabolism, energy levels, and balancing immunity.

— Thyromin strengthens the thyroid (see THYROID).

12. Use antioxidants.

— Longevity is the highest antioxidant supplement.

— Berry Young Juice is the highest antioxidant juice.

— Super C contains vitamin C and bioflavonoids and acts as a strong immune support.

— Essential Manna contains an extremely wide variety of natural antioxidants.

13. Reduce candida and fungal overgrowth in the body. These can seriously impair and overload immune function. Alkaline ash whole foods and FOS (fructoligosaccharides) can minimize fungal growth.

— Essential Manna is a whole food complex of alkaline-ash nutrients.

(See BODY pH ACID/ALKALINE BALANCE)

14. Increase intake of antioxidants when exposed to radiation. If you know you have been exposed to radiation, feeling fatigued from it, or if you are flying with commercial airlines (because of the greater exposure to radiation due to the high altitude) an increased daily amount of antioxidant supplements is needed. When flying, increase intake 10 days before the trip and continue this higher dosage for 10 days after the trip.

Guidelines for the Healthiest Diet

Breakfast is the most important meal of the day. Some people work for an hour or two prior to having breakfast to promote appetite and prime the digestive system.

Eat breakfast between 6 and 7 a.m. Do not consume any fruit, sugar, or high glycemic index foods. The exception to this is strawberries or raspberries with cereal. Sugar-free yogurt is a good source of acidophilus and bifidobacteria cultures essential of proper intestinal flora. Cereals can include oatmeal, millet, wheat, barley, triticale, or a mixture of these, with coconut milk, rice milk, soy milk, whey powder, or goat milk. Since we do not have enough enzymes to handle multiple foods, it is best to not mix over 3 grains or different foods at a time. Bread should always be toasted; this changes it from a wet food to a dry food, making it more digestible. But eat sparingly. A and B blood types will gain weight eating any type of bread simply because the grains are all hybrid today.

As a rule, breakfast is the best meal of the day for eating proteins, such as beans, rice, eggs, fish, etc. Avoid meat after the noon meal. This will provide more energy and stamina in the afternoon. Always consume Polyzyme with high protein meals. Lunch should consist of carbohydrates and complex carbohydrates and proteins in the form of pasta (a high gylcemic index food, eat sparingly), mixed vegetables, particularly greens and light meats—freshwater fish, cage-free chicken. Drink water with the meal.

For the person engaged in body-building, consume proteins before 3 p.m. by having it at breakfast, mid-morning, lunch, and mid-afternoon. Eat carbohydrates and complex carbohydrates for the evening meal, and have fresh fruit for a snack.

Dinner should be eaten as close to 3 p.m. as possible. It is better not to eat late at night. Both fruit and solid vegetables are suitable for evening meals. If one must eat a large, heavy meal late in the day or evening, an extra portion of Essentialzyme or Polyzyme is needed to promote proper digestion, reduce gas, and prevent putrefaction and fungal growth in the intestines.

Be patient. It may take 2 to 2 1/2 years of very diligent work to establish good digestive function. Listen to your body and modify the program as your body changes.

Hering's Four Laws of Healing

Constantine Hering, a German homeopath who emigrated to the United States in the 1830s, is considered the father of American homeopathy. He formulated four fundamental principles of healing:

1. Healing progresses from the deepest part of the organism—the mental and emotional levels and the vital organs—to the external parts, such as the skin and extremities.

2. As healing progresses, symptoms appear and disappear in the reverse of their original chronological order of appearance.

3. Healing progresses from the upper to the lower parts of the body. This means that head symptoms may clear before stomach symptoms. Deep toxins in the colon or liver will be released before the more surface areas.

4. The most recent illnesses will be the first to leave. This means that flu symptoms experienced a month ago will leave earlier in the healing than the bronchitis suffered two years before.

Radiation Treatments

Restoring proper flora in bowels

If taking antibiotics or undergoing chemotherapy or radiation: Take a full dose of a good probiotic (acidophilus and bifidus) daily for one week after finishing with antibiotics or medical intervention.

Yogurt taken before lighter meals also helps provide friendly bacteria. The need for yogurt is sometimes indicated by an intolerance of dairy products.

For patients undergoing radiation, saturate the site 10 days prior to treatment with melaleuca alternifolia and melaleuca ericifolia. Take 4 double 00 capsules per day, before, during radiation, and for 30 to 60 days following the treatment.

26

Liver Health and pH Balance

Liver and pH

The pH of the blood is very tightly controlled by the body. When serum pH becomes too acidic, then calcium is robbed from the bones and biochemical changes begin to slowly tax and stress liver tissues.

The Importance of Liver Health

Proper liver function is essential for life. The liver is responsible for removing and neutralizing toxins and germs from the blood, promoting digestion, maintaining hormone balance, regulating blood sugar levels, and making proteins that regulate blood clotting.

Cumulative liver stress caused by toxins, poor diet, or disease inevitably lead to irreversible liver damage and death. The first stage is known a condition known as fatty liver in which fat deposits accumulate and poison the liver. It has been estimated that 5% of the general population and 25% of patients with obesity and diabetes suffer from fatty liver. With time, fatty liver eventually progresses to cirrhosis, a condition in which non-functioning scar tissue replaces working tissue; it is the 8th leading cause of death by disease, killing over 22,000 people a year.

Signs of an Overloaded or Toxic Liver

- Loss of appetite
- Nausea
- Weakness
- Weight loss
- Edema and ascites. When the liver stops making albumin, water increases in the leg (edema) and abdomen (ascites).

- Bruising and bleeding. Caused when liver slows production of clotting proteins.
- Jaundice. Yellowing of the skin and eyes.
- Itching. Bile products deposited in the skin may cause intense itching
- Gallstones
- Forgetfulness, poor concentration, or disturbed sleep
- Sensitivity to medication. Because the liver does not remove drugs from the blood at the usual rate, drugs act longer than expected.
- Portal hypertension. The flow of blood through the portal vein is slowed, which increases the pressure inside.
- Varices. Blood from the intestines and spleen backs up into blood vessels in the stomach and esophagus. These vessels swell and are more likely to burst.
- Lowered immunity. Cirrhosis can result in immune system dysfunction, leading to infection.

Liver Dangers

- Exposure to Chemicals, Toxins, Pharmaceutical Drugs, and Parasites. Many pesticides, petro-chemicals, and environmental toxins are potent liver stressors. Acetaminophen can also stress the liver as can reactions to prescription drugs. Parasitic infection (schistosomiasis) can also contribute to cirrhosis.

- Poor Diet. Excess intake of refined carbohydrates, transfatty acids, and sugars can cause fatty liver or liver degeneration over time.

- Iron Overload. Excess iron in the diet can stress the liver, especially in individuals who are genetically unable to dispose of or sequester dietary iron (hemochromatosis). Creates a haemo-type liver pathology.

- Diabetes, Protein Malnutrition, Obesity, and Corticosteroid Use. Any of these can cause Non-alcoholic Steatohepatitis (NASH). NASH results in deadly fat buildup and eventual cirrhosis in the liver.

- Viruses. The hepatitis B and C viruses are major causes of chronic liver disease and cirrhosis in the United States. Hepatitis viral infections cause inflammation and low-grade damage to the liver that eventually leads to cirrhosis and death.

A 2003 study conducted by Roger Lewis MD at the Young Life Research Clinic in Provo, Utah evaluated the efficacy of helichrysum, ledum, and celery seed in treating cases of advanced Hepatitis C. In one case of a male age 20 diagnosed with a Hepatitis C viral count of 13,200. After taking two capsules (approx. 750 mg each) of a blend of helichrysum, ledum, and celery seed (JuvaCleanse) per day for a month with no other intervention, patients showed that viral counts dropped to 2,580, an over 80 percent reduction.

- Inherited diseases. Alpha-1 antitrypsin deficiency, Wilson's disease, galactosemia, and glycogen storage diseases are inherited disorders that result in malproduction, malprocessing, and malstorage by the liver of enzymes, proteins, and metals.

- Blocked bile ducts. When the ducts that carry bile out of the liver are blocked, bile backs up and damages liver tissue (biliary cirrhosis).

The Importance of Alkalinity to Health

As the liver's filtered ability becomes impaired the blood becomes increasing acidic. Unfriendly bacteria and fungi that populate our intestinal tracts thrive in an acid environment and are responsible for secreting mycotoxins, which are the root cause of many debilitating human conditions. In fact, many researchers believe that most diseases can be linked to blood and intestinal acidity, which contributes to an acid-based yeast and fungus dominance.

The symptoms of excess internal acidity include:

- Fatigue / low energy
- Unexplained aches and pains
- Overweight conditions
- Low resistance to illness
- Allergies
- Unbalanced blood sugar
- Headaches
- Irritability / mood swings
- Indigestion
- Colitis / ulcers
- Diarrhea / constipation
- Urinary tract infections
- Rectal itch / vaginal itch

The ideal pH for human blood is between 7.4 and 7.6. Preserving this alkalinity (pH balance) is the bedrock on which sound health and strong bodies are built. When the blood loses its alkalinity and starts to become more acidic, the foundation of health is undermined. This creates an environment where we become vulnerable to disease and runaway yeast and fungus overgrowth.

The naturally occurring yeast and fungi in the body thrive in an acidic environment. These same yeast and fungi are responsible for secreting a large number of poisons called mycotoxins, which are believed to be one of the root causes of many diseases and debilitating conditions.

When yeast and fungus decline in the body, so does their production of mycotoxins, the poisonous waste products and byproducts of their life cycles. There are numerous varieties of these mycotoxins, many of which are harmful to the body and must be neutralized by our immune systems. When our bodies are overwhelmed by large quantities of these toxins, our health becomes impaired, and we become susceptible to disease and illness.

Many cancers have been linked to mycotoxins. For example, the fungus *Aspergillus flavus*, which infests stored peanuts, not only generates cancer in laboratory animals but has been documented as the prime culprit in many liver cancers in humans.

By balancing the body's pH and creating a more alkaline environment, you can rein in the microbial overgrowth and choke off the production of disease-producing mycotoxins. With pH balance restored, the body can regain newfound vigor and health.

How to Restore Alkalinity

An alkaline environment is hostile to fungi, which require acidity to survive and thrive. Lowered yeast and fungus populations translate into lower levels of body-damaging, disease-inducing mycotoxins.

Some of the most common varieties of pathogenic bacteria, yeast, and fungi that live in the intestines are inactive. However, when the body is weakened by illness, stress, and excess acidity caused by stress, these bacteria become harmful and active, changing into an invasive mycelic form.

1. **Carefully monitor your diet.** Avoiding yeast- and fungus-promoting foods is a crucial factor in combating excess acidity and fungus over-growth. Meats, sugars, dairy products, pickled and malted products can be especially acidic. On the other hand, garlic is excellent for controlling fungi and yeast. Other high-alkaline, fungus-inhibiting foods include green and yellow vegetables, beans, and whole uncracked nuts.

   The natural ratio between alkaline and acid foods in the diet should be 4:1—four parts alkaline foods to one part acid. JuvaPower and JuvaSpice are mixtures of extremely alkaline and high-antioxidant foods that nourish the liver and combat toxic acidity.

   The pH of a raw food does not always determine its acidity or alkalinity in the digestive system. Some foods, like lemons, might be acidic in their natural state but when consumed and digested are converted into alkaline residues. Thus, the true determinant of a food's pH is whether it is an alkaline-ash or acid-ash food. In this case, lemons are an alkaline-ash food.

2. **Avoid the use of antibiotics.** The overuse of antibiotics for incidental, minor, or cosmetic conditions not only increases the resistance of pathogenic microorganisms, but it kills the beneficial bacteria in your body, leaving the mycotoxin-generating yeast and fungi intact. This is why many women suffer outbreaks of yeast infections after antibiotic use.

3. **Use essential oils.** Many essential oils possess important antimicrobial, antibacterial and anti-fungal properties. Clove and Thyme essential oils have been documented to kill over 15 different strains of fungi.

Essential oils work best when blood and tissues are alkaline. When our systems become acidic—due to poor diet, illness, or emotional stress—essential oils lose some of their effects. So the best way to enhance the action of essential oils is to alkalize your body.

4. **Using alkaline minerals.** Increasing intake of calcium can dramatically boost blood and intestinal alkalinity. Calcium and magnesium-rich supplements such as SuperCal and MegaCal can help alkalinize both blood and body tissues. AlkaLime is an outstanding source of alkaline salts that can help reduce internal acidity. JuvaPower and JuvaSpice are also rich in minerals and yeast-fighting phytonutrients.

5. **Lower stress.** Emotional and psychological tension can be especially damaging to bodily systems and act as a prime promoter of acid formation in the body. To properly appreciate how acidic stress can be, just think back to the last time you were seriously stressed-out and had to reach for an antacid tablet to soothe your heartburn or stomach discomfort.

   Blends of essential oils high in sesquiter-penes, such as frankincense, myrrh, and sandal-wood, can produce profound balancing and calming effects on emotions. They work by affecting the limbic system of our brain, the seat of our emotions.

6. **Boost friendly flora.** From three to four pounds of beneficial bacteria permanently reside in the intestines of the average adult. Not only are they the first line of defense against foreign invaders, but they are absolutely essential for health, energy, and optimum digestive efficiency. These intes-tinal houseguests not only control mucus and debris, but they produce B vitamins, vitamin K, and main-tain the all-important pH balance of the body.

   These friendly flora are also important in counteracting and opposing yeast and fungus overgrowth. When our natural cultures are compromised or disrupted by taking antibiotics or by poor dietary practices, yeast and fungus start growing unopposed and begin colonizing and invading larger swaths of our internal terrain, secreting ever-increasing volumes of poisonous mycotoxins.

Using an acidophilus or bifidus supplement may be especially valuable in boosting levels of naturally occurring beneficial bacteria in the body and preventing fungal and yeast overgrowth. They also help the body maintain proper pH balance for nutrient digestion and absorption. Ideally, the lactobacillus acidiphilus and bifidobacterium bifidus cultures must be combined with plantain to promote implantation on the intestinal wall.

Research indicates a significant proportion of bacteria from many acidophilus supplements do not reach the lower intestine alive, or they arrive in such a weakened state that they are not of much benefit. This is why combining the acidophilus and bifidus cultures with plantain is so important because plantain helps these cultures adhere to the intestinal walls.

An even more effective means of fortifying the friendly flora in our intestines is by consumption of fructooligosaccharides (also known as FOS). FOS is one of the most powerful natural agents for feeding our friendly flora. FOS is made up of medium-chain sugars that cannot be used by pathogenic yeast and fungi. The end result is that FOS starves fungi while feeding the acidophilus and bifidus cultures that are our main defense against disease.

But FOS is far more than just an outstanding means of rebuilding and protecting the beneficial bacteria inside the body. Over a dozen clinical studies have documented the ability of fructooligosaccharides to prevent constipation, lower blood sugar and cholesterol levels, and even prevent cancer. (Hidaka et al., 1991; Briet et al., 1995); Bouhnik et al., 1996; Kawaguchi et al., 1993; Luo et al., 1996); Rochat et al., 1994; Tokunaga et al., 1993).

Testing Your pH

You can easily test your pH at home by purchasing small litmus-paper strips at your drug store or pharmacy. To get the most accurate reading, expose the strip to a sample of your saliva immediately after awakening in the morning and before eating breakfast. Color changes on the litmus paper will determine pH; check the instructions of your kit for specific details on how to read the litmus paper.

27

Health Issues

Many of today's health concerns are caused by so-called modern conveniences. Increased use of sugars, artificial sweeteners, contaminated water, and even microwave ovens can all be harmful to health.

Sugars and Sweeteners

Nothing stresses the human body as much as refined sugar. Called a "skeletonized food" and a "castrated carbohydrate" by Edward Howell, Ph.D., and a "metabolic freeloader" by Ralph Golan, M.D., sugar actually drains the body of vitamins, minerals, and nutrients in the process of being burned for energy. Sugar also stresses the pancreas, forcing it to pump out a surge of unneeded digestive enzymes.

Sugars also undermine and retard immune response. One study measured the effects of 100 grams of sugar (sucrose) on neutrophils, a form of white blood cell that comprises a central part of immunity. Within one hour of ingestion, neutrophil activity dropped 50 percent and remained below normal for another four hours (Castleman, 1997).

Population studies have also linked sugar consumption with diabetes and heart disease. According to researcher John Yudkin, the reason sugar elevates the risk of heart disease is due to an automatic built-in safety switch inside the body. To protect itself from being immediately poisoned from excess sugar, the body converts it into fats, like triglycerides. So instead of killing you quickly, the body defends itself by clogging its arteries, thereby killing you on the installment plan.

The worst dangers, though, are not found in natural sugars but in the use of artificial sweeteners. Seventy-five percent of the adverse reactions reported to the U. S. Food and Drug Administration come from a single substance: the artificial sweetener, aspartame.

Aspartame is marketed today as NutraSweet, Equal, Spoonful and Equal-Measure. With so many Americans on one diet or another, the market for aspartame is simply enormous. And it matters not that aspartame users are suffering from symptoms ranging from headaches, numbness and seizures to joint pain, chronic fatigue syndrome, multiple sclerosis, and epilepsy.

This toxic artificial sweetener is made up of three chemicals: aspartic acid, phenylalanine and methanol. What these chemicals do in our bodies is anything but sweet.

Aspartame

A recent book by Dr. Russell L. Blaylock, professor of neurosurgery at the Medical University of Mississippi, *Excitotoxins: The Taste That Kills,* explains that aspartame is a neurotransmitter facilitating the transmission of information from one neuron to another. Aspartame allows too much calcium into brain cells, killing certain neurons, earning aspartame the name of "excitotoxin." With aspartame now in over 9,000 products such as instant breakfasts, breath mints, cereals, frozen desserts, "lite" gelatin desserts and even multivitamins, it is no surprise that there is a virtual epidemic of memory loss, Alzheimer's disease, and multiple sclerosis. In a move much like a telephone company selling your phone number to telephone solicitors and then charging you to block their calls, G. D. Searle (the Monsanto company that manufactures aspartame) is searching for a drug to combat memory loss caused by excitatory amino acid damage most often caused by aspartame.

Phenylalanine

The chemical phenylalanine, a by-product of aspartame metabolism, is an amino acid normally found in the brain. You may have heard of testing infants for phenylketonuria (PKU), a condition where phenylalanine cannot be metabolized, which can lead to death. It has been shown that excessive amounts of phenylalanine in the brain can cause serotonin levels to decrease. Does it seem that half the people you know are on Prozac? Perhaps the flooding of American foods and soft drinks with aspartame is contributing to this need for drugs like Prozac and Zoloft.

But depression is not the most worrisome result of excessive phenylalanine levels in the brain. Dr. Blaylock writes that schizophrenia and susceptibility to seizures can occur as a result of these high levels. The Massachusetts Institute of Technology surveyed 80 people who suffered seizures following the ingestion of aspartame. The Community Nutrition Institute concluded that these cases met the FDA's own definition of an imminent hazard to the public health, but the FDA made no move to remove this dangerous product from the market.

Do you fly the friendly skies? You may be interested to know that both the Air Force's magazine, *Flying Safety,* and *Navy Physiology,* the Navy's publication, detailed warnings about pilots being more susceptible to seizures after consuming aspartame. The Aspartame Consumer Safety Network notes that 600 pilots have reported acute reactions to aspartame including grand mal seizures in the cockpit. Many other publications have warned about aspartame ingestion while flying, including a paper presented at the 57th Annual Meeting of the Aerospace Medical Association.

Methanol

Another by-product of aspartame is methanol. Free methanol results when aspartame is heated higher than 86 degrees F. If you cook a sugar-free pudding that contains aspartame, you are creating free methanol. If methanol were a criminal in a police lineup, it would wear a sign saying, "aka wood alcohol." For those desperate enough to drink it, wood alcohol can lead to blindness and even death. One quart of aspartame-sweetened beverage contains about 56 mg of methanol. The EPA states that methanol is "considered a cumulative poison due to the low rate of excretion once it is absorbed."

Methanol is truly criminal after it enters your body. It breaks down into formic acid and formaldehyde. Formaldehyde is a known carcinogen and can cause birth defects by interfering with DNA replication. Our Desert Storm troops were treated to free diet drinks that sat in the hot sun of Saudi Arabia. Many of the unusual symptoms found in Desert Storm veterans are similar to those of people chemically poisoned by formaldehyde.

The artificial sweetener aspartame would certainly not sell if people knew what kind of a toxic chemical stew they were ingesting.

Natural Low-Glycemic Sweeteners

Blue Agave Nectar (Organic)

The blue agave cactus grows in Central America. It produces a sweetener that is about 68 percent fructose, 22 percent glucose, 4 percent fructoligosaccharides. Because of its heavy fructose concentration, blue agave is 32 percent sweeter than table sugar but has a low glycemic index (about 34). This means that when consumed, blue agave has a minimal impact on blood sugar levels following consumption. It is much better suited for people with candida infections.

Grade B Maple Syrup

The US and Canada have slightly different grading systems for maple syrup. What is classified as Grade B maple syrup in the US is the same as grade C maple syrup in Canada. This grade is the best sweetener and the most balanced sugar. It is processed from the last tapping of the maple sap, so it is richer in invert sugars and minerals.

Grade B Maple Syrup is also a lower glycemic index food, resulting in a slow, gradual rise in blood sugar levels. The best maple syrup is currently produced in Vermont because it is strictly regulated for purity and authenticity by government law. Some unscrupulous marketers in other areas have been known to add refined sugars to colored diluted genuine maple syrup to produce a cheaper product. Also, a number of years ago, there was a problem with some Canadian and US producers inserting formaldehyde pellets in their sugar maples trees to keep tap holes open longer, increasing yields.

28

Longevity/Anti-aging Therapies

Essential oils and aromatics were some of the most highly prized natural medicines of the ancient world. References to cassia, clove, frankincense, myrrh, spikenard, cinnamon, and rosemary appear in many historical writings, including the Old and New Testaments as well as the writings of Hippocrates, Avicenna, and ancient Egyptian hieroglyphics.

Intriguing new research offers a tantalizing glimpse into the far-reaching potential of essential oils like thyme (Thymus vulgaris) to reverse or slow the aging process by acting as powerful antioxidants that protect tissues and organs from oxidative stress and damage. Other oils, such as clove (Syzygium aromaticum) and lemon (Citrus limon) have not only been shown to act as powerful antioxidants, but also to protect cellular DNA from damage and to act as potent antiseptics with broad-spectrum germ-killing properties.

What Causes Aging?

There is still some controversy concerning the cause of aging and premature death. Some researchers believe that declining levels of hormones from the pituitary and hypothalamus are the culprits. Others point an accusing finger at the crosslinking of collagen, a key protein of the soft tissues that constitutes a third of all protein in the body. Still others blame the buildup of lipofuscin, a brownish pigment that accumulates inside the cells, particularly nerve and heart muscle cells.[1]

However, the oxidative stress/free radical theory of aging is the most persuasive and substantiated. This rationale posits that aging is caused by cumulative oxidative stress to the cell walls, receptors, and DNA. Rogue electrons that are generated from normal metabolic and immune functions attack proteins and disrupt DNA, eventually overwhelming the natural repair abilities of the body and sometimes leading to disease and death.[2,3,4]

While many researchers have focused on damage to the DNA (the blueprint for cellular operations) as the cause of aging, few have appreciated how devastating free radical damage can be to fats—especially the unstable polyunsaturated fatty acids (PUFAs) that form the phospholipid membranes of almost every cell in the body. When these fatty membranes are attacked by free radicals, ion transport and hormone receptors are disrupted.[5] As cell membranes become less fluid, they lose their ability to function normally. This can hasten the onset of tissue and organ damage and lead to premature death.

One of the most easy-to-understand examples of the detrimental effects of cell membrane brittleness occurs in the blood vessel walls. As the blood vessels lose their flexibility, the risk of hypertension (high blood pressure) increases, as does the incidence of arteriosclerosis.

Why does free radical damage escalate with age? Because antioxidant protection declines as we grow older. Free radical scavengers such as superoxide dismutase (SOD) and glutathione peroxidase chart a steady decline along with other antioxidants. This means that the older body is less efficient in neutralizing free radicals and combating the oxidative damage that gradually weakens and eventually destroys key organs.

1. Hayflick, L. *How and Why We Age*. Ballantine Books, New York, 1994.

2. Harmon, D, Ageing: a theory based on free radical and radiation chemistry. *J. Gerontology* 11, (1956): 298-300.

3. Harmon, D, Free radical theory of ageing: Effect of free radical inhibitors on the mortality rate of male LAFmice. *J. Gerontology* 23 (1968): 476-482.

4. Harmon, D, Free radical theory of ageing: Effect of the amount and degree of unsaturation of dietary fat on mortality rate. *J. Gerontology* 26 (1971): 451-457.

5. Stubbs CD & Smith AD, The modification of mammalian membrane polyunsaturated fatty acid composition in relation to membrane fluidity and function. *Biochimica et Biophysica Acta* 779, (1984)89-137.

Essential Oils vs. Fatty Oils

Fatty oils are very different from essential oils. Fatty oils, such as cottonseed, almond, olive, corn, sunflower, and canola oil, are usually pressed from a seed or fruit. They are greasy in texture and have little odor, being simple mixtures of several different fatty acids (ie., capric, stearic, and oleic).

In contrast, essential oils are usually steam distilled from leaves, flowers, roots, and bark. They have strong odors and are not greasy. Because many are lighter than water, they float and tend to evaporate very easily. Essential oils are complex mosaics of hundreds of aromatic molecules (ie., terpenes, sesquiterpenes, and phenols) that usually have a ring-like structure.

THYMOL
(from thyme ess. oil)

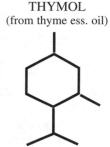

CAPRIC FATTY ACID
(from coconut oil)

Methyl end   Acid end

H-C-C-C-C-C-C-C-C-C-C $\overset{\displaystyle O}{\underset{\displaystyle OH}{\diagup}}$

Levels of polyunsaturated fats such as DHA (decosahexaenoic acid) are also crucial for healthy brain and eye function. DHA occurs in unusually high concentrations in the cerebral cortex—the most advanced part of the brain structure where logic and reasoning take place. When DHA becomes oxidized and loses its double bonds because of free radical attacks, brain and cognitive function can deteriorate. This can lead to memory loss, dementia, and even *death. By protecting* fats like DHA from free radical attack, hydrolysis, or oxidation, brain health can be significantly improved.[6,7,8,9]

The crux of the problem is that DHA and other long chain PUFAs are very unstable and are vulnerable to chemical alteration and oxidation. This means that the antioxidant systems of the body must work overtime to protect them in order to sustain health. An even greater problem is that the liver slows down PUFA production with age, so it becomes less and less able to replace through desaturase activities the dwindling supply of PUFA needed to sustain the brain, tissues, and other organs.[10]

Thus the longevity of the organism is strongly linked to preserving the integrity of the polyunsaturated fats that comprise cells, nerves, and other tissues. Preventing the degradation of these fats from free radical damage can forestall the signs of accelerated aging.

Preserving the Integrity of Fats *In Vitro*

In the late 1980s, Dr. Radwan Farag of the biochemistry department of the University of Cairo was among the first to show in vitro how selected essential oils were able to significantly slow the rancidity (oxidation) of fatty oils such as cottonseed oil. He dosed samples of cottonseed oil with 200 ppm of thyme oil (55.7% thymol and 36% p-cymene) and 400 ppm of clove oil (85.3% eugenol). After comparing the essential oil-treated samples with untreated control samples, he found that both thyme and clove oil afforded significant protection against rancidity to the cottonseed oil as determined by lowered peroxide and TBA values. Thyme oil generated a 20% reduction in rancidity while clove oil triggered almost a 30% drop.[11]

A second study by Dr. Farag and his colleagues showed that essential oils such as thyme, clove, rosemary (Rosmarinus officinalis), and sage (Salvia officinalis) arrested the oxidation of linoleic acid, a polyunsaturated omega-6 fatty acid.[12]

In addition, Dr. Farag demonstrated the safety of these essential oils in vivo. When he added thyme and clove oils to rat feed rations at up to six times

6. Barja de Quiroga G, et al., Antioxidant defences and peroxidation in liver and brain of aged rats. *Biochemical Journal* 272 (1990), 247-250.

7. Lamptey MS & Walker BL, A possible dietary role for linolenic acid in the development of the young rat. Journal of Nutrition 106, (1976) 86-93.

8. Okuyama H, Minimum requirements of n-3 and n-6 essential fatty acids for the function of the central nervous system and for the prevention of chronic disease. *Proceedings of the Society for Experimental Biology and Medicine* 200, (1992) 174-176.

9. Yamamoto N, et al, Effects of dietary alpha-linolenate/linolenate balance of brain lipid composition and learning ability of rats. *Journal of Lipid Research* 28, (1987) 144-151.

10. Bourre et al., Function of dietary polyunsaturated fatty acids in the nervous system. *Prostaglandins, Leukotrienes, and Essential Fatty Acids* 48 (1993): 5-15.

11. Farag et al., Antioxidant activity of some spice essential oils on linoleic acid oxidation in aqueous media. *JAOCS* June 1989;66: 792-799.

12. Farag et al., Inhibitory effects of individual and mixed pairs of essential oils on the oxidation and hydrolysis of cottonseed oil and butter. *FASC*, 1989; 40: 275-279.

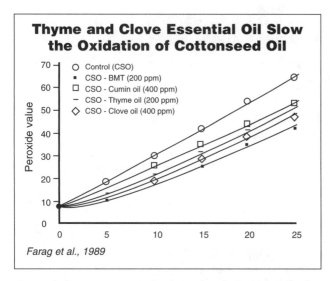

Thyme and Clove Essential Oil Slow the Oxidation of Cottonseed Oil

Farag et al., 1989

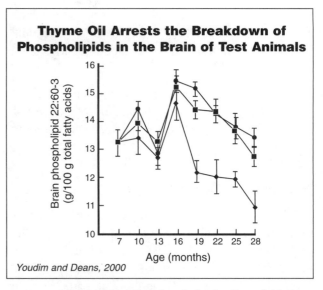

Thyme Oil Arrests the Breakdown of Phospholipids in the Brain of Test Animals

Youdim and Deans, 2000

the minimum concentration needed to stall fat oxidation, none of the rats studied suffered any negative side effects. Essential oil-fed rats exhibited no difference in protein, cholesterol, and liver enzyme levels (SGPT, SGOT) when compared with a control group.[13]

Protecting Fats and Phospholipids in Animals

Almost a decade after Farag's groundbreaking research, another series of more intensive in vivo studies were begun at the Scottish Agricultural College in the United Kingdom and the Semmelweis University of Medicine in Hungary. In these clinical trials, researchers found that daily lifelong feeding of thyme and clove oils to laboratory animals

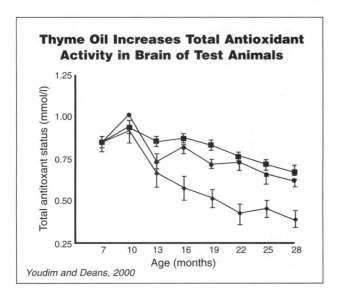

Thyme Oil Increases Total Antioxidant Activity in Brain of Test Animals

Youdim and Deans, 2000

preserved key antioxidant levels in the liver, kidneys, heart, and brain. Even more importantly, essential oils arrested the oxidation and destruction of long-chain PUFAs throughout the organism.

One of the first studies to document these remarkable antioxidant effects was conducted at the Semmelweis University of Medicine in 1993. Researchers fed different groups of mice with daily doses of 0.72 mg of essential oils including thyme (Thymus vulgaris), clove (Syzygium aromaticum), nutmeg (Myristica fragrans), and pepper (Piper nigrum). Groups of younger mice (6 months old) were treated for five weeks, while groups of 22 month-old mice were treated for 21 weeks. Following treatment, the livers of the animals were examined for levels of C20 and C22 polyunsaturated fatty acids, which declines substantially during the animal's lifetime.

The results were phenomenal. According to the researchers, "dietary administration of the volatile oils to the aging mice had a marked effect on fatty acid distribution by virtually restoring the proportions of the polyunsaturated fatty acids within the phospholipids to the levels observed in young mice."

Another randomized, controlled animal study at Semmelweis University in 1997 showed that these same essential oils—thyme, clove, nutmeg, and pepper—restored DHA in the eyes to much younger levels. As a long-chain polyunsaturated fatty acid (PUFA) that is very fragile and easily oxidized,

---

13. Farag et al., Safety evaluation of thyme and clove essential oils as natural antioxidants. *Afr J Agr Sci.* 1991;18: 169-17.

DHA is absolutely crucial for normal eye health. Declining levels of DHA have been directly linked to heightened risk of age-related macular degeneration, the leading cause of blindness in old age.[14,15]

In this case, dietary supplementation of just 3.9 mg per day of essential oils to laboratory animals over a 17-month period was sufficient to markedly slow DHA loss in their eyes.

Preserving Brain Function

The brain is another organ where DHA is essential to health. Karesh Youdim and his colleagues at the Scottish Agricultural College tested the ability of essential oils to preserve DHA levels in the brain of 100 animal subjects. Feeding them a daily dose (42.5 mg/K of body weight) of thyme oil (48% thymol) over the course of their lifetime (28 months), the researchers achieved stunning results: Thyme oil dramatically slowed age-related DHA and PUFA degradation in the brain. In other words, the essential oil of thyme was able to partially prevent brain aging through protection of essential fatty acids. An analysis of the data showed that the DHA levels in 28 month-old animals' brains was almost the same as that of 7 month-olds. In human terms, this was equivalent to an 80-year-old having the brain chemistry of a 20-year-old![16]

Thyme oil supplements also slowed the decline of total brain antioxidant levels that occurs with age. Lifelong supplementation with thyme oil in laboratory rats resulted in antioxidant levels dropping by only 29%, compared with a 45% fall for untreated animals.

Even more startling is the fact that thyme essential oil also preserved levels of PUFAs in the animals' hearts, livers, and kidneys, while at the same time raising total antioxidant levels—including key antioxidants such as glutathione peroxidase and superoxide dismutase. This was accomplished by feeding laboratory rats daily thyme oil supplements (42.5 mg/K of body weight) throughout their lives.[17]

Clove Oil Affords Protection Against Cancer

Clove oil also has potent antioxidant-boosting properties. Animal studies conducted at LKT Laboratories in Minneapolis, Minnesota, found that five compounds within clove oil significantly increased levels of GST (glutathione S-transferase), one of the most important detoxifying enzymes in the human body that is critical for neutralizing potential cancer-causing chemicals. Just 60 mg of each of the five compounds (b-caryophyllene, b-

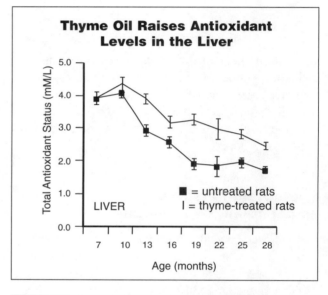

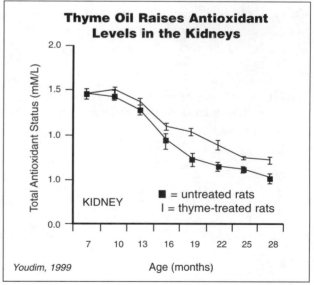

14. Rotstein et al., Effects of aging on the composition and metabolism of docosahexaenoate-containing lipids of retina. Lipids, 1987 Apr;22(4):253-60.

15. Neuringer M & Connor WE, N-3 fatty acids in the brain and retina: evidence for their essentiality. *Nutrition Reviews* 44, 285-294.

16. Youdim KA, et al., Effect of thyme oil and thymol dietary supplementation on the antioxidant status and fatty acid composition of the ageing rat brain. *Br J Nutr.* 2000 Jan;83(1):87-93.

17. Youdim KA, Deans SG., Dietary supplementation of thyme (Thymus vulgaris L.) essential oil during the lifetime of the rat: its effects on the antioxidant status in liver, kidney and heart tissues. *Mech Ageing Dev.* 1999 Sep 8;109(3):163-75.

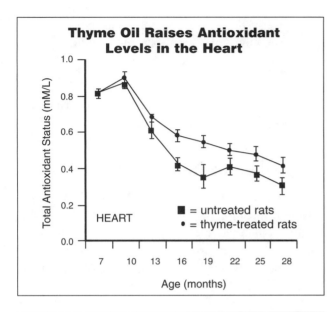

Thyme Oil Raises Antioxidant Levels in the Heart

Y-axis: Total Antioxidant Status (mM/L)
X-axis: Age (months)

HEART
■ = untreated rats
● = thyme-treated rats

How 5 Constituents in Clove Oil Raise Glutathione Levels

Compound	Liver Levels of GST	Small Bowel Levels of GST
Control	0.74	0.25
Compound 1	1.92	0.75
Compound 2	2.13	1.20
Compound 3	1.47	0.63
Compound 4	1.54	0.81
Compound 5	1.26	0.59

Zheng et al., 1992.

caryophyllene oxide, a-humulene, a-humulene epoxide I, and eugenol) fed to rats over the course of six days (3 doses of 20 mg each) resulted in a doubling of GST activity in the liver and a quadrupling of GST level in the small bowel mucosa. The authors concluded that "these sesquiterpenes show promise as potential anticarcinogenic agents."[18]

Many other researchers have shown that clove essential oil exhibits pronounced antitumoral and DNA-protectant effects.[19,20]

Essential oils may do more than just raise antioxidant levels and block damage to PUFAs. They may also protect cellular DNA from damage that can eventually lead to mutations and subsequent tumor growth. In a 1986 study, Yokota et al., found that a diet including 5% eugenol (the chief constituent in clove oil) helped protect test animals against the mutagenic and cancer-causing affects of the chemical benzo-a-pyrene.[21]

Potent Weapons Against Microbes

Another method by which aromatics and essential oils may exert a life-lengthening effect is through their ability to inhibit the growth of bacteria, fungi, and viruses. Some bacteria, such as Chlamydia pneumoniae have been implicated as one of the true causes of heart disease. Viruses, such as HIV and hepatitis, have resulted in liver failure and premature death. Fungi like Candida albicans have been implicated in cancer due to their secretion of mycotoxins.

One of the most comprehensive studies to probe the powerful antimicrobial effects of essential oils was conducted with D. Gary Young and Sue Chao at Weber State University. Using disc diffusion assays, they tested the killing power of 67 different essential oils against a variety of yeast, molds, gram negative bacteria, and gram positive bacteria. Cinnamon, clove, thyme, peppermint, oregano, and mountain savory exerted the strongest antimicrobial properties.[22]

The following year they tested the ability of thyme, oregano, and clove essential oils to destroy colonies of Streptococcus pneumoniae, the bacteria responsible for many types of throat, sinus, and lung infections.[23]

Essential Oils: Treatments for Arthritis, Heart Disease, and More

A growing body of clinical research during the last several decades indicates that essential oils have enormous potential to treat conditions ranging from acne to obesity.

18. Zheng GQ, et al. Sesquiterpenes from clove (Eugenia caryophyllata) as potential anticarcinogenic agents. *J Nat Prod.* 1992 Jul;55(7):999-1003.

19. Rompelberg et al. Antimutagenicity of eugenol in the rodent bone marrow micronucleus test. *Mutat Res.* 1995 Feb;346(2):69-75.

20. Sukumaran et al. Inhibition of tumour promotion in mice by eugenol. *Indian J Physiol Pharmacol.* 1994 Oct;38(4):306-8.

21. Yokota H, et al., Suppressed mutagenicity of benzo[a]pyrene by the liver S9 fraction and microsomes from eugenol-treated rats. *Mutat Res.* 1986 Dec;172(3):231-6.

22. Chao, et al., Screening for Inhibitory Activity of Essential Oils on Selected Bacteria, Fungi, and Viruses. *Journal of Essential Oil Research*, 1997.

23. Chao et al., Antimicrobial Effects of Essential Oils on Streptococcus pneumoniae. *JEOR*, 2001.

Peppermint (Mentha piperita) has been reviewed for its ability to block pain, relieve headaches [24], combat indigestion [25], boost mental alertness [26,27], induce weight loss [28], kill lice [29], and inhibit tumor growth. [30]

Melaleuca (Melaleuca alternifolia) has been used to treat acne [31], kill fungi [32], and inhibit bacteria growth. [33,34]

Lavender (Lavandula angustifolia) fights travel sickness [35], reduces atherosclerosis [36], protects blood vessels [37], acts as a local anaesthetic [38], and has anticonvulsant properties. [39]

Clove (Syzygium aromaticum) has been researched for its action against tooth decay [40] as well as its antifungal [41] and anticonvulsant activities. [42]

Rosemary (Rosmarinus officinalis) has been shown to enhance alertness [43], combat fungi such as Candida albicans, and act as an antioxidant. [44]

Orange (Citrus aurantium) halts fungus infection [45,46] and inhibits tumor formation. [47] Limonene, an important component of orange and lemon oil has demonstrated similar tumor-suppressing effects in studies at Indiana University. [48]

Basil (Ocimum basilicum) has been shown to have anticancer properties. [49]

Eucalyptus (Eucalyptus radiata) has been studied for reducing inflammation [50], improving cerebral blood flow [51], inhibiting Candida growth [52], and treating bronchitis. [53]

Many other documented benefits of aromatics have been recorded in recent medical literature. [54-66]

Longevity Nutrition

During the last five years, D. Gary Young has traveled throughout the world investigating the regions inhabited by most long-lived peoples on earth: the Ningxia province in China, Hunzaland in Pakistan, southern Ecuador, the Talish Mountain region of Azerbaijan, and the Copper Canyon of central Mexico. After intensively examining the dietary habits of these cultures, he found one common denominator: an active lifestyle and a mineral-rich diet exceptionally high in antioxidant foods, such as wolfberries and apricots.

In particular, he found that Chinese wolfberries (Ningxia variety) and potassium-rich apricots were two foods consumed by people routinely reaching 110 and 120 years of age.

D. Gary Young's book, *Longevity Secrets,* discusses the scientific reasons why these foods may confer important anti-aging properties. This is certainly due to their extremely high content of

24. Gobel et al. Effect of peppermint and eucalyptus oil preparations on neurophysiological and experimental algesimetric headache parameters. *Cephalalgia.* 1994 Jun;14(3):228-34; 182.

25. Dalvi et al. Effect of peppermint oil on gastric emptying in man: a preliminary study using a radiolabelled solid test meal. *Indian J Physiol Pharmacol.* 1991 Jul;35(3):212-4.

26. Dember WN, et al., Olfactory Stimulation and Sustained Attention, *Compendium of Olfactory*, (Avery N. Gilbert, Editor) pp. 39-46.

27. Miltner et al. Emotional qualities of odors and their influence on the startle reflex in humans. *Psychophysiology.* 1994 Jan;31(1):107-10.

28. Hirsch, Alan. A Scentsational Guide to Weight Loss. Rockport, MA: Element, 1997.

29. Veal L. The potential effectiveness of essential oils as a treatment for headlice, Pediculus humanus capitis. *Complement Ther Nurs Midwifery.* 1996 Aug;2(4):97-101.

30. Russin, et al. Inhibition of rat mammary carcinogenesis by monoterpenoids. *Carcinogenesis.* 1989 Nov;10(11):2161-4.

31. Bassett et al. A comparative study of tea-tree oil versus benzoylperoxide in the treatment of acne. *Med J Aust.* 1990 Oct 15;153(8):455-8.

32. Nenoff et al. Antifungal activity of the essential oil of Melaleuca alternifolia (tea tree oil) against pathogenic fungi in vitro. *Skin Pharmacol.* 1996;9(6):388-94.

33. Cox et al. The mode of antimicrobial action of the essential oil of Melaleuca alternifolia (tea tree oil). *J Appl Microbiol.* 2000 Jan;88(1):170-5.

34. Carson et al. Antimicrobial activity of the major components of the essential oil of Melaleuca alternifolia. *J Appl Bacteriol.* 1995 Mar;78(3):264-9.

35. Bradshaw et al. Effects of lavender straw on stress and travel sickness in pigs. *J Altern Complement Med.* 1998 Fall;4(3):271-5.

36. Nikolaevskii et al. Effect of essential oils on the course of experimental atherosclerosis. *Patol Fiziol Eksp Ter.* 1990 Sep-Oct;(5):52-3.

37. Siurein S A. Effects of essential oil on lipid peroxidation and lipid metabolism in patients with chronic bronchitis]. *Klin Med* (Mosk). 1997;75(10):43-5.

38. Ghelardini et al. Local anaesthetic activity of the essential oil of Lavandula angustifolia. *Planta Med.* 1999 Dec;65(8):700-3

39. Elisabetsky et al. Anticonvulsant properties of linalool in glutamate-related seizure models. *Phytomedicine.* 1999 May;6(2):107-13.

40. Cai and Wu .Compounds from Syzygium aromaticum possessing growth inhibitory activity against oral pathogens. *J Nat Prod.* 1996 Oct;59(10):987-90.

41. Covello et. al. Determination of eugenol in the essence of "Eugenia caryophyllata". Titration in non-aqueous solvent and comparison with other methods of analysis. *Boll Chim Farm.* 1966 Nov;105(11):799-806.

42. Pourgholami M.H. et.al. Evaluation of the anticonvulsant activity of the essential oil of Eugenia caryophyllata in male mice. *J Ethnopharmacol.* 1999 Feb;64(2):167-71.

43. Diego Migul A. et al. Aromatherapy positively affects mood, EEG patterns of alertness and math computations. *Int J Neurosci.* 1998 Dec;96(3-4):217-24.

44. Lopez-Bote et. al. Effect of dietary administration of oil extracts from rosemary and sage on lipid oxidation in broiler meat. *Br Poult Sci.* 1998 May;39(2):235-40.

45. Ramadan W. et. al. Oil of bitter orange: new topical antifungal agent. *Int J Dermatol.* 1996 Jun;35(6):448-9.

46. Alderman G, and Elmer H., Inhibition of Growth and Aflatoxin Production of Aspergillus Parasiticus by Citrus Oils. Z. Leb. Unt-Forsch 1976: 353-58.

essential minerals such as magnesium and potassium, as well as a their rich supply of potent natural antioxidants.

Research also indicates that foods high in anti-oxidants, such as wolfberries, blueberries, straw-berries, raspberries, and spinach can dramatically increase glutathione levels and actually reverse the signs of aging.

A new test developed by USDA researchers at Tufts University in Boston, Massachusetts, has been able to identify the highest known antioxidant foods. Known as ORAC (oxygen radical absorbance capacity), this test is the first of its kind to measure both time and degree of free radical inhibition.

The Ningxia wolfberry was documented to have the highest ORAC score of any food tested. A special variety grown on the Yellow River in the Ningxia Province of central China, the Ningxia cultivar is very different from any other type of wolfberry. Among the 17 types of wolfberry identified, the Ningxia wolfberry has by far the highest levels of immune-stimulating polysaccharides. It also possesses over 33 times the antioxidant power of oranges and an incredible 120 times the antioxidant potential of carrots. In addition, the Chinese wolfberry is one of the most nutrient-dense foods known, rich in many vitamins and minerals including calcium, magnesium, B vitamins, and vitamin C.

A diet high in antioxidants can combat the free radical damage in the body that is associated with premature aging and degenerative diseases.

The Hunza People—
Limited Caloric Intake

The Hunzakuts living in the remote Hunza Valley in northern Pakistan are renowned for their longevity. The Hunzakuts (as they call themselves) routinely live past ages 100, 110 and even 120. They also share another remarkable trait: the near absence of degenerative disease.

It is known that the diet of the Hunza people is high in potassium and low in sodium. Apricots, barley, millet, and buckwheat are the main staples of their diet along with mineral-rich water with a pH of 8.5. But there is yet another unusual factor that may protect the health of the Hunza people and increase their longevity: their limited food intake.

Because the land provides just enough food to cover their basic caloric expenditures, the Hunzakuts rarely indulge in overeating. In fact, prior to the construction of the Korakoram High-way, they annually endured near-fasting conditions for several weeks each spring, a time when the previous year's food was depleted and the current year's harvests had not yet begun.

47. Wattenberg L.W. et. al. Inhibitory effects of 5-(2-pyrazinyl)-4-methyl-1,2-dithiol-3-thione (Oltipraz) on carcinogenesis induced by benzo[a]pyrene, diethylnitrosamine and uracil mustard. *Carcinogenesis*. 1986 Aug;7(8):1379-81.

48. Crowell P. L. Prevention and therapy of cancer by dietary monoterpenes. *J Nutr*. 1999 Mar;129(3):775S-778S.

49. Aruna, K. and V.M. Sivaramakrishnan. "Anticarcinogenic Effects of the Essential Oils from Cumin, Poppy and Basil." Food Chem Toxicol. 1992;30(11):953-56.

50. Juergens et. al. The anti-inflammatory activity of L-menthol compared to mint oil in human monocytes in vitro: a novel perspective for its therapeutic use in inflammatory diseases. *Eur J Med Res*. 1998 Dec 16;3(12):539-45.

51. Nasel et.al. Functional imaging of effects of fragrances on the human brain after prolonged inhalation. *Chem Senses*. 1994 Aug;19(4):359-64.

52. Steinmetz et. al.,Transmission and scanning electronmicroscopy study of the action of sage and rosemary essential oils and eucalyptol on Candida albicans. *Mycoses*. 1988 Jan;31(1):40-51.

53. Ulmer et. al., [Chronic obstructive bronchitis. Effect of Gelomyrtol forte in a placebo-controlled double-blind study]. Fortschr Med. 1991 Sep 20;109(27):547-50.

54. Cao G, et al, Antioxidant capacity in different tissues of young and old rats. *Proceedings of the society for Experimental Biology and Medicine* 211(1996), 359-365.

55. Chao et al., Antimicrobial Effects of Essential Oils on Streptococcus pneumoniae. *JEOR*, 2001.

56. Deans SG, et al, Natural antioxidants from aromatic and medicinal plants. *Role of Free Radicals in Biological Systems*, pp. 159-165 (1993a) [J Feher, A Blazovics, B Matkovics and M Mezes, editors]. Budapest: Akademiai Kiado.

57. Farag et. al. Acute hepatic damage in rats impairs metharbital metabolism. *Pharmacology*. 1987;34(4):181-91.

58. Halliwell B & Gutteridge JMC, *Free Radicals in Biology and Medicine*, 2nd Edition. (1989), Oxford: Clarendon Press.

59. Inhibition of growth and aflatoxin production of Aspergillus parasiticus by citrus oils. *Z Lebensm Unters Forsch*. 1976 Apr 28;160(4):353-8.

60. Kaplan RJ & Greenwood CE, Dietary saturated fatty acids and brain function. *Neurochemistry Research* 23, (1989)615-626.

61. Ramadan W. et. al. Oil of bitter orange: new topical antifungal agent. *Int J Dermatol*. 1996 Jun;35(6):448-9.

62. Recsan Z, et al, Effect of essential oils on the lipids of the retina in the aging rat: a possible therapeutic use. *J Ess Oil Res* 9, (1997) 53-56.

63. Scott BL & Bazan NG, Membrane docosahexaenoate is supplied to the developing brain and retina by the liver. *Proceedings of the National Academy of Sciences USA* 86, (1989) 2903-2907.

64. Socci DJ, et al, Chronic antioxidant treatment improves the cognitive performance in aged rats. *Brain Research* 693, (1995) 88-94.

65. Wahnon R, et al, Age and membrane fluidity. *Mechanisms of Ageing and Development* 50, (1989) 249-255.

66. Youdim KA, et al., Effect of thyme oil and thymol dietary supplementation on the antioxidant status and fatty acid composition of the ageing rat brain. *Br J Nutr*. 2000 Jan;83(1):87-93.

Restricted caloric intake such as fasting can have powerful effects on longevity because it increases blood levels of growth hormone which is one of the most significant anti-aging hormones to be identified during the last two decades. Secreted by the pituitary gland, growth hormone production steadily declines with age. By age 70, the human body produces less than one-tenth of the growth hormone it did at age 20.

Clinical studies have repeatedly shown that growth hormone production is stimulated by low glucose levels. Because fasting depresses glucose levels, it leads to a surge in natural growth hormone production (Khansari et al., 1991).

Other studies have shown that the practice of caloric restriction (providing all necessary nutrients but limiting calorie intake) results in increased longevity and postponement of disease. Clive McCay at Cornell University showed that rats fed a diet low in calories but high in vitamins, minerals, and nutrients lived up to twice as long as rats fed on a regular diet (McCay et al., 1939). Ray Walford of the University of California in Los Angeles found that in studies on mice, the greater the reduction in calories, the longer the animal lived—as long as the vitamin and mineral content remained constant and the calories consumed did not drop below 40 percent of the normal (Walford et al., 1987).

29

Enzyme Therapy

Importance of Enzymes

Digestive enzymes are absolutely vital to human health. They break down and digest food in order to liberate the essential nutrients, vitamins, and minerals that sustain life. Some digestive enzymes are present in the food we eat; some are produced by the body itself.

A lack of digestive enzymes in the diet forces the body to overproduce its own digestive enzymes and limits its ability to produce metabolic enzymes which are also crucial for health and normal metabolism. This limitation occurs because both digestive enzymes and metabolic enzymes are created from the same enzyme precursors. The production of these precursors is limited in the human body, so when the digestive system must overproduce digestive enzymes (due to an enzymeless diet), it causes a harmful underproduction of metabolic enzymes.

How important are metabolic enzymes? Metabolic enzymes are involved in every process of the human body. The immune system, circulatory system, liver, kidneys, spleen, pancreas, and even our ability to see, breathe, and think, depend upon metabolic enzymes.

When the diet is supplemented with digestive enzymes that are naturally present in whole, raw, or uncooked foods, two powerful benefits are unleashed:

1. The body can extract maximum nutritional value from food

2. The body can reduce its internal production of digestive enzymes, which allows for higher production of metabolic enzymes, crucial for daily metabolism, health, and detoxification.

Categories of Enzymes:

Metabolic enzymes

These enzymes work in the blood, tissues, and organs. Our organs are run by metabolic enzymes. These enzymes convert food substances into healthy cells. One researcher found over 98 enzymes carrying out metabolic functions in the arteries alone.

Digestive enzymes produced by the body

These include trypsin, chymotrypsin, and pepsin, which contain a broad spectrum of protein, starch, and fat-digesting enzymes. Some typical animal-derived enzymes include pancrelipase (from pigs) and pancreatin (from cows).

Protein digesting enzymes

- protease 4.5 (this number refers to the pH environment that the enzyme works best in)
- protease 6.0
- protease 3.0
- peptidase

Fat-digesting enzymes

- lipase

Starch-, sugar-, and carbohydrate-digesting enzymes

- alpha-galactosidase
- sucrase
- maltase
- invertase
- lactase
- cellulase,
- amylase
- glucomylase
- hemicellulase
- phytase
- malt diastase

Digestive enzymes found in food

These are present naturally in raw food and jump start the digestive process. They are broadly classified into proteases (protein-digesters), lipases (fat-digesters), and amylases (starch digesters). There are also many different subcategories of enzymes.

Broad-spectrum plant enzymes

- papain
- bromelain

Amylase is the only digestive enzyme that does not exist in a newborn infant. It can only be obtained through mother's milk. Children who use formulas and cow's milk do not receive this enzyme. This may be the reason some children are born with allergies or develop allergies as they begin growing.

In the food chain, nature has strategically placed enzymes in many raw or whole foods to assist our own body's enzymes in the digestive process.

Ancient cultures prized the natural enzymes in foods—especially meats. They worked hard to conserve the natural enzymes present in their foodstuffs because they knew how valuable they were for strength and health. This is why many ancient cultures "aged" or cured meats. This allowed the natural enzymes present in the flesh to predigest it, thereby easing the burden on their own digestive system and conserving their own limited pool of enzymes.

When meat is predigested, it places less stress on the body's own enzyme bank. Predigestion also enhances the breakdown of peptide chains and proteins into free form amino acids, the building blocks of every major body function, from immunity to growth.

Every protein that enters the human body via digestion has to be broken down into amino acids before it can be fully utilized. Meats that are not completely digested contain large protein fragments that cannot benefit the body. In fact, these protein fragments can cause allergic reactions if the body's antibodies mistake them for foreign microorganisms. Even worse, these protein fragments can become trapped in the intestines where they will ferment and promote parasite infestation.

Cathepsin is a natural enzyme present in all animal flesh. The aging or "curing" process allows cathepsin, an enzyme that is within the flesh, to slowly digest the meat. This is not unlike the process that ripens bananas. A green banana starts out high in starch. As it ages or ripens, the natural amylase in the banana converts the starches into sugar. In effect, the amylase is digesting the banana, eventually turning it brown.

As soon as an animal is dead, cathepsin begins to predigest the meat. It begins splitting large peptide (protein) chains into smaller, more digestible ones. When this meat is eaten after it has been hung for two to three weeks, the digestive system now has a far easier job completing its breakdown and liberating the vital free-form amino acids, the building blocks of all bodily processes.

The remarkable physical strength and endurance exhibited by the pioneers and Native Americans may have been due to their consumption of enzyme-rich raw and unprocessed foods, despite the sometimes meager rations of less than four ounces of food a day. We have been taught that you must eat to have strength. But there is more to it than that. You must be able to digest and assimilate the nutrients that you take in, in order to sustain health and strength.

On the average, only 8 percent of the food we consume is metabolized to sustain normal bodily function. The remainder passes through us undigested. Even worse, only 1 to 2 percent of the nutrient value of the food that we consume reaches our cells.

Many people today suffer wheat and grain allergies. This may be due to the fact that grains are not grown and prepared as they used to be.

Egyptian hieroglyphics depict the ancient process of grain harvesting. The grain was cut with a scythe, tied into sheaves and left to stand in the field for several days. It was then loaded into ox carts, hauled to the threshing site and thrown into a big stone grinder operated by an ox team. The stone rolled around on the grain, cracking the hulls. With the sifting of the wind, the chaff was blown off, and the grain picked up by slaves and carried in baskets to the storehouse.

Stone-ground, whole-wheat bread which is rich in enzymes, vitamin E, and other nutrients, sadly, is a thing of the past. Today, modern technology brings grain to us via a machine called a combine. The combine cuts the grain, almost instantly separates the kernel from the husk and delivers the grain ready for market on the same day it was cut. It is then further processed to strip out the vitamin E and other oils. Most of it is then bleached leaving only a tiny fraction of the grain's initial enzymes.

To maximize the enzymes in a food, the fruit of the plant needs to mature on the stalk/stem to the point of 'ripening,' or readiness to sprout. This is when the enzyme content of the food is the highest. Unfortunately, many fruits, vegetables and grains are harvested when they are immature and assumed to ripen "in transit." This results in a food that has a far lower enzyme content.

In order for grains to fully digest in the human body, they must contain a full complement of their natural enzymes. Every food has its own specific enzymes. In order for a grain to have viable enzymes, it must have time to germinate. Once it germinates, its enzymes are released from the bondage of enzyme inhibitors. This is why sprouted grains are so health-giving, because the enzyme inhibitors have been deactivated and can no longer counteract the natural enzymes present in the food.

What are some of the early signs of enzyme deficiency? Digestive complaints, heartburn, gas, bloating, fatigue, headaches, stomach aches, diarrhea, constipation, chronic fatigue, yeast infections, nutritional deficiencies, pain, joint stiffness; colon, liver, pancreas, and intestinal problems, skin eruptions, psoriasis, and eczema.

Many enzymes are not only deficient but also inactive. At the Young Life Research Clinic in Springville, Utah, Gary Young tested over 21 different enzyme products from 21 different manufacturers and did not find a single one that was effective in a clinical environment. The patients were closely monitored, their food intake measured; their blood and digestive systems regularly measured and analyzed. The clinic staff found that patients were simply not obtaining value from their foods because their enzymes were inactive.

How are enzymes destroyed or rendered inactive?

1. Chemical cultivation. When natural food is grown in an artificial, chemical environment created by chemical fertilizers, herbicides and pesticides, enzyme content suffers.

2. Heat. Enzymes begin breaking down at 118° F and are totally destroyed at 129° F.

3. Pasteurization, Sterilization, Freezing, Microwaving. All these modern processes render enzymes inactive.

D. Gary Young has traveled the world studying cultures renowned for their longevity: The Vilcabamba in Ecuador, the Aszerbijani people of the Talish Mountains, the Georgian people in the Caucasus region, the Inner-Mongolian people in the province in Ningxia, and the Hunzakut people in Northern Pakistan. All these people share two common traits: They practice fasting on a regular basis and they live to be over 120 years of age. Fasting allows the body to slow down the secretion of digestive enzymes, thereby permitting an increase in metabolic enzymes that help the body to repair and rejuvenate tissue that has been damaged or destroyed. In effect, the fasting process rebuilds the body.

In addition, fasting spurs an increase in growth hormone release, which is important for preventing premature aging.

The human body has the potential to live for 120 years and beyond. However, devitalized, enzyme-deficient foods deplete our enzyme stores and unduly stress the organs and major physical processes. This can hasten the onset of many degenerative diseases. Hence, one of the most effective ways of preventing disease is to maintain an ample reserve of enzymes in the body.

Medical research shows that food enzyme supplements can fight illness, slow the development of life-threatening diseases, and slow the effects of aging.

Dr. Francis Pottinger conducted an amazing study with over 900 cats. He fed one group of cats raw milk and meat. They lived healthy and disease free. They produced healthy litters generation after generation. He fed another group of cats pasteurized milk and cooked food. After the first generation, this group became lethargic and began to suffer from allergies, infections, and other diseases, including heart, kidney, and lung diseases. Each succeeding generation of cats that ate cooked food suffered more diseases. By the third generation, the cats were unable to reproduce.

Another study showed that after eating cooked food, the human body reacted just as if suffering an acute illness. Within 30 minutes of eating cooked food, white blood cell counts increased dramatically, as though the body were fighting an infectious disease.

In a very interesting experiment, one group of pigs was fed enzyme-rich raw potatoes and another group enzyme-deficient cooked potatoes. The pigs eating cooked potatoes gained weight rapidly. The pigs that were eating raw potatoes did not get fat.

An area of deep concern is obesity. Dr. David Galton at the Tufts University School of Medicine tested people weighing 230-240 pounds. He found that almost all of them were lacking lipase enzymes in their fatty tissues. Lipase, found abundantly in raw foods, is a fat-splitting enzyme that aids the body in digestion. Lipase activity breaks down and dissolves fat throughout the body. Without lipase, fats are kept and stored in tissues. We see this manifest around the waistline, hips, and thighs.

It is astounding to see the obesity levels of America's children. According to 1998 statistics, a minimum of 25 percent of our children are overweight today—an increase of 33 percent since 1978. This obesity may be due to chronic enzyme deficiency.

30

Personal Usage Reference

How Essential Oils Work

Essential oils can work through inhalation, ingestion, topical application, or rectal/vaginal retention.

Although topical use is perhaps best known, dietary use of essential oils may be one of the most effective ways of unlocking their health benefits. Many essential oils have been used as food flavorings or as a part of patent medicines for centuries, endowing them with a long history of safe use. Recent research suggests that certain high ORAC essential oils act as potent antioxidants that can actually raise antioxidant levels in the body and prevent premature aging.

Many of the oils listed in this section are classified as "GRAS" by the U.S. Food and Drug Administration. This means they are "generally regarded as safe" for human consumption. An appendix of GRAS oils appears in Appendix C.

Topical application is probably the most common means of using essential oils. According to researcher Jean Valnet, M.D., an essential oil that is directly applied to the skin can pass into the bloodstream and diffuse throughout the tissues in 20 minutes or less. More recent studies have also documented the ability of essential oils to penetrate the stratum corneum (the upper layer of skin) to reach the subdermal tissues and blood vessels beneath.[1,2]

Some of the compounds in essential oils that work synergistically to enhance permeation include alpha-pinene (frankincense, valerian, basil, cistus), beta-pinene (galbanum, hyssop, fir, rosemary), alpha-terpineol (bay laurel, *Melaleuca ericifolia*, ravensara), 1,8-cineole (*Eucalyptus globulus*, *E. radiata, E. dives*, rosemary) and d-limonene (white fir, tangerine, orange, lemon, grapefruit).

Inhalation is an effective means of therapeutically using and delivering an essential oil. The fragrance of an essential oil can have a direct influence on both the body and mind due to its ability to stimulate the brain's limbic system (a group of subcortical structures including the hypothalamus, the hippocampus, and the amygdala). This can produce powerful effects that can effect everything from emotional balance and energy levels to appetite control, heart, and immune function.

Some researchers believe that the inhalation of an essential oil can also enhance the body's frequency, which can have a direct impact on disease. Disease and emotional trauma foster a negative frequency that may be disrupted or broken by essential oils. Oils with higher frequencies can elevate the entire frequency of the body whether topically or orally administered, thereby creating an internal environment that opposes the establishment of some disease conditions.

When to Mix Oils and Blends

The essential oils and blends that are listed for a specific condition can be used either separately or together. By combining a single oil with another recommended single oil or blend, a synergistic or additive effect is produced that results in stronger total effect than the sum of the actions produced by each oil or blend separately.

As a rule, when a list of oils or blends is recommended and does not list specific quantities, usually 1-3 drops of each oil should be used. For example, if the list reads, "Lavender, lemongrass, marjoram, ginger," this means that 1 drop of lavender

---

1. Taiwan Huang, Fang, Hung, Wu, Tsai "Cyclic monoterpene extract from cardamom oil as a skin permeation enhancer for indomethacin: in vitro and in vivo studies." *Biological and Pharmaceutical Bulletin* 1999 Jun;22(6):642-6.

2. Ogiso, Iwaki, Paku "Effect of various enhancers on transdermal penetration of indomethacin and urea, and relationship between penetration parameters and enhancement factors." *Journal of Pharmaceutical Sciences.* 1995 Apr;84(4):482-8.

should be mixed with one drop of any 2-4 of these oils for a synergetic blend. Normally it is best to avoid using more than 3 oils in any given blend at a time.

How to Choose an Essential Oil

The essential oils listed for a specific condition are not designed to be a comprehensive or complete list; they are merely a starting point. Other oils that are not listed can also be effective.

In addition, essential oils are not listed in any particular order. This is because one oil might be more compatible with one person's unique body chemistry than another's for aromatic purposes and skin sensitivity, not necessarily for physical response. If results are not felt within several minutes, try another oil, blend, or combination, on the next application.

How to Use Essential Oils

Essential oils should be used in moderation as they are highly concentrated. Use with VITA FLEX, contact, or acupuncture-point applications. In most cases, one or two drops is sufficient to produce significant effects. It is strongly recommended that most essential oils be diluted in vegetable oil prior to either topical or internal application (particularly if you have not used essential oils previously). Specific directions for each oil are listed in Appendicies E, P, Q and R.

When using essential oils topically, first do a skin test with 1 drop of essential oil on the inside of the upper arm. Use no more than 10 to 20 drops during one topical application.

Many essential oils can be used as dietary supplements, and a list of these oils appears in Appendix C. All essential oils should be diluted prior to oral use unless directed by a physician or one trained in the oral use of essential oils. No more than 2-4 drops should be consumed at one time (in a single serving) unless indicated otherwise. The simplest way to dilute essential oils for ingestion is to mix a drop in a teaspoon of honey (do not give honey to children age

Address the overall health of the body when considering a specific solution. Although essential oils have powerful therapeutic effects, they are not, by themselves, a total solution. They must be accompanied by a program of internal cleansing, proper diet, and supplementation. This may also include lifestyle changes, such as exercise, meditation/yoga, and stress-free situations.

Step 1. Cleanse

Cleansing the colon and liver is the first and most important step to take when dealing with any disease. Many imbalances can be corrected by cleansing alone. Products that cleanse the body include: Cleansing Trio (Essentialzyme, ComforTone, and ICP), Chelex, ParaFree, JuvaTone, and JuvaFlex (See Cleansing programs in Chapter 25).

Step 2. Balance and Build

Once the body has been cleansed, various systems of the body can be balanced and nourished. This includes rebuilding and nourishing beneficial intestinal flora, and remineralizing the blood and tissues. Products that build the body include: Mineral Essence, Essential Manna, Master Formula vitamins, WheyFit, VitaGreen, Power Meal, and Super Cal.

Step 3. Support

Supporting the endocrine and immune system comprises the third phase. Products include: ImmuPro, ImmuneTune, Exodus, Be-Fit, Wolfberry Crisp bars, Super C, Essential Omegas, Super B, Ultra Young.

NOTE: Infants or children under 8 should not undergo a colon and liver cleanse. Instead, use 3 drops of Di-Tone in a tsp. of V-6 Mixing Oil or Massage Oil Base, rub around the navel, and place warm hot packs over the stomach. Also apply Di-Tone or fennel on bottom of the feet.

Consult Your Health Care Professional

Consult your health care professional about any serious disease or injury. Do not attempt to self-diagnose or prescribe any natural substances such as essential oils for health conditions that require professional attention.

1 or under) or a cup of almond or rice milk. If taste is a problem, oils can be diluted 50-50, placed in a gelatin capsule and swallowed.

When using essential oils always increase fluid intake because the oils can accelerate the detoxification process in the body. If you are not taking in adequate fluids, toxins could recirculate causing nausea, headaches, etc.

Avoid Petrochemicals

Exercise caution when applying essential oils to skin that has been exposed to cosmetics, personal care products, or soaps and cleansers containing synthetic or petroleum-based chemicals. Essential oils may react with such chemicals and cause skin irritation, nausea, or headaches.

Essential oils can also react with toxins built up in the body from chemicals in food, water, and the work environment. If you experience a reaction to essential oils, temporarily discontinue their use and start an internal cleansing program (30 days using the Cleansing Trio) before resuming regular use of essential oils.

Tip on Safe Use:

Skin-test the diluted essential oil on a small patch of skin. If any redness or irritation results, cleanse skin thoroughly and reapply. If skin irritation persists, discontinue using that oil or oil blend.

How to Use This Reference Guide

This Guide has two parts, which must be used together in order to correctly and safely develop regimens for essential oil application.

The first part of the guide is a list of 18 standard application methods found on the next two pages. For each of these applications, dilution rates, mixtures and procedures are listed in detail. These applications are listed in five basic groups: TOPICAL, RETENTION, ORAL, INGESTION and INHALATION. The details of each application method are listed here at the beginning of this chapter to avoid unnecessary repitition throughout the remainder of the chapter. It is recommended that you read through all these application methods to familiarize yourself with them before using this guide.

How to Convert		
1 drop	=	approximately 60 mg
1 ml	=	1/5 teaspoon
1 ml	=	approximately 20 drops
1 ml	=	fills one 00 capsule
5 ml	=	1 teaspoon
5 ml	=	approximately 80 drops
15 ml	=	1 tablespoon
15 ml	=	1/2 fluid ounce
240 ml	=	1 cup (depends on product)
30 ml	=	1 fluid ounce
28 grams	=	1 ounce

The second part of the guide, comprising the rest of the chapter, includes application suggestions for over 300 different illnesses and injuries with single essential oils, blends, dietary supplements and topical treatments, which are appropriate for those conditions. Each topic contains some or all of the following headings pointing to the products to use and how to use them:

Singles
Blends
EO Applications
Dietary Supplements
Topical Treatments
Other

Within each 'EO Applications' heading is a listing of keywords indicating which of the 18 application methods are appropriate and effective for that condition. It is important to note that abbreviated keywords are listed in the body of this guide. Readers must return to the application methods explanations on the next two pages to get the full detail of how to use the oils in each particular application method.

As explained in earlier sections of this book, essential oils are very concentrated natural substances —easily 100 times more concentrated than the natural herbs they come from. So dilution of an essential oil is a very important aspect of using it therapeutically. Some essential oils are so mild that dilution is simply not necessary, even for use on infants. Others are so strong that dilution is mandatory. (See Appendix E for a list of recommended safe dilutions for all the oils mentioned in this book).

A Sample Lookup

Here is an example of how to develop an application program using the two parts of the guide. Let's say that you are experiencing a sore throat and want to know what you can do to treat that condition with the products in this reference book.

Step 1: Locate the disease/injury topic alphabetically in the Personal Usage Guide

In this case, the heading you are looking for is a subhead located under the main heading of THROAT INFECTIONS. It is found on page 412.

Step 2: Note the recommended essential oils – both singles and blends – to be used.

In this case, the section on Sore Throat lists 10 single oils, 3 standard blends, and 2 custom blends that all may be helpful when used according to the methods listed in the EO Applications section.

Although this listing shows 15 possible oils, only 1-3 oils or blends should be used at any given time. You will need to select 1-3 oils or blends that you will use based on availability, budget and aroma (for example, some oils are strong enough that you may not want to be using or wearing them at work.)

Step 3: Make a list of the recommended essential oil (EO) applications listed for the illness/injury you are checking.

In this case, under the THROAT INFECTIONS heading, quite a variety of methods is listed. Altogether 10 different application methods are listed, ranging from Direct Inhalation to Raindrop Technique. (Not all conditions have this many application methods. Most recommend only one or two.) The 10 listed application methods for a sore throat are intended to show all possible application methods for using essential oils in treating that condition.

Normally, only 1-3 different applications should be used at any given time. This is a matter of both convenience and safety. If someone were to attempt all 10 applications for a sore throat at once, it would require an enormous investment of time, be extremely inconvenient and would put more essential oil in that person's body than is needed or helpful.

Again, cross check the keyword application method descriptions under each disease heading with the detailed application descriptions on this page an the next. This will provided important additional information, such as dilution rates and frequency of application.

Step 4: Note any additional dietary supplements and topical treatments listed for the condition.

The recommended usage for these products can be found in the product listings in chapters 10-17.

Step 5: Make a written personal regimen that includes the 1-3 oils you have selected, the 1-3 EO application methods you will be using, the dietary supplements and the topical treatments, if any.

This will save you from having to look up everything again each time you do your applications.

Step 6: Make sure you understand the proper essential oil dilution levels.

If you do not properly link oils with their application method details, you could make a mistake here. For example, one of the applications for sore throat is Direct Inhalation, in which the oils are used in their 'neat,' or undiluted state. However, for Topical Application to the skin, the dilution rate is 50-50 or 1 part essential oil to 1 part vegetable oil. (V6 Oil Complex)

Step 7: Be faithful with your regimen.

Therapeutic-grade essential oils are wonderful, natural, healing substances, and they work extremely well with the body's own defenses to solve problems. However, they are not drugs, and they may not always work in seconds, or even minutes. Essential Oils will enhance and speed up the benefits of dietary supplements, but it is still a 'natural' process. Sometimes it can take hours or even days to see the improvement.

The 18 Basic Essential Oil Application Methods

NOTE: Please read this information carefully as all directions in the following personal guide section will refer to the 18 methods outlined here.

TOPICAL APPLICATION (On the skin surface)
- NEAT: Apply neat (undiluted) as directed to affected area. (See Appendix E)

- DILUTE 50-50: 1 part essential oil (s) to 1 part V6 Oil Complex. (See Appendix E)

- DILUTE 20-80: 1 part essential oil(s) to 4 parts V6 Oil Complex. (See Appendix E)

- VITA FLEX: Apply 1-3 drops neat to the Vita Flex points on the feet as directed. See Vita Flex chart found in Chapter 20 for point locations.

- COMPRESS: Dilute 1 part essential oil(s) with 4 parts V6 Oil Complex and apply 8-10 drops on affected area. Cover with a HOT, moist hand towel. Then cover the moist towel with a dry towel for 10-15 minutes. Can also use a cool, moist hand towel instead of a hot one, to create a COLD compress.

- BATH SALT: Mix thoroughly 10-15 drops of essential oil into 2 tablespoons of Epsom salts or baking soda. Dissolve in warm bathwater as tub is filling and soak for at least 20 minutes before using soap or shampoo; or place in special shower head designed to hold salt/essential oil mixture and shower for 10 minutes.

- BODY MASSAGE: Apply diluted in a 20:80 ratio (1 part essential oils to 4 parts V6 Oil Complex) in a full-body massage.

- RAINDROP Technique: (See Chapter 21)

RETENTION

- RECTAL: Dilute the recommended essential oil(s) in 40:60 ratio (4 parts essential oil to 6 parts V6 Oil Complex), insert 1-2 tablespoons in rectum with a bulb syringe and retain up to 8 hours or overnight.

- TAMPON: Dilute the recommended essential oil(s) in 40:60 ratio (4 parts essential oil to 6 parts V6 Oil Complex). Apply 1-2 tablespoons to a tampon and insert into vagina (for internal infection) OR apply to a sanitary pad (for external lesions). Retain up to 8 hours or overnight. Use only tampons or sanitary pads made with non-perfumed, non-scented organic cotton.

ORAL

- GARGLE: Add 2-3 drops essential oil with 4 tablespoons purified water, shake or mix vigorously. Gargle for 30 seconds.

- TONGUE: Apply 1 drop of essential oil neat to the back of the tongue with cotton swab or fingertip. Retain, allowing oil to combine with saliva, for at least 1 minute, then swallow. Note: this should NOT be done with essential oils which have a **20-80** application code. (See Appendix E)

INHALATION

- DIFFUSION: Diffuse neat in a cold-air diffuser (cold air diffusers are not designed to handle vegetable oils because they are thicker and may clog the diffuser mechanism).

- DIRECT: Apply 2-3 drops of essential oil(s) to the palm of one hand; rub palms together; cup hands over nose and mouth (being careful not to touch the skin near your eyes) and inhale vapors deeply 6-8 times.

- VAPOR: Run hot, steaming water into a sink or large bowl. Water should be at least 2 inches deep to retain heat for a few minutes. Drape a towel over your head, covering the hot water also, enclosing your face over the steaming water. Add 3-6 drops of essential oils(s) into the hot water. Inhale vapors as deeply as possible several times, through the nose, as they rise with the steam. Recharge vapors with additional hot water.

INGESTION

- CAPSULE: Unless directed otherwise, use a clean medicine dropper to fill the larger half of an empty gelatin capsule (available at health food stores) half-way with essential oil(s); then fill the remainder with V6 Advanced Oil Complex or a high quality cold-pressed vegetable oil, seal with the other half of the gel cap and take as directed.

  There are two basic dosages used for capsules, indicated by capsule size. '00' size capsules (which contain a 400 mg dose when filled with a 50-50 dilution of essential oil) and '0' size capsules (which contain a 200 mg dose when filled with a 50-50 dilution of essential oil). If '0' size capsules are not readily available, you can half fill '00' size capsules.

- RICE MILK: Add the essential oil to rice milk and take as directed. Use 3-5 drops in 1/2 cup of rice milk. Goat milk may be substituted for rice milk.

- SYRUP: Add the essential oil to Blue Agave nectar or Grade B Maple Syrup. Use 3 drops in 1 tsp. maple syrup. Hold in mouth for 30 seconds before swallowing. Blue Agave nectar (a low-glycemic natural sweetener derived from the Agave plant) seems to work more effectively than maple syrup.

ABSCESS (Skin)

(See SKIN DISORDERS)

ABSENTMINDEDNESS

Clinical studies on Ningxia wolfberry *(Lycium barbarum)* have shown that it has an anti-senility effect. Clinical studies at University of Colorado Health Sciences Center found that high antioxidant foods such as spinach (found in JuvaPower) and blueberry (found in Berry Young Juice) dramatically improved learning and cognition.[3, 4]

(See BRAIN DISORDERS)

Single Oils:
Peppermint, cardamom, vetiver, frankincense, sandalwood, rosemary, basil

Blends:
Clarity, Brain Power, M-Grain

EO Applications:
INHALATION:
DIFFUSION, 15 min every 2 hours, as needed
DIRECT, 2-4 times daily, as needed
TOPICAL:
NEAT, 1-2 drops on temples and/or back of neck, as needed.

Dietary Supplementation:
Power Meal, Ultra Young, Sulfurzyme, VitaGreen, Essential Omegas, Mineral Essence, JuvaPower/Spice, Berry Young Juice.

ABUSE (mental and physical)

The trauma from mental and physical abuse can result in self-defeating behavior that can undermine success later in life. Through their powerful effect on the limbic system of the brain (the center or stored memories and emotions), essential oils can help release pent-up trauma, emotions, or memories.

Single Oils:
Geranium, sandalwood, or melissa.

Blends:
SARA, Trauma Life, Release, Acceptance, Forgiveness, Surrender, Humility, Joy, White Angelica, Inner Child, Harmony, Hope, Brain Power, Citrus Fresh, Christmas Spirit, Valor

EO Applications:
INHALATION:
DIFFUSION, 15 min. every 2 hours as needed
DIRECT, 2-3 times daily, as needed
TOPICAL:
NEAT, 1-2 drops on temples and/or back of neck as needed. Also apply 2-3 drops on the Vita Flex liver point of the right foot. Also apply a trace under the nose.

Dietary Supplementation:
Power Meal, Super C, Super C Chewable, Super B

Other:

Physical Abuse: Begin with application of 2-3 drops Forgiveness, unless suicidal. It is most effective around the navel. Follow with 1-2 drops Release over the Vita Flex points, especially the liver point of right foot, and under the nose.

Parental, Sexual or Ritual Abuse: 1-3 drops SARA over the area where abuse took place; then Forgiveness, Trauma Life, Release, Joy, or Present Time.

Spousal Abuse: Use Forgiveness, Trauma Life, Acceptance, Release, Valor, Joy, or Envision.

Feelings of Revenge: 1-2 drops of Surrender on the sternum over the heart, 2-3 drops of Present Time on the thymus, and 2-3 drops Forgiveness over navel.

Suicidal: 2 drops Hope on rim of ears. Melissa, Brain Power, or Present Time may be beneficial also.

Protection/Balance: 1-2 drops of White Angelica on each shoulder, 1-2 drops Harmony over thymus and on energy centers or chakras of the body.

---

3. Galli RL et al., "Fruit polyphenolics and brain aging: nutritional interventions targeting age-related neuronal and behavioral deficits." *Ann N Y Acad Sci.* 2002 Apr; 959: 128-32.

4. Bickford PC et al., "Antioxidant-rich diets improve cerebellar physiology and motor learning in aged rats." *Brain Res.* 2000 Jun 2; 866(1-2): 211-7.

ACID/ALKALINE BALANCE

(See FUNGAL INFECTIONS, ACIDOSIS, and ALKALOSIS)

ACIDOSIS

(See FUNGAL INFECTIONS)

Acidosis is a condition where the pH of the intestinal tract and the blood serum become excessively acidic. This can promote the growth of pathogenic fungi like candida and exacerbate yeast infections. Acidic blood can stress the liver and eventually lead to many forms of chronic and degenerative diseases.

To raise pH, avoid acid-ash foods, overuse of antibiotics, and monitor the pH of the saliva (6.4-6.5) and blood (7.3-7.6). (See APPENDIX B)

Single Oils:
Peppermint, lemon

Blends:
Di-Tone

EO Applications:
INGESTION:
> CAPSULE, 00 Size, 2 daily between meals, if possible, otherwise with meals

Dietary Supplementation:
AlkaLime, Mega Cal, JuvaPower/Spice, Essentialzyme, Polyzyme, VitaGreen, Wolfberry Crisp

Other Regimens:
Take Polyzyme with peppermint until acid level is balanced, then add Essentialzyme.

To reduce acid indigestion and prevent fermentation that can contribute to bad dreams and interrupted sleep: 1 tsp. AlkaLime in water before bedtime.

To raise pH, take 2-6 capsules of VitaGreen 3 times daily and take 1 tsp. AlkaLime in water one hour before or two hours after meals each day. For maintenance, take 1 tsp. AlkaLime once per week.

To stimulate enzymatic action in the digestive tract: Mix together or use individually, raw carrot juice, alfalfa, trace minerals, and papaya.

ACNE

(See SKIN DISORDERS)

A.D.D.

(See ATTENTION DEFICIT DISORDER)

ADDICTIONS

Many food and chemical dependencies, such as addictions to tobacco, caffeine, drugs, alcohol, and sugar may originate in the liver. Cleansing and detoxifying the liver is a crucial first step toward breaking free of these addictions. Increasing intake of alkaline calcium can help bind bile acids and prevent fatty liver. A colon and tissue cleanse is also important.

Using stevia, stevioside, or FOS can help reduce sugar cravings. Stevia is a supersweet noncaloric extract derived from an ancient South American herb, while FOS is a sweet-tasting indigestible sugar derived from chicory roots and Jerusalem artichokes with no calories and important health benefits. (See APPENDIX P)

Trace mineral and mineral deficiencies can also play a part in some addictions. Magnesium, potassium, calcium, and zinc should all be included in the diet.

Blends:
Harmony, Peace & Calming, JuvaCleanse, JuvaFlex

EO Applications:
INHALATION:
> DIFFUSION, 15 min every 2 hours as needed
> DIRECT, 2-3 times daily, as needed

TOPICAL:
> NEAT, 1-2 drops on temples and/or back of neck 4 times daily
> COMPRESS, warm, over liver

Dietary Supplementation:
JuvaTone, JuvaPower/Spice, Stevia, Wolfberry Crisp, Mineral Essence, SuperCal, Mega Cal, ComfortTone, Essentialzyme, ICP

(See LIVER and SMOKING CESSATION)

ADDISON'S DISEASE

(See ADRENAL GLAND IMBALANCE)

ADRENAL GLAND IMBALANCE

The adrenal glands consist of two sections: An inner part called the medulla produces stress hormones and an outer part called the cortex secretes critical hormones called glucocorticoids and aldosterone. Because of these hormones, the cortex has a far greater impact on overall health than the medulla does.

Why are aldosterone and glucocorticoids so important? Because they directly affect blood pressure and mineral content and help regulate the conversion of carbohydrates into energy.

Addison's Disease

In cases like Addison's disease, adrenal cortex hormones are no longer produced or severely limited. This can lead to life-threatening fluid and mineral loss unless these hormones are replaced.

Because Addison's disease is an autoimmune disease in which the body's own immune cells destroy the adrenal glands, it may be treated with MSM. MSM is an important source of organic sulfur that has been shown to have positive effects with many types of autoimmune diseases, including lupus, arthritis, and fibromyalgia.

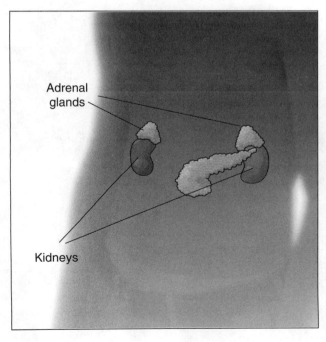

Adrenal glands

Kidneys

Supporting the Adrenal Glands

Add essential oils to 1/4 teaspoon of massage oil and apply as a warm compress over the adrenal glands (located on top of the kidneys).

- 3 drops clove
- 3 drops nutmeg
- 7 drops rosemary

If adrenal insufficiency is accompanied by a lack of thyroid hormone, the condition is known as Schmidt's syndrome.

Symptoms:
- Severe fatigue
- Lightheadedness when standing
- Nausea
- Depression/irritability
- Craving salty foods
- Loss of appetite
- Muscle spasms
- Dark, tan-colored skin

Essential oils can play a part in correcting deficiencies in adrenal cortex function. Nutmeg, for example, has adrenal-like activity that raises energy levels.

Single Oils:
Nutmeg, sage, clove, rosemary, basil

Blends:
EndoFlex, Joy, En-R-Gee

EO Applications:
TOPICAL:
    COMPRESS, warm, over the adrenal
    gland area (on back, over the kidneys)
INGESTION:
    CAPSULE, 00 size, 2 daily

Other:
The following essential oil blend recipe is designed to be used with a compress over the adrenal area:
- 3 drops clove
- 3 drops nutmeg
- 7 drops rosemary
- 20 drops massage oil or V-6 Mixing Oil.

Dietary Supplementation:
Thyromin, VitaGreen, Royal Essence, Super B, Master Formula, Mineral Essence

Other:

Supplementation regimen for adrenal support
- Thyromin: 1 immediately after awakening.
- Super B: 1 after meals. If you experience a niacin flush (skin becoming red and itchy for about 15 minutes), use only 1/2 of a tablet.
- Master Formula: 2-6 tablets, 3 times daily according to blood type and need.

Cushing's disease

Cushing's disease is the opposite of Addison's disease. It is characterized by the overproduction of adrenal cortex hormones. While these hormones are crucial to sound health in normal amounts, their unchecked overproduction can cause as much harm as their underproduction. This results in the following symptoms:

- Slow wound healing
- Low resistance to infection
- Obesity
- Acne
- Moon-shaped face
- Easily-bruised skin
- Weak or wasted muscles
- Osteoporosis

Although Cushing's disease can be caused by a malfunction in the pituitary, it is usually triggered by excessive use of immune-suppressing corticosteroid medications—such as those used for asthma and arthritis. Once these are discontinued, the disease often abates.

Single Oils:
Lemon, peppermint, fleabane, nutmeg

Blends:
ImmuPower, Thieves, Endoflex

EO Applications:
TOPICAL:
COMPRESS, warm, over adrenal area (on back, over kidneys)
INGESTION:
CAPSULE, 00 size, 2 daily

Dietary Supplementation:
Exodus, ImmuPro, ImmuneTune

AGE-RELATED MACULAR DEGENERATION (AMD)

AMD is one of the most common causes of blindness among people over 60 years of age. In fact 30% of all people over 70 years of age suffer to some degree from this disease. The most common form of the disease is DRY in which macular cells degenerate irreversibly. The WET form of the disease is marked by abnormal blood vessel growth that results in macula-damaging blood leaks. The disease results in a steady loss of central vision until eyesight is totally impaired.

For dry AMD, the best prevention will be foods rich in antioxidants and carotenoids. The Ningxia wolfberry, the highest known antioxidant food, is also extremely high in lutein, which is vital for preserving eye health. Other foods rich in carotenoids that are also powerful antioxidants include blueberries and spinach. Clove oil, the highest known antioxidant nutrient, can also be a front line treatment.

Single Oils:
Clove

Blends:
Longevity

EO Applications:
Capsule, 00 size, 1 daily

Dietary Supplementation:
Longevity Capsules, ImmuPro, Berry Young Juice, Wolfberry Crisp, Super C Chewable

AGENT ORANGE EXPOSURE

Single Oils:
Ledum, German chamomile, carrot seed

Blends:
JuvaFlex, JuvaCleanse, EndoFlex

EO Applications:
TOPICAL:
NEAT, 4-6 drops JuvaFlex, JuvaCleanse over liver area and 2-4 drops of EndoFlex over adrenal gland area, 2 times daily
COMPRESS, warm, over liver area, 1-2 times daily

Dietary Supplementation:
ImmuPro, ImmuneTune, Cleansing Trio, JuvaTone, Thyromin

Other:
The following is a regimen for liver cleansing support to aid in relieving effects of toxic exposure:

- Essentialzyme: 3 servings daily
- ComforTone, ICP, and JuvaTone: 3 servings daily
- ImmuneTune: 4 servings daily
- Rub 3 drops EndoFlex on the thyroid (hollow at base-front of neck) and 3 drops over the kidneys 3 times daily. Also rub 3 drops on the thyroid and kidney Vita Flex points of the feet.
- After 90 days on the program, gradually reduce the above amounts but stay on the program for a full year.
- Add 1 cup Epsom salts and 4 ounces of 35 percent food-grade hydrogen peroxide to bath water once daily.
- Take a 30-minute bath with 6 cups of Epsom salts per tub of water. Drink 3 glasses of Master Cleanse lemonade (see Chapter 24) and 1 ounce of Berry Young Juice while bathing.

AGITATION

Single Oils:
Lavender, orange, Roman chamomile

Blends:
Peace & Calming, Forgiveness, Surrender, Joy

EO Applications:
INHALATION:
DIFFUSION, 15 min. every 2 hours, as needed
DIRECT, 2-3 times per day, as needed
TOPICAL:
NEAT, 1-2 drops on temples and/or back of neck
VITA FLEX, 1-2 drops on brain and heart points

Dietary Supplementation:
Super B, Super C, Super C Chewable, Super Cal.

AIDS (Acquired Immune Deficiency Syndrome)

The AIDS virus attacks and infects immune cells that are essential for life.

Essential oils such as lemon, cistus, thyme, and lavender have immune building properties. Other oils like cumin *(Cuminum cyminum)* have an inhibitory effect on viral replication. In May 1994, Dr. Radwan Farag of Cairo University demonstrated that cumin seed oil had an 88 to 92 percent inhibition effect against HIV, the virus responsible for AIDS. Other antiviral essential oils include oregano, frankincense, sandalwood, grapefruit, and tsuga.

Single Oils:
Cistus, lemon, cumin, blue cypress, sandalwood, tsuga, grapefruit, myrrh, frankincense

Blends:
Brain Power, Exodus II, Valor, Thieves, ImmuPower

EO Applications:
Essential oil regimen:
1. Valor and Thieves: 4-6 drops on feet daily for 3 weeks
2. Exodus II: 6-8 drops along spine 3 times weekly
3. ImmuPower: 6 drops daily in a capsule
4. Raindrop Technique: 2 times weekly

Dietary Supplementation:
Cleansing Trio, JuvaTone, Rehemogen, Thyromin, ImmuPro, ImmuneTune, VitaGreen, Sulfurzyme, Exodus, Super B, Berry Young Juice, Ultra Young, Mighty Mist

Other:
Supplementation regimen:
1. ImmuPro: Chew 4-8 tablets before going to bed; also take 2 in morning and 2 in afternoon.
2. Cleansing Trio for 120 days with JuvaTone.
3. ImmuGel: 1/2 tsp., 3 times daily. Hold in mouth for better absorption, swallow slowly.
4. Thyromin: Start with 2 at night, 1 in morning.
5. ImmuneTune: 6-8 capsules daily.
6. VitaGreen: 6-10 capsules daily.
7. Sulfurzyme: 1 tablespoon.
8. Exodus: Up to 18 capsules daily.
9. Super B: 1 tablet daily with a meal.

10. Ultra Young: 3 sprays on inside of each cheek, 4-5 times daily.
11. Eat 5-6 mini-meals daily, primarily Power Meal (3 times daily) and fish for protein. Do not eat beef or chicken for first 3-4 weeks to allow more energy for immune building.

ALCOHOLISM

(See also ADDICTIONS)

Single Oils:
Lavender, Roman chamomile, orange, helichrysum, elemi, rosemary

Blends:
JuvaFlex, JuvaCleanse, Forgiveness, Acceptance, Surrender, Motivation, Joy

EO Applications:
INHALATION:
DIFFUSION, 15 min every 2 hours as needed
DIRECT, 2-3 times daily, as needed
TOPICAL:
NEAT, 1-2 drops on temples and/or back of neck 4 times daily
COMPRESS, warm, over liver

Dietary Supplementation:
JuvaTone, JuvaPower/Spice, Cleansing Trio, Thyromin, Power Meal, Detoxyme, Mega Cal, Mineral Essence

ALKALOSIS

(See also ACIDOSIS)

Alkalosis is a condition where the pH of the intestinal tract and the blood becomes excessively alkaline. While moderate alkalinity is essential for good health, excessive alkalinity can cause problems and result in fatigue, depression, irritability, and sickness.

The best solution is to lower, or acidify, the internal pH of the body using a high protein diet. Ultrafiltered whey is the best solution for excess alkalinity (it is contained in Wheyfit). Rudolf Wiley, Ph.D., recommends courses of action to accomplish this in *BioBalance: The Acid/Alkaline Solution to the Food-Mood-Health Puzzle.*

Single Oils:
Ginger, tarragon, anise

Blends:
Di-Tone

EO Applications:
INGESTION:
CAPSULE, 00 Size, 2 daily between meals, if possible, otherwise with meals

Dietary Supplementation:
Essentialzyme, Sulfurzyme, WheyFit, Wolfberry Crisp

ALLERGIES

Allergies can be triggered by food, pollen, environmental chemicals, dander, dust, and insect bites and can impact:

Respiration—wheezing, labored breathing
Mouth—swelling of the lips or tongue, itching lips
Digestive tract—diarrhea, vomiting, cramps
Skin—rashes, dermatitis
Nose—sneezing, congestion

Food Allergies

Food *allergies* are different from food *intolerances*. The former involve an immune system reaction, whereas the latter involves a gastrointestinal reaction (and is far more common). For example, peanuts often produce a lifelong allergy in adults due to peanut proteins being targeted by immune system antibodies as foreign invaders. In contrast, intolerance of pasteurized cow's milk that causes cramping and diarrhea is due to the inability to digest lactose (milk sugar) because of a lack of the enzyme lactase.

Food allergies are often associated with the consumption of peanuts, shellfish, nuts, wheat, cow's milk, eggs, and soy. Infants and children are far more susceptible to food allergies than adults, due to the immaturity of their immune and digestive systems.

A thorough intestinal cleansing is one of the best ways to combat most allergies. Start with the Cleansing Trio and JuvaTone.

Hay fever (allergic rhinitis)

Hay fever is an allergic reaction triggered by airborne allergens (pollen, animal hair, feathers, dust mites) that cause the release of histamines and subsequent inflammation of nasal passages and sinus-related areas. Allergies resemble asthma, which manifests in the chest and lungs.

Symptoms: Inflammation of the nasal passages, sinuses, and eyelids that causes sneezing, runny nose, watery, red, itchy eyes, and wheezing.

Single Oils:
Lavender, ledum, German chamomile, Roman chamomile

Blends:
Harmony, Valor, Juva Cleanse

EO Applications:
INHALATION:
>DIFFUSION, 15 min every 2 hours, as needed
>DIRECT, 2-4 times daily, as needed

INGESTION:
>CAPSULE, 00 size, 2 times daily

Dietary Supplementation:
Sulfurzyme, Detoxzyme, Essentialzyme, Polyzyme, VitaGreen, Cleansing Trio, JuvaTone

ALOPECIA AREATA (Hair Loss)

Alopecia is an inflammatory hair-loss disease that is the second-leading cause of baldness in the U.S. A randomized, double-blind study at the Aberdeen Royal Infirmary in Scotland found that certain essential oils were extremely effective in combating this disease. [5,6]

Single Oils:
Thyme, rosemary, lavender, cedarwood

EO Applications:
TOPICAL:
>DILUTE 20-80, (5 drops essential oils in 20 drops olive, grapeseed or fractionated coconut oil). Massage into scalp before sleep nightly

2-4 drops in 1-2 tsp shampoo

ALUMINUM TOXICITY

(See METAL TOXICITY, Aluminum)

ALZHEIMER'S

(See BRAIN DISORDERS)

ANALGESIC

An 'analgesic' is defined as a compound that binds with a number of closely related specific receptors in the central nervous system to block the perception of pain or affect the emotional response to pain. A number of essential oils have analgesic properties.

Single Oils:
Peppermint, elemi, wintergreen, clove, lavender, lemongrass, Idaho tansy

Blends:
PanAway, Thieves

Additional simple blends for pain relief:
1. Equal parts helichrysum and clove
2. Equal parts tea tree and rosemary
3. Equal parts wintergreen, spruce and black pepper
4. 3 parts tea tree with 5 parts rosemary

EO Applications:
TOPICAL:
>DILUTE 50-50, apply 4-6 drops on location, as needed

Topical Treatments:
Peppermint Cedarwood Moisturizing Bar Soap can be a topical treatment for mild pain.

ANEMIA

(See BLOOD DISORDERS)

ANEURYSM

(See also CARDIOVASCULAR CONDITIONS)

Aneurysms are weak spots on the blood vessel wall which balloon out and may eventually rupture. In cases of brain aneurysms, a bursting

5. Hay, Jamieson, Ormerod "Randomized trial of aromatherapy. Successful treatment for alopecia areata." *Archives of Dermatology.* 1998 Nov;134(11):1349-52.

6. Kalish, Gilhar "Alopecia areata: autoimmunity--the evidence is compelling." *The Journal of Investigative Dermatology Symposium Proceedings* 2003 Oct;8(2):164-7.

blood vessel can cause a hemorrhagic stroke, which can result in death or paralysis (with a fatality rate of over 50 percent).

See your physician for treatment immediately if you have, or suspect you have, an aneurysm.

Some essential oils and nutritional supplements support the cardiovascular system. Cypress strengthens capillary and vascular walls. Helichrysum helps dissolve blood clots.

Single Oils:
Helichrysum, sandalwood, Idaho tansy, cypress

Blends:
Aroma Life, Brain Power

Aneurysm blend:
- 5 drops of frankincense
- 1 drop helichrysum
- 1 drop cypress

EO Applications:
TOPICAL:
 DILUTE 50-50, on affected area 3-5 times daily
INHALATION:
 DIFFUSION, 15 minutes, 4-6 times daily
INGESTION:
 CAPSULE, 00 size, 2 times daily

Dietary Supplementation:
Ultra Young, Essential Manna, Rehemogen

ANGINA

(See HEART)

ANOREXIA

(See ADDICTIONS)

While psychotherapy remains indispensable, the inhalation of essential oils may alter emotions enough to effect a change in the underlying psychology or disturbed-thinking patterns which supports this self-destructive behavior. This is accomplished by the ability of fragrance to directly impact the emotional hub inside the brain known as the limbic system. Essential oils such as lemon and ginger when inhaled regularly can combat the emotional addiction that leads anorexics to premature death.

Many people with anorexia believe they don't deserve to be healthy or loved unless they are "slender."

Anorexia nervosa is an eating disorder characterized by total avoidance of food and virtual self-starvation. It may or may not be accompanied by bulimia (binge-purge behavior).

Many anorexics suffer life-threatening nutrient and mineral deficiencies. The lack of magnesium and potassium can actually trigger heart rhythm abnormalities and cardiac arrest. Replacement of calcium, magnesium, potassium, and other minerals is absolutely essential for this condition.

Single Oils:
Tarragon, mandarin, orange, lemon, ginger

Blends:
Christmas Spirit, Valor, Citrus Fresh, Motivation, Brain Power

EO Applications:
INHALATION:
 DIFFUSION, 15 minutes every 2 hours
 DIRECT, 2-3 times daily, as needed
TOPICAL:
 NEAT, 1-2 drops on temples and/or back of neck 4 times daily
 COMPRESS, warm, over liver area

Dietary Supplementation:
Ultra Young, Super Cal, BodyGize, Mineral Essence

ANTHRAX

(See INFECTIONS)

Caused by the bacteria *Bacillus anthracis,* anthrax is one of the oldest and deadliest diseases known. There are three predominant types: the **external** form acquired from contact with infected animal carcasses, the **internal** form is obtained from breathing airborne anthrax spores, and **battlefield anthrax**, which is a far more lethal variety of internal anthrax that was developed for biological warfare. When the airborne variety of anthrax invades and lungs, it is 90 percent fatal unless antibiotics are administered at the very beginning of the infection. Often anthrax goes undiagnosed until it is too late for antibiotics.

External varieties of anthrax may be contracted by exposure to animal hides and wool. While vaccination and antibiotics have stemmed anthrax infection in recent years, new strains have developed that are resistant to all counter measures.

According to Jean Valnet, M.D., thyme oil is effective for killing the anthrax bacillus.[7] Two highly antimicrobial phenols in thyme, carvacrol and thymol, are responsible for this action.

Single Oils:
Thyme, oregano, clove, cinnamon, rosewood

Blends:
Thieves, Exodus II

EO Applications:
TOPICAL:
　　DILUTE 20-80, on hands and exposed
　　skin areas
INHALATION:
　　DIFFUSION, 5 minutes 4-6 times daily to
　　purify air
INGESTION:
　　CAPSULE, 00 size, 4 times daily

Dietary Supplementation:
Exodus, ImmuneTune, Super C Chewable

Other:
Topical treatments to help prevent contracting or spreading anthrax include Thieves Cleansing Bar Soap, Thieves Household Cleaner, Thieves Spray and Thieves Wipes.

ANTIBIOTIC REACTIONS

Synthetic antibiotic drugs indiscriminately kill both beneficial and harmful bacteria. This can result in yeast infections (including candida), diarrhea, poor nutrient assimilation, fatigue, degenerative diseases, and many other conditions and symptoms.

The average adult has 3-4 pounds of beneficial bacteria permanently residing in the intestines. These beneficial flora:
• Constitute the first line of defense against bacterial and viral infection
• Produce B vitamins
• Maintain pH balance

• Combat yeast and fungus overgrowth
• Aid in the digestive process

Dietary Supplementation:
Wolfberry Crisp bars.

During antibiotic treatment, take 2-3 servings of acidophilus daily on an empty stomach before meals. After completing antibiotic treatment, continue using acidophilus for 10-15 days.

ANTISEPTIC

Antiseptics prevent the growth of pathogenic microorganisms. Many essential oils have powerful antiseptic properties. Clove and thyme essential oils have been documented to kill over 50 types of bacteria and 10 types of fungi. Other potent antiseptics include, cinnamon/cassia oil, tea tree, oregano, and mountain savory.

Single Oils:
Thyme, clove, oregano, rosemary, manuka, tea tree, mountain savory, eucalyptus (all types), lavandin, cinnamon, cassia, ravensara

Blends:
Purification, Melrose, Christmas Spirit, Thieves, ImmuPower, Raven, R.C.

EO Applications:
TOPICAL:
　　DILUTE, According to application code
　　(see Appendix E) and apply to affected
　　area 2-10 times daily as needed

Other:
Skin Care: Thieves Bar Soap, Melaleuca Rosewood Bar Soap, Thieves Antiseptic Spray, Thieves Wipes, Rose Ointment

APNEA

Apnea is a temporary cessation of breathing during sleep. It can degrade the quality of sleep resulting in chronic fatigue, lowered immune function, and lack of energy.

Blends:
Clarity, Surrender, Valor

7.　Jean Valnet, MD, "The Practice of Aromatherapy: A Classic Compendium of Plant Medicines & Their Healing Properties," *Healing Arts Press*, 1990, p. 197.

EO Applications:
INHALATION:
DIFFUSION, in the bedroom throughout the night while sleeping
TOPICAL:
NEAT, 2-4 drops on soles of feet just before bedtime

Dietary Supplementation:
VitaGreen, Super B, Thyromin

Supplementation regimen for apnea:
- Three VitaGreen capsules 2 times daily.
- One Super B 3 times daily with meals.
- Two Thyromin capsules at bedtime.

APPETITE, LOSS OF

Ginger has been shown to stimulate digestion and improve appetite.

Single Oils:
Ginger, spearmint, orange, nutmeg

Blends:
Inner Child, Citrus Fresh, Christmas Spirit

EO Applications:
INHALATION:
DIFFUSION, 10 min., 3-5 times daily
DIRECT, 3-5 times daily, as needed
INGESTION:
CAPSULE, 00 size, 1 times daily

Supplements:
Essentialzyme, Polyzyme, ComforTone

ARTERIOSCLEROSIS

This condition is defined as any one of a group of diseases which causes a thickening and a loss of elasticity of arterial walls. It can be caused by inflammation and is frequently an underlying cause of heart attack or stroke.

Single Oils:
Helichrysum, clove, nutmeg, cypress, frankincense

Blends:
Longevity, Aroma Life

EO Applications:
INGESTION:
CAPSULE, 00 size, 2 times daily

Dietary Supplementation:
AD&E, Longevity Capsules, Essential Omegas, Chelex, JuvaTone, JuvaPower/Spice, Rehemogen

ARTHRITIS

Osteoarthritis

Osteoarthritis involves the breakdown of the cartilage that forms a cushion between two joints. As this cartilage is eaten away, the two bones of the joint start rubbing together and wearing down. In contrast, rheumatoid arthritis is caused from a swelling and inflammation of the synovial membrane, the lining of the joint.

Natural anti-inflammatories (blue chamomile, wintergreen) combined with cartilage builders (glucosamine/chondroitin) are powerful natural cures for arthritis. The best natural anti-inflammatories include fats rich in omega-3s (like flax seed oil, the key ingredient in Essential Omegas) and essential oils such as nutmeg, wintergreen, German (blue) chamomile, and balsam fir. The best cartilage builders include Type II collagen and glucosamine (contained in BLM powder).

Nutmeg, a source of myristicin, has been researched for its anti-inflammatory effects in several studies. It works by inhibiting pro-inflammatory prostaglandins when taken internally or applied topically. Clove exhibits similar action.

Chamazulene, the blue sesquiterpene in German chamomile, also shows strong anti-inflammatory activity when used both topically and orally.

Methyl salicylate, a major component of wintergreen, is a chemical cousin to the active agent in aspirin and also has strong anti-inflammatory and analgesic properties.

Glucosamine and chondroitin are the two most powerful natural compounds for rebuilding cartilege and are the key ingredients in the supplement BLM.

Single Oils:
Wintergreen, nutmeg, clove, German chamomille, helichrysum, Idaho balsam fir, Douglas fir, white fir, spruce, pine, cypress, peppermint, vetiver, marjoram, rosemary CT cineol, *Eucalyptus citriodora*, basil, oregano, lemongrass, Idaho tansy, black pepper, elemi, lavander

Blends:
PanAway, Relieve It, Aroma Siez, Ortho Ease, Ortho Sport. (PanAway and Relieve It have cortisone-like action, which give relief of arthritic pain without the cortisone side effects.)

EO Applications:
Dilute 5-10 drops essential oils in 1 tsp. V6 Oil Complex and apply on location. Essential oils can also be applied neat, then followed by application of V6 Oil Complex or AromaSilk Satin Body Lotion.

Dietary Supplementation:
BLM, Essential Omegas, Super Cal, Longevity Capsules, ArthroTune, ImmuneTune, Sulfurzyme, Mega Cal

Supplementation regiment of osteoarthritis:
- BLM: 2-4 capsules, 2 times daily
- Super Cal: 2-3 capsules, 2 times daily
- Essential Omegas: 2 droppers, 3 times daily
- ArthroTune: 2-6 capsules, 3 times daily
- ImmuneTune: 2-3 capsules, 3 times daily

Detoxification of the body and strengthening the joints is important. Cleanse the colon and liver. Rehemogen cleans and purifies the blood which may have toxins blocking nutrient and oxygen absorption into cells (see CIRCULATION).

Apply oils on location followed by massage oil or AromaSilk Satin Body Lotion.

Other:
Regenolone is an excellent companion personal care product to support the joints.

Rheumetoid Arthritis

Rheumatoid arthritis is a painful inflammatory condition of the joints marked by swelling, thickening, and inflammation of the synovial membrane lining the joint. (In contrast, osteoarthritis is characterized by a breakdown of the joint cartilage without any swelling or inflammation.)

Rheumatoid arthritis is classified as an autoimmune disease because it is caused by the body's own immune system attacking the joints.

Other factors can aggravate arthritis such as:
- Deficiencies of minerals and other nutrients
- Microbes and toxins
- Lack of water intake

Essential oils constitute some of the most effective treatments for combating arthritis pain and combating infection in cases where it is present. Peppermint has been studied for its ability to kill pain by blocking substance P and calcium channels.[8]

In cases where arthritis is caused by infectious organisms, such as *Borrelia burgdorferi, (Lyme Disease) Chlamydia,* and *Salmonella,* essential oils may counteract and prevent infection, especially when diffused or applied topically. Highly antimicrobial essential oils include: mountain savory, rosemary, *Melaleuca alternifolia* (tea tree), and oregano. The oils can pass into the bloodstream when applied topically.

Additionally, MSM has been documented to be one of the most effective natural supplements for reducing the pain associated with rheumatism and arthritis. The subject of a number of clinical studies, MSM was used extensively by Ronald Lawrence, M.D., in his clinical practice to successfully treat rheumatism and arthritis. MSM is the key ingredient in the supplement Sulfurzyme.

Also, glucosamine and chondroitin are some of the most powerful natural compounds for reducing inflammation, halting the progression of arthritis and rebuilding cartilage. These are the key ingredients in the supplement BLM.

---

8. Gobel et al., "Effect of peppermint and eucalyptus oil preparations on neurophysiological and experimental algesimetric headache parameters." Cephalalgia. 1994 Jun;14(3):228-34; discussion 182.

Single Oils:
Peppermint, wintergreen, oregano, Idaho balsam fir, helichrysum, nutmeg, clove, vetiver, marjoram, cypress, mountain savory, Idaho tansy, valerian,

Blends:
PanAway, Relieve It, Aroma Siez, Peace & Calming, Sacred Mountain, Melrose

EO Applications:
TOPICAL:
> DILUTE according to application code (see Appendix E) and apply to affected area 1-3 times daily, as needed
> COMPRESS, Cold, 1-2 times daily

INGESTION:
> CAPSULE, 00 size, 2 times daily

Dietary Supplementation:
Sulfurzyme, BLM, Essential Omegas, Super Cal, Longevity Caps, ArthroTune, Mega Cal

Topical Treatments:
Regenolone, Peppermint Cedarwood and Morning Start Bar Soap, Ortho Ease, Ortho Sport Massage Oil, Morning Start Bath Gel

ASTHMA

During an asthma attack, the bronchials (air tubes) in the lungs become swollen and clogged with a thick, sticky mucus. The muscles of the air tubes will also begin to constrict or tighten. This results in very difficult or labored breathing. If an attack is severe, it can actually be life-threatening.

Many asthma attacks are triggered by an allergic reaction to pollen, skin particles, dandruff, cat or dog dander, dust mites, and foods such as eggs, milk, flavorings, dyes, and preservatives. Asthma can also be triggered by respiratory infection, exercise, stress, and psychological factors.

(See ALLERGIES)

Single Oils:
ravansara, Roman chamomile, *Eucalyptus polybractea, Eucalyptus radiata*, Idaho balsam fir, spruce, pine, myrtle, peppermint, thyme, lemon, lavender, juniper, frankincense, marjoram, rose, mountain savory

Blends:
Melrose, Di-Tone, Purification, Thieves, Raven, R.C., Inspiration, Sacred Mountain

EO Applications:
TOPICAL:
> NEAT, 2-4 drops to soles of feet
> 2-3 times daily

INGESTION:
> CAPSULE, 00 size, 2 times daily

Essential oils should not be inhaled for asthma-related problems. The oils should be applied to the soles of the feet or ingested (if they are GRAS – Generally Regarded As Safe--see Appendix C)

Dietary Supplementation:
ImmuGel, VitaGreen, ImmuneTune, Ultra Young, Essentialzyme, Carbozyme

ATHLETE'S FOOT

(See FOOT PROBLEMS)

ATTENTION DEFICIT DISORDER (ADD and ADHD)

Terry Friedmann, MD has recently completed pioneering studies using essential oils to combat ADD and ADHD. Using twice a day inhalation of essential oils including vetiver, cedarwood, and lavender, Dr. Friedmann was able to achieve clinically significant results in 60 days. Researchers postulate that essential oils mitigate ADD and ADHD through their stimulation on the limbic system of the brain.

Because attention deficit disorder may be caused by mineral deficiencies in the diet, increasing nutrient intake and absorption of magnesium, potassium, and other trace minerals can also have a significant beneficial effect in resolving ADD.

Single Oils:
Vetiver, lavender, sandalwood, cardamom, cedarwood, peppermint, ledum,

Blends:
Brain Power, Joy, Peace & Calming, Clarity, Longevity

EO Applications:
INHALATION:
> DIFFUSION, 15 min. 4-8 times daily
> DIRECT, 4-8 times daily

Dietary Supplementation: Mineral Essence, Essential Manna, Wolfberry Crisp, Essential Omegas, Berry Young Juice, Power Meal.

AUTISM

(See Attention Deficit Disorder)

Improving diet can be the key to ameliorating cases of autism. Replacing high glycemic sweeteners (ie. sugar) with low-glycemic sweeteners (ie. Blue Agave nectar,) has produced outstanding results in numerous cases of autism.

Autism is a neurologically based developmental disorder that is four times more common in boys than girls. It is characterized by:

- Social ineptness (loner)
- Nonverbal and verbal communication difficulties
- Repetitive behavior (rocking, hair twirling)
- Self injurious behavior (head-banging)
- Very limited or peculiar interests
- Reduced or abnormal responses to pain, noises, or other outside stimuli

Autism is being increasingly linked to certain vaccinations, the MMR being most often cited by researchers. British researcher Andrew Wakefield, MD, suggests single shots for children for measles, mumps and rubella (instead of the combined MMR shot) until further research is done.

Until very recently, children were receiving large doses of mercury (from thimerosal, a vaccine preservative that contains 49.6% mercury) that were well above the limit recommended by the EPA, through vaccination. Some success in reversing autism has resulted through mercury detoxification along with nutritional supplementation.

Some researchers believe that gastrointestinal disorders may be linked to the brain dysfunctions that cause autism in children (Horvath et al., 1998). In fact, there have been several cases of successful treatment of autism using pancreatic enzymes.

Stimulation of the limbic region of the brain may also help treat autism. Aromas from essential oils have a powerful ability to stimulate this part of the brain since the sense of smell (olfaction) is tied directly into the mind's emotional and hormonal centers. As a result the aroma of an essential oil has the potential to exert a powerful influence on disorders such as ADD and autism.

Single Oils:
Vetiver, frankincense, sandalwood, *Eucalyptus globulus*, melissa, cedarwood

Blends: Valor, Brain Power, Clarity, Peace & Calming

EO Application:
INHALATION:
DIFFUSION, 15 min. 4-6 times daily
DIRECT, 4-6 times daily

Dietary Supplementation:
Essentialzyme, Essential Omegas, Polyzyme, ImmuPro, Berry Young Juice, Wolfberry Crisp Bar, Power Meal

BACK INJURIES AND PAIN

(See SPINE INJURIES AND PAIN)

BALDNESS

(see also ALOPECIA AREATA)

Male pattern baldness is often a result of excess conversion of testosterone to dihydrotestosterone through the enzyme 5-alpha reductase. It can also be caused by an inflammatory condition called alopecia areata.

Single Oils:
Fleabane, rosemary, peppermint, black pepper

EO Applications:
TOPICAL:
DILUTE 20-80, massage into scalp before retiring. (For this application, fractionated coconut oil is recommended as the diluting oil. It's finer structure is more readily absorbed into the scalp.)

BED WETTING

Blends:
Valor, Acceptance, Harmony

EO Applications:
INHALATION:
DIFFUSION, during then night, as needed
TOPICAL:
NEAT, 2-4 drops on soles of feet before bedtime

Dietary Supplementation:
K&B

Use K&B tincture once in the afternoon and once before bedtime (2 droppers maximum).

BELL'S PALSY

(See NERVE DISORDERS)

BENIGN PROSTATE HYPERPLASIA (BPH)

(See PROSTATE PROBLEMS)

BITES

(See INSECT BITES or SNAKE BITES)

BLADDER INFECTION

(See URINARY/BLADDER INFECTION)

BLEEDING

(See HEMORRHAGING)

BLEEDING GUMS

(See ORAL CARE)

BLISTERS and BOILS

Blisters are created when fluid is trapped under the skin. They can be caused by physical injury (ie., chemical burns, sunburns) or microbial infestation (ie., fungal and viral diseases such as Herpes simplex, athlete's foot, etc.).

Boils (carbuncles are groups of boils) are caused by bacterial infection which creates a pus-filled hair follicle. They are easily treated with antiseptic essential oils including melaleuca and clove.

Blisters

Single Oils:
Lavender, sandalwood, melissa, cistus, tea tree, frankincense, lavender, Roman or German chamomile

Blends:
Purification, Inspiration, Melrose

EO Applications:
TOPICAL:
DILUTE 50-50, apply to blistered area 3-5 times daily, as needed

Topical Treatments:
Lavaderm.

Boils

Single Oils: Clove, thyme, oregano, tea tree, melaleuca ericifolia, manuka, cassia, cinnamon bark.

Blends:
Purification, Melrose, Exodus II, Thieves

EO Applications:
TOPICAL:
DILUTE 50-50, 2-3 drops on location 3-6 times daily

BLOATING

(See also MENSTRUAL CONDITIONS)

Bloating is usually a result of hormonal or mineral imbalances that trigger excess fluid retention in the body. One of the best natural remedies is progesterone, which is added to creams and absorbed transdermally.

Single Oils:
Tarragon, peppermint, juniper, fennel, clary sage

Blends:
Di-Tone

EO Applications:
TOPICAL:
> NEAT, 2-4 drops on soles of feet 2-3 times daily

INGESTION:
> Capsules, 00 size, 1 times daily

Dietary Supplementation:
Essentialzyme, Polyzyme, PD80/20

Other:
Progessence Cream

BLOOD CLOTS

(See also CIRCULATION DISORDERS and CARDIOVASCULAR CONDITIONS)

As people age, the viscosity or thickness of the blood increases and also the tendency of the blood to clot excessively.

If blood clots (also known as embolisms) occur in the brain, they cause strokes; if they obstruct a coronary artery, they cause ischemic heart attacks.

People with diabetes or high blood pressure are far more likely to die from blood clots.

Natural blood thinners, such as clove oil, wintergreen oil, and nutmeg oil can be highly effective. These oils also are some of the most powerful antioxidants known and can slow the formation of oxidized cholesterol and foam cells that are implicated in atherosclerosis. Helichrysum is also effective for preventing blood clot formation and promoting the dissolution of clots.

Foods rich in vitamin E and omega-3 fats are vital for regular use in the diet.

Single Oils:
Helichrysum, clove, nutmeg, lemon, orange, grapefruit, tangerine, lemon. cistus

Blends:
Thieves, PanAway, Longevity

EO Applications:
TOPICAL:
> DILUTE 50-50, on location 4-6 times daily
> COMPRESS, warm, 15 min., 2 times daily
> Massage equal parts lemon, lavender and helichrysum on location, with or without hot packs

INGESTION:
> CAPSULE, 00 size, 2 times daily between meals (this works especially well with helichrysum and cistus
> RICE MILK, 2 times daily

Dietary Supplementation:
AD&E, Essential Omegas, Longevity Caps, Thieves, Essential Manna, Berry Young Juice

Other:
Dentarome Toothpastes (all varieties) contain clove oil, a natural blood thinner

BLOOD DISORDERS

(See also CIRCULATION DISORDERS and CARDIOVASCULAR CONDITIONS)

Anemia

Anemia is a condition caused from the lack of red blood cells (or a lack of properly functioning ones). Nutritional deficiencies such as the lack of adequate iron or vitamin B12 can contribute to this disorder.

Anemia also may be caused by improper liver function. In such cases, a liver cleanse and liver nutritional support may be effective for rebuilding red blood cell counts.

There can be many different causes of anemia. You should see your physician for proper diagnosis if you suspect anemia.

Single Oils:
Lemon, lemongrass, spikenard, helichrysum

Blends:
Aroma Life, JuvaFlex, Juva Cleanse

EO Applications:
TOPICAL:
> NEAT, 2-3 drops on Vita Flex points of feet, or on inside of wrists, 2-3 times daily

INGESTION:
> CAPSULE, 00 size, 2 times daily

Dietary Supplementation:
Super B, Master Formula Vitamins, Rehemogen, Mineral Essence, JuvaTone, JuvaPower/Spice, VitaGreen, Chelex

Blood Platelets (Low)

Dietary Supplementation:
Rehemogen

To enhance effects of Rehemogen use with JuvaTone, JuvaPower/Spice

Blood Detoxification

Detoxified blood results in better nutrient and oxygen flow and is the key to begin combating many diseases.

Single Oils:
Helichrysum, German chamomile, Roman chamomile, rosemary, geranium, orange, lemon, cardemom

Blends:
Di-Tone, JuvaFlex, JuvaCleanse, Exodus, EndoFlex

EO Applications:
TOPICAL:
NEAT, 2-3 drops on Vita Flex points of feet, or on inside of wrists, 2-3 times daily
INGESTION:
CAPSULE, 00 size, 2 times daily

Dietary Supplementation:
VitaGreen, Rehemogen, Chelex, JuvaPower/Spice, AlkaLime, Sulfurzyme

Rehemogen helps with most types of blood disorders including toxemia and blood toxicity.

Chelex helps remove heavy metals from the blood system. Use with cardamom and JuvaTone.

MSM (found in Sulfurzyme) purifies the body and blood.

Blood Circulation (Poor)

Single Oils:
Helichrysum, lemongrass, clove, nutmeg, balsam fir, orange, lemon, cistus

Blends:
Citrus fresh, Longevity, R.C., Valor, Thieves

EO Applications:
TOPICAL:
NEAT, 2-3 drops on Vita Flex points of feet, or on inside of wrists, 2-3 times daily

INGESTION:
CAPSULE, 00 size, 2 times daily

Dietary Supplementation:
Super B, Longevity Caps, Wolfberry Crisp

Essential oils when used regularly can improve circulation as much as 20 percent.

BLOOD PRESSURE, HIGH (Hypertension)

(See CARDIOVASCULAR CONDITIONS)

BLOOD PRESSURE, LOW (Hypotension)

(See CARDIOVASCULAR CONDITIONS)

BONE (Bruised, Broken)

Single Oils:
Helichrysum, wintergreen, peppermint, spruce, Idaho balsam fir, white fir, pine, cypress, rosemary, basil, elemi, Idaho tansy, lemongrass, clove, ginger

Blends:
Aroma Siez, PanAway, Peace & Calming, Aroma Life, Relieve It, Melrose, Sacred Mountain

Another blend for bone health and healing:
- 8 drops Idaho balsam fir
- 6 drops helichrysum
- 1 drop oregano
- 1 drop vetiver

Seeing the Big Picture Can Produce Big Results

When selecting oils, particularly for injuries, think through the cause and type of injury and select oils for each segment. For instance, a broken bone could encompass muscle damage, nerve damage, ligament strain or tear, inflammation, infection, bone injury, and possibly an emotion. Select an oil or oils for each perceived problem and apply in rotation or prepare a blend to cover all of them. The emotion may be shock, anger, guilt, or the person may have had pain for a long time and needs to release or relieve it. They may need some joy in their lives, etc. Work through all factors of the injury.

EO Applications:
TOPICAL:
> NEAT or DILUTE 50-50, 2-4 drops on location, 2-4 times daily as needed
> Note: Apply extremely gently if bone break is suspected

Dietary Supplementation:
PD 80/20, Super Cal, Mineral Essence, ArthroTune. Mega Cal, BLM

Other:
Ortho Ease, Ortho Sport, Regenolone, Progessence Cream

Bone Pain (See also ARTHRITIS)

Single Oils:
Wintergreen, spruce, pine, balsam fir, helichrysum

EO Applications:
TOPICAL:
> NEAT, 2-4 drops on location, 2-5 times daily as needed

Dietary Supplementation:
Ultra Young, ArthroTune, Essential Manna, BodyGize, Power Meal, Super Cal, Sulfurzyme. Mega Cal, BLM

Poor bone and muscle development can indicate HGH and/or potassium deficiency.

Broken Bones

A health professional should always be involved in the diagnosis and setting of a broken bone or a suspected broken bone.

Blend:
The following recipe is for a blend which can help speed the bone mending process:
- 10 drops wintergreen
- 3 drops helichrysum
- 2 drops lemongrass
- 3 drops pine
- 4 drops ginger
- 4 drops vetiver

EO Applications:
Prior to casting the broken bone, mix the above oils and very gently apply 2-8 drops (depending on size of area) to break area, neat. If there are any signs of skin sensitivity or irritation, be prepared to apply a small amount of V-6 Oil Complex.

Dietary Supplementation:
ArthroTune, Super Cal, BLM, AD&E, Mega Cal

BRAIN DISORDERS

(See NEUROLOGICAL DISEASES)

The fragrance of many essential oils exerts a powerful stimulus on the limbic system—a part of the brain located on the margin of the cerebral cortex, including the amygdala, hippocampus, and hypophysis which interact directly with the thalamus and hypothalamus. Acting together, these glands and brain components combined are the seat of memory, emotions, and sexual arousal, They also govern aggressive behavior.

The ability of essential oils to pass the blood-brain barrier gives them enormous therapeutic potential against such neurological diseases like Parkinson's, Alzheimer's, Lou Gehrig's, and MS.

Alzheimer's Disease

Over 4 million Americans suffer from Alzheimer's. Alzheimer's was found to nearly double in subjects with high levels of homocysteine in the Framingham Study. Aluminum continues to be linked to Alzheimer's yet older Americans are urged to get yearly flu shots which contain aluminum as an adjuvant. Pepper, grapefruit and fennel oils have been found to stimulate brain activity[9]. Peppermint oil has been helpful in protecting against stresses and toxins in brain cells.[10]

Dr. Richard Restick, a leading neurologist in Washington, D.C., stated that maintaining normal synaptic firing would forestall many types of neurological deterioration in the body.

---

9. Haze S, Sakai K, Gozu Y, "Effects of fragrance on sympathetic activity in normal adults," *Jpn J Pharmacol* 2002 Nov;903):247-53.

10. Koo HN et al., "Inhibition of heat shock-induced apoptosis by peppermint oil in astrocytes," *J Mol Neurosci* 2001 Dec;17(3):391-6.

Right Brain vs. Left Brain

The left brain is logical, rational, and judgmental. The right brain is artistic and creative.

Essential oils are believed to heighten right brain activity while increasing left brain integration.

Essential oils high in sesquiterpenes, such as vetiver, cedarwood, patchouli, German chamomile, myrrh, melissa, and sandalwood, are known to cross the blood-brain barrier. The following oils are general cerebral stimulants:

Single Oils:
Cedarwood, vetiver, sandalwood, ginger, nutmeg, myrrh, German chamomile, spikenard, *Eucalyptus globulus*, frankincense, melissa, patchouli, fleabane, helichrysum

Helichrysum increases neurotransmitter activity. Nutmeg is a general cerebral stimulant and also has adrenal cortex-like activity.

Blends:
Brain Power, Valor, Aroma Life

EO Applications:
TOPICAL:
> NEAT, As needed, apply 1-2 drops directly onto the brain reflex center. These points include the forehead, temples, and mastoids (the bones just behind the ears). Apply oils and mild direct pressure to the brainstem area (center top of neck at base of skull) and work down the spine.
> VITA FLEX, apply 1-2 drops to brain points on feet 1-2 times daily
> RAINDROP Technique once every two weeks. You can also apply 3-6 drops essential oils to a natural bristle brush (essential oils may dissolve plastic bristles). Rub and brush vigorously along the brain stem and spine.

Dietary Supplementation: JuvaTone, JuvaPower/Spice, VitaGreen, Chelex, AD&E, Power Meal, AminoTech, Essential Omegas, WheyFit, Sulfurzyme

Impaired Concentration

Single Oils:
Basil, lemon, peppermint, bergamot, cardomom, rosemry, clary sage, frankincense

Blends:
Brain Power, Clarity, Harmony, Valor

EO Applications:
TOPICAL:
> NEAT, apply 1-2 drops to brain reflex centers (see above application), as needed

INHALATION:
> DIRECT, 2-4 times daily, as needed

Impaired Memory

Single Oils:
Peppermint, rosemary, basil, vetiver, rose, lemon, lemongrass, cardamom

Peppermint improves mental concentration and memory. Dr. Dember conducted a study at the University of Cincinnati in 1994 showing that inhaling peppermint increased mental accuracy by 28 percent.[11]

The fragrance of diffused oils, such as lemon, have also been reported to increase memory retention and recall.

Blends:
Brain Power, Clarity, M-Grain, En-R-Gee

Memory blend Recipe #1:
- 5 drops basil
- 10 drops rosemary
- 2 drops peppermint
- 4 drops helichrysum

Memory blend Recipe #2:
- 4 drops lavender
- 3 drops geranium
- 3 drops rosewood
- 3 drops rosemary
- 2 drops tangerine
- 1 drops spearmint
- 2 drops Idaho tansy

---

11. Dember, Warm, 1994. USA. Parasuraman, Compendium of Olfactory Research

EO Applications:
TOPICAL:
> DILUTE 50-50, apply 2-3 drops on temples, forehead, mastoids (bone behind ears) and/or brainstem (back of neck), as needed

INHALATION:
> DIRECT, 2-6 times daily, as needed

Dietary Supplementation:
Longevity Caps, Essential Manna, Essential Omegas, Ultra Young, VitaGreen, Mineral Essence

Other:
Vascular cleansing may improve mental function by supporting improved blood flow, boosting distribution of oxygen and nutrients (see VASCULAR CLEANSING).

Mental Fatigue

Single Oils:
Cardamom, rosemary, vetiver, cedarwood, peppermint, frankincense.

Blends:
Brain Power, Acceptance, Clarity.

EO Applications:
TOPICAL:
> NEAT, apply 1-2 drops to brain reflex centers (forehead, temples, mastoids), and/or brain stem (back of neck) as needed

INHALATION:
> DIRECT, as needed

Dietary Supplementation:
Essential Omegas

Stimulate Pineal/Pituitary Gland

Single Oils:
Sandalwood, vetiver, cedarwood, lavender, frankincense.

Blends:
Dream Catcher, Forgiveness, Gathering, Harmony, Humility, 3 Wise Men, ImmuPower

These blends contain frankincense and sandalwood, which help oxygenate the pineal/pituitary gland, thus improving attitude and frequency balance.

Dietary Supplementation:
Ultra Young

Stroke

Two principal kinds of strokes can damage the brain: thrombotic strokes and hemorrhagic strokes. Thrombotic strokes are caused from a blood clot lodging in a cerebral blood vessel and cutting blood supply to a part of the brain. A hemorrhagic stroke is caused by an aneurysm, or a weakness in the blood vessel wall that balloons out and ruptures, spilling blood into the surrounding brain tissue. Strokes are very serious events and if you suspect that you may be susceptible, immediately see a physician.

To reduce your risk of stroke, essential oils can be used topically or as supplements. In particular, the essential oils of clove and nutmeg were found to exert anti-clotting action in clinical trials, and can be used as a preventative measure to reduce the risk of thrombotic stroke.

Thrombotic Strokes

(See BLOOD CLOTS in BLOOD DISORDERS)

Single Oils:
Helichrysum, cypress, juniper, peppermint, clove, lemon, grapefruit, orange, tangerine, nutmeg, cistus

Blends:
Thieves, Longevity, ImmuPower, Aroma Life, Clarity, Brain Power

EO Applications:
TOPICAL:
> DILUTE 50-50, apply 1-3 drops on temples, forehead, mastoids, back of neck and at base of throat just above clavicle notch
> VITA FLEX, apply 1-3 drops on brain points of feet

INGESTION:
> CAPSULE, 00 size, 2 times daily
> RICE MILK, 2 times daily

Dietary Supplementation:
Sulfurzyme, Essential Omegas, Essential Manna, Super Cal

These supplements are rich in essential minerals, fatty acids, and nutrients necessary for regenerating and rebuilding damaged nerve tissues.

Hemorrhagic Strokes

(See also HEMORRHAGING or BRUISING)

The essential oil of cypress may help strengthen vascular walls.

Single Oils: Cypress, helichrysum

EO Applications:
INGESTION:
> CAPSULE, 00 size, 2 times daily
> RICE MILK, 2 times daily

Dietary Supplementation:
Sulfurzyme, Essential Omegas, Essential Manna, Super Cal

BREASTFEEDING

Dry, Cracked Nipples

Single Oils:
Lavender, myrrh, geranium, sandalwood, helichrysum

Blends:
Valor

EO Applications:
TOPICAL:
> DILUTE 50-50 and massage over breast and on Vita Flex points of the feet

Improve Lactation

Single Oils:
Geranium, fennel, sage

Blends:
Joy

EO Applications:
TOPICAL:
> DILUTE 50-50, massage 2-4 drops over breasts and on Vita Flex points of the feet.

Mastitis (Infected Breast)

Single Oils:
Roman chamomile, clove, thyme, rosemary, lavender

EO Applications:
TOPICAL:
> DILUTE 20-80 and massage over breast and on Vita Flex points of the feet.

Breast blend #1:
- 8 Roamn Chamomile
- 8 drops lavender
- 3 drops cypress

Breast blend #2:
- 10 drops tangerine
- 10 drops lavender
- 1 tsp V6 Oil Complex

Massage on the breasts and under armpits twice daily.

BRUISING

(See also BLOOD CLOTS in BLOOD DISORDERS)

Some people bruise easily because the capillary walls are weak and break easily, particularly in the skin. Those who bruise easily may be deficient in vitamin C.

Essential oils can help speed the healing of bruises and reduce the risk of blood clot formation. Oils like cypress help to strengthen capillary walls, while oils like helichrysum help speed the reabsorption of the blood that has collected in the tissue.

Single Oils:
Cypress, helichrysum, white fir, lavender, Roman chamomille, geranium

Blends:
Bruise blend Recipe 1:
- 5 drops helichrysum
- 4 drops lavender
- 3 drops cypress
- 3 drops lemongrass
- 3 drops geranium

Bruise blend Recipe 2:
- 6 drops clove
- 4 drops black pepper
- 3 drops peppermint
- 2 drops marjoram
- 2 drops geranium
- 2 drops cypress

EO Applications:
TOPICAL:
> NEAT or DILUTE 50-50, 1-3 drops on bruised area, 2-5 times daily. Helichrysum is especially beneficial in healing bruises when applied neat on location.
> COMPRESS, cold, on location, 2-4 times daily, as needed

Dietary Supplementation:
Master Formula Vitamins, VitaGreen, JuvaTone, JuvaPower/Spice, Super C

Regimen:
- Apply 2-3 drops of helichrysum on location neat or put in 2 oz. water and take as a dietary supplement, 2 times daily
- Super C Chewable: 2-6 tablets, 3 times daily.
- Master Formula Vitamin: 2-6 tablets, 3 times daily
- VitaGreen: 2-6 capsules 3 times daily.

BURNS

(See also SKIN DISORDERS and SHOCK)

There are three types of burns:

- First-degree burns only damage the outer layer of the skin. Sunburn is typically a first-degree burn.

- Second-degree burns damage both the outer layer and the underlying layer known as the dermis. It is manifested by blisters.

- Third-degree burns not only destroy or damage skin but can even damage underlying tissues.

Burns can be caused by sunlight, chemicals, electricity, radiation, or heat. Thermal burns are the most common type.

Aloe vera gel (contained in LavaDerm) has been extensively used in the treatment of burns and has been studied for its anti-inflammatory and tissue-regenerating properties. Helichrysum, lavender, and Idaho balsam fir oils support tissue regeneration and reduce scarring and skin discoloration.

The Deadly Dehydration of Burns

The reason that burns tend to swell and blister is due to fluid loss from the damaged blood vessels. This is why it is important to keep the burn well hydrated and to drink plenty of water.

In cases of serious burns, fluid loss can become so severe that it sends the victim into shock and requires intravenous transfusions of saline solution to bring up blood pressure.

Severe burns can result in dehydration and mineral loss. Inflammation often accompanies burns, so dietary protocols should be used to lessen inflammation.

NOTE: All burns can be serious, therefore, seek medical attention if necessary. If the burn is large or severe, the individual may go into shock. Inhaling oils may help reduce the shock. (See SHOCK)

After a burn has started to heal and is drying and cracking, use Rose Ointment or body lotion with a few drops of lavender oil to keep skin soft and to promote faster healing.

Dietary Supplementation:
Essential Omegas, Longevity Capsules, Sulfurzyme, Super Cal

First-Degree Burns (Sunburn)

The best prevention for sunburn is to avoid prolonged exposure to the sun. When you do go outdoors, always wear sunblock or lotion with an SPF greater than 15—especially during the summer and when you expect to be outdoors for a prolonged period of time.

In the event of a sunburn, lavender essential oil can offer excellent pain-relieving and healing benefits.

Single Oils:
Lavender, Idaho balsam fir, helichrysum, blue cypress, rose, *Melaleuca ericifolia*

Blends:
Gentle Baby, Australian Blue, Melrose, Highest Potential

EO Applications:
TOPICAL:
NEAT or DILUTE 50-50, 1-3 drops on burn location to cool tissue and reduce inflammation. Apply 3-6 times daily or as needed.

Topical Treatments:
LavaDerm Cooling Mist, Tender Tush Ointment, Rose Ointment, Lavender-Rosewood Bar Soap, Peppermint-Cedarwood Bar Soap

For fast relief of first-degree burns, spray burn immediately with LavaDerm Cooling Mist and continue misting as necessary to cool the area.

Spray as often as 4-5 times and hour for the first two hours and follow with 2-3 drops of lavender or Idaho balsam fir oil.

Use Lavender-Rosewood Soap or Peppermint-Cedarwood soap only after burn has started to heal (24-48 hours).

Second-Degree Burns (Blisters)

(see also BLISTERS)

Spray burn immediately with LavaDerm Cooling Mist and continue misting when necessary to cool the area. Spray 4-5 times every hour and follow with 2-3 drops of lavender oil.

Thereafter, apply LavaDerm every 15-30 minutes during the first day. (Keep LavaDerm refrigerated.) Apply 2-4 drops of lavender oil as needed immediately after each LavaDerm misting.

On days 2 through 5, mist every hour and follow with 2-4 drops lavender oil.

Continue using cooling mist 3 to 6 times daily until healed. Apply Rose Ointment to keep tissue soft.

Third-Degree Burns

For third-degree burns, seek immediate medical attention and follow the health professional's advice.

Spraying LavaDerm on the burn every few minutes for the first 24 hours will help tissue rehydrate. Applying a few drops of lavender oil after misting, will also help the healing process.

BURSITIS

Bursitis is an inflammation of the bursa, which are small, fluid-filled sacs located near the joints. Bursa act as shock absorbers when muscles or tendons come into contact with bone. As the bursa become swollen, they result in pain, particularly when the affected joint is used.

Bursitis can be caused by injury, infection, or arthritis, and usually involves the joints of the knees, elbows, shoulders, and Achilles tendon. Occasionally bursitis can occur in the base of the big toe. Bursitis may signal the beginning of arthritis.

Single Oils:
Idaho balsam fir, marjoram, basil, lavender, black pepper, peppermint, wintergreen, Idaho tansy, elemi, oregano

Blends:
Relieve It, Sacred Mountain, PanAway.

EO Applications:
TOPICAL:
NEAT or DILUTE 50-50, 2-4 drops on affected area/joint 3-5 times daily, or as needed to soothe pain
COMPRESS, cold, around affected join, 1-3 times daily

Dietary Supplementation:
Essential Omegas, Sulfurzyme, ArthroTune, AlkaLime, Super Cal, Mega Cal, BLM

Topical Treatment: Ortho Ease, Ortho Sport Massage Oil, Sacred Mountain Bar Soap, and Peppermint-Cedarwood Bar Soap.

CANCER

NOTE: No cancer treatment should be undertaken without consulting a licensed medical practitioner. The essential oil applications listed here can be used to complement the effectiveness of conventional cancer therapies. These essential oil applications should continue until the cancer is in remission.

Groundbreaking research slated to be published in 2004 at Brigham Young University for the first time identified essential oils which effectively kill cancer cells while being non-toxic to normal cells (non neoplastic cells). Some of the most effective oils studied included sandalwood essential oil which inhibited growth by up to 90% of several different types of cancer cells (cervical, breast, skin and prostate) while having little or no harmful effect on normal cells. Sandalwood showed excellent action even at very small concentrations (100 ppm). Tsuga, thyme, grapefruit, and thyme linalool also showed low normal cell toxicity and strong anticancer action.

Oils rich in limonene, such as lemon, orange, tangerine, and Idaho balsam fir have been shown in clinical studies to have potent anticarcinogenic effects. According to a study at the University of Indiana[12], "monoterpenes would appear to act through multiple mechanisms in the chemoprevention and chemotherapy of cancer." Studies using 1-15 grams a day of limonene in very advanced cancer patients resulted in almost 20% of the patients going into remission.

To enhance the action of essential oils, strong cleansing and nutritional building programs are required. The three programs below can be tailored to fit your particular needs and can have a profound effect on any cancer treatment.

1. Intensive cleanse with Cleansing Trio and JuvaTone.

2. Modified Burrough's Cleanse using cayenne pepper, lemon juice, and blue agave nectar. (See Cleansing and Diets, Chapter 25)

3. The Essentialzyme Ramping Program (see box below).

Essentialzyme Ramping Program for cancer

This program should be monitored by a health care professional:

Phase 1: Start with 3 tablets, 3 times daily. Increase amount by 1 tablet every day until nauseous. At this point, discontinue Essentialzyme for 24-36 hours.

Phase 2: Start again with 4 tablets, 3 times daily. Increase daily amount until nausea starts again. Stop and rest for 24-36 hours.

Phase 3: Start with 5 tablets, 3 times daily. Increase amount by one tablet every day until nausea starts. Rest for 24-36 hours.

Phase 4: Go back to the amount taken before nausea occurred the third time. Continue this amount for 6 weeks.

Phase 5: Start enzyme saturation again.

How Pollutants Contribute to Cancer

The pollutants to which we are exposed accumulate in tissues such as the breasts, thyroid, ovaries, and uterus. Some of these chemicals can mimic or imitate natural hormones, thereby activating hormone receptors that over-stimulate glands. This can increase the risk of hormone-dependent cancers, such as breast and uterine cancer.

All cancers are best treated in the early stages by alternating and varying the essential oils used each week, so the cancer cells do not build up a resistance to the treatment.

The following are regarded generally as anti-cancerous oils:

Single Oils:
Helichrysum, lemon, orange, tangerine, ledum, sandalwood, lavender, clove, thyme, Idaho balsam fir, tsuga, frankincense, myrtle

Blends: ImmuPower, Longevity

When people suffer terminal illness, their minds can be fractured, and they can have difficulty focusing and collecting their thoughts. The Valor, Gathering and Grounding blends promote greater focus and the ability to gather feelings and deal constructively with emotions related to cancer.

Another simple anti-cancer recipe:
- 12 drops frankincense
- 5 drops lavender
- 6 drops helichrysum

EO Applications:
TOPICAL:
NEAT or DILUTE 50-50, 1-3 drops applied directly on skin cancers or cancerous nodes, 2-5 times daily
VITA FLEX, 1-3 drops neat on foot reflex points relevant for internal cancers
RAINDROP Technique, 2-3 times monthly, substituting anti-cancerous oils for the five optional Raindrop oils (see Chapter 21)

---

12. Crowell P. Prevention and therapy of cancer by dietary monoterpenes. J Nutr. 1999 Mar;129(3):775S-778S.

INGESTION:
> CAPSULE, 00 size, 2 capsules,
> 2-4 times daily

RETENTION:
> RECTAL, 3 times weekly, using
> 20-80 dilution

Dietary Supplementation:
ImmuPro, VitaGreen, Super C Chewable,
ImmuneTune, Essential Manna, Power Meal,
Thyromin, Exodus, Sulfurzyme, Mineral
Essence, Essential Omegas, Rehemogen, Berry
Young Juice

Gary Young's Daily Anti-Cancer Program

- Master Formula: 4-6 tablets daily
- VitaGreen: 8-10 capsules daily
- Super C: 8-10 tablets daily
- ImmuPro: 6-10 tablets at night; 4 morning and afternoon
- Power Meal: 2 scoops, 3 times daily
- WheyFit: 2 scoops daily
- Essentialzyme: 2-6 tablets, 3 times daily according to blood type
- Thyromin: Start 1 before bedtime and increase as needed.
- Exodus: 6-8 capsules daily
- Sulfurzyme: Begin with 1 tsp., 3 times daily and increase to 1-3 Tbsp. daily
- Super B 2-4 tablets daily. Super B is a good source of all B vitamins including pantothenic acid (vitamin B5). Many cancer patients evidence a deficiency in vitamin B5

Brain Tumor

Single Oils: Frankincense, grapefruit, clove, tsuga, blue cypress

EO Applications:
TOPICAL:
> NEAT or DILUTE 50-50, if needed, 2-4
> drops to temples, forehead, mastoids and
> back of neck, 2-6 times daily

INGESTION:
> CAPSULE, 00 size, 2 capsules,
> 2-4 times daily

Dietary Supplementation: ImmuPro, Berry
Young Juice, Longevity Caps

Brain Tumor regimen:
- Take 15 to 20 tablets of ImmuPro, 15 capsules of Exodus, and 10 tablets of Super C Chewable daily.
- Maintain a concentrated carrot juice diet. Potassium is critical. Drink plenty of dandelion tea (diuretic) and yellow dock tea (iron), and take milk thistle for the liver.

To increase blood flow to the brain:
- Mix 4 drops frankincense and 5 drops ImmuPower and massage 3-5 drops on the neck 3-5 times daily.
- Mix 15 drops frankincense and 6 drops clove in 1/2 oz. V-6 Mixing Oil or Massage Oil Base and rub 5-7 times daily on the brain stem (spine at base of skull), temples, mastoids (behind the ears), forehead, and crown (top of head).
- Put 10 drops frankincense and 1 drop clove in diffuser. Sit in front of the diffuser and breathe vapors for 1/2 hour, 3 times daily. If you get a headache or feel nauseous, reduce to what is tolerable, but do not quit.
- AlkaLime: Take 1 tsp. in a glass of distilled or purified water 1 hour before or after each meal to help restore pH balance.

Bone Cancer

Single Oils:
Frankincense, sandalwood, clove, tsuga

Blends:
ImmuPower

EO Applications:
TOPICAL:
> DILUTE 50-50, massage 4-6 drops on
> location and on spine 2-4 times daily
> NEAT, apply 2-3 drops each of frankincense
> and ImmuPower along the spine,
> 3 times daily

INGESTION:
> CAPSULE, 00 size, 2 capsules
> 1-3 times daily
> RICE MILK, 4-6 times daily

Bone Cancer blend:
- 15 drops frankincense
- 6 drops clove
- 1 Tbsp. V6 Oil Complex

Massage 4-6 drops on location 3-5 times daily

Dietary Supplementation:
Cleansing Trio. Longevity Caps, Berry Young Juice, Essential Omegas

Breast Cancer

The use of topically applied natural progesterone (20 mg per day) can dramatically reduce the risk of breast cancer. (See Progessence Cream, Chapter 11) Eighty-five percent of all breast cancers are ductal cancers, and natural progesterone has been shown to slow the growth of ductal cells that promote cancer growth. In addition, new research indicates that some essential oils can dramatically inhibit cancer growth while leaving normal cells unharmed.

Studies at the Young Life Research Institute of Natural Medicine show that ledum, Idaho balsam fir, tsuga, lavender, clove, and frankincense may be effective in treating breast cancer.

For a cancer preventative, dilute up to 20 drops of either orange, sandalwood, myrtle, or tsuga in 1 tablespoon of olive oil, put in 00-size capsule and take one daily as a dietary supplement.

Lignans in flax seeds have also been shown to prevent breast cancer growth.

Single Oils:
Orange, sandalwood, frankincense, ledum, myrtle, clove, lemon, orange, tangerine, tsuga

Blends:
Brain Power, Present Time

EO Applications:
TOPICAL:
> DILUTE 50-50, apply 4-10 drops on location daily
> VITA FLEX, apply 1-3 drops to breast Vita Flex points (see location in breast cancer regimen below)

INGESTION:
> CAPSULE, 00 size, 1 capsule 2-4 times daily
> RICE MILK, 2-4 times daily

Specific breast cancer regimen:

A. Massage 1-3 drops frankincense on breast Vita Flex point on feet, which is on top of the foot at the base of the three middle toes. Continue massaging the Vita Flex areas after applying the oil (see Vita Flex Technique in chapter 20).

B. Layer on location 15 drops frankincense, 10 drops lavender, and 3 drops clove. Apply oils and massage daily for 4 days, then rest for 4 days. Repeat as necessary.

C. Put 6 drops of frankincense and 4 drops ledum in a 00-size capsule, fill remainder with vegetable oil. Take 1-3 capsules daily.

D. Diffuse frankincense and Brain Power for 15 minutes 2-5 times daily.

Dietary Supplementation:
Cleansing Trio, JuvaTone, JuvaPower/Spice, Longevity Caps, Power Meal, ImmuPro, Essential Omegas, AminoTech, WheyFit, Super Cal, Berry Young Juice, BodyGize

Topical Treatments:
Cel-lite Magic, Progessence Cream

Other:
1. Keep lymphatics open with deep breathing exercise and aerobics.

2. Have a body massage with Cel-lite Magic, once per month to work the lymph nodes in the abdomen and the thoracic region.

3. The soy in BodyGize helps balance estrogen hormones. Take 2-3 Tbsp. BodyGize with water or juice 1-2 times daily.

    Note: *Do not use for estrogen-receptor positive cancers.*

4. Discontinue use of antiperspirants (not deodorant) and monitor calcium levels.

Cervical Cancer

The use of topically applied natural progesterone creams can dramatically reduce the risk of cervical cancer, especially in postmenopausal women. In addition, new research indicates that some essential oils can significantly inhibit cancer growth while leaving normal cells unharmed.

Single Oils:
Tsuga, thyme, galbanum, patchouli, sandalwood, Douglas fir, hyssop, nutmeg, sage

EO Applications:
INGESTION:
CAPSULE, 00 size, 2-4 times daily
RETENTION:
TAMPON, 3 times per week

Dietary Supplementation:
(See listing under main Cancer heading)

Colon Cancer

To enhance the action of essential oils, cancer requires strong cleansing and fasting programs. Cancer is best treated in its early stages by alternating and varying the essential oils used each week, so the cancer cells do not build up a resistance to the treatment.

For a cancer preventative, mix up to 20 mg of these essential oils in 1 tablespoon of vegetable oil, and put in 00 size gel caps. Take one per day.

The gastritis associated with *H. pylori* infection is closely associated with gastric cancers.[13] Highly antiseptic oils can kill *Helicobacter pylori* that causes the infection. These oils include oregano, mountain savory, tea tree, and thyme.

Single Oils:
Clove, frankincense, ledum, orange, tsuga, lavender

EO Applications:
INGESTION:
CAPSULE, 00 size, 2-4 times daily
RICE MILK, 2-4 times daily

Colon Cancer Regimen:

Day 1: Put 10 drops of frankincense, 10 drops tsuga in a vegetable capsule and swallow 3-4 times daily.

Day 2: Mix 16 drops frankincense and 3 drops clove, and put in vegetable capsule. Take orally 3-4 times daily.

Day 3: Mix equal parts frankincense and lavender in a vegetable capsule and take 3-4 times daily.

Day 4: Take frankincense capsules 3-4 times daily.

Days 5-8: Repeat the above 4-day cycle.

Days 9-12: Rest for 4 days.

Day 13: Restart the regimen.

Dietary Supplementation:
EssentialZyme, ComforTone, ICP, Detoxzyme

Supplementation Regimen:

1. Begin with EssentialZyme to digest toxic waste.

2. Take 2 capsules ComforTone, 3 times daily. Increase by one daily until the bowels move. Then begin reducing. If diarrhea occurs, reduce amount of ComforTone used and increase ICP fiber beverage. Drink plenty of purified or distilled water.

3. ICP fiber cleanse: Begin with 1 Tbsp. in water, 3 times daily. Increase to 2 Tbsp. 3 times daily or as needed until bowels are moving regularly.

Hodgkin's Disease

Reed-Sternberg cells are a hallmark trait of lymphatic cancers of this type.

Single Oils:
Clove, lavender, frankincense, cistus

Blends:
Longevity

EO Applications:
TOPICAL:
NEAT or DILUTE 50-50 on location 2-4 times daily or as needed

INGESTION:
CAPSULE, 00 size, 3-5 times daily

Dietary Supplementation:
(See listing under main Cancer heading)

---

13. Uemura N, Okamoto S, Yamamoto S, "H. pylori infection and development of gastric cancer," *Keio J Med* 2002 Dec;51 Suppl 2:63-8.

Leukemia

Single Oils:
Frankincense, clove, lavender.

Blends:
Thieves, Longevity.

EO Applications:
TOPICAL:
VITA FLEX, 1-3 drops on soles of feet 2 times daily
BODY MASSAGE, apply very gently, do not do deep tissue massage.

Dietary Supplementation:
Longevity Caps, Rehemogen, Super C, ImmuPro, ImmuneTune, VitaGreen, Berry Young Juice, Longevity Caps

Supplementation regimen:

Take the following daily, for 30-40 days:
- ImmuPro: 10 tablets before retiring; 2-4 tablets morning and afternoon
- Rehemogen: 3 droppers, 3 times daily
- Super C: 12 tablets daily
- ImmuneTune: 15 capsules daily
- VitaGreen: 9 capsules daily
- Longevity Caps: 3 capsules 3 times daily
- Fresh carrot juice: 1/2 gallon daily

Liver Cancer

Cleansing is extremely important since an optimally functioning liver is necessary to rid the body of toxins. Anger and hate affect the liver and cause extreme toxicity, eventually triggering disease.

Single Oils:
Frankincense, lavender, lemon, orange, tangerine, thyme

Blends: JuvaFlex, JuvaCleanse

EO Applications:
TOPICAL:
NEAT or DILUTE 50-50 if needed, 2-6 drops over liver area 2-4 times daily
COMPRESS, warm, over liver area nightly
VITA FLEX, massage 1-3 drops on liver Vita Flex points of feet

INGESTION:
CAPSULE, 00 size, 3-5 times daily
RICE MILK, 3-5 times daily

Liver Cancer blend:
- 30 drops frankincense
- 20 drops lavender
- 10 drops tsuga
- 10 drops ledum
- 4 tablespoons castor oil

Apply 20-30 drops of this mixture over the liver area, then cover with a warm moist towel for 20 minutes as a compress, 5 nights per week.

Also, fill 00-size capsules with this mixture and take 1 capsule 3-5 times daily

Supplements: JuvaTone, JuvaPower/Spice, Essential Omegas, Berry Young Juice, alpha lipoic acid, Ultra Young

Lung Cancer

Single Oils:
Ledum, orange, frankincense, Idaho balsam fir, ravensara, sage

Blends:
Raven, R.C., Longevity, ImmuPower

Lung cancer blend #1:
- 4 drops frankincense
- 3 drops sage
- 3 drops myrrh
- 3 drops clove
- 2 drops ravensara
- 2 drops hyssop

Lung cancer blend #2:
- 6 drops R.C.
- 5 drops clove
- 4 drops myrrh
- 5 drops frankincense
- 2 drops sage

EO Applications:
INHALATION:
DIFFUSION, 15 minutes 3-5 times daily
INGESTION:
CAPSULE, 00 size, 1 capsule 3 times daily
RETENTION:
RECTAL, nightly, retain for 8 hours

Lung Cancer Regimen:

Day 1: Diffuse frankincense and R.C. for 1 hour three times a day. Make a rectal implant by diluting 10 drops of each of these two oils with 1 tbsp V6 Oil Complex and retain overnight.

Day 2: Same as day 1, using frankincense and R.C. in rectal implant.

Day 3: Same as day 1, using frankincense and lavender in rectal implant.

Day 4: Same as day 1, using 20 drops frankincense in a rectal implant.

Rest 2 days before continuing. If no improvement is detected, omit rest days and begin again.

Alternate oils for retention enema use (add any one of the following oils to 1 teaspoon of olive oil):

- *Eucalyptus globulus*: 10 drops
- Frankincense: 10 drops
- Peppermint and frankincense: 5 drops
- Idaho balsam fir: 20 drops
- Cypress: 10 drops

Diffuse regularly during the day the same oil combinations (neat) that are used in the retention enema for that night.

Rub ImmuPower up the spine, daily. Apply warm compress on back and chest twice daily.

Dietary Supplementation:
Super C, ImmuPro, Super Cal, Berry Young Juice, alpha lipoic acid, Essential Manna, K & B

Supplementation regimen:
Take 10 to 20 Super C Chewable daily, dandelion tea, raw lemon juice, red clover tea, and K & B.

If edema is a problem, include: Super Cal, Essential Manna, Berry Young Juice, Mega Cal, or organic bananas.

Lymphoma (Cancer of Lymph Nodes)

Both Hodgkin's disease and non-Hodgkin's disease are characterized by swollen lymph gland nodes, generally first appearing on the neck, armpit or groin.

Lymphoma may be caused from petrochemical pollution in the air and water. After prolonged exposure, toxins such as benzene, styrene, and toluene begin to accumulate in the lymphatic system, eventually triggering cellular mutations and cancer.

Symptoms for non-Hodgkin's lymphoma
- Generally ill, loss of appetite, loss of weight, fever, and night sweats

Symptoms of Hodgkin's lymphoma
- Fever, fatigue, weakness, itching

Single Oils:
Frankincense, myrrh, clove, sage, sandalwood, lavender

Blends:
ImmuPower

Recipe 1:
- 10 drops frankincense
- 5 drops clove or myrrh
- 3 drops sage

Recipe 2: (for massage):
- 15 drops frankincense
- 6 drops clove

EO Applications:
TOPICAL:
    NEAT or DILUTE 50-50 if needed, 2-4 drops on swollen nodes 2 times daily. Rub along spine 2-3 times daily
    BODY MASSAGE, 2-3 times weekly
    RAINDROP Technique, 2 times monthly
RETENTION:
    RECTAL, nightly, will bring faster results than topical applications

Dietary Supplementation:
ImmuPro, ImmuneTune, Super C, VitaGreen, Cleansing Trio

Supplementation regimen
- ImmuneTune: 4 capsules, 3 times daily
- Super C: 6 tablets, 3 times daily
- VitaGreen: 6 capsules, 3 times daily
- ImmuPro: 3 tablets, 4 times daily.

Follow this program for one month, then gradually reduce. If lymphoma goes into remission, continue program for another month, then gradually reduce. It is best to eat a total vegetarian diet. O-blood types, who need more protein, should eat fresh stream trout or wild Arctic salmon.

Melanoma (Skin Cancer)

Melanoma is the most lethal form of skin cancer. It tends to aggressively spread and metastasize, quickly colonizing the lymph nodes and internal organs. It has a high rate of fatality.

A sudden change in the appearance of an old mole or the appearance of red lesions, may indicate melanoma. If you suspect that you have melanoma or any skin cancer, you should immediately contact your physician.

Single Oils:
Sandalwood, orange, blue cypress, tangerine, myrrh, lavender, Idaho tansy, tsuga, tea tree, lemongrass

Blends:
Longevity, Release, JuvaFlex, JuvaCleanse, EndoFlex, Purification, Thieves

Melanoma blend:
• 3 drops lavender
• 4 drops frankincense

EO Applications:
TOPICAL:
NEAT, apply 2-5 drops on location 3-5 times daily
INGESTION:
CAPSULE, 00 size, 2 times daily
RICE MILK, 2-4 times daily

Dietary Supplementation:
ImmuPro, Essential Omegas

Ovarian Cancer

Single Oils:
Sandalwood, lemon, orange, blue cypress, myrrh, frankincense, geranium

Blends: Protec, Longevity, ImmuPower

EO Applications:
TOPICAL:
NEAT, 3-5 drops up the spine, on the feet, just below the navel and on the throat.
Do this application 1-2 times daily
INGESTION:
CAPSULE, 00 size, 3 times daily
RICE MILK, 2-4 times daily
RETENTION:
TAMPON, nightly

Daily Regimen for Ovarian Cancer:
• Mix the blend below and use in alternating rectal and vaginal retention. Use vaginal retention with tampon one night and rectal retention the second night, and so on.
  • 15 drops frankincense
  • 5 drops myrrh
  • 6 drops geranium
  • 1 Tbsp. V-6 Oil Complex

• Rub 3-4 drops ImmuPower up the spine, on the feet, and on the throat, daily.

• Rub 1/2 tsp. Protec topically over each of the following locations: abdomen, ovaries, the reproductive Vita Flex points on hands and feet.

• Use Protec for nightly vaginal retention. Start with 1/2 tsp. and build up to 1 Tbsp. If irritation occurs, discontinue for 3 days and start again with a smaller amount.

To increase Protec's strength, add extra oils and use in alternating applications:

• *NIGHT 1: Add 3 to 4 drops of frankincense.*
• *NIGHT 2: Add 3 to 4 drops of clove.*
• *NIGHT 3: Add 3 to 4 drops of myrrh.*

Dietary Supplementation:
ImmuPro, BodyGize, Essential Omegas, alpha lipoic acid, ArthroTune

Prostate Cancer

Many prostate cancers may be testosterone-dependent, so it may be necessary to avoid taking anything that can raise testosterone levels, such as DHEA or androstenedione. Research by Dr. John Lee, MD, suggests that a quality progesterone cream may be the most potent therapy for preventing prostate cancer. Neurogen and Progessence creams provide natural progesterone.

Single Oils:
Orange, tangerine, ledum, Idaho balsam fir, frankincense, myrrh, cumin, sage, tsuga

Blends: Protec, Mister, Longevity, Juva Cleanse

EO Applications:
TOPICAL:
> DILUTE 50-50, 1-3 drops between the rectum and scrotum 1-3 times daily
> VITA FLEX, 1-3 drops, neat. on reproductive points on feet (sides of ankles)

INGESTION:
> CAPSULE, 00 size, 3 times daily
> RICE MILK, 2-4 times daily

RETENTION:
> RECTAL, nightly

Prostate blend Regimen:
The blend below helped to reduce PSA (prostate specific antigen) counts over 70 percent in a 2 months period:

- 10 drops frankincense
- 5 drops myrrh
- 3 drops sage

1. Mix the above oils in 1 Tbsp. V-6 Oil Complex for rectal retention, nightly
2. Rub 1-3 drops of the above blend, neat, on the Vita Flex reproductive points (ankles) on both feet, 2 times daily.
3. Dilute the blend 50-50 and apply 2-4 drops on the area between the rectum and scrotum 2 times daily.

Also, use Protec for nightly rectal retention. Start with 1/2 tsp. and build up to 1 Tbsp. If irritation occurs, discontinue for 3 days and start again with a smaller amount.

To increase Protec's strength, add extra oils and use for alternating applications:

- *NIGHT 1: Add 3 to 4 drops of frankincense.*
- *NIGHT 2: Add 3 to 4 drops of clove.*
- *NIGHT 3: Add 3 to 4 drops of tsuga.*

Dietary Supplementation:
Super B, ProGen, ImmuPro, Cleansing Trio, JuvaTone, JuvaPower/Spice

Topical Treatments:
Neurogen and Progessence creams. Apply 1/2 tsp 2 times daily to the area between the scrotum and the rectum.

Uterine Cancer

Environmental pollutants become lodged in tissues, such as the breasts, thyroid, ovaries, and uterus. Many chemicals mimic or imitate our natural hormones and can fit the hormone receptors, thus tricking and over-stimulating these organs. This can become a major source of cancer of the breast, uterus, ovaries, and lymph nodes.

(Same program as OVARIAN CANCER above.)

CANDIDA

(See FUNGAL INFECTIONS)

CANKER SORES

(See also COLD SORES)

These are technically known as aphthous ulcers and are not regarded as an infectious disease and are not caused by the Herpes virus.

Canker sores tend to occur because of stress, illness, weakened immune system, and injury caused by such things as hot food, rough brushing of teeth, or dentures. They appear under the tongue more commonly than cold sores.

Single Oils:
Melissa, clove, lavender, niaouli, sandalwood

Blends:
Thieves, Australian Blue

Topical/Oral Treatments
Thieves Antiseptic Spray, Fresh Essence Plus

EO Applications:
TOPICAL:
> NEAT, 1 drop applied gently with fingertip to canker sore 4-8 times daily

ORAL:
> GARGLE, 2-4 times daily

INGESTION:
> SYRUP, Maple, 2-4 times daily

Dietary Supplementation:
ImmuPro, goldenseal root powder

CARBON MONOXIDE POISONING

Almost everyone who lives in a large metropolitan area will suffer varying degrees of subtle carbon monoxide poisoning. The more polluted or stagnant the air, the more likely that carbon monoxide levels in the blood may be elevated.

IMPORTANT: Anyone who has suffered serious carbon monoxide poisoning should be immediately exposed to fresh air while a doctor, paramedic, or other emergency health professional is summoned.

Singles:
Ravansara, *Eucalyptus radiata*, myrtle

Blends:
Longevity, R.C., Purification, Inspiration, Valor, Sacred Mountain

EO Applications:
Re-oxygenation regimen (perform every 3-4 hours)
- Massage Valor on the bottom of feet.
- Apply Purification on the spine and back, Raindrop style
- Diffuse Purification, rub 2-4 drops on the feet.
- Massage 2-4 drops of R.C., Purification, Inspiration, or Sacred Mountain, and massage on the lung Vita Flex areas on bottom of the feet and on top of the feet at the base of the toes.

Dietary Supplementation:
Master Formula Vitamins, VitaGreen, Super B, Super C Chewable

CARDIOVASCULAR CONDITIONS

(See also BLOOD CLOTS, BLOOD DISORDERS, HEART, DIABETES, ORAL CARE)

Hardening of the Arteries

Singles:
Helichrysum, lavender, cypress, cistus

Blends:
Aroma Life, Longevity.

EO Applications:
TOPICAL:
BODY MASSAGE, 2 times weekly

INGESTION:
CAPSULE, 00 size, 3 times daily

Dietary Supplementation:
Essential Omegas, Longevity Caps, Wolfberry Crisp, mega Cal, AD&E

Blood Pressure, High (Hypertension)

Single Oils:
Lavender, marjoram, rosemary, ylang ylang, cypress, rosemary, jasmine absolute

Blends:
Aroma Life, Aroma Siez, Peace & Calming, Citrus Fresh, Joy

EO Applications:
TOPICAL:
DILUTE 20-80, full body massage daily
INHALATION:
DIFFUSION, 20 minutes, 3 times daily
INGESTION:
CAPSULE, 00 size, 1-2 times daily

Additional essential oil regimens:
1. For 3 minutes, massage 1-2 drops each of Aroma Life and ylang ylang on the heart Vita Flex point and over the heart and carotid arteries alon the neck. Blood pressure will begin to drop within 5 to 20 minutes. Monitor the pressure and reapply as required. Lemon and helichrysum can also be used.
2. Inhalation of jasmine reduces anxiety and therefore, lowers blood pressure.

Dietary Supplementation:
HRT, CardiaCare, Essential Manna, ImmuPro, ImmuneTune, Super B, Mineral Essence, Super Cal, Stevia

Supplementation regimen:
1. Increase intake of magnesium which acts as a smooth-muscle relaxant and acts as a natural calcium channel blocker for the heart, lowering blood pressure and dilating the heart blood vessels. Mineral Essence, Essential Manna, and Super Cal are good sources of magnesium.
2. Take 20 mg daily of vitamin B3 (niacin) an excellent vasodilator (found in Super B).

3. Use therapeutic-grade Hawthorne berry extracts. Hawthorne berry (contained in HRT tincture provides powerful cardiovascular support.
4. Do a colon and liver cleanse.

Blood Pressure, Low (Hypotension)

Single Oils:
Sage, pine, rosemary

Blends:
Aroma Life, EndoFlex, Joy

EO Applications:
TOPICAL:
   DILUTE 20-80, full body massage daily
INHALATION:
   DIFFUSION, 20 minutes, 3 times daily
INGESTION:
   CAPSULE, 00 size, 1-2 times daily

Additional essential oil regimens:
1. Use 1-2 drops each of Aroma Life and rosemary on heart Vita Flex points; for massage, dilute with few drops of V6 Oil Complex.
2. Place 3 drops each of Aroma Life and rosemary in a capsule and take 2 times daily

High Cholesterol

Helichrysum lowers and regulates cholesterol and reduces blood clotting. Aroma Life regulates and lowers blood pressure and breaks down plaque on the blood vessel walls.

Single Oils:
Rosemary, clove, German and Roman chamomile, spikenard, helichrysum, geranium, fennel

Blends:
Aroma Life, Longevity, JuvaFlex, JuvaCleanse, Di-Tone, EndoFlex, ImmuPower

Cholesterol reducing blend:
• 2 to 5 drops rosemary
• 5 drops Roman chamomile
• 3 drops helichrysum
• 5 drops lemongrass

EO Applications:
TOPICAL:
   NEAT or DILUTE 50-50 if needed, 2-4 drops at pulse points where arteries are close to the surface (wrists, inside elbows, base of throat), 2-3 times daily. Also rub 6-10 drops along spine 3 times daily
   BODY MASSAGE, 2 times weekly
INGESTION:
   CAPSULE, 00 size, 3 times daily
   RICE MILK, 1-2 times daily

Dietary Supplementation:
CardiaCare, JuvaPower/Spice, VitaGreen, Super C Chewable, Super Cal, Longevity Caps, Mineral Essence, Essential Omegas, ICP, Polyzyme, Essentialzyme

Supplementation regimens:
1. Do a colon and liver cleanse using the Cleansing Trio, JuvaTone, JuvaPower/Spice, and JuvaFlex and JuvaCleanse. JuvaTone is particularly useful for high cholesterol. ICP helps break down plaque.
2. Mix 25 drops of HRT in 6 ounces of distilled water, and drink 3 times daily. Supports blood system and circulation deficiency.
3. Magnesium acts as a smooth muscle relaxant and supports the cardiovascular system. It acts as a natural calcium channel blocker for the heart, lowering blood pressure and dilating the heart blood vessels (*Dr. T. Friedmann*). Mineral Essence, Super Cal and Mega Cal are good sources of magnesium.

Phlebitis (Inflammation of Veins)

Single Oils:
Helichrysum, German chamomile, nutmeg, Roman chamomile, geranium, lavender, cistus

Blends:
Longevity, Aroma Life

EO Applications:
TOPICAL:
   NEAT, 2-4 drops on location 2-4 times daily
   COMPRESS, cold on location 2-4 times daily

Dietary Supplementation:
Essential Omegas, Longevity Caps

313

CARPAL TUNNEL SYNDROME

(See NERVE DISORDERS)

CATARACTS/GLAUCOMA

(See EYE DISORDERS)

CELLULITE

Cellulite is one of the harder types of fats to dissolve in the body. Cellulite is an accumulation of old fat cell clusters that solidify and harden as the surrounding tissue loses its elasticity.

Excess fat is undesirable for two reasons:

1. The extra weight puts an extra load on all body systems, particularly the heart and cardiovascular system, as well as the joints (knees, hips, spine etc).

2. Toxins and petrochemicals (pesticides, herbicides, metallics) tend to accumulate in fatty tissue. This can contribute to hormone imbalance, neurological problems, and a higher risk of cancer.

Essential oils such as ledum, tangerine and grapefruit may help reduce fat cells. Cypress enhances circulation to support the elimination of fatty deposits. The essential oils of lemongrass and spearmint also may help fat metabolism. Cel-Lite Magic Massage Oil contains many of these oils and may help reduce cellulite deposits.

Cellulite is slow to dissolve, so target areas should be worked for a month or more in conjunction with weight training, a weight loss program, and drinking purified water—one-and-a-half times the body weight in ounces each day. Be patient. You should begin to see results in 4 to 6 weeks when using the oils in combination with a muscle-building and weight-loss regimen.

Single Oils:
Rosemary, grapefruit, lemon, tangerine, cypress, fennel, juniper, spearmint, lemongrass

Blends:
EndoFlex, Citrus Fresh

Cellulite blend #1:
• 5 drops rosemary
• 10 drops grapefruit
• 2 drops cypress

Cellulite blend #2:
• 10 drops grapefruit
• 5 drops lavender
• 3 drops helichrysum
• 3 drops patchouli
• 4 drops cypress

Cellulite blend #3: (Bath):
• 5 drops juniper
• 3 drops orange
• 3 drops cypress
• 3 drops lemon

Mix the above recipe together with 2 tablespoons Epsom salts or Bath Gel Base and dissolve in warm bath water. Massage with Cel-Lite Magic after bath.

EO Applications:
TOPICAL:
DILUTE 50-50, massage 3-6 drops vigorously on cellulite locations at least 3 times daily, especially before exercising. BATH SALTS, 2-4 times weekly Apply 3-5 drops of grapefruit, neat, 1-2 x daily to increase fat-reducing action in areas of fat rolls, puckers, and dimples.

Dietary Supplementation:
Thyromin, ThermaBurn, ThermaMist, Essential Omegas, Power Meal, Wheyfit, AminoTech

Thyromin, ThermaBurn, and ThermaMist balance and boost metabolism.

Topical Treatments:
Cel-Lite Magic Massage Oil

CEREBRAL PALSY

(See MUSCLES, NEUROLOGICAL DISORDERS)

CHEMICAL SENSITIVITY REACTION

Environmental poisoning and chemical sensitivity are becoming a major cause of discomfort and disease. Strong chemical compounds, such as insecticides, herbicides, and formaldehyde found in paints, glues, cosmetics, and finger nail polish, enter the body easily. Symptoms include indigestion, upper and lower gas, poor assimilation, poor electrolyte balance, rashes, hypoglycemia, allergic reaction to foods and other substances, along with emotional mood swings, fatigue, irritability, lack of motivation, lack of discipline and creativity.

Single Oils:
Frankincense, sandalwood

Blends:
Purification, Clarity, Brain Power, JuvaFlex, JuvaCleanse, M-Grain

EO Applications:
TOPICAL:
DILUTE 50-50, on affected areas, 2-4 times daily
INGESTION:
CAPSULE, 00 size, 1-3 times daily

Dietary Supplementation:
ImmuPro, ImmuneTune, Exodus, Rehemogen, Chelex, JuvaTone, JuvaPower/Spice, Cleansing Trio

For headache relief:
• 4 Essentialzyme
• 1/8 tsp M-Grain diluted 50/50 in vegetable oil

Drink 2-3 large glasses of water immediately after using these products.

(See also VASCULAR CLEANSING)

Toxic Chemical Absorption

Handling refuse or any type of contaminant without protective gloves may cause discoloration of hands, as well as chemical exposure.

Use good rubber gloves and change them often or at least wash them out with strong soap, rinse well, and dry well. If hands become discolored through chemical absorption, soak them in a solution of 3 percent hydrogen peroxide, available at most drug stores. This helps remove chemicals from the skin.

Single Oils:
Lavender, lemon

Blends:
Purification

EO Applications:
TOPICAL:
NEAT, rub 3-7 drops lavender, lemon or Purification on hands, then cover with clean cotton gloves or wrap lightly with cotton bandage all night.

CHICKEN POX (Herpes Zoster)

(See also COLD SORES, BLISTERS)

Chicken pox (also known as shingles, *Varicella Zoster*, or *Herpes zoster*) is caused by a virus that is closely related to the Herpes simplex virus. This virus is prone to hiding along nerves under the skin and may cause recurring infection through life.

When *Herpes zoster* infection occurs in children it is known as chicken pox; when infection occurs or reoccurs in adults, it is known as shingles.

A childhood bout with chicken pox may leave the virus dormant in sensory (skin) nerves. If the immune system is taxed by severe emotional stress, illness, or long-term use of cortico-steroids, the dormant viruses may become active and start to infect the pathway of the skin nerves.

Single Oils:
Lavender, tea tree, sandalwood, niaouli, melissa, clove

Blends:
Australian Blue, Thieves

EO Applications:
TOPICAL:
Add 20 drops of essential oils (using any of the above oils) to 1 tablespoon of calamine lotion or V6 Oil Complex and lightly dab on spots (lesions)

Dietary Supplementation:
ImmuPro, Essential Omegas

Topical Treatments:
Thieves Antiseptic Spray, Ortho Ease, LavaDerm Cooling Mist, Shower Mate with Filter (filled with lavender oil and Epsom salts), Lavender-Rosewood Bar Soap, Melaleuca Geranium Bar Soap

Shingles

Shingles is a short-lived viral infection of the nervous system that starts with fatigue, fever, chills, and intestinal upset. The affected skin areas become sensitive and prone to blistering. One attack usually provides immunity for life. However, for many people, particularly the elderly, pain can persist for months, even years.

NOTE: Occurrences of shingles around the eyes or on the forehead can cause blindness. Consult an ophthalmologist (eye doctor) immediately if such outbreaks occur.

Single Oils:
Elemi, Idaho tansy, tea tree, ravensara, oregano, mountain savory, blue cypress, sandalwood, thyme, peppermint, tamanu (a fatty acid oil)

Blends:
Thieves, Australian Blue, Exodus II

Shingles blend #1:
- 10 drops German chamomile
- 5 drops lavender
- 4 drops sandalwood
- 2 drops geranium

Shingles blend #2:
- 10 drops sandalwood
- 5 drops blue cypress
- 4 drops peppermint
- 2 drops ravensara

EO Applications:
TOPICAL:
DILUTE 50-50, apply 6-10 drops on affected area, back of neck and down the spine 1-3 times daily.
COMPRESS, alternating warm and cold, on spine, 1-3 times daily

Shingles regimen:
A. Layering in Raindrop Technique style, apply 3-4 drops each of oregano, mountain savory and thyme along the spine
B. Apply 15-20 drops V6 Oil Complex to the spine, massage briefly over the other oils, then cover the skin with a dry towel and apply a warm pack for 15-20 minutes). NOTE: Be cautious about warming.

If the back becomes too hot, remove the warm pack immediately and add more V6 Oil Complex to cool.
C. Remove the warm pack and towel, then layer 4-8 drops each of tea tree, elemi and peppermint along the spine
D. Put the dry towel back over the skin and apply an ice pack for 30 minutes.

Dietary Supplements:
ArthroTune, Super Cal, AD&E, Essential Omegas, Sulfurzyme

CHOLECYSTITIS

(See GALLBLADDER INFECTION)

Inflammation of the gallbladder due to obstruction of the gallbladder (bile) outlet with symptoms ranging from mild edema and congestion to severe infection and perforation.

CHOLERA

Cholera is an acute diarrheal disease caused by an interotoxin produced by a gram negative bacteria called *Vibrio cholerae*. Severe cases are marked by vomiting, muscle cramps and constant watery diarrhea which can result in serious fluid loss, saline depletion, acidosis and shock. The disease is typically found in India and Southeast Asia and is spread by feces-contaminated water and food. If you suspect cholera, you should immediately seek professional medical advice.

A recent study shows that lemon—freshly squeezed juice, peel, and essential oil—act as a biocide against *Vibrio cholerae* with no harmful side effects.[14]

Single Oils:
Lemon, clove, thyme, rosemary, oregano

EO Applications:
INGESTION:
CAPSULE, 00 size, 3 times daily with meals

CHOLESTEROL

(See CARDIOVASCULAR CONDITIONS)

---

14. de Castillo et al., "Bactericidal activity of lemon juice and lemon derivatives against Vibrio cholerae," *Biol Pharm Bull* 2000 Oct;23(10):1235-8.

CHRONIC FATIGUE SYNDROME

(See EPSTEIN-BARR VIRUS)

CIRCULATION DISORDERS

(See also BLOOD CLOTS, BLOOD DISORDERS and CARDIOVASCULAR CONDITIONS)

Good circulation is undoubtedly the foundation of good health; however, sluggish or inadequate circulation can result in tissue toxicity, starvation, and eventually, cellular death. The damage that poor or inadequate circulation can cause is best illustrated in the gangrene that often develops in the legs and arms of many advanced diabetic patients. Because the blood cannot efficiently circulate through these areas, parts of the tissues literally rot away.

Niacin (nicotinic acid) is effective for dilating blood vessels and increasing circulation. The amino acid L-arginine and cayenne pepper have similar properties.

Essential oils may be extremely useful for promoting circulation. Myrtle, lemon, and cypress have been used to strengthen and dilate capillaries and increase circulation. Helichrysum, clove and citrus oils are natural blood thinners, balancing the viscosity or thickness of the blood, and they amplify the effects of cypress. Marjoram relaxes muscles and dilates blood vessels, while nutmeg acts as a circulatory stimulant and anti-inflammatory. Goldenrod is a vein decongestant.

Single Oils:
Goldenrod, helichrysum, marjoram, cypress, myrtle, orange, grapefruit, clove, peppermint, geranium, nutmeg, cistus

Blends:
Aroma Life, Pan Away, En-R-Gee, Longevity, Citrus Fresh, Di-Tone, Harmony

EO Applications:
TOPICAL:
DILUTE 50-50, 2-4 drops on affected area 2-3 times daily. Also apply over carotid arteries and pulse points, wherever arteries are close to the skin surface.
BODY MASSAGE, 2-3 times weekly, start at feet and work up to heart

INGESTION:
CAPSULE, 0 size, 2 times daily

Dietary Supplementation:
Super B, Cel-Lite Magic, HRT, CardiaCare, VitaGreen, Longevity Caps, Rehemogen, and JuvaTone, JuvaPower/Spice

Circulation support regimen:
1. Put 25 drops HRT in 1 oz. distilled water and take 3 times daily
2. Rub 2-4 drops Aroma Life on the carotid arteries and pulse points, wherever an artery comes close to the skin, 2 times daily
3. Apply 2-4 drops Harmony over areas of poor circulation, 1-3 times daily as needed
4. Take 1/4 tsp of cayenne pepper with a full glass of pure water daily. Avoid using at bedtime.

To Improve Circulation

Blends:
Circulation blend #1:
• 5 drops basil
• 8 drops marjoram
• 10 drops cypress
• 3 drops peppermint

Circulation blend #2:
• 3 drops basil
• 2 drops peppermint
• 4 drops cypress
• 8 drops marjoram
• 10 drops wintergreen

EO Applications:
TOPICAL:
DILUTE either of the above recipes in 1 tsp V6 Oil Complex and massage on location, 1-3 times daily

Varicose Veins (Spider Veins)

The blue color of varicose veins is congealed blood in the surrounding tissue from hemorrhaging of capillaries around the veins. This blood has to be dissolved and re-absorbed.

Helichrysum helps dissolve the coagulated blood in the surrounding tissue.

Cypress strengthens capillary walls.

Single Oils:
Helichrysum, cypress, wintergreen, basil, peppermint, lemon, lavender

Blends:
Citrus Fresh, Aroma Life, Aroma Siez

Varicose vein blend #1:
- 3-4 drops basil
- 1 drop wintergreen
- 1 drop cypress
- 1 drop helichrysum

Varicose vein blend #2:
- 2 drops helichrysum
- 2 drops of cypress.

EO Applications:
TOPICAL:
> NEAT, apply 2-4 drops on location, massaging toward the heart, 3-6 times daily

Nightly Varicose Vein Regimen (legs):
A. Apply 1-3 drops varicose vein blend #1, neat on location. Rub very gently towards heart with smooth strokes along the vein, then up and over the vein until the oil is absorbed. Repeat with blend #2.
B. Apply 6 drops tangerine and 6 drops cypress to the area. Gently massage until absorbed.
C. Do the lymphatic pump procedure described in Chapter 22.
D. Follow with a soft massage of the whole leg using 10-15 drops of Aroma Life, diluted 50-50
E. Wrap and elevate the leg. It is best to do this at night before retiring and to gradually elevate the foot off the bed, an inch more each night, until it is 4 inches higher than the head.
F. Wear support hose during the daytime. It may take up to a year to achieve desired results.

Dietary Supplementation:
VitaGreen, Super B, Longevity Caps

Topical Treatment:
OrthoEase, Cel-Lite Magic, Thieves Spray

COLD SORES (Herpes Simplex Type 1)

Cold sores are also known as *Herpes labialis.* Diets high in the amino acid lysine can reduce the incidence of herpes. Conversely, the amino acid arginine can worsen herpes outbreaks.

Studies have shown neat applications of melissa to be effective against Herpes Simplex type I and Herpes Labialis. The healing period was shortened, the spread of infection prevented, and symptoms such as itching, tingling and burning were lessened.[15,16]

Peppermint and tea tree oils have also been studied for positive effects on the pain of herpes.[17,18]

Single Oils:
Melissa, tea tree, peppermint, lavender, sandalwood, mountain savory, ravensara, oregano, thyme

Blends:
Thieves, Melrose, Purification

EO Applications:
TOPICAL:
> NEAT, apply one drop as soon as a cold sore starts. Repeat 5-10 times daily.
> DILUTE 50-50, dilution in V6 Oil Complex will help to reduce discomfort or drying of the skin when applying essential oils to an open sore.

Dietary Supplementation:
ImmuPro, Super C, Longevity Caps, VitaGreen, ImmuneTune, Stevia, Cleansing Trio, JuvaTone, JuvaPower/Spice

Topical Treatments:
Thieves Antiseptic Spray, Thieves Lozenges, ImmuGel

Apply ImmuGel with 1 drop each of sandalwood and tea tree.

15. Dimitrova et al., "effect of Melissa officinalis L. extracts," Acta Microbiol Bulg 1993;29-:65-72.

16. Koytchev R, et al., "Balm mint extract (Lo-701) for topical treatment of recurring herpes labialis," Phytomedicine 1999 Oct;6(4):225-30.

17. Davies SJ, Harding LM, Baranowski AP, "A novel treatment of postherpetic neuralgia using peppermint oil," Clin J Pain 2002 May-Jun;18(3):200-2

18. Carson CF et al., "Melaleuca alternifolia (tea tree) oil gel (6%) for the treatment of recurrent herpes labialis," J Antimicrob Chemother 2001 Sep;48(3):450-1.

COLDS

(See also INFECTION, SINUS INFECTIONS, THROAT INFECTIONS, and LUNG INFECTIONS)

The best treatment for a cold or flu is prevention. Because many essential oils have strong antimicrobial properties, they can be diffused to prevent the spread of airborne bacteria and viruses. Antiviral essential oils (such as basil, hyssop, rosemary, tea tree, clove, oregano and thyme) and blends (such as Thieves, Purification, R.C., Raven, and Sacred Mountain (as well as many of the oils in the Oils of Ancient Scripture kit) are very effective as preventative aids in avoiding colds as well as in helping the body defenses fight colds, once an infection has started. ImmuPro tablets are a powerful immune stimulant that can also increase infection resistance.

Single Oils:
Peppermint, thyme, bay laurel, oregano, rosewood, *Eucalyptus radiata*, tea tree, ravensara, rosemary, mountain savory

Blends:
Melrose, Thieves, Australian Blue, Purification, ImmuPower, Sacred Mountain, Exodus II, Raven, R.C., Christmas Spirit

Cold blend #1:
- 2 drops lemon
- 4 drops Eucalyptus radiata
- 5 drops rosemary
- 4 drops peppermint
- 3 drops cypress

Cold blend #2:
- 5 drops rosemary
- 4 drops R.C.
- 4 drops frankincense
- 1 drops oregano
- 2 drops peppermint

EO Applications:
INHALATION:
    DIRECT, 3-5 times daily, or as needed
    VAPOR, 2-3 times daily, as needed
INGESTION:
    SYRUP, 3-6 times daily
ORAL:
    GARGLE, 3-6 times daily

TOPICAL:
    DILUTE 50-50, massage 1-3 drops on each of the following areas: forehead, nose, cheeks, lower throat, chest and upper back, 1-3 times daily
    VITA FLEX, massage 1-3 drops on Vita Flex points on the feet, 1-2 times daily
    RAINDROP Technique, 1-2 times weekly
    BATH SALTS, (see below)

Bath blend for relief of cold symptoms:
- 2 drops Eucalyptus radiata
- 6 drops frankincense
- 3 drops helichrysum
- 6 drops spruce
- 15 drops ravensara
- 1 drop wintergreen

Stir above essential oils into 1/2 cup Epsom salt or baking soda, then add the mixture to hot bath water while tub is filling. Soak in hot bath until water cools.

Dietary Supplementation:
ImmuPro, Thieves Lozenges, Super C, Super C Chewables, Longevity Caps, VitaGreen, ImmuneTune, Rehemogen, Power Meal, Exodus

Oral Treatment:
Thieves Antiseptic Spray

Congestive Cough

Single Oils:
Eucalyptus globulus, goldenrod, ledum, spruce, ravensara, cedarwood, marjoram, hyssop

Blends:
Thieves, Melrose, Peace & Calming, Raven, R.C., Idaho balsam fir

EO Applications:
INGESTION:
    SYRUP, 2-4 times daily
INHALATION:
    DIRECT, 3-6 times daily, as needed
    VAPOR, 1-3 times daily, as needed
ORAL:
    GARGLE, 4-6 times daily
TOPICAL:
    COMPRESS, warm, 1-2 times daily over chest, over throat and on upper back

Dietary Supplementation:
ImmuPro, Super C, Super C Chewables, Exodus, Thieves lozenges, Thieves Antiseptic Spray

Other:
Gargle 3-6 times daily with Fresh Essence Plus mouthwash

Excess Mucus

(See MUCUS)

Head Cold / Sinus Congestion

(See also SINUS INFECTIONS)

Single Oils:
Ledum, German chamomile, *Eucalyptus radiata*, frankincense, pine, Idaho balsam fir, peppermint, rosemary, ravensara, lemon

Blends:
R.C., Raven, Melrose, Sacred Mountain, Christmas Spirit

EO Applications:
INHALATION:
  DIRECT, 3-5 times daily, or as needed
  VAPOR, 2-3 times daily, as needed
INGESTION:
  SYRUP, 3-6 times daily
ORAL:
  GARGLE, 3-6 times daily
TOPICAL:
  DILUTE 50-50, massage 1-3 drops on each of the following areas: forehead, nose, cheeks, lower throat, chest and upper back, 1-3 times daily
  VITA FLEX, massage 1-3 drops on Vita Flex points on the feet, 1-2 times daily
  RAINDROP Technique, 1-2 times weekly
  BATH SALTS, daily

COLITIS, Ulcerative

Also known as ileitis or proctitis, ulcerative colitis is marked by the inflammation of the top layers of the lining of the large intestine (colon) It is different from both irritable bowel syndrome (which has no inflammation) and Crohn's disease (which occurs deeper in the colon wall).

The inflammation and ulcerous sores that are characteristic of ulcerative colitis occur most frequently in the lower colon and rectum and occasionally throughout the entire colon.

Symptoms include: fatigue, nausea, weight loss, loss of appetite, bloody diarrhea, loss of body fluids and nutrients, frequent fevers, abdominal cramps, arthritis, liver disease, skin rashes

Single Oils:
Peppermint, spearmint, tarragon, anise, fennel

Blends: Di-Tone, Thieves

EO Applications:
INGESTION:
  CAPSULE, 00 size, 2-3 times daily
  SYRUP, 3-4 times daily
TOPICAL:
  DILUTE 50-50, massage 4-6 drops over lower abdomen area 2-4 times daily

Dietary Supplementation:
ICP, ComforTone, AlkaLime, Polyzyme, Essential Omegas, Detoxzyme, Mega Cal

COLITIS, Viral

In cases where colitis is caused by a virus rather than a bacteria, the following treatments are recommended:

Single Oils:
Blue cypress, melissa, oregano, cumin, tea tree, lemongrass, tarragon, niaouli, thyme, Roman chamomile, German chamomile, rosemary, peppermint, clove, cinnamon

Blends:
Thieves, Longevity, Di-Tone, Melrose, Purification, 3 Wise Men

EO Applications:
INGESTION:
  CAPSULE, 00 size, 2-3 times daily
TOPICAL:
  DILUTE 50-50, massage 4-6 drops over colon area 2-4 times daily
  VITA FLEX, 1-3 drops on colon Vita Flex points
  RAINDROP Technique, 1-2 times weekly

COMPRESS, warm, diluted 20-80, using equal parts helichrysum and Di-Tone over colon area

RETENTION:

RECTAL, use the formula below in a rectal implant 3 times weekly

Viral colitis retention blend:

- 2 drops oregano
- 2 drops thyme
- 3 drops Purification
- 2 drops Roman chamomile
- 2 drops clove or cinnamon
- 2 drops Di-Tone

Mix above oils with 1 tablespoon V6 Advanced Oil Complex

Dietary Supplementation:

Polyzyme, ImmuPro, VitaGreen, Master Vitamin Formula

Colon and Liver Cleanse:

Cleansing Trio, JuvaTone, JuvaFlex, JuvaCleanse

Take Polyzyme, along with ComforTone. Wait about 2 weeks or more before adding ICP. Start with a small amount of the ICP and increase slowly. If any discomfort is experienced, reduce the amount taken.

COMA

Single Oils:

Frankincense, vetiver, sandalwood, cypress, black pepper, peppermint, Idaho balsam fir

Blends:

Trauma Life, Hope, Valor, Surrender

EO Applications:
INHALATION:

DIFFUSION, 15 minutes, 4-7 times daily

TOPICAL:

DILUTE 50-50, 3-5 drops on temples, neck and shoulders

Dietary Supplementation:

Mineral Essence, Ultra Young

CONFUSION

Single Oils:

Peppermint, lemon, rosemary, basil, cardamom

Blends:

Clarity, Brain Power, M-Grain, Legacy, Gathering

Dietary Supplementation:

Mineral Essence, Super Cal, Super B, Ultra Young.

CONGESTIVE HEART FAILURE

(See HEART)

Coenzyme Q10 is one of the most effective supplements for supporting the heart muscle.

Single Oils:

Helichrysum, cypress, goldenrod

Blends:

Aroma Life, Longevity

Dietary Supplementation:

HRT, CardiaCare, Super Cal, Mineral Essence, Essential Omegas

CONNECTIVE TISSUE TRAUMA
(Ligaments, Tendons)

Tendonitis, (often called Tennis Elbow and Golfer's Elbow), is a torn or inflamed tendon. Tenosynovitis, sometimes called "Trigger Finger," is an inflamed tendon being restricted by its sheath (particularly thumbs and fingers). Repetitive use or infection may be the cause.

Super Cal and BLM provide critical nutrients for connective tissue repair. Sulfurzyme, an outstanding source of organic sulfur, equalizes water pressure inside the cells and reduces pain.

How to Speed Healing

With any damaged tissue, circulation should be increased to promote healing. The essential oil of cypress can increase circulation.

Anytime there is tissue damage, there is always inflammation which should be addressed first.

PanAway reduces pain and lemongrass promotes the repair of connective tissue. Lavender with lemongrass, and marjoram with lemongrass work well together for inflamed tendons.

When selecting oils for injuries, think through the cause and type of injury and select appropriate oils. For instance, tendonitis could encompass muscle damage, nerve damage, ligament strain/tear, inflammation, infection, and possibly an emotion. Therefore, select an oil or oils for each potential cause and apply in rotation or prepare a blend to address multiple causes. The emotional distress may be anger or guilt.

The oils in Ortho Sport and Ortho Ease Massage Oils reduce pain and promote healing.

Single Oils:
Basil, lemongrass, marjoram, helichrysum, wintergreen, cypress, peppermint, rosemary, *Eucalyptus radiata*

Blends:
PanAway, Aroma Life, R.C., Relieve It, Release, Citrus Fresh

The following lists show singles and blends best suited to the specific trouble spots involved with connective tissue:

BONE:
Wintergreen, spruce, Idaho balsam fir, PanAway, Relieve It

MUSCLE:
Basil, marjoram, lavender, Relieve It, PanAway

LIGAMENT:
Lemongrass, helichrysum, lavender, PanAway, Relieve It, elemi, Idaho tansy

TENDONS:
Lavender, lemongrass, marjoram

SPASMS:
Aroma Siez with Ortho Ease or Ortho Sport Massage Oils

EO Applications:
TOPICAL:
NEAT or DILUTE 50-50 as required. Gently massage 4-6 drops on affected areas 2-4 times daily. For swelling, elevate and apply ice packs
COMPRESS, cold, 2-4 times daily

Dietary Supplementation:
Master Formula, ArthroTune, Super Cal, Super B, Super C, VitaGreen, Longevity Caps, Mineral Essence, Sulfurzyme (capsules or powder)

Topical Treatment: Ortho Ease, Regenolone, Neurogen, Ortho Sport Massage Oils

Knee Cartilage Injury

Single Oils:
Peppermint, Idaho balsam fir, Douglas fir, wintergreen, white fir

Blends:
Cartilage blend:
- 9 drops lemongrass
- 10 drops marjoram
- 12 drops ginger

Sprain/Torn Ligament

NOTE: For sprains, use cold packs. For any serious sprain or constant skeletal pain, always consult a health care professional. Any time there is tissue damage, there is always inflammation. Reduce this first.

Single Oils:
Idaho tansy, valerian, vetiver,

Blends:
PanAway

Sprain blend:
- 5 drop lemongrass
- 15 drops Aroma Siez

Tendonitis

Tendonitis blend #1:
- 8 drops vetiver
- 8 drops valerian
- 4 drops Idaho tasny

Tendonitis blend #2 (for pain relief):
- 10 drops rosemary
- 10 drops *Eucalyptus radiata*
- 10 drops peppermint

Topical Treatment: Ortho Ease, Regenolone, Neurogen, Mega Cal, BLM

CONSTIPATION

The principle causes of constipation are inadequate fluid intake and low fiber consumption. Constipation can eventually lead to diverticulosis and diverticulitis, conditions common among older people. Certain essential oils have demonstrated their ability to improve colon health through supporting intestinal flora, stimulating intestinal motility and peristalsis, fighting infections and eliminating parasites.

(see also DIVERTICULOSIS and DIVERTICULITIS)

Single Oils:
Ginger, peppermint, fennel, tarragon, anise seed.

Blends:
Di-Tone

EO Applications:
INGESTION:
> CAPSULE, 00 size, 2-3 times daily
> RICE MILK, 2-4 times daily

Dietary Supplementation:
Essentialzyme, Cleansing Trio, AlkaLime, Polyzyme, BodyGize, Longevity Caps, Wolfberry Crisp, Power Meal

Regimen:
- Essentialzyme: 3 to 6 capsules, 3 times daily
- AlkaLime: 1 Tbsp. in water, 2 times daily before or after meals
- ComforTone: Start with 1 capsule and increase next day to 2 capsules. Continue to increase 1 capsule each day until bowels start moving.

Why Constipation Can Produce Problems Later in Life

The reason constipation creates diverticulosis is due to the fact that the muscles of the colon must strain to move an overly-hard stool, which puts excess pressure on the colon. Eventually weak spots in the colon walls form, resulting in the creation of abnormal pouches called diverticula.

These pouches can also be created by parasites which burrow and embed in the lining of the colon wall and lay eggs there. It's always wise to consider treating for parasites when diverticula are present.

- ICP: One week after beginning ComforTone, start with 1 Tbsp., 2 times daily and then increase to 3 times daily, up to 2 Tbsp., 3 times daily.
- Drink aloe vera juice, water, prune juice, unsweetened pineapple juice, and other raw fruit and vegetable juices, regularly.

CONVULSIONS

(See also BRAIN DISORDERS)

Monitor diet. Discontinue sugar and dairy products, fried and processed foods.

Blends:
Brain Power, Valor

Dietary Supplementation:
Master Formula, Ultra Young

EO Applications:
INHALATION:
> DIRECT, 4-6 times daily
> DIFFUSION, 20 minutes, 2-3 times daily
TOPICAL:
> NEAT, apply 2-4 drops at base of skull, across the neck and top of spine (C1-C6 vertebrae) and on bottom of feet (for relief only)

CORNS

(See FOOT PROBLEMS)

COUGHS

(See LUNG INFECTIONS and COLDS)

CRAMPS (Abdominal)

(See DIGESTIVE PROBLEMS)

CRAMPS (Muscle)

(See MUSCLES)

CROHN'S DISEASE

Crohn's disease creates inflammation, sores, and ulcers on the intestinal wall. These sores occur deeper than ulcerative colitis. Moreover, unlike other forms of colitis, Crohn's disease can also occur in other areas of the body including the large intestine, appendix, stomach, and mouth.

Symptoms include:
- Abdominal cramping
- Lower right abdominal pain
- Diarrhea
- A general sense of feeling ill

Attacks may occur once or twice a day for life. If the disease continues for years, it can cause deterioration of bowel function, leaking bowel, poor absorption of nutrients, loss of appetite and weight, intestinal obstruction, severe bleeding, and increased susceptibility to intestinal cancer.

Some researchers believe that Crohn's disease is caused by an overreacting immune system and is actually an autoimmune disease (where the immune system mistakenly attacks the body's own tissues). MSM has been extensively researched for its ability to treat many autoimmune diseases, and is the subject of research by University of Oregon researcher Stanley Jacobs. (MSM is a key ingredient in Sulfurzyme).

Single Oils:
Peppermint, nutmeg

Blends:
Di-Tone

EO Applications:
INGESTION:
    CAPSULE, 00 size, 3 times daily
    RICE MILK, 2-4 times daily
TOPICAL:
    RAINDROP Technique, 1-2 times weekly, using ImmuPower

Dietary Supplementation:
Sulfurzyme, Polyzyme, ImmuGel, AlkaLime, ICP, VitaGreen, Cleansing Trio, Power Meal, and Mineral Essence

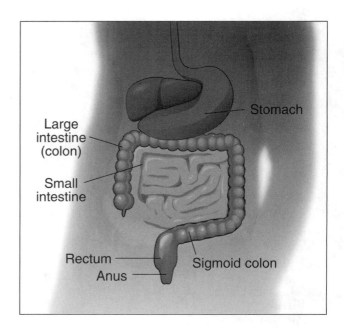

Regimen for Crohn's disease:

- Polyzyme: 1-2 capsules, 3 times daily.
- ImmuGel: 1/2 tsp., 5 times daily.

Each phase lasts 1 week and should be added to the previous phases.

Phase I: Take Polyzyme in yogurt or liquid acidophilus, and charcoal tablets. Do not use ICP, ComforTone, or Essentialzyme.

Phase II: Add AlkaLime if no diarrhea, and BodyGize.

Raw juices (5 oz. celery and 2 oz carrot).

Phase III: VitaGreen

Phase IV: (Start only after a week with no sign of bleeding).
- ComforTone (1 capsule morning and night) until stools loosen.
- ICP: Start with 1 level tsp., 2 times daily and gradually increase.
- Essentialzyme: Start 1 tablet, 3 times daily. If irritation occurs, discontinue Cleansing Trio for a few days and start again.
- Mineral Essence: Start the second week: 1 dropper, 2 times daily.

CUSHING'S DISEASE

(See ADRENAL GLAND IMBALANCE)

CUTS

(See WOUNDS, SCRAPES AND CUTS)

CYST (Ganglion)

Singles:
Oregano, thyme

EO Applications:
TOPICAL:
NEAT, 2 drops oregano first day, 2 drops thyme second day, apply on location as often as needed

CYSTITIS

(See URINARY TRACT/BLADDER INFECTION)

DANDRUFF

(See HAIR AND SCALP PROBLEMS)

DECONGESTANTS

(See MUCUS)

DENTAL PROBLEMS

(See ORAL CARE)

DEODORANT

(See FUNGAL INFECTIONS)

Excessive body odor indicates putrefaction in the system and possibly poor digestion from the lack of enzymes in the digestive tract. It can also be caused by hormone imbalances and candida infections.

The essential oils of lavender, lavandin, citronella, geranium, and melaleuca inhibit proliferation of odor-causing bacteria on the skin.

Single Oils:
Lavender, geranium, bergamot, cypress, blue cypress, *Eucalyptus globulus*, myrtle

Blends:
Aroma Siez, Dragon Time, EndoFlex, Joy, Mister, R.C., Melrose

EO Applications:
TOPICAL:
DILUTE 50-50, apply 2-4 drops under arms or on the skin. Put 2 drops on a washcloth when washing.
BATH SALTS, daily

Deoderant Powder Recipe:
- 4 ounces of unscented talcum powder
- 2 ounces of baking soda
- 3 drops lavender oil or geranium oil

Mix well. Use under arms, on the feet (or in shoes).

Topical Treatment:
Aromaguard Deodorant, Fresh Essence Plus, Progessence Cream, Thieves Antiseptic Spray

DEPRESSION

(See also INSOMNIA)

Diffusing or directly inhaling essential oils can have an immediate positive impact on mood. Olfaction is the only sense that can have direct effects on the limbic region of the brain. Studies at the University of Vienna[19] have shown that some essential oils and their primary constituents (cineol) can stimulate blood flow and activity in the emotional regions of the brain.

Clinical studies at the Department of Psychiatry at the Mie University of Medicine showed that lemon not only reduced depression but reduced stress when inhaled. [20]

Single Oils:
Jasmine absolute, lemon, sage, frankincense, peppermint

Blends:
Joy, Valor, Passion, Hope

---

19. Nasel et al., Functional imaging of effects of fragrances on the human brain after prolonged inhalation, *Chem Senses,* 1995 Jun;20(3):349-50.

20. Komori, Fujiward, Tanida, Nomura, Yokoyama "Effects of citrus fragrance on immune function and depressive states". *Neuroimmunomodulation.* 1995 May-Jun;2(3):174-80.

EO Applications:
INHALATION:
> DIFFUSION, 20 minutes, 3 times daily
> DIRECT, 4-6 times daily

Dietary Supplementation:
Essential Omegas, AD&E, Vitagreen, Royaldolphus

Postpartum Depression

Single Oils:
Vetiver, lemon, cedarwood, sandalwood, St. John's wort

Blends:
Trauma Life, Joy, Peace & Calming, Transformation

EO Applications:
INHALATION:
> DIFFUSION, 20 minutes, 3 times daily
> DIRECT, 4-6 times daily

TOPICAL:
> NEAT, 2-4 drops on temples and/or back of neck 2-4 times daily, as needed

Dietary Supplementation:
Ultra Young

DERMATITIS
(see Eczema/Dermatitis in SKIN DISORDERS)

DIABETES (Blood Sugar Imbalance)

Diabetes is the leading cause of cardiovascular disease and premature death in westernized countries today. Diabetes causes low energy and persistently high blood glucose.

Type I Diabetes usually manifests by age 30 and is often considered to be genetic. Type II Diabetes generally manifests later in life and may have a nutritional origin.

Single Oils:
Coriander, cinnamon, fennel, dill, cypress, rosemary, clove

Blends:
Thieves, EndoFlex, JuvaFlex, JuvaCleanse, Di-Tone

EO Applications:
INGESTION:
> CAPSULE, 0 size, 3 times daily

Dietary Supplementation:
VitaGreen, Stevia, Master His/ Hers, Essentialzyme, Carbozyme, Super B, BodyGize, Power Meal, Longevity Caps, Mineral Essence, Sulfurzyme, Wolfberry Crisp Bars

Regimen for diabetes:
- BodyGize and Power Meal, at least one serving of each daily
- VitaGreen: 8 to 16 capsules daily.
- Sulfurzyme: 1 to 4 Tbsp. daily.
- Mix equal amounts of Thieves, coriander, fennel and dill and massage this blend on pancreas Vita Flex points of the feet 2-4 times daily. Alternatively, this same blend can be applied in a warm compress over pancreas area.
- Cleansing Trio, JuvaTone, JuvaFlex, JuvaCleanse, JuvaCleanse. Use these as recommended to help the body detoxify

VitaGreen is high in plant protein, which helps balance blood glucose. The MSM/sulfur found in the Sulfurzyme promotes insulin production.

Essentialzyme supports enzyme production, which helps keep the pancreas from premature wasting and enlargement, a condition linked to diabetes and premature aging.

Super B is a good source of B vitamins to support pancreas function.

The Stevia leaf extract is one of the most health-restoring plants known. It is a natural sweetener, has no calories, and does not have the harmful side effects of processed sugar or sugar substitutes. Stevia increases glucose tolerance and helps normalize blood sugar fluctuations.

Wolfberry balances the pancreas and is a detoxifier and cleanser. Diabetes is not common in certain regions of China, where wolfberry is consumed regularly.

An East Indian herbal formula was shown in a *Journal of the National Medical Association* study to possess hypoglycemic activity. The herbs are: *Cinnamomum tamale*, *Pterocarpus marsupeum*, *Momordica charantia*, *Azardichta indica*, *Tinospora cordifolia*, *Aegle marmelose*, *Gymnema sylvestre*, *Syzygium cumini*, *Trigonella foenum graecum*, and *Ficus racemosa*.

DIGESTION PROBLEMS

Any of the following indicate that the digestive system is not digesting properly:
- Rumbling or gurgling sounds in the abdomen.
- Heartburn (may be a possible indication of candida).
- Constipation and/or diarrhea.
- Constant hunger or fatigue after eating.
- Food intolerance or food allergies.
- Intestinal parasites.

Poor bowel function is linked to enzyme deficiency, low fiber, insufficient liquid, bad diet, and stress.

Cramps (Stomach)

Single Oils:
Rosemary, ginger, basil, peppermint

EO Applications:
INGESTION:
CAPSULE, 0 size, 2 times daily
RICE MILK, 1-3 times daily
TOPICAL:
DILUTE 50-50, apply 6-10 drops over stomach area 2 times daily
COMPRESS, warm, 1-2 times daily
VITA FLEX, 1-3 drops on stomach Vita Flex points of feet

Diarrhea

Single Oils:
Peppermint, nutmeg, ginger, oregano, mountain savory, clove, lemon

Blends:
Di-Tone, Thieves

Diarrhea detox blend:
- 4 drops lemon
- 3 drops mountain savory
- 2 drops oregano

EO Applications:
INGESTION:
CAPSULE, 0 size, 2 times daily
RICE MILK, 1-3 times daily

TOPICAL:
DILUTE 50-50, apply 6-10 drops over stomach area 2 times daily
COMPRESS, warm, 1-2 times daily
VITA FLEX, 1-3 drops on stomach Vita Flex points of feet

Dietary Supplementation:
Essential Omegas, ComforTone, ICP, Essentialzyme, JuvaTone, JuvaPower/Spice

A maintenance dosage of ComforTone has protected travelers going to other countries from diarrhea and other digestive discomforts.

Nutmeg has been shown to have powerful action against diarrhea in a number of medical studies.[21,22]

Gas, Flatulence:

Single Oils:
Peppermint, tarragon, nutmeg, anise seed, fennel, ledum, carrot seed

Blends: Di-Tone

EO Applications:
INGESTION:
CAPSULE, 0 size, 2 times daily
TOPICAL:
DILUTE 50-50, apply 6-10 drops over stomach area twice daily
COMPRESS, warm, 1-2 times daily
VITA FLEX, 1-3 drops on stomach Vita Flex points of feet

Dietary Supplementation:
Essentialzyme, Polyzyme, AlkaLime, Super Cal, mega Cal

Heartburn

Lemon juice is one of the best remedies for heartburn. Mix the juice of 1/2 squeezed lemon in 8 oz. water and slip slowly upon awakening each morning.

By ingesting lemon juice and/or essential oils the stomach stops excreting digestive acids. Therefore alleviating heartburn or other stomach ailments.

21. Weiss HJ, et al., "The effect of salicylates on the hemostatic properties of platelets in man," *J Clin Invest* 1968 Sep;47(9):2169-80.

22. Fawell WN, Thompson G, "Nutmeg for diarrhea of medullarly carcinoma of thyroid," *N Eng J Med* 1973 Jul 12;289(2):108-9.

Single Oils:
Peppermint, ginger, spearmint, lemon

Blends:
Di-Tone, EndoFlex, JuvaFlex, JuvaCleanse

Heartburn blend:
- 2 drops basil
- 1 drop Idaho tansy
- 8 drops sage
- 3 drops sandalwood

EO Applications:
INGESTION:
    CAPSULE, 0 size, 2 times daily
TOPICAL:
    DILUTE 50-50, apply 6-10 drops over
    stomach area twice daily
    COMPRESS, warm, 1-2 times daily
    VITA FLEX, 103 drops on stomach Vita
    Flex points of feet

Dietary Supplementation:
ICP, ComforTone, Essentialzyme, Polyzyme,
Detoxzyme, Alkalime, Juva Power

Hiccups

(See HICCUPS)

Indigestion

Singles:
Peppermint, nutmeg, fennel, ginger, cumin,
spearmint, orange, grapefruit

Blends:
Di-Tone

EO Applications:
INGESTION:
    CAPSULE, 0 size, 2 times daily
    RICE MILK, 1-3 times daily, as needed
TOPICAL:
    DILUTE 50-50, apply 6-10 drops over
    stomach area twice daily
    VitaFlex, 1-3 drops on stomach Vita
    Flex points of feet

Dietary Supplementation:
Stevia, ICP, ComforTone, Essentialzyme,
Polyzyme, Carbozyme, Lipozyme, Stevia

Polyzyme, Essentialzyme or Detoxzyme taken
before eating helps with digestion and upset
stomach. When heaviness is felt in the stomach,
Polyzyme is a beneficial companion to Di-Tone.

Nausea

(See NAUSEA)

Ulcers, Stomach

Ulcers may be caused by *Helicobacter pylori*
(bacteria). Several gastroduodenal diseases
include gastritis and gastric or peptic ulcers.

Single Oils:
Clove, cinnamon, tea tree, oregano, thyme

Blends:
Thieves, R.C., Exodus II, Legacy

EO Applications:
INGESTION:
    CAPSULE, 0 size, 1 capsule
    3 times a day for 20 days

DIPTHERIA

An acute infectious disease caused by toxigenic
strains of *Corynebacterium diphtheriae,* acquired
by contact with an infected person or carrier. It is
usually confined to the upper respiratory tract,
and characterized by the formation of a tough
false membrane attached firmly to the underlying
tissue that will bleed if forcibly removed. In the
most serious infections the membrane begins in
the tonsil area and may spread to the uvula, soft
palate and pharyngeal wall, followed by the
larynx, trachea, and bronchial tree where it may
cause life-threatening bronchial obstructions.

Single Oils:
Goldenrod, thyme, clove, *Eucalyptus radiata*

EO Applications:
INHALATION:
    DIRECT, 6-8 times daily
INGESTION:
    CAPSULE, 00 size, 2 times daily

DISINFECTANT

(See ANTISEPTIC)

DIVERTICULOSIS / DIVERTICULITIS

Diverticulosis is one of the most common conditions in the U.S. It is caused by a lack of fiber in the diet. Diverticulosis is characterized by small, abnormal pouches (diverticula) that bulge out through weak spots in the wall of the intestine. It is estimated that half of all Americans from age 60 to 80 have diverticulosis.

Symptoms:
• Cramping
• Bloating
• Constipation

One of the easiest ways to resolve this condition is by increasing fiber intake to 20-30 grams daily. Peppermint oil stimulates contractions in the colon.

While diverticulosis involves the condition of merely having colon abnormalities, diverticulitis occurs when these abnormalities or diverticula become infected or inflamed. Diverticulitis is present in 10 to 25 percent of people with diverticulosis.

Symptoms:
• Tenderness on lower left side of abdomen
• Fever and chills
• Constipation
• Cramping

Many of these symptoms are similar to those of irritable bowel syndrome.

(See also IRRITABLE BOWEL SYNDROME)

Single Oils:
Patchouli, anise seed, tarragon, rosemary, fennel, peppermint, mountain savory, oregano, thyme, nutmeg, frankincense

Blends: Di-Tone. Melrose

Recipe 1:
• 15 drops Di-Tone
• 5 drops Melrose

Recipe 2:
• 10 drops Di-Tone
• 15 drops frankincense

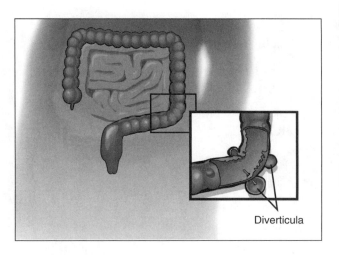

Diverticula

EO Applications:
INGESTION:
> CAPSULE, enteric coated, 0 size, 2-3 times daily
> SYRUP, 2-3 times daily

TOPICAL:
> DILUTE 50-50, 3-5 drops on lower abdomen 2 times daily
> VITA FLEX, 2-4 drops on intestinal Vita Flex points on feet, 2-3 times daily
> COMPRESS, warm, 2 times daily

RETENTION:
> RECTAL, nightly before retiring, retain overnight

Dietary Supplementation:
ICP, Essential Manna, products in the Cleansing Trio, Mineral Essence, ImmuPro, ImmuneTune, Essential Omegas, Exodus, Immugel, Stevia, Comfortone, Immugel, Juva Power

DIZZINESS

Single Oils:
Cypress, tangerine, peppermint, basil, cardamom, frankincense

Blends:
Aroma Life, Clarity, Brain Power, Thieves

EO Applications:
INHALATION:
> DIRECT, 1-2 minutes, as needed

TOPICAL:
> NEAT, 1-3 drops on temples, back of neck and shoulders, as needed
> VITA FLEX, 1-3 drops on brain Vita Flex points of feet, as needed

329

Dietary Supplementation:
VitaGreen, Essential Manna

Topical Treatment:
Cel-Lite Magic Massage Oil

If blood circulation is a factor, see
CIRCULATION.

DYSENTERY

Single Oils:
Lemon, mountain savory, oregano, peppermint

Blends: Thieves, Di-Tone

Mix Thieves with 5 drops of peppermint and
take orally.

EO Applications:
INGESTION:
   CAPSULE, 00 size, 3 times daily

Dietary Supplementation:
Polyzyme, Detoxzyme, ImmuPro,
Essentialzyme, ICP, Mineral Essence, Juva
Power

DYSPEPSIA

(See DIGESTIVE PROBLEMS)

EAR PROBLEMS

Ear Ache

Single Oils:
Thyme, lavender, tea tree, rosemary,
helichrysum, Roman chamomile, ravensara,
peppermint, *Eucalyptus radiata*

Blends:
Melrose, Purification, PanAway, Thieves
(diluted), Immupower

Other:
Thieves Antiseptic Spray

EO Applications:
TOPICAL:
   DILUTE 50-50 in warm olive or
   fractionated coconut oil. Apply 2 drops to a
   cotton swab. Using the swab, apply traces
   to the skin AROUND the opening of the ear,
   but not in it. Put 2-3 drops of the diluted

essential oil on a piece of cotton and place it
carefully over the ear opening. Leave in
overnight. Additional relief may be obtained
by placing a warm compress over the ear
VITA FLEX, massage 1-2 drops on ear lobes
and on ear Vita Flex points of the feet

CAUTION: Never put essential oils directly
into the ear. Ear pain can be very serious.
Always seek medical attention if pain persists.

Dietary Supplementation:
Super C, Longevity Caps, ImmuPro, VitaGreen,
ImmuneTune, Rehemogen, Cleansing Trio,
JuvaTone, JuvaPower/Spice

Ear Mites

Single Oils:
Eucalyptus radiata, tea tree

Blends:
Purification

EO Applications:
TOPICAL:
   DILUTE 50-50 in warm olive oil. Apply 2
   drops to a cotton swab. Using the swab,
   apply traces to the skin AROUND the
   opening of the ear, but not in it. Put 2-3
   drops of the diluted essential oil on a piece
   of cotton and place it carefully over the ear
   opening. Leave in overnight. Additional
   relief may be obtained by placing a warm
   compress over the ear
   VITA FLEX, massage 1-2 drops on ear lobes
   and on ear Vita Flex points of the feet

CAUTION: Never put essential oils directly into
the ear. Ear pain can be very serious. Always
seek medical attention if pain persists.

Perforated Eardrum

Single Oils:
Lavender

Blends:
Melrose

EO Applications:
TOPICAL:
   DILUTE 50-50 in warm olive oil. Apply 2
   drops to a cotton swab. Using the swab,
   apply traces to the skin AROUND the

opening of the ear, but not in it. Put 2-3 drops of the diluted essential oil on a piece of cotton and place it carefully over the ear opening. Leave in overnight.

CAUTION: Never put essential oils directly into the ear. Ear pain can be very serious. Always seek medical attention if pain persists.

ECZEMA

(See ECZEMA/PSORIASIS in SKIN DISORDERS)

EDEMA (Swelling)

(See also KIDNEY DISORDERS, WATER RETENTION)

Swelling--particularly around the ankles--is noticeable when fluids accumulate in the tissue. This puffiness under the skin and around the ankles is more apparent at the end of the day when fluids settle to the lowest part of the body. A potassium deficiency can make swelling worse, so the first recourse is to increase potassium intake.

Single Oils:
Ledum, German chamomile, cedarwood, wintergreen, peppermint, lavender, clove grapefruit, juniper, orange, fennel, geranium,

Blends:
Aroma Life, EndoFlex, DiTone

Edema blend #1:
- 10 drops tangerine
- 5 drops cypress
- 10 drops lemon or 3 drops juniper

Edema blend #2:
- 10 drops wintergreen
- 6 drops fennel
- 2 drops idaho tansy
- 3 drops patchouli
- 10 drops tangerine

EO Applications:
TOPICAL:
DILUTE 50-50, massage 3-5 drops into affected area 2-3 times daily
COMPRESS, cold, 1-2 times daily
VITA FLEX, massage 1-3 drops on bladder Vita Flex point on foot

INGESTION:
CAPSULE, 0 size, 2 times daily

Morning and Evening Edema regimen:

Morning blend:
- 10 drops tangerine
- 10 drops cypress

Evening blend:
- 8 drops geranium
- 5 drops cypress
- 5 drops helichrysum

Dilute each blend 50-50 in vegetable or massage oil and rub 6-10 drops on legs working from the feet up to the thighs. Do this for one week

Dietary Supplementation:
Essential Manna, nutmeg oil, Super Cal, Super C, K & B, Master Formula Vitamins

EMOTIONAL TRAUMA

(See Chapter 14)

The effect of heavy emotional trauma can disrupt the stomach and digestive system. (See DIGESTION)

Single Oils:
Idaho balsam fir, frankincense, lavender, lemon, German chamomile, *Citrus hystrix*, rose, galbanum, valerian

Blends:
Present Time, Valor, Release, Peace & Calming, Trauma Life, Sacred Mountain, White Angelica, Christmas Spirit, 3 Wise Men, Citrus Fresh

Dietary Supplementation:
JuvaTone, JuvaPower/Spice

EO Applications:
INHALATION:
DIRECT, 3-4 times daily, as needed
TOPICAL:
NEAT, apply 1-2 drops to crown of head and forehead as needed. Best if applied in a quiet, darkened room
VITA FLEX, massage 1-3 drops on heart Vita Flex points, 2-3 times daily
INGESTION:
SYRUP, 1-2 times daily

Additional regimens:

Place 1-3 drops of Release over the thymus and rub in gently. Apply up to 3 times daily as needed.

Blend equal parts frankincense and Valor and apply 1-2 drops neat on temples, forehead, crown and back of neck before retiring. Use for 3 nights.

ENDOCRINE SYSTEM

The endocrine system encompasses the hormone-producing glands of the body. These glands cluster around blood vessels and release their hormones directly into the bloodstream. The pituitary gland exerts a wide range of control over the hormonal (endocrine) system and is often called the master gland. Other glands include the pancreas, adrenals, thyroid and parathyroid, ovaries, and testes. The limbic system lies along the margin of the cerebral cortex (brain) and is the hormone-producing system of the brain. It includes the amygdala, hippocampus, pineal, pituitary, thalamus, and hypothalamus.

Essential oils increase circulation to the brain. This better enables the pituitary and other glands to secrete neural transmitters and hormones that support the endocrine and immune systems.

The thyroid is one of the most important glands for regulating the body systems. The hypo-thalamus plays an even more important role, since it not only regulates the thyroid, but the adrenals and the pituitary gland as well.

The following oils are endocrine supportive:

Single Oils:
Fleabane, helichrysum, lemon verbena, nutmeg, clove, rosemary, spearmint, spruce

Blends:
EndoFlex, En-R-Gee, Humility, Lady Sclareol, SclarEssence

EO Applications:
INGESTION:
    CAPSULE, 0 size, 2 times daily
INHALATION:
    DIRECT, 3 times daily
    DIFFUSION, 15 minutes 3 times daily
TOPICAL:
    VITA FLEX, massage 1-3 drops on Vita
    Flex points for the glands on feet

Additional regimen:

Place 1-2 drops of EndoFlex on the tongue, the roof of the mouth, the thyroid and adrenals, and the Vita Flex points for these glands on the feet.

Dietary Supplementation:
Thyromin, Ultra Young, PD 80/20, Ultra Young+

EPILEPSY

Single Oils:
Clary sage, jasmine absolute

Blends:
Valor, Brain Power

EO Applications:
INHALATION:
    DIRECT, 4 times per day as needed.
TOPICAL:
    DILUTE 50-50, apply 1-3 drops on back of
    neck and behind ears 2-3 times daily
    VITA FLEX, massage 2-4 drops on brain
    Vita Flex points on feet, 2-3 times daily

Dietary Supplementation:
Cleansing Trio, Essential Omegas, Juva Power, Blue Agave Nectar (no processed sugars)

EPSTEIN-BARR VIRUS

(See also HYPOGLYCEMIA, FATIGUE, THYROID, ADRENAL GLAND IMBALANCE)

Also known as Chronic Fatigue Syndrome, the Epstein-Barr virus is a type of herpes virus that also causes mononucleosis.

Symptoms include indigestion, upper and lower gas, poor assimilation, poor electrolyte balance, allergic reaction to foods and other substances, emotional mood swings, fatigue, irritability, and a lack of motivation, discipline, and creativity.

Hypoglycemia is a precursor and can render the body susceptible to the Epstein-Barr virus. Treat the hypoglycemia, and the symptoms of the Epstein-Barr virus may begin to disappear.

Single Oils:
Thyme, clove, sandalwood, grapefruit, nutmeg, blue tansy, mountain savory, oregano, tea tree, rosemary

Blends:
ImmuPower, EndoFlex, Thieves, Longevity Di-Tone, Exodus II

EO Applications:
INGESTION:
CAPSULE, 00 size, 3 times daily
TOPICAL:
RAINDROP Technique, weekly with ImmuPower
INHALATION:
DIRECT, 4-5 times daily

Dietary Supplementation:
Super C Chewable, ImmuPro, Thyromin, ImmuneTune, Cleansing Trio, Berry Young Juice, JuvaTone, JuvaPower/Spice, ImmuGel Power Meal, Mineral Essence, Detoxyme, Mega Cal

Mononucleosis

Infectious mononucleosis is a disease caused by the Epstein-Barr virus (EBV) which is a type of herpes virus. Symptoms usually last four weeks or more. The spleen enlarges and may even rupture in severe cases.

Single Oils:
Ravensara, hyssop, thyme, mountain savory, frankincense

Blends:
Thieves, R.C., Raven

Mononucleosis blend:
• 3 drops Thieves
• 3 drops thyme
• 3 drops mountain savory
• 2 drops ravensara

EO Applications:
INGESTION:
CAPSULE, 00 size, 1 capsule twice daily
TOPICAL:
RAINDROP Technique twice a week
VITA FLEX, massage 3-6 drops on bottom of feet twice daily

Dietary Supplements:
ImmuPro, Super C Chewable, Cleansing Trio

EXPECTORANT

(See MUCUS)

EYE DISORDERS

(See AGE-RELATED MACULAR DEGENERATION)

In 1997 Dr. Terry Friedmann, MD, eliminated his need for glasses after applying sandalwood and juniper on the areas around his eyes--above the eyebrows and on the cheeks (being careful never to get oil into eyes.) He also used the supplements of Chelex, VitaGreen, the Cleansing Trio, and JuvaTone for a complete colon and liver cleanse.

CAUTION: Never put any essential oils in the eyes or on eyelids.

Blocked Tear Ducts

Single Oils: Lavender.

EO Applications:
1 drop lavender oil rubbed over the bridge of the nose has been reported to work in seconds.

Cataracts and Glaucoma

Cataracts are a clouding of the eye lens that often comes with aging. Glaucoma is a condition caused by an abnormal buildup of intraocular pressure in the eye.

Single Oils:
Clove, lavender

Clove oil is the most powerful known antioxidant and when taken internally it can slow or prevent both cataracts and glaucoma.

EO Application:
INGESTION:
CAPSULE, 0 size 2-3 times daily

Blends:
Eye blend #1:
• 10 drops lemongrass
• 5 drops cypress
• 3 drops *Eucalyptus radiata*

Eye blend #2:
- 10 drops lemon
- 5 drops cypress
- 3 drops *Eucalyptus radiata*

EO Applications:
TOPICAL:

DILUTE 20-80, apply 2-4 drops in a wide circle around the eye, being careful not to get any oil in the eye or on the eyelid, 1-3 times daily. This may also help with puffiness. Also apply on temples and eye Vita Flex points on the feet and hands (the undersides of your two largest toes and your index and middle fingers.)

NOTE: If essential oils should ever accidentally get into the eyes, dilute with V-6 Advanced Oil Complex or other pure vegetable oil. NEVER rinse with water.

Dietary Supplementation:
Alpha lipoic acid, Essential Omegas, Mineral Essence, Longevity Caps, AD&E, VitaGreen

Selenium supports the eyes. Mineral Essence is a good source of all minerals, including selenium. AD&E is beneficial for all eye problems.

Topical Treatment:
NeuroGen

Blurred Vision

Single Oils:
Idaho Tansy, helichrysum, lavender, peppermint

Blends:
Aroma Life, PanAway

Dietary Supplementation:
Longevity Caps, Alpha lipoic acid, Mineral Essence, AD&E, Master Formula Vitamins, VitaGreen, Sulfurzyme, Super B, Essential Omegas, Super Cal, Power Meal, Mega Cal

Pink Eye

Blends:
Purification, 3 Wise Men, ImmuPower

EO Applications:
INHALATION:

DIFFUSER, at night while sleeping

FAINTING

(See SHOCK)

Single Oils:
Melissa, peppermint, sandalwood, cardamom, spearmint.

Blends:
Clarity, Brain Power, Trauma Life

EO Applications:
INHALATION:

DIRECT, 1-2 times as needed

FATIGUE

(See DIABETES, EPSTEIN-BARR VIRUS, HEART, THYROID, ADRENAL GLAND IMBALANCE)

Hormone imbalances may play a large role in fatigue as well as latent viral infections (Herpes virus and/or Epstein-Barr Virus). Also mineral deficiencies (especially magnesium) can play a large part in low energy.

Natural progesterone for women and DHEA for men can be instrumental in helping combat the fatigue that comes with age and declining hormone levels. Because pregnenolone is a precursor for all male and female hormones, both men and women can benefit from its supplementation.

Physical Fatigue

A lack of energy can be due to a host of factors, including poor thyroid function or adrenal imbalance. Other factors may also play a part, including diabetes, cancer and other conditions.

Single Oils:
Lemongrass, juniper, basil, lemon, peppermint, rosemary, nutmeg, black pepper, thyme, melissa, cypress

Blends:
Motivation, Valor, En-R-Gee, Hope, Clarity, Citrus Fresh, Awaken, Joy

VitaGreen is a plant-derived high-protein energy formula that athletes use to boost endurance. Longevity Caps increase energy and endurance.

Digestion and colon problems may cause fatigue. A colon and liver cleanse unburdens the digestive system and increases energy.

EO Applications:
INHALATION:
> DIRECT, 2-5 times daily
> DIFFUSION, 10 minutes 3 times daily

TOPICAL:
> DILUTE 50-50, 2-4 drops on temples, in clavicle notch (over thyroid), and behind ears, 2-4 times daily as needed

Dietary Supplementation:
VitaGreen, Power Meal, Master Formula, Mineral Essence, WheyFit, Wolfberry Crisp bars, Longevity Caps, Super B, Thyromin

Mental Fatigue

Single Oils:
Black pepper, sage, peppermint, nutmeg, spearmint, pine

Blends:
En-R-Gee, Clarity, Live With Passion, Envision, Valor, Motivation

EO Applications:
TOPICAL:
> DILUTE 50-50, 2-4 drops at base of throat, temples, back of neck, as needed
> VITA FLEX, massage 1-3 drops on relevant Vita Flex points on feet
> 1-3 times daily

INHALATION:
> DIRECT, 2-4 times daily

INGESTION:
> SYRUP, 1-3 times daily

Dietary Supplementation:
Thyromin, Power Meal, VitaGreen, Master Formula Vitamins, Essential Omegas, Mineral Essence, Longevity Caps, Ultra Young, Berry Young Juice

Topical Treatments:
Morning Start Bath Gel, Peppermint/ Cedarwood Bar Soap, Morning Start Bar Soap, Ortho Ease Massage oil

FERTILITY

Single Oils:
Clary sage, sage, anise seed, fennel, yarrow, geranium

Blends:
Dragon Time, Acceptance, Passion, Mister, Sensation, Lady Sclareol, SclarEssence

EO Applications:
TOPICAL:
> NEAT or DILUTE 50-50, as desired, 2-4 drops on the reproductive Vita Flex points of hands and feet (inside of wrists, around the front of the ankles in line with the anklebone, on the lower sides of the anklebone, and along the Achilles tendon.) 1-3 times daily.

Dietary Supplementation:
PD 80/20, VitaGreen, Essential Manna

Use VitaGreen 3-8 capsules, 2-3 times daily, and Essential Manna

Topical Treatments:
Protec, Progessence, Prenolone

> **Women**: Rub daily 1/2 tsp Prenolone or Progessence on lower back area and the lower bowel area near the pubic bone.

> **Men**: Take 2-4 ProGen capsules daily to nourish the reproductive system. Also rub 4-6 drops Protec on the lower abdomen near the pubic bone and in the area between the scrotum and the rectum. (Alternatively, use 1 tablespoon of Protec in overnight rectal retention.)

FEVER

(See INFECTION)

Fevers are one of the most powerful healing responses orchestrated by the human body, and are especially valuable in fighting infectious diseases. However, if fever raises body temperature excessively (over 104° F) then neurological damage can occur.

Some essential oils are very cooling when applied to the skin and can help reduce fevers. Because of its menthol content, peppermint is used predominately for fever control.

Single Oils:
Peppermint, *Eucalyptus radiata*, rosemary, ledum, Idaho balsam fir

Blends:
ImmuPower, Melrose

EO Applications:
TOPICAL:
DILUTE 50-50, apply 2-3 drops to forehead, temples and back of neck.
INGESTION:
RICE MILK, sip slowly, 1-2 times as needed
CAPSULE, 00 size, 1-2 capsules, as needed
SYRUP, dissolve 1 tsp of the syrup/essential oil mixture in an 8 oz glass of cool water and sip slowly.
INHALATION:
DIRECT, 3-4 times as needed

Dietary Supplementation:
Super C Chewable, ImmuPro, ImmuneTune, Exodus, Essential Omegas, Longevity Caps, Fresh Essence Plus

Topical Treatments:
Cinnamint Lip Balm

FIBRILLATION

(See HEART)

FIBROIDS

(See MENSTRUAL CONDITIONS)

Fibroids are fairly common benign tumors of the female pelvis that are composed of smooth muscle cells and fibrous connective tissue. Fibroids are not cancerous and neither develop into cancer nor increase a women's cancer risk in the uterus.

Fibroids can have a diameter as small as 1 mm or as large as 8 inches. They can develop in clusters or alone as a single knot or nodule.

Fibroids frequently occur in premenopausal women and are seldom seen in young women who have not begun menstruation. Fibroids usually stabilize or even regress in women who have been through menopause.

Single Oils:
Frankincense, cistus, lavender, Idaho tansy, oregano, pine, helichrysum

Blends:
Valor, EndoFlex, Cel-Lite Magic, Protec

EO Applications:
INGESTION:
CAPSULE, 0 size, 2 times daily
TOPICAL:
COMPRESS, warm on lower abdomen, daily

Dietary Supplementation:
Ultra Young, Thyromin, VitaGreen, AlkaLime, Essential Omegas, Power Meal, Prenolone, PD 80/20, and Essentialzyme

FIBROMYALGIA

Fibromyalgia is an autoimmune disorder of soft tissues. (By contrast, arthritis occurs in the joints.) Symptoms include general body pain, in some parts worse than others, usually brought on by short periods of exercise.

The pain is ubiquitous and continuous. It interrupts sleep patterns so that the fourth stage of sleep is never attained, and thus the body cannot rejuvenate and heal. Fibromyalgia is an acid condition in which the liver is toxic (see LIVER DISORDERS).

The best natural treatments for fibromyalgia are omega-3 fats such as flax seed, proteolytic enzymes such as bromelain and pancreatin, and MSM.

According to UCLA researcher, Ronald Lawrence, M.D. Ph.D., supplementation with MSM offers a breakthrough in the treatment of fibromyalgia.

Single Oils:
German chamomile, nutmeg, Idaho balsam fir

Blends:
PanAway, Relieve It, ImmuPower, Ortho Ease, Ortho Sport

Fibromyalgia blend #1:
• 8 drops Idaho balsam fir
• 6 drops white fir
• 4 drops wintergreen
• 2 drops spruce

Fibromyalgia blend #2:
- 10 drops PanAway
- 8 drops wintergreen
- 8 drops marjoram
- 6 drops spruce

EO Applications:
TOPICAL:
> DILUTE 50-50, gently massage 2-4 drops on pain locations
> COMPRESS, warm, on location, 3 x weekly
> BODY MASSAGE, weekly
> Raindrop, adding Immune blend, weekly

INGESTION:
> CAPSULE, 0 size, 2 times daily

Dietary Supplementation:
Sulfurzyme, Polzyme, Essential Omegas, Super C Chewable, VitaGreen, Essentialzyme, ImmuneTune, Super Cal

Topical Treatment:
Regenolone

Fibromyalgia Regiment:

1. Start cleansing by using Cleansing Trio.
2. Use 2 Tbsp. Sulfurzyme daily
3. Eat less acidic-ash foods and more alkaline-ash foods such as wheat sprouts or barley sprouts. The following is a list of alkalinizing supplements:
   - VitaGreen: up to 4 times daily.
   - Super C: 4-6 tablets daily.
   - ImmuneTune: 2-6 times daily.
   - Mineral Essence: 2-3 droppers, 2 times daily in water or cold apple juice will supply the trace minerals needed without increasing the acid condition.
   - Super Cal or Mega Cal: 2-4 capsules daily, or as needed
   - ImmuPower: Apply 4-6 drops along the spine and back along with Raindrop Technique (See chapter 21 on RAINDROP TECHNIQUE).

FLATULENCE (GAS)

(See DIGESTIVE PROBLEMS)

Flatulence (gas) can be caused by a lack of digestive enzymes and the consumption of indigestible starches that promote bifidobacteria production in the colon. Although increasing bifidobacteria production can lead to gas, it is highly beneficial to long term health, as the increase of beneficial flora crowds out disease-causing microorganisms such as Clostridium perfringens. Consumption of FOS (fructooligosaccharides), an indigestible sugar, can create short term flatulence even as it drastically improves bifidobacteria production in the small and large intestine and increases mineral absorption.

Dietary Supplementation:
Carbozyme, Essentialzyme Detoxzyme, Wolfberry Crisp, Cleansing Trio, Alkalime

FLU (Influenza)

(See INFLUENZA)

FOOD POISONING

Single Oils:
Tarragon, patchouli, rosemary

Blends:
Di-Tone, Exodus II, Thieves

EO Applications:
INGESTION:
> CAPSULE, 00 size, 2 capsules, 2-3 times per day

Dietary Supplementation:
ComforTone, JuvaTone, AlkaLime, Polyzyme, Detoxzyme, Essentialzyme

FOOT PROBLEMS

Athlete's Foot

(see FUNGAL INFECTIONS)

Blisters on Feet

(see BLISTERS and BOILS)

Bunions

Bunions are caused from bursitis at the base of a toe. (See BURSITIS)

Blends:
Bunion Recipe:
- 6 drops *Eucalyptus radiata*
- 3 drops lemon
- 4 drops raven
- 1 drop wintergreen

EO Applications:
TOPICAL:
> NEAT or DILUTE 50-50, as needed. Apply 2-4 drops over bunion area 2-3 times daily

Corns

Single Oils:
Lemon, tangerine, grapefruit, oregano, myrrh

Blends: Citrus Fresh

EO Applications:
TOPICAL:
> NEAT, 1 drop directly on the corn 2-3 times daily

Sore Feet

Single Oils:
Peppermint, white fir, lavender, patchouli, myrrh, frankincense, sandalwood, vetiver

Blends:
Melrose, PanAway, Relieve It

EO Applications:
TOPICAL:
> DILUTE 50-50, massage 6-9 drops onto each foot at night
> COMPRESS, warm, for added effect and penetration
> BATH SALTS, mix 10 drops essential oils in 1 Tbsp. Epsom salts and add to hot water in a basin large enough for footbath

Topical Treatment:
Ortho Sport or OrthoEase Massage Oils, Fresh Essence Plus mouthwash (used on the feet)

FRIGIDITY

(See SEXUAL DYSFUNCTIONS)

FUNGAL INFECTIONS

Fungi and yeast feed on decomposing or dead tissues. They exist everywhere: inside our stomachs, on our skin, and out on the lawn. When kept under control, the yeast and fungi populating our bodies are harmless and digest what our bodies cannot or do not use.

When we feed the naturally-occurring fungi in our bodies too many acid-ash foods, such as sugar, animal proteins, and dairy products, the fungal populations grow out of control. This condition is known as systemic candidiasis and is marked by fungi invading the blood, gastrointestinal tract, and tissues.

Fungal cultures such as candida excrete large amounts of poisons called mycotoxins as part of their life cycles. These poisons must be detoxified by the liver and immune systems. Eventually they can wreak enormous damage on the tissues and organs and are believed to be an aggravating factor in many degenerative diseases, such as cancer, arteriosclerosis, and diabetes.

Insufficient intake of minerals and trace minerals like magnesium, potassium, and zinc may also stimulate candida and fungal overgrowth in the body.

Symptoms of Systemic Fungal Infection:

- Fatigue/low energy
- Overweight
- Low resistance to illness
- Allergies
- Unbalanced blood sugar
- Headaches
- Irritability
- Mood swings
- Indigestion
- Colitis and ulcers
- Diarrhea/constipation
- Urinary tract infections
- Rectal or vaginal itch

Athlete's Foot

(See RINGWORM in this section).

Tinea pedis or athlete's foot is a fungal infection of the skin that infects the feet. (it is identical to ringworm which infects the skin in the rest of the body). This fungus thrives in the warm, moist environment to which many feet are subjected.

The best remedy is to keep feet cool and dry and avoid wearing tight-fitting shoes or heavy natural (ie. cotton) socks. Wear sandals, shoes, and socks woven from a light, breathable fabric.

It is especially important to control this fungus infection during showering or bathing, since the moist, warm environment favors the growth of the *Tinea* culture responsible for athlete's foot. Antifungal essential oils such as melaleuca and Melrose can be added to bath salts or Epsom salts and used in a the RainSpa shower head to create a mild, antifungal shower.

Single Oils:
Tea tree, niaouli (MQV), *Melaleuca ericifolia*, blue cypress, lemongrass (always dilute), Idaho balsam fir, lavender, peppermint, thyme, mountain savory

Blends:
Melrose, Thieves, Purification, ClaraDerm

Athlete's foot blend #1:
• 8 drops tea tree
• 2 drop lavender

Athlete's foot blend #2:
• 8 drops tea tree
• 4 drops peppermint
• 2 drops mountain savory

EO Applications:
TOPICAL:
NEAT or DILUTE 50-50 as needed.
Apply 5-7 drops to affected areas between toes and around toenails
BATH SALTS, daily

Topical Treatments:
Thieves Antiseptic Spray, Ortho Ease Massage Oil. Fresh Essence Plus Mouthwash (used on the feet), Peppermint-Cedarwood Bar Soap, Rose Ointment

Candida Albicans (Intestinal)

Two of the most powerful weapons for fighting intestinal fungal infections such as candida are FOS (fructooligosaccharides) and *L. acidophilus* cultures.

FOS has been clinically documented in dozens of peer-reviewed studies for its ability to build up the healthy intestinal flora in the colon and combat the overgrowth of negative bacteria and fungi (See APPENDIX P).

Acidophilus cultures have also been shown to combat fungus overgrowth in the gastrointestinal tract.

Single Oils:
Tea tree, juniper, ravensara, thyme, cumin, peppermint,cistus, lavender, lemongrass, rosemary, geranium, palmarosa, rosewood

Blends:
Melrose, Raven, R.C., ImmuPower

EO Applications:
TOPICAL:
Dilute 50-50 or 20-80, as needed, massage 3-4 drops on thymus (at clavical notch, center of collarbone at base of throat) to stimulate the immune system. Also apply 3-6 drops on bottoms of the feet and on the chest. Also apply 5-10 drops on stomach. Do these applications 2 times daily.
VITA FLEX, massage 2-4 drops on relevant Vita Flex points of feet 2-4 times daily.
BATH SALTS, daily
INGESTION:
CAPSULE, 0 size, 2-3 times daily between meals
RICE MILK, 3 times daily between meals
Dietary Supplementation:
Essentialzyme, ImmuPro, ImmuneTune, VitaGreen, Thyromin, Super C Chewable, AlkaLime, Exodus

Combating Ringworm

Using antifungal essential oils while bathing or showering is especially important because fungal infections thrive in moist, warm environments. Essential oils like tea tree or Melrose can easily be added to bath salts or Epsom salts to combat fungal infections.

There are specially designed shower heads that can be filled with bath salts and essential oils. As the water passes over the mixture, it disperses the essential oils and salts into the shower spray, creating an antiseptic spa.

Ringworm and Skin Candida

The ringworm fungus infects the skin causing scaly round itchy patches. It is infectious and can be spread from an animal or human host alike. Skin candida is a fungal infection that can erupt almost anywhere on the skin. It shows up in various places, such as behind the knees, inside the elbows, behind the ears, on temple area, and between the breasts.

Single Oils:
Tea tree, niaouli (MQV), *Melaleuca ericifolia*, blue cypress, lavender, rosemary, geranium, rosewood, myrrh

Blends:
Melrose, Raven, R.C., Ortho Ease, Clara Derm

Ringworm blend:
• 3 drops tea tree
• 3 drops spearmint
• 1 drop peppermint
• 1 drop rosemary

Skin Candida blend:
• 2 drops Idaho tansy
• 10 drops tea tree
• 1 drop oregano
• 2 drops patchouli

EO Applications:
TOPICAL:
   NEAT, massage 2-4 drops over affected area, then layer on Rose ointment, 2-4 times daily. In severe cases, use 35 percent food-grade hydrogen peroxide to

clean infected areas before applying essential oils. Saturate a gauze with essential oils and apply to affected area and wrap to hold in place.

Topical Treatment:
Thieves Antiseptic Spray, Ortho Sport or OrthoEase Massage Oils, Fresh Essence Plus (used topically), Rose Ointment

Thrush

Thrush is a fungal infection of the mouth and throat marked by creamy, curd-like patches in the oral cavity. Even though it appears in the mouth, thrush is usually a sign of systemic fungal overgrowth throughout the body. Thrush can usually be treated locally through the use of antifungal essential oils such as clove, cinnamon, rosemary CT cineol, peppermint, and rosewood.

Single Oils:
Cinnamon, clove, peppermint, rosemary cineol, geranium, rosewood, orange, lavender

Blends:
Thieves, Melrose, Purification, ImmuPower

EO Applications:
ORAL:
   GARGLE, 3-5 times daily
TOPICAL:
   Dilute 50-50 or 20-80, as needed, massage 3-4 drops on thymus (at clavical notch, center of collarbone at base of throat) to stimulate the immune system. Also apply 3-6 drops on bottoms of the feet and on the chest. Also apply 5-10 drops on stomach. Do these applications 2 times daily
   VITA FLEX, massage 2-4 drops on relevant Vita Flex points of feet, 2-4 times daily
INGESTION:
   CAPSULE, 0 size, 2-3 times daily between meals
   RICE MILK, 3 times daily between meals

NOTE: These applications are for adults, not infants. In cases of infants with thrush, consult a medical professional first.

Oral Hygiene:
Fresh Essence Plus Mouthwash, Thieves Lozenges

Vaginal Yeast Infection

Essential oils like tea tree have been documented to have highly antifungal activity. Positive results have been obtained on vaginal yeast infections using these oils in douches.

Single Oils:
Lavender, tea tree, rosemary, Roman chamomile, geranium, rosewood, peppermint, spearmint, mountain savory, thyme, bay laurel

Blends:
Melrose, Purification, R.C., Di-Tone, Aroma Siez, Dragon Time, Mister, Clara Derm

Vaginal yeast infection blend #1:
- 7 drops Purification
- 2 drops frankincense
- 5 drops mountain savory

Vaginal yeast infection blend #2:
- 12 drops tea tree
- 12 drops Purification
- 12 drops juniper

EO Applications:
RETENTION:
    TAMPON, nightly for 5-10 days, as needed
INGESTION:
    CAPSULE, 00 size, 3 times daily

Topical Treatment:
Fresh Essence Plus mouthwash

GALLBLADDER INFECTION

The gallbladder stores bile created by the liver and releases it through the biliary ducts into the duodenum to promote digestion. Bile is extremely important for fat digestion and the absorption of vitamins such as A, D, and E.

When bile flow is obstructed due to gallstones or inflamed due to infection, serious consequences can ensue, including poor digestion, jaundice, and severe abdominal pain.

Single Oils:
Lemon, ledum, carrot seed, celery seed, juniper, German chamomile

Blends:
JuvaFlex, Juva Cleanse, PanAway, Release

EO Applications:
INGESTION:
    CAPSULE, 00 size, 1 capsule 3 times daily
TOPICAL:
    NEAT, apply 6-10 drops over gallbladder area, 2-3 times daily
    COMPRESS, warm, 2-3 times daily
    VITA FLEX, massage 1-3 drops on liver Vita Flex points of the feet, 2-3 times daily

Dietary Supplementation:
Sulfurzyme, JuvaTone, Essentialzyme, Polyzyme

GALLSTONES

When bile contains excessive cholesterol, bilirubin, or bile salts, gallstones can form. Stones made from hardened cholesterol account for the vast majority of gallstones, while stones made from bilirubin, the brownish pigment in bile, constitute only about 20 percent of gallstones.

Gallstones can block both bile flow and the passage of pancreatic enzymes. This can result in inflammation in the gallbladder (cholecystitis) or pancreas (pancreatitis) and jaundice. In some cases, gallstones can be life-threatening, depending on where they are lodged.

Several Japanese studies show that limonene (a key constituent in orange, lemon, and tangerine oils) can effectively dissolve gallstone with no negative side effects.

Single Oils:
Lemon, orange, grapefruit, mandarin, tangerine, juniper, nutmeg, rosemary

Blends:
JuvaFlex, Juva Cleanse

Gallbladder blend:
- 2 drops ledum
- 1 drop Roman chamomile
- 1 drop lavender
- 1 drop rosemary
- 1 drop helichrysum
- 1 drop juniper

EO Applications:
INGESTION:
>   Capsule: 0 size, 2 times daily for 2 weeks

TOPICAL:
>   DILUTE 50-50, massage 6-10 drops over gallbladder twice daily
>   COMPRESS, 2-3 times daily
>   VITA FLEX, massage 1-3 drops on liver Vita Flex points of feet, 2-3 times daily

GANGRENE

Gangrene is the death or decay of living tissue caused by a lack of blood supply. A shortage of blood can result from a blood clot, arteriosclerosis, frostbite, diabetes, infection, or some other obstruction in the arterial blood supply. Gas gangrene (also known as acute or moist gangrene) occurs when tissues are infected with *Clostridium* bacteria. Unless the limb is amputated or treated with antibiotics, the gangrene can be fatal.

The part of the body affected with gangrene displays the following symptoms:

- Coldness
- Dark in color
- Looks rotten/decomposed
- Putrid smell

Other symptoms include:
- Fever
- Anemia

Dr. René Gattefossé suffered gas gangrene as a result of burns from a chemical explosion at the turn of the century. He successfully engineered his own recovery solely with the use of pure lavender oil.

NOTE: as with all serious medical conditions, consult your health care professional immediately if you suspect gangrene.

Single Oils:
Oregano, lavender, mountain savory, thyme, ravensara, cistus, blue cypress

Blends:
Exodus II, Thieves, ImmuPower, Melrose

EO Applications:
TOPICAL:
>   DILUTE 20-80, apply 2-4 drops on affected area, 3-5 times daily
>   COMPRESS, warm, 3 times daily, every other day

Dietary Supplementation:
Exodus, PD 80/20, Essential Omegas, ImmuPro, ImmuneTune, Super C

Topical Treatment:
Regenolone, NeuroGen

GASTRITIS

(See DIGESTIVE PROBLEMS)

Gastritis occurs when the stomach's mucosal lining becomes inflamed and the cells become eroded. This can lead to bleeding ulcers and severe digestive disturbances. Gastritis may be caused by excess acid production in the stomach, alcohol consumption, stress, and fungal or bacterial infections.

Symptoms of gastritis:
- Weight loss
- Abdominal pain
- Cramping

Single Oils:
Tarragon, peppermint, fennel

Blends:
Di-Tone, Thieves

EO Applications:
INGESTION:
>   CAPSULE, 0 size, 2 times daily for 7 days

TOPICAL:
>   COMPRESS, warm, over stomach area, as needed

Dietary Supplementation:
Mineral Essence, Essentialzyme, Polyzyme

Supplementation regimen for gastritis
- Essentialzyme: 3-4 capsules, 3 times daily
- Polyzyme: 3-4 capsules, 3 times daily
- Mineral Essence: 2-3 droppers, 3 times daily
- ComforTone and ICP: Begin after 2 weeks of using the products listed above.
- Alkalime: 1/2 tsp. each morning
- Mega Cal: 1 Tbsp. each morning in 8 oz. warm water

GINGIVITIS

(See ORAL CARE)

Essential oils are one of the best treatments against gum diseases such as gingivitis and pyorrhea. Clove oil, for example, is used as dental disinfectant; and the active principle in clove oil, eugenol, is one of the best-studied germ-killers available.

GLAUCOMA

(See EYE DISORDERS)

Common among people over 30 years of age, glaucoma is an eye disease in which escalating pressure within the fluid of the eye eventually damages the optic nerve and causes blindness. Many people are unaware of that they have the disease until their peripheral vision is permanently lost.

Glaucoma usually develops in middle age or later, although glaucoma in newborns, children, and teenagers can occur.

GOUT

(See also KIDNEY DISORDERS)
(for pain, see JOINT STIFFNESS & PAIN)

Gout is a disease marked by abrupt, temporary bouts of joint pain and swelling that are most evident in the joint of the big toe. It can also affect the wrist, elbow, knee, ankle, hand, and foot. As the disease progresses, pain and swelling in the joints becomes more frequent and chronic, with deposits called tophi appearing over many joints, including the elbows and on ears.

Gout is characterized by accumulation of uric acid crystals in the joints caused by excess uric acid in the blood. Uric acid is a byproduct of the breakdown of protein that is normally excreted by the kidneys into the urine. To reduce uric acid concentrations, it is necessary to support the kidneys, adrenal, and immune functions. It is also necessary to detoxify by cleansing and drinking plenty of fluids.

Excess alcohol, allergy-producing foods, or strict diets can cause outbreaks of gout. Foods rich in purines, such as wine, anchovies, and animal liver, can also cause gout.

Single Oils:
Geranium, ledum, carrot seed, celery, juniper, Roman chamomile, lemon

Blends:
PanAway, JuvaFlex, Juva Cleanse

Gout blend:
- 10 drops geranium
- 8 drops juniper
- 5 drops rosemary
- 3 drops Roman chamomile
- 4 drops lemon
- 8 drops tea tree

EO Applications:
INGESTION:
CAPSULE, 0 size, 3 times daily for 10 days, then rest 4 days, repeat as needed
RICE MILK, 3 times daily
TOPICAL:
NEAT, gently massage 1-3 drops o affected joints 2-3 times daily

Dietary Supplementation:
Thyromin, Essential Manna, Mineral Essence, Super C, Super Cal, ArthroTune, VitaGreen, Sulfurzyme, Cleansing Trio, JuvaTone, JuvaPower/Spice

Supplementation regimen for gout:
- Mineral Essence: 3 droppers, 3 times daily
- ArthroTune: 3 capsules, 3 times daily
- JuvaTone: up to 10 tablets daily, reduce after 2 weeks.
- Super Cal: 2-4 capsules, 2 times daily

- Super C: 2-4 tablets, 2 times daily
- VitaGreen: 2-6 capsules, 2 times daily

Topical Treatment:
Ortho Ease Massage Oil, Ortho Sport Massage Oil

GRAVE'S DISEASE

(See THYROID)

GUM DISEASE

(See ORAL CARE)

HAIR AND SCALP PROBLEMS

Sulfur is the single most important mineral for maintaining the strength and integrity of the hair and hair follicle.

Single Oils:
Rosemary, lavender, clary sage, sage, cedarwood, basil, sandalwood, juniper, ylang ylang, sandalwood, lemon, cypress, rosewood

Rosemary adds body and conditions the hair.

Blends:
Blend for dry hair:
- 2 drops ylang ylang
- 8 drops rosewood
- 4 drops geranium

Blend for oily hair:
- 6 drops patchouli
- 2 drops lavender
- 6 drops lemon

Blend to help with split ends:
- 1 drop rosemary
- 3 drops sandalwood
- 1 drop ylang ylang

EO Applications:
TOPICAL:
> DILUTE 20-80, massage 1 tsp into the scalp vigorously and thoroughly for 2-3 minutes; leave on scalp for 60-90 minutes. (An excellent time to do this would be during an exercise routine). Mix 2-4 drops of essential oils with 1-2 teaspoons of shampoo to wash hair after exercising.

A rinse to help restore the acid mantle of the hair:
- 1 drop rosemary
- 1 tsp. pure apple cider vinegar
- 8 oz. water.

Use as a final rinse on hair. Rub 1 or 2 drops on as hairdressing or on hairbrush to prevent static electricity.

NOTE: Quality shampoos containing essential oils do not lather up as much as other shampoos because they do not contain harmful, foaming agents.

Dietary Supplementation:
ParaFree, Thyromin, Super B, Master Formula, Longevity Caps, Sulfurzyme

Topical Treatment:
Lavender Volume Hair and Scalp Wash, Lemon Sage clarifying Hair and Scalp Wash, Rosewood Moisturizing Hair and Scalp Wash

Premature Graying

This condition is thought to be from a deficiency of biotin, an important B vitamin.

Sandalwood helps retard greying. Rosewood may lighten hair color.

Dandruff

Dandruff may be caused by allergies, parasites (fungal), and/or chemicals.

Melaleuca alternifolia (tea tree) has been shown to be effective in treating dandruff and other fungal infections.[23]

Single Oils:
tea tree, rosemary, cedarwood

Blends:
Citrus Fresh, Melrose

Dandruff blend:
- 5 drops lemon
- 1 drop rosemary or sage
- 1 drop lavender

---

23. "Antifungal activity of the essential oil of *Melaleuca alternifolia* (tea ree oil) against pathogenic fungi in vitro." Skin Pharmacol. 1996;9(6):388-94.

EO Applications:
TOPICAL:

DILUTE 50-50, massage 1 tsp into the scalp vigorously and thoroughly for 2-3 minutes; leave on scalp for 60-90 minutes. (An excellent time to do this would be during an exercise routine). Mix 2-4 drops of essential oils with 1-2 teaspoons of shampoo to wash hair after exercising.

Topical treatment:
Lavender Volume Hair and Scalp Wash, Lemon-Sage Clarifying Hair and Scalp Wash

Hair Loss

(See ALOPECIA AREATA)

Hair loss is caused by hormonal imbalances (such as increase in testosterone), or inflammatory conditions (as in the case of alopecia areata).

Essential oils are excellent for cleansing, nourishing, and strengthening the hair follicle and shaft. Rosemary (cineol chemotype) encourages hair growth.

Single Oils:
Lavender, rosemary, cedarwood, sandalwood, clary sage

Blends:
Hair loss prevention blend #1:
- 3 drops rosemary
- 5 drops lavender
- 4 drops cypress
- 2 drops clary sage
- 2 drops juniper

Add 10 drops of the above blend to 1 tsp. of fractionated coconut oil and massage into the scalp where it is balding; then rub gently into the remainder of the scalp. This works best when done at night.

Hair loss prevention blend #2:
- 10 drops cedarwood
- 8 drops rosemary
- 10 drops sandalwood
- 10 drops lavender

Hair loss prevention blend #3:
- 6 drops rosemary cineol
- 8 drops ylang ylang
- 12 drops cedarwood
- 12 drops clary sage

EO Applications:
TOPICAL:

DILUTE 50-50, massage 1 tsp. into the scalp vigorously and thoroughly for 2-3 minutes; leave on scalp for 60-90 minutes. (An excellent time to do this would be during an exercise routine). Mix 2-4 drops of essential oils with 1-2 teaspoons of shampoo to wash hair after exercising

Dietary Supplementation:
Super B, Essential Omegas, Thyromin, Sulfurzyme.

Topical Treatment:
EndoBalance

HALITOSIS (Bad Breath)

(See alsoDIGESTION PROBLEMS and ORAL CARE).

(See also CANDIDA in FUNGAL INFECTIONS)

Persistent bad breath or gum disease, may be a sign of poor digestion, candida/yeast infestation, or other health problems.

Single Oils:
Nutmeg, peppermint, spearmint, lemon, mandarin, cinnamon, tarragon

Blends:
Thieves

Bad breath blend:
- 4 drops spearmint
- 2 drops mandarin
- 2 drops cinnamon

Disinfectant mouthwash:
- 3 drops peppermint
- 2 drops lemon
- 2 drops clove
- 1 drop tea tree oil

Thoroughly stir the above essential oil blend into one bottle of Fresh Essence Plus Mouthwash or dilute blend in 2 tsp. blue agave nectar and 4 oz. of hot water. Gargle as needed.

EO Applications:
ORAL:

GARGLE, 2-4 times daily as needed
TONGUE, 2-4 times daily as needed

Oral Treatment:
Fresh Essence Plus Mouthwash, Dentarome Ultra Toothpaste, Thieves Antiseptic Spray, Thieves Lozenges

HASHIMOTO'S THYROIDITIS

(See THYROID)

HEAD LICE

The most common remedy for lice (pediculosis) and their eggs (nits) is lindane (gamma benzene hexachloride) a highly toxic polychlorinated chemical that is structurally very similar to hazardous banned pesticides such as DDT and chlordane. It is so dangerous that Dr. Guy Sansfacon, head of the Quebec Poison Control Centre in Canada, has requested that lindane be banned.

Essential oils represent a safe and effective alternative. A 1996 study by researchers in Iceland showed the effectiveness against headlice of the essential oils of anise seed, cinnamon leaf, thyme, tea tree, peppermint, and nutmeg in shampoo and rinse solutions.[24]

Single Oils:
Eucalyptus radiata, lavender, peppermint, thyme, geranium, nutmeg, rosemary

Blends:
Head lice blend:
- 4 drops Eucalyptus radiata
- 2 drop lavender
- 2 drop geranium

EO Applications:
TOPICAL:

DILUTE 50-50, 1 tsp. applied to scalp. Massage into entire scalp, cover with disposable shower cap and leave for at least 1/2 hour. Then shampoo and rise well. Use the rinse below.

Head lice rinse:
- 2 drops Eucalyptus radiata
- 2 drops lavender
- 2 drops geranium
- 1/2 oz. vinegar
- 8 oz. water

Mix into a container with a watertight lid. Shake vigorously, then pour over hair making sure every strand is rinsed. This should be done leaning over bathtub or sink. This is not recommended if you are still in the bathtub as lice may cling to other body hairs. Dry naturally. Repeat daily until lice and eggs are gone.

Head lice rinse 2:
- 2 drops rosemary
- 2 drops clove
- 2 drops peppermint
- 1 Tbsp. fractionated coconut oil

Massage into scalp and let sit for 20 minutes. Remove with dry towel.

Head lice rinse 3

1 cup Fresh Essence Plus massaged into hair and scalp. Retain for 30 minutes before rinsing out.

Topical Treatment:
Ortho Ease, Ortho Sport

HEADACHES

(See also STRESS, HYPOGLYCEMIA)

Headaches are usually caused by hormone imbalances, circulatory problems, stress, sugar imbalance (hypoglycemia), structural (spinal) misalignments, and blood pressure concerns

Placebo-controlled double-blind crossover studies at the Christian-Albrechts University in Kiel, Germany, found that essential oils were just as effective in blocking pain from tension-type headaches as acetominophen (ie., Tylenol).[25, 26]

Essential oils also promote circulation, reduce muscle spasms, and decrease inflammatory response.

24. Veal L, "The potential effectiveness of essential oils as a treatment for headlice, Pediculus humanus capitis," *Complement Ther Nurs Midwifery* 1996 Aug;2(4):97-101.

25. Gobel H, et al., *Effectiveness of Oleum menthae piperitae and paracetamol in therapy of headache of the tension type.* Nervenarzt. 1996 Aug; 67(8): 672-81.

26. Gobel H, Schmidt G, Soyka D. *Effect of peppermint and eucalyptus oil preparations on neurophysiological and experimental algesimetric headache parameters.* Cephalalgia. 1994 Jun; 14(3): 228-34; discussion 182.

Headache from Diffusing
(Clarity and Brain Power)

People who get an instant headache from diffusing usually have a blockage related to heavy metals or synthetic chemicals from cosmetics and other topical chemicals.

Single Oils: Helichrysum, rosemary

Blends: Aroma Life, M-Grain, and Clarity.

Apply helichrysum, rosemary, Aroma Life, and M-Grain to the arteries in the neck or along upper parts of wrists or on other pulse points where arteries are closest to the surface of the skin.

Continue to diffuse Clarity or the offending oil, for short periods of time, until headaches cease.

Single Oils:
Peppermint, Idaho balsam fir, Roman chamomile, German chamomile, lavender, basil, spearmint, valerian, clove, rosemary, *Eucalyptus globulus*

Blends:
M-Grain, Brain Power, Clarity, Relieve It, PanAway, Thieves

Headache blend #1:
* 4 drops Idaho tansy
* 5 drops Roman chamomile
* 2 drops peppermint
* 2 drops lavender
* 1 drop basil
* 3 drops rosemary

Headache blend #2:
* 2 drops Idaho tansy
* 1 drop Roman chamomile
* 3 drops spearmint
* 7 drops lavender

EO Applications:
INHALATION:
> DIFFUSION, 15 minutes 3-5 times daily
> DIRECT, 3-8 times daily as needed

TOPICAL:
> DILUTE 50-50, apply 1-3 drops on back of neck, behind ears, on temples, on forehead, and under nose. Be careful to keep away from eyes and eyelids.

ORAL:
> TONGUE, place a drop on the tongue then push against the roof of the mouth

Dietary Supplementation:
VitaGreen, Essential Omegas, Power Meal, BodyGize, Essentialzyme

Topical Treatment:
Prenolone, Prenolone+, Progessence

Children's Headache

Single Oils:
German chamomile, grapefruit, peppermint, lavender, rosemary

Blends:
Peace & Calming, PanAway

Children's Headache blend:
* 1 drop German chamomile
* 10 drops grapefruit
* 5 drops peppermint
* 3 drops rosemary

EO Applications:
TOPICAL:
> DILUTE 50-50, apply 2-4 drops on temples, forehead, and brainstem. Also massage on thumbs and big toes.

Hormone Imbalance Headache

(See MENSTRUAL CONDITIONS)

Migraines (Vascular-type Headache)

The vast majority of migraine headaches may be due to colon congestion or poor digestion. The Cleansing Trio is most important for cleansing the colon. Eye strain and decreased vision can accompany migraine headaches. AD&E contains large amounts of lutein, which is vital for healthy vision.

Single Oils:
Helichrysum, sandalwood, basil, rosemary, peppermint, lavender, marjoram, melissa, German chamomile, *Eucalyptus radiata*

Blends:
M-Grain, Clarity

M-Grain is specially formulated for migraine headaches.

EO Applications:
TOPICAL:
> NEAT, Apply 1-2 drops to temples, at base of neck, in center of forehead, and at nostril openings. Also massage on thumbs and big toes

INHALATION:
> DIRECT, as needed

Dietary Supplementation:
AD&E, Polyzyme, Cleansing Trio, Essentialzyme

Sinus Headache

(See also SINUS INFECTION)

Single Oils:
Rosemary, tea tree, *Eucalyptus radiata*, lavender, lemon, geranium

Blends:
Melrose, R.C., Purification

Sinus headache blend:
- 5 drops *Melaleuca ericifolia*
- 9 drops rosemary
- 2 drops bergamot
- 7 drops lavender
- 3 drops lemon
- 4 drops geranium

EO Applications:
INHALATION:
> DIFFUSION, 10 min. 2-5 times daily and at night
> DIRECT, 2-5 times daily as needed

Dietary Supplementation:
Super C Chewable, AD&E, Essential Omegas, Master Formula Vitamins, ImmuPro

Tension Headache

(See also STRESS)

Single Oils:
Idaho balsam fir, peppermint, lavender, marjoram, lemongrass, rosemary, valerian, cardamom

Blends:
Valor, Aroma Siez, M-Grain

EO Applications:
TOPICAL:
> DILUTE 50-50, apply 1-2 drops around the hairline, on the back of the neck, and across the forehead. Be careful not to use too much, as it will burn if any oil drips near eyes. If this should occur, dilute with a pure vegetable oil. Never with water.

HEARING IMPAIRMENT

Single Oils:
Helichrysum, juniper, geranium, peppermint, lavender, basil

Blends:
Melrose, ImmuPower, Purification

EO Applications:
TOPICAL:
> NEAT, (1) apply 1 drop essential oil on a cotton ball, then place it carefully in the opening of the ear canal. Retain overnight. Do NOT place oils directly in the ear canal. NEAT, (2) massage 1-2 drops on each ear lobe, behind the ears, and down the jaw line (along the Eustachian tube).

Hearing Vita Flex Regimen
- Apply 1-2 drops neat helichrysum to the area OUTSIDE the opening to the ear canal with fingertip or cotton swab. Do NOT put oil inside the ear canal
- After applying the helichrysum, hold ear lobes firmly and pull in circular motion 10 times to help stimulate absorption and circulation in the ear canal.

Tinnitus (ringing in the ears)

Single Oils:
Helichrysum, juniper, geranium, peppermint, lavender, basil

EO Applications:
TOPICAL:
> NEAT, massage 1-2 drops on temples and forehead and back of neck. Additionally, apply 1 drop each on tips of toes and fingers, so that the oils get into the Vita

Flex pathways. (A change in hearing can often be noticed within 15-20 minutes.) VITA FLEX, Do the hearing Vita Flex regimen described above

HEART

(See CARDIOVASCULAR CONDITIONS and CONGESTIVE HEART FAILURE)

Many people do not understand how someone who is relatively healthy, with low cholesterol levels, suffers a heart attack with no explanation. The explanation is actually inflammation, the fundamental cause of heart disease.

Inflammation of the heart is caused when blood vessels leading to the heart are clogged and damaged. This releases a protein into the bloodstream called C-reactive protein. The level of this protein indicates the degree of inflammation in the linings of the arteries. Certain essential oils have been documented to be excellent for reducing inflammation. German chamomile contains azulene, a blue compound with highly anti-inflammatory properties. Peppermint is also highly anti-inflammatory. Other oils also have anti-inflammatory properties such as helichrysum, spruce, wintergreen, and valerian. Clove, nutmeg and wintergreen are natural blood thinners and help reduce blood clotting.

Magnesium, the most important mineral for the heart, acts as a smooth muscle relaxant and supports the cardiovascular system. Magnesium will act as a natural calcium channel blocker for the heart, lowering blood pressure and dilating the heart blood vessels (according to Terry Friedmann, MD).

Heart Vita Flex

The foot Vita Flex point related to the heart is on the sole of the left foot, on the ring toe (second toe) and behind the knuckle. Massaging this point is as effective as massaging the hand and arm together.

The hand Vita Flex point related to the heart is in the palm of the left hand, one inch below the ring finger joint (at the lifeline). A secondary heart point is on the bottom of the left arm in line with the inside of the up-turned arm (approximately 2

inches up the arm from the funny bone), not on the muscle but up under the muscle. Have another person use thumbs and firmly press these two points alternately for 3 minutes, in a kind of pumping action. Work all 3 points when possible. Start with the foot first; then go to the hand and arm.

Angina

Single Oils:
Ginger, goldenrod, orange, melissa

Blends:
Aroma Life, Peace & Calming

EO Applications:
TOPICAL:
NEAT, massage 1-3 drops over heart area 1-3 times daily. Also apply to left chest, left shoulder and back of neck
VITA FLEX, massage 1 drop each of 2 or 3 of the recommended oils on heart Vita Flex points on foot, hand, and arm, as needed

Fibrillation

This is a specific form of heart arrhythmia that occurs when the upper heart chambers contract at a rate of over 300 pulsations per minute. The lower chambers cannot keep this pace, so efficiency is reduced and not enough blood is pumped. Palpitations, a feeling that the heart is beating irregularly, more strongly, or more rapidly than normal, are the most common symptoms.

Single Oils:
Goldenrod, ylang ylang, marjoram, valerian, lavender, rosemary, Idaho tansy

Blends:
Aroma Life, Peace & Calming, Joy

EO Applications:
TOPICAL:
NEAT, massage 1-3 drops over heart area 1-3 times daily. Also apply to left chest, left shoulder and back of neck
VITA FLEX, massage 1 drop each of 2 or 3 of the recommended oils on heart Vita Flex points on foot, hand, and arm, as needed

INHALATION:
DIRECT, as often as needed to bring calm

Dietary Supplementation:
HRT, CardiaCare, Mineral Essence, Super Cal, Wolfberry Crisp, Sulfurzyme

Heart Attack (Myocardial Infarction)

A heart attack is a circulation blockage resulting in an interruption of blood supply to an area or the heart. Depending on the size of the area affected, it can be mild or severe.

NOTE: Contact your physical immediately if you suspect a heart attack.

Single Oils:
Goldenrod, thyme, lavender, Roman chamomile, helichrysum, Idaho tansy, clove nutmeg

Blends:
Longevity, Aroma Life, Peace & Calming, PanAway, Relieve It, Harmony, Valor

EO Applications:
TOPICAL:
NEAT, apply 1-2 drops to heart Vita Flex points on foot, hand, and arm as described under the 'Heart Vita Flex' section at the beginning of this heading. If there is not enough time to remove shoes to get at the feet, apply the 'pumping' action to left hand and arm points. Using 1-2 drops of Aroma Life on each point will increase effectiveness and may even revive an individual having a heart attack while waiting for medical attention.

Dietary Supplementation:
CardiaCare, HRT Tincture, Longevity Caps, CardiaCare, Mineral Essence, Essential Omegas, AD&E, Super Cal, Power Meal, Berry Berry Young Juice, Sulfurzyme

Tachycardia

Another form of heart arrhythmia in which the heart rate suddenly increases to 160 beats per minute or faster.

Single Oils:
Marjoram, ylang ylang, lavender, goldenrod, Idaho tansy

Blends:
Aroma Life, Peace & Calming, Joy

EO Applications:
TOPICAL:
NEAT, massage 1-3 drops over heart area 1-3 times daily. Also apply to left chest, left shoulder and back of neck
VITA FLEX, massage 1 drop each of 2 or 3 of the recommended oils on heart Vita Flex points on foot, hand, and arm, as needed
INHALATION:
DIRECT, as often as needed to bring calm

Dietary Supplementation:
CardiaCare, HRT Tincture, Sulfurzyme

Tonic-Stimulant

Single Oils:
Goldenrod, anise seed, mandarin, rosemary, peppermint, thyme, marjoram

Blends:
Aroma Life

EO Applications:
TOPICAL:
NEAT, massage 1-3 drops over heart area 1-3 times daily
VITA FLEX, massage 1 drop each of 2 or 3 of the recommended oils on heart Vita Flex points on foot, hand, and arm, as needed
INHALATION:
DIRECT, as often as needed to bring calm

HEARTBURN

(See Heartburn in DIGESTION PROBLEMS)

HEAVY METALS

(See also METAL TOXICITY, Aluminum)

We absorb heavy metals from air, water, food, skin care products, mercury fillings in teeth, etc. These chemicals lodge in the fatty tissues of the body, which, in turn, give off toxic gases that may cause allergic symptoms. Cleansing the body of these heavy metals is extremely important to have a healthy immune function, especially if one has amalgam fillings.

Drink at least 64 ounces of distilled water daily to flush toxins and chemicals out of the body.

Single Oils:
Helichrysum, cypress, frankincense, German chamomile, lemongrass, geranium

Blends:
Juva Cleanse

EO Applications:
TOPICAL:
DILUTE 50-50, apply 4-6 drops to under arms, kidney area and bottoms of feet, 1-3 times daily
RAINDROP Technique, 1-3 times monthly
INGESTION:
CAPSULE, 0 size, 1 capsule once a day

(See CIRCULATION PROBLEMS)

Dietary Supplementation:
JuvaTone, JuvaPower/Spice, VitaGreen, Super C, ImmuPro, ImmuneTune, ImmuGel, Longevity Caps, Chelex, K&B Tincture, HRT tincture, Rehemogen, AD&E, Essentialzyme

(See also CHEMICAL SENSITIVITY REACTION)

Vascular Cleansing

This regimen is to help cleanse the blood and tissues of heavy metal toxins. Certain essential oils and supplements can have a very beneficial effect in ridding the body of these toxins.

1. Chelex: Take 1 full dropper in 4 ounces of water 2 times daily to remove heavy metals. Cardamom essential oil and VitaGreen enhance this action.

2. Massage the body with Aroma Life and 1-2 drops of helichrysum, followed by Cel-Lite Magic Massage oil.

3. Vascular Cleansing blend:
   - 10 drops juniper
   - 10 drops cypress
   - 10 drops lemongrass
   - 1 Tbsp V6 Oil Complex

Rub 2-4 drops under arms, on arms, on skin above kidneys and on bottoms of feet 1-3 times daily.

4. To remove dental mercury from gum tissue, mix 3 drops helichrysum and 4 drops Thieves and put on a rolled gauze and place next to the gums. Only apply to one area at a time; for example, apply on lower left gum on the first night, the upper left the second night and so on.

NOTE: *For young or very sensitive gums, dilute with V-6 Oil Complex.*

(See CIRCULATION PROBLEMS)

HEMATOMA

A hematoma is a tumor-like mass of coagulated blood, caused by a break in the blood vessel or capillary wall. Essential oils, such as helichrysum or geranium, are excellent for balancing blood viscosity and dissolving clots. Clove oil and citrus rind oils, such as lemon and grapefruit, exert a blood-thinning effect that can help speed the dissolution of the clot.

Those who bruise easily are usually low in vitamin C, which may be caused by insufficient intake or poor absorption.

Single Oils:
Cypress, cistus, helichrysum, lemon, grapefruit, clove, nutmeg, wintergreen

Blends:
Aroma Life, PanAway

Dietary Supplementation:
Super C Chewable, Mineral Essence

HEMORRHAGES

Some essential oils, when topically applied or used on pressure bandages, are excellent for slowing bleeding and initiating healing.

Single Oils:
Helichrysum, geranium, cistus, cypress, lavender, myrrh, hyssop

Blends:
Aroma Life, PanAway

EO Applications:
TOPICAL:
COMPRESS, cold, as needed
NEAT, 1-2 drops on location for small wounds

HEMORRHOIDS

Single Oils:

Cypress, cistus, helichrysum, myrrh, lemon, spikenard, basil, peppermint

Blends:

Aroma Siez, Aroma Life, PanAway

Hemorrhoid blend #1:
- 3 or 4 drops of basil
- 1 drop of wintergreen
- 1 drop of cypress
- 1 drop of helichrysum

Hemorrhoid blend #2:
- 3 drops cypress
- 2 drops helichrysum
- 10 drops myrtle

EO Applications:
TOPICAL:

DILUTE 50-50, apply 3-5 drops on location. This may sting, but usually brings relief with one or two applications.

RETENTION:

RECTAL, once every other day for 6 days.

Dietary Supplementation:

Cel-Lite Magic, Essentialzyme, Polyzyme, VitaGreen, Super B, Longevity Caps

Cleanse using the Cleansing Trio

Topical Treatment:

Cel-Lite Magic

HEPATITIS

(See HEPATITIS in LIVER DISORDERS)

HERPES SIMPLEX

(See SEXUALLY TRANSMITTED DISEASES for Herpes Type II, COLD SORES for Herpes Type I, and CHICKEN POX for Herpes Zoster)

HICCUPS

Hiccups are usually caused by irritated nerves of the diaphragm, possibly caused from a full stomach or indigestion.

(See also DIGESTIVE PROBLEMS)

One technique for stopping hiccups that often works when others fail is to stimulate the Vita Flex point for hiccups by placing one drop of cypress and one drop of tarragon on the end of the index finger; then place that finger against the esophagus in the clavicle notch in the center, and curl inward and down, like you're curling down inside the throat, and release.

Cypress or tarragon either topically applied or taken as a dietary supplement may relax intestinal spasms, nervous digestion, and hiccups.

Single Oils:

Cypress, tarragon, peppermint

EO Applications:
TOPICAL:

DILUTE 50-50, apply 3-5 drops to chest and stomach areas.

INGESTION:

CAPSULE, 0 size, 1 capsule 2 times daily
RICE MILK, 2-4 times daily

HIVES

(See ITCHING in SKIN DISORDERS and LIVER DISORDERS)

Hives is a generalized itching or dermatitis that can be due allergies, damaged liver, chemicals, or other factors.

Single Oils:

Peppermint, patchouli, myrrh

EO Applications:
TOPICAL:

DILUTE 50-50, 2-4 drops on location as needed
COMPRESS, cold, as needed

Dietary Supplementation:

Super Cal, Mega Cal, Mineral Essence, AD&E

Topical Treatment:

Tender Tush Ointment

HORMONE IMBALANCE

(See Hormone Imbalance under MENSTRUAL CONDITIONS)

HOT FLASHES

(See MENSTRUAL CONDITIONS)

HUNTINGTON'S CHOREA

(See NEUROLOGICAL DISEASES)

HYPERACTIVITY

Single Oils:
Lavender, cedarwood, vetiver, Roman chamomile, peppermint, valerian

EO Applications:
INHALATION:
DIRECT, 5 times daily for up to 30 days, then off 5 days, then repeat if necessary
TOPICAL:
NEAT, 2-4 drops on toes and balls of feet, as needed

HYPERPNOEA

Abnormally fast, labored breathing

Single Oil:
Ylang Ylang

EO Applications:
TOPICAL:
NEAT, 2-3 drops on solar plexus, base of throat and back of neck, as needed

HYPERTENSION

(See CARDIOVASCULAR CONDITIONS)

HYPOGLYCEMIA

Hypoglycemia may also be caused by low thyroid function (See THYROID).

Excessive consumption of sugar or honey will also cause reactive hypoglycemia, in which a rapid rise in blood sugar is followed by a steep drop to abnormally low levels.

In some cases, hypoglycemia may be a precursor to candida, allergies, chronic fatigue syndrome, depression, and chemical sensitivities.

Signs of hypoglycemia (low blood sugar) include:
- Fatigue, drowsiness, and sleepiness after meals.
- Headache or dizziness if periods between meals are too long.
- Craving for sweets.
- Allergic reaction to foods.
- Palpitations, tremors, sweats, rapid heart beat.
- Inattentiveness, mood swings, irritability, anxiety, nervousness, inability to cope with stress, and feelings of emotional depression,
- Lack of motivation, discipline, and creativity.
- Hunger that cannot be satisfied.

Often people with some of these symptoms are misdiagnosed as suffering either chronic fatigue or neurosis. Instead, they may be hypoglycemic.

To treat chronic hypoglycemia, it may be necessary to first treat the underlying candida or yeast overgrowth (See FUNGAL INFECTIONS).

Essential oils may reduce hypoglycemic symptoms by helping to normalize sugar cravings and supporting and stabilizing sugar metabolism in the body.

Single Oils:
Lavender, cinnamon, cumin, clove, thyme, coriander, lemon, dill

Blends:
Thieves, JuvaFlex, JuvaCleanse, Di-Tone, Exodus II

EO Applications:
INGESTION:
CAPSULE, 00 size, 1 times daily (coriander, dill and thyme work best through ingestion)
INHALATION:
DIRECT, 2-5 times daily as needed

Dietary Supplementation:
Power Meal, BodyGize, VitaGreen, Stevia, ThermaMist, ThermaBurn, Exodus, Mineral Essence, Essential Manna, Berry Young Juice

HYSTERECTOMY

(See Hysterectomy in MENSTRUAL CONDITIONS)

IMPOTENCE

(See also SEXUAL DYSFUNCTIONS)

Impotence (the inability to perform sexually) can be caused by physical limitations (an accident or injury) or psychological factors (inhibitions, trauma, stress, etc). In males, impotence is often linked to problems with the prostate or prostate surgery

(See also PROSTATE PROBLEMS)

If impotence is related to psychological trauma or unresolved emotional issues, it may be necessary to deal with these issues before any meaningful progress can be made.

(See also TRAUMA)

There is an extensive historical basis for the ability of fragrance to amplify desire and create a mood that can overcome frigidity or impotence. In fact, aromas such as rose and jasmine have been used since antiquity to attract the opposite sex and create a romantic atmosphere.

Modern research has shown that the fragrance of some essential oils can stimulate the emotional center of the brain. This may explain why essential oils have the potential to help people overcome impotence based on emotional factors or inhibitions.

Single Oils:
Ylang ylang, clary sage, sandalwood, jasmine frankincense, myrrh, ginger, nutmeg, rose,

Blends:
Valor, Joy, Lady Sclareol, SclarEssence

Dietary Supplementation:
ProGen (for men)

INDIGESTION

(See DIGESTIVE PROBLEMS)

INFECTION (Bacterial and Viral)

Diffusing essential oils is one of the best ways to prevent the spread of airborne bacteria and viruses. Many essential oils, such as oregano, mountain savory, and rosemary, exert highly antimicrobial effects and can effectively eliminate many kinds of pathogens.

To Kill Airborne Viruses and Bacteria

Periodically alternate diffusing ImmuPower and Thieves.

Topically apply 1 drop *Melaleuca alternifolia* and 1 drop rosemary to stem infection.

Single Oils: Tea Tree, cinnamon, clove, thyme, oregano, ravensara, or frankincense.

Blends: Thieves, Melrose, Purification

Viruses and bacteria have a tendency to hibernate along the spine. The body may hold a virus in a suspended state for long periods of time. When the immune system is compromised, these viruses may be released and then manifest into illness. Raindrop Technique along the spine helps reduce inflammation and kill the microorganism.

Oregano and thyme are generally used first for the Raindrop application. However, other oils may also be used and may be more desirable for some people. ImmuPower, R.C., and Purification all work well in the Raindrop application method.

Mountain savory, ravensara, and thyme applied during Raindrop Technique on the spine are beneficial for most infections, particularly chest-related.

(See also COLDS, LUNG-, SINUS-, and THROAT INFECTION)

Single Oils:
Mountain savory, rosemary lemongrass, spruce, clove, thyme, oregano, rosewood, sage, cistus, tea tree

Blends:
Purification, Melrose, R.C., Thieves, ImmuPower, Exodus II, 3 Wise Men

EO Applications:
TOPICAL:
> DILUTE 20-80, 4-6 drops on location
> 2-3 times daily
> RAINDROP Technique, 1-2 times weekly

INGESTION:
> CAPSULE, 00 size, 1 capsule twice daily

Dietary Supplementation:
Super C Chewable, Exodus, Berry Young Juice, Longevity Caps, VitaGreen, ImmuPro, ImmuneTune, Rehemogen

INFERTILITY

Natural progesterone creams when used at the beginning of the cycle (immediately following the cessation of menstruation) can improve fertility. Some essential oils have hormone-like qualities that can support or improve fertility processes.

Single Oils:
Clary sage, anise seed, fennel, blue yarrow, geranium

Blends:
Dragon Time, Mister, EndoFlex, SclarEssence

EO Applications:
INGESTION:
  CAPSULE, 0 size, 2 times daily
TOPICAL:
  NEAT, for females, apply 2-4 drops to the lower back and lower abdomen areas, 2 times daily
  VITA FLEX, 1-3 drops applied to the reproductive Vita Flex points on hands and feet (These are the inside of wrists, inside and outside of the upper foot on either side of the anklebone, and along the achilles tendon) 2 times daily

Dietary Supplementation:
VitaGreen, Mineral Essence, Super Cal, Essential Manna, Ultra Young, Thyromin

Topical Treatment:
Progessence, Prenolone, Prenolone+, EndoBalance.

INFLAMMATION

Inflammation can be caused by a variety of conditions, including bacterial infection, poor diet, chemicals, hormonal imbalance, and physical injury.

Certain essential oils have been documented to be excellent for reducing inflammation. German chamomile contains azulene, a blue compound with highly anti-inflammatory properties. Peppermint is also highly anti-inflammatory. Other oils with anti-inflammatory properties include helichrysum, spruce, wintergreen, and clove.

Some oils are better suited for certain types of inflammation. For example:

- Myrrh and helichrysum work well for inflammation due to tissue/capillary damage, and bruising.

- German chamomile and lavender are helpful with inflammation due to bacterial infection.

- Ravensara, hyssop, and thyme are appropriate for inflammation caused by viral infection.

Single Oils:
Wintergreen, helichrysum, clove, nutmeg, lavender, ravensara, thyme, German chamomile, Roman chamomile, cypress, myrrh, hyssop, peppermint, spruce

Blends:
Purification, PanAway, Aroma Siez, Melrose, ImmuPro, Relieve It, Exodus II

Anti-inflammation blend #1:
- 10 drops fir
- 6 drops tea tree
- 4 drops German chamomile
- 2 drops peppermint
- 2 drops lemongrass

Anti-inflammation blend #2:
- 6 drops frankincense
- 6 drops fir
- 6 drops *Eucalyptus citriodora*
- 4 drops ravensara
- 3 drops wintergreen
- 1 drop peppermint

EO Applications:
TOPICAL:
  DILUTE 50-50, 2-4 drops on inflamed area, 2 times daily
  COMPRESS, cold, 1-3 times daily as needed
INGESTION:
  CAPSULE, 0 size, 2 times daily

Topical Treatment:
Ortho Ease, Relaxation, Ortho Sport

INFLUENZA

(See COLDS)

Single Oils:
Idaho tansy, lemon, blue cypress, mountain savory, oregano, *Eucalyptus radiata*, myrtle, peppermint

Blends:
ImmuPower, Di-Tone, Exodus II, Thieves, ParaFree, Essentialzyme, Polyzyme

EO Applications:
INGESTION:
RICE MILK, 2-4 times daily
CAPSULE, 00 size, 1 capsule 3 times daily
INHALATION:
DIRECT, 2-4 times daily
TOPICAL:
DILUTE 50-50, 2-4 drops on chest, stomach or lower back, as needed, 2- times daily
RAINDROP Technique, 1-2 times weekly
COMPRESS, warm, over lower abdomen, 1-2 times daily
BATH SALTS, (see below)

Influenza Recipe for bath
- 2 drops Eucalyptus radiata
- 6 drops frankincense
- 3 drops helichrysum
- 6 drops spruce
- 15 drops ravensara
- 1 drop wintergreen

Stir above essential oils thoroughly into 1/4 cup Epsom salt or baking soda, then add salt/oil mixture to hot bath water while tub is filling. Soak in hot bath until water cools.

Dietary Supplementation:
ParaFree, Essentialzyme, Polyzyme, ImmuPro, ImmuneTune, ImmuGel, Exodus, Essential Omegas

INSECT BITES

(See INSECT REPELLENT)

Because of their outstanding antiseptic and oil-soluble properties, essential oils are ideal for treating most kinds of insect bites. Essential oils such as lavender and peppermint reduce insect-bite-induced itching and infection.

Singles oils:
Lavender, eucalyptus globulus, citronella, tea tree, peppermint, rosemary

Blends:
Purification, Melrose, PanAway

Blend for stings and bites:
- 1 drop thyme
- 10 drops lavender
- 4 drops *Eucalyptus radiata*
- 3 drops Roman or German chamomile

EO Applications:
TOPICAL:
NEAT or DILUTE 50-50, apply 1-2 drops on bite location 2-4 times daily

Bee Stings

Single Oils:
Lavandin, Idaho tansy

Blends:
Purification, Melrose, PanAway

Bee Sting blend:
- 2 drops lavender
- 1 drop helichrysum
- 1 drop German chamomile
- 1 drop wintergreen

Bee Sting Regimen:
- Flick or scrape stinger out with credit card or knife, taking care not to squeeze the venom sack.
- Apply 1-2 drops Purification, Melrose, lavender, or Idaho tansy on location. Repeat until the venom spread has stopped.
- Apply lavandin with or without one or more of the single oils listed, 2-3 times daily until redness abates. PanAway may be substituted for Purification.

Black Widow Spider Bite

Get victim to an emergency care facility immediately. Rub 1 drop lavender every 2-3 minutes over the bite until you reach the hospital.

Brown Recluse Spider Bite

The bite of this spider causes a painful redness and blistering which progresses to a gangrenous slough of the affected area. Seek immediate medical attention.

Blends:
Purification, Thieves

Spider Bite blend:
- 1 drop lavandin
- 1 drop helichrysum
- 1 drop Melrose

EO Applications:
TOPICAL:
NEAT, 1 drop of either of the two above blends every minute until you reach professional medical treatment.

Chiggers (Mites)

Single Oils:
Tea tree, lavender

Blends:
R.C., Purification

EO Applications:
TOPICAL:
NEAT, 2-6 drops, depending on size of affected area, 3-5 times daily

Ticks

Single Oils:
Thyme, oregano, peppermint

Blends:
R.C., Purification

EO Applications:
TOPICAL:
NEAT, apply 1 drop neat thyme or oregano to tick to loosen from skin. Apply 1 drop neat Purification on site to detoxify wound. Apply 1 drop neat peppermint every 5 minutes for 5 minutes to reduce pain and infection

---

Using Essential Oils As Insect Repellents

Mosquito-repellent: Lemon, peppermint, *Eucalyptus radiata*, lemongrass.

Moth repellent: Patchouli.

Horse-fly repellent: Idaho tansy floral water.

Aphids repellent: Mix 10 drops spearmint and 15 drops orange essential oils in 2 quarts salt water, shake well, and spray on plants.

Cockroach repellent: Mix 10 drops peppermint and 5 drops cypress in 1/2 cup salt water. Shake well and spray where roaches live.

Silverfish repellent: *Eucalyptus radiata*, citriadora

To repel insects, essential oils can be diffused or put on cotton balls or cedar chips (for use in closets or drawers).

INSECT REPELLENT

Single Oils:
Peppermint, *Eucalyptus radiata,* lemon, lime, lavender, tea tree, cedarwood, geranium, Idaho tansy, rosemary, patchouli, citronella, lemongrass, thyme

Blends:
Purification, Thieves, Melrose

Insect Repellent blend:
- 6 drops peppermint
- 6 drops tea tree
- 9 drops *Eucalyptus radiata*

EO Applications:
TOPICAL:
DILUTE 20-80, apply to exposed skin as needed

INSOMNIA

After age 40, sleep quality and quantity deteriorates substantially as melatonin production in the brain declines. Supplemental melatonin has been researched to dramatically improve sleep/wake cycles and combat age-related insomnia.

To Relax Before Sleep:

Rub Peace & Calming or Dream Catcher across the shoulders along with a little lavender or Roman chamomile if needed.

Put 1 drop of Harmony on energy meridians to help balance the energy flow in the body. (1 drop on stomach, navel, thymus, throat, forehead, and crown of head).

Insomnia may also be caused by bowel or liver toxicity, poor heart function, negative memories and trauma, depression, mineral deficiencies, hormone imbalance, or underactive thyroid.

The fragrance of many essential oils can exert a powerful calming effect on the mind through their influence on the limbic region of the brain. Historically, lavender sachets or pillows were used.

Single Oils:
Valerian, lavender, cedarwood, lemon, German chamomile, Roman chamomile, mandarin, St. John's wort, Idaho balsam fir, rosemary, cypress

Blends:
Peace & Calming, Citrus Fresh, Harmony, Dream Catcher, Valor, Present Time, Gentle Baby, Citrus Fresh, 3 Wise Men

Insomnia blend #1:
- 12 drops orange
- 8 drops lavender
- 4 drops citrus hystrix
- 3 drops geranium
- 2 drops Roman chamomile

Insomnia blend #2:
- 15 drops lavender
- 15 drops Peace & Calming

EO Applications:
INHALATION:
> DIFFUSION, 30-60 min. at bedtime. Or apply 1-3 drops on a cotton ball and place on or near your pillow.

TOPICAL:
> NEAT, apply 1-3 drops to shoulders, stomach and on bottoms of feet.
> BATH SALTS, just before retiring at night

Dietary Supplementation:
ImmuPro, Super Cal, Thyromin, HRT tincture, CardiaCare, PD80/20, PowerMeal

Take one 00 capsule of lavender oil 1 hour before bedtime.

Topical Treatment:
Progessence, Prenolone

Insomnia from Bowel Toxicity

(See also DIGESTIVE PROBLEMS)

Dietary Supplementation:
Essentialzyme, Comfortone, ICP

A fasting or cleansing program is important for combating insomnia caused by excess toxins accumulating in the liver and the gastrointestinal tract. Excessive toxins may also produce recurring migraine headaches, skin eruptions, discoloration, changes in pigmentation, acne, or bumpy skin.

Insomnia from Depression

(See also DEPRESSION)

Depression is a major cause of insomnia. St. John's wort has been proven highly effective in reducing depression. A lack of adequate mineral intake (ie., magnesium, zinc, copper, selenium, potassium) can also contribute to clinical depression.

Single Oils:
St. John's wort, melissa, frankincense, lemon

EO Applications:
TOPICAL:
> NEAT, apply 1-3 drops to shoulders, stomach and on bottoms of feet.

Dietary Supplementation:
Mineral Essence, Essential Manna, Wolfberry Crisp, Berry Young Juice, Master Formula Vitamins, Essential Omegas, Super B, Ultra Young, AD&E.

Insomnia from Thyroid Imbalance

(See also THYROID)

Hyperthyroidism (having an overactive thyroid) is caused by chlorine in the drinking water and can trigger insomnia.

Single Oils:
Myrrh, myrtle

EO Applications:
TOPICAL:
>   NEAT, apply 1-3 drops to shoulders, stomach and on bottoms of feet.

Dietary Supplementation:
Thyromin

IRRITABLE BOWEL SYNDROME

(See DIGESTIVE PROBLEMS)

Irritable bowel syndrome (IBS) is a common disorder of the intestines marked by the following symptoms:

- Cramps
- Gas and bloating
- Constipation
- Diarrhea and loose stools

IBS may be caused by a combination of stress and a high-fat diet. Fatty foods worsen symptoms by increasing the intensity of the contractions in the colon, thereby increasing symptoms. Chocolate and milk products, in particular, seem to have the most negative effect on IBS sufferers.

IBS is not the same as colitis, mucous colitis, spastic colon, and spastic bowel. Unlike colitis, IBS does not involve any inflammation and is actually called a "functional disorder" because it presents no obvious, outward signs of disease.

A number of medical studies have documented that peppermint oil (in enteric-coated capsules) is beneficial in treating irritable bowel syndrome and decreases pain.[27,28,29]

Single Oils:
Peppermint, anise seed, fennel, tarragon

Blends:
Di-Tone, Juva Cleanse

EO Applications:
INGESTION:
>   CAPSULE, 0 size, 2 times daily
>   RICE MILK, 2-4 times daily
>   SYRUP, 2-4 times daily

Dietary Supplementation:
ICP, ComforTone, Polyzyme, Essentialzyme, Lipozyme, Juva Power, Immugel

ITCHING

(See SKIN DISORDERS or FUNGAL INFECTIONS)

JAUNDICE

(See LIVER DISORDERS)

Jaundice refers to the yellowing of the skin that is a result of a stressed or damaged liver.

Single Oils:
Ledum, amyris, carrot seed, German chamomile, thyme, geranium

Blends:
JuvaFlex, JuvaCleanse, Release

EO Applications:
INGESTION:
>   CAPSULE, 0 size, once a day, using JuvaFlex, JuvaCleanse
TOPICAL:
>   COMPRESS, warm, 2-3 times daily over the liver

Dietary Supplementation:
Cleansing Trio, JuvaTone, milk thistle, Rehemogen

27. Weydert JA, et al., "Systematic review of treatments for recurrent abdominal pain," *Pediatrics* 2003 Jan;111(1):e1-11.

28. Logan AC, Beaulne TM, "The treatment of small intestinal bacterial overgrowth with enteric-caoated peppermint oil: a case report," *Altern Med Rev,* 2002 Oct;7(5):410-7.

29. Sagduyu K, "Peppermint oil for irritable bowel syndrome," *Psychosomatics* 2002 Nov-Dec;43(6):508-9.

JOINT STIFFNESS AND PAIN

(See also PAIN, ARTHRITIS and CONNECTIVE TISSUE)

Single Oils:
Spruce, Douglas fir, elemi, Idaho balsam fir, wintergreen, German chamomile, cypress, peppermint, helichrysum, pine

Blends:
PanAway, Aroma Siez, Aroma Life, Relieve It

Joint Pain blend #1:
- 10 drops black pepper
- 2 drops rosemary
- 5 drops marjoram
- 5 drops lavender

Joint Pain blend #2:
- 8 drops spruce
- 8 drops sandalwood
- 7 drops fir
- 5 drops hyssop
- 4 drops lemongrass
- 5 drops helichrysum
- 4 drops wintergreen
- 2 drops blue chamomile
- 3 drops vetiver
- 1 drop Idaho tansy

EO Applications:
TOPICAL:
> DILUTE 50-50, massage 3-6 drops on location, repeat as needed to control pain VITA FLEX, apply to appropriate Vita Flex points on the feet. Repeat as needed

Dietary Supplementation:
Sulfurzyme, Power Meal, Ultra Young, ArthroTune, ArthroPlus

Topical Treatment:
Regenolone, Ortho Ease, Ortho Sport, Morning Start Bath Gel, Peppermint-Cedarwood Bar Soap, Melaleuca/Geranium Bar Soap

JUVENILE DWARFISM

Dwarfism is caused by insufficient production of growth hormone by the pituitary. The essential oil *Conyza canadensis* (Fleabane) was used by Daniel Pénoël, M.D., in his clinical practice for reversing retarded maturation. This essential oil is included in Ultra Young.

Singles:
Fleabane

Blends:
Brain Power

Brain Power stimulates the limbic system.

Dietary Supplementation:
Ultra Young, Ultra Young+, PD 80/20

Topical Treatment:
Prenolone+, EndoBalance

KIDNEY DISORDERS

The kidneys remove waste products from the blood, control blood pressure. The kidneys filter over 200 quarts of blood each day and remove over 2 quarts of waste products and water which flow into the bladder as urine through tubes called ureters.

Strong kidneys are essential for good health. Inefficient or damaged kidneys can result in wastes accumulating in the blood and causing serious damage.

High blood pressure can be a cause and a result of chronic kidney failure, since kidneys are central to blood regulation (see BLOOD PRESSURE, HIGH).

Symptoms of poor kidney function:
- Infrequent or inefficient urinations.
- Swelling, especially around the ankles.
- Labored breathing due to fluid accumulation in chest.

Case History

It was reported that a man had a heart bypass using a vein removed from his leg. The leg swelled up from fluid retention and could be moved around like jelly. The leg was first massaged from the foot up with 4 drops cypress mixed into Cel-Lite Magic Massage Oil. The massage was repeated with 4 drops each of fennel and geranium mixed into the same massage oil. After 20 minutes of massaging the swelling had dissipated.

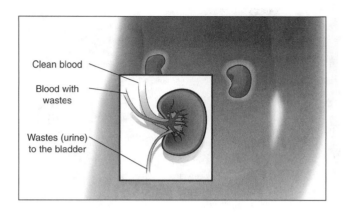

Clean blood

Blood with wastes

Wastes (urine) to the bladder

Diuretic (To Increase Urine Flow)

Single Oils:
Ledum, rosemary, juniper, fennel, anise seed, lemongrass, grapefruit, geranium, sage

Blends:
JuvaFlex, JuvaCleanse, EndoFlex, Di-Tone, Acceptance

Dietary Supplementation:
K & B Tincture, Cleansing Trio, and JuvaTone, JuvaPower/Spice

EO Applications:
INGESTION:
CAPSULE, 0 size, 3 times daily
TOPICAL:
DILUTE 50-50, massage 6-8 drops over kidney area on back, 1-2 times daily
COMPRESS, warm, 1-2 times daily

Topical Treatment:
Cel-Lite Magic Massage Oil

Edema (Swelling)

(See EDEMA, WATER RETENTION)

A Simple Way To Strengthen the Kidneys

• Take 3 droppers K & B Tincture in 4 oz. distilled water, 3 times daily.

• Drink 8 oz. water with about 10 percent cranberry juice and the fresh juice of 1/2 lemon.

• Drink plenty of other liquids, preferably distilled water.

Kidney Inflammation/Infection (Nephritis)

Kidney inflammation can be caused by structural defects, poor diet, or bacterial infection from *Escherichia coli, Staphylococcus aureus, Enterobacter, and Klebsiellabacteri.*

Abnormal proteins trapped in the glomeruli can also cause inflammation and damage to these tiny filtering units. This is called *glomerulonephritis.* This disease can be acute (flaring up in a few days), or chronic (taking months or years to develop). The mildest forms may not show any symptoms except through a urine test. At more advanced stages, urine appears smokey (as small amounts of blood are passed) and eventually red as more blood is excreted—the signs of impending kidney failure. As with all serious conditions, you should immediately consult a health care professional if you suspect a kidney infection of any kind.

Symptoms include:
• Feeling of discomfort in lower back
• Drowsiness
• Nauseous
• Smokey or red-colored urine

Damage to the glomeruli (tiny filtering units in the kidneys) caused by bacterial infections is called *pyelonephritis.* To reduce infection, drink a gallon of water mixed with 8 oz. of cranberry juice daily and use the following products:

Single Oils:
Myrrh, cypress, juniper, geranium, tangerine, marjoram

Blends:
Thieves, JuvaFlex, JuvaCleanse, Aroma Life, EndoFlex

EO Applications:
INGESTION:
CAPSULE, 00 size, 2 times daily for 10 days
RICE MILK, 2-4 times daily
TOPICAL:
COMPRESS, cold, 1-2 times daily over kidney area
VITA FLEX, massage 1-3 drops on kidney Vita Flex points on feet

Dietary Supplementation:
K & B tincture

Kidney Compress regimen:
    Kidney Compress blend:
- 5 drops juniper
- 5 drops tangerine
- 3 drops geranium
- 1 drop helichrysum

Mix the above oils with 1/2 tsp V6 Oil Complex or massage oil and massage 6-10 drops of the mixture on the back over the kidney area. Apply a COLD compress over the kidneys for one night.

The following night do another COLD compress over the kidneys using 10 drops ImmuPower in 1/4 tsp. V6 Oil Complex. Each night, massage the kidney Vita Flex points on the feet. Repeat, if needed. Take 3 droppers of K & B three times daily.

Three Phase Kidney Support regimen:

Phase I:
Perform a colon and liver cleanse

Phase II:
Daily Regimen:
- 4 servings of Power Meal and 6 capsules VitaGreen
- 3 droppers Rehemogen 3 times daily
- Apply 2-4 drops Aroma Life, JuvaFlex, or JuvaCleanse over the kidneys, on kidney Vita Flex points of the feet, and around the navel.
- After 10 days, add ImmuneTune and Super C.

Phase III:
Drink a gallon of water mixed with 8 oz. of unsweetened cranberry juice daily.

Kidney Stones

A kidney stone is a solid piece of material that forms in the kidney from mineral or protein-breakdown products in the urine. Occasionally, larger stones can become trapped in a ureter, bladder, or urethra, which can block urine flow causing intense pain.

There are four types of kidney stones: Stones made from calcium (the most common type), stones made from magnesium and ammonia (a struvite stone), stones made from uric acid, and stones made from cystine (the most rare).

Detoxifing the Kidneys

The Chinese Wolfberry has been used in China for centuries as a kidney tonic and detoxifier. Essential oils can also assist in the detoxification due to their unique lipid-soluble properties.

Blends:
- Helichrysum with juniper or fennel.
- Helichrysum with Di-Tone, JuvaFlex or Juva Cleanse.

Place 1-3 drops in water and take as a dietary supplement three times a day. Apply as a compress over kidneys and bladder

Supplements: K & B tincture, Cleansing Trio, JuvaTone, VitaGreen, and Sulfurzyme.

Some of the symptoms of kidney stones include:
- Persistent, penetrating pain in side
- A burning sensation during urination
- Blood in the urine
- Bad-smelling or cloudy urine
- Fainting

It is important to drink plenty of water *(at least 12 eight-ounce glasses daily)* to help pass or dissolve a kidney stone.

Single Oils:
Wintergreen, geranium, juniper, helichrysum, fennel, lemongrass

Blends:
Kidney stone compress blend:
- 10 drops *Eucalyptus radiata*
- 10 drops geranium
- 10 drops juniper
- 1 Tbsp. V6 Oil Complex

EO Applications:
TOPICAL:
    COMPRESS, warm, use 6-10 drops of
    above blend, over kidney area
    1-2 times daily
    VITA FLEX, massage 2-3 drops on
    kidney Vita Flex points of feet
INGESTION:
    CAPSULE, 00 size, 2 times daily
    RICE MILK, 2-4 times daily

Dietary Supplementation:
Cleansing Trio, Juvatone, K & B, Polyzyme, Essentialzyme, Detoxzyme, ComforTone

Other options for helping the body pass a stone:

Kidney Stone drink #1
- 5 drops rosemary
- 5 drops geranium
- 5 drops juniper
- 1 Tbsp. blue agave nectar
- juice from 1/2 lemon
- 8 oz. warm distilled water

Emulsify the three essential oils in the blue agave nectar, then add the lemon juice, stir briskly into 8 ounces of warm water and drink on empty stomach. Do this 2-3 times daily until stone passes.

Kidney Stone drink #2:
- 2 Tbsp. virgin olive oil
- 8 oz. organic apple juice
  Mix the above in a sealed container, shake vigorously, then drink, 2-3 times daily until stone passes.

Cleansing regimen to aid in passing a stone:
1. Start with colon cleanse using Cleansing Trio.
2. Support the liver by using JuvaTone. 1 tablet 3 times daily during the first week; 2 tablets 3 times daily during succeeding weeks.
3. Take one dropper K & B in 8 oz pure water every 2 hours.
4. Drink as much extra water as you can comfortably consume to help flush kidneys.

Ureter Infection

The ureter is the duct from the kidney to the bladder.

Single Oils:
Lemon, myrtle

EO Applications:
INGESTION:
    CAPSULE, 00 size, twice daily for 10 days
    RICE MILK, 2-4 times daily
TOPICAL:
    VITA FLEX, massage 1-3 drops on kidney Vita Flex points on feet

Dietary Supplementation:
Super C, AlkaLime

KNEE CARTILAGE INJURY

(See CONNECTIVE TISSUE)

LEUKEMIA

(See CANCER)

LEG ULCERS

(See SKIN DISORDERS)

LIVER DISORDERS

The liver is one of the most important organs in the body, playing a major role in detoxifying the body. When the liver is damaged, due to excess alcohol consumption, viral hepatitis, or poor diet, an excess of toxins can build up in the blood and tissues that can result in degenerative disease and death.

Symptoms of a stressed or diseased liver include:
- Jaundice (abnormal yellow color of the skin). This may be the only visible sign of liver disease.
- Nausea
- Loss of appetite
- Dark-colored urine
- Yellowish or grey-colored bowel movements
- Abdominal pain or ascites, a unusual swelling of the abdomen caused by an accumulation of fluid
- Itching, dermatitis, or hives
- Disturbed sleep caused by the build up of unfiltered toxins in blood
- General fatigue and loss of energy
- Lack of sex drive

Detoxification of Liver and Gall Bladder

Single Oils:
Ledum, *Citrus hystrix*, celery seed, helichrysum, mandarin, cardamom, geranium, carrot seed, German chamomile, Roman chamomile

Blends:
JuvaFlex, JuvaCleanse, Release, ImmuPower, Thieves, Di-Tone, EndoFlex

Liver blend:
- 2 drops German chamomile
- 3 drops helichrysum
- 10 drops orange
- 5 drops rosemary

Gall Bladder blend:
- 2 drops Roman chamomile
- 2 drops German chamomile

EO Applications:
INGESTION:
> CAPSULE, 0 size, 2 times daily
> RICE MILK, 2-4 times daily

TOPICAL:
> COMPRESS, warm, over the liver
> 1-2 times daily
> VITA FLEX, massage 1-3 drops on liver
> Vita Flex point of foot, 1-2 times daily
> RAINDROP Technique, 1-2 times weekly

Dietary Supplementation:
JuvaTone, JuvaPower/Spice, Rehemogen,
Sulfurzyme, Cleansing Trio, Power Meal, Chelex

Hepatitis

Viral hepatitis is a serious, life-threatening disease of the liver which results in scarring (cirrhosis) and eventual organ destruction and death. There are several different kinds of hepatitis: Hepatitis A (spread by contaminated food, water, or feces) and hepatitis B and C (spread by contaminated blood or semen).

A 2003 study conducted by Roger Lewis MD at the Young Life Research Clinic in Provo, Utah evaluated the efficacy of helichrysum, ledum, and celery seed in treating cases of advanced Hepatitis C. In one case of a male age 20 diagnosed with a Hepatitis C viral count of 13,200. After taking two capsules (approx. 750 mg each) of a blend of helichrysum, ledum, and celery seed (JuvaCleanse) per day for a month with no other intervention, patients showed that viral counts dropped to 2,580, an over 80 percent reduction.

Symptoms include jaundice, weakness, loss of appetite, nausea, brownish or tea colored urine, abdominal discomfort, fever and whitish bowel movements.

Single Oils:
Ledum, celery seed, ravensara, German chamomile, thyme, clove

---

How to Protect Your Liver

- Use supplements such as schizandra, milk thistle, and N-acetyl cysteine
- Avoid alcoholic beverages.
- Avoid unnecessary use of prescription drugs. Even some common over-the-counter pain relievers can have toxic effects on the liver in moderately high doses.
- Consume a diet high in selenium.
- Avoid mixing pharmaceutic drugs. Be especially cautious in mixing prescription drugs with alcohol.
- Avoid exposure to industrial chemicals whenever possible.
- Eat a healthy diet.
- The Chinese wolfberry (Ningxia variety) is widely used in China as a liver tonic and detoxifier.

Blends:
JuvaFlex, JuvaCleanse, Di-Tone, ImmuPower, Thieves, Release, Exodus II

EO Applications:
INGESTION:
> CAPSULE, 0 size, 3 times daily
> RICE MILK, 2-4 times daily

TOPICAL:
> DILUTE 50-50, apply 1-3 drops on carotid arteries (on right and left side of throat just under jaw bone on either side), 2-5 times daily. (Carotid arteries are an excellent place to apply oils for fast absorption.)
> COMPRESS, warm, over liver
> 1-2 times daily
> VITA FLEX, massage 1-3 drops on liver
> Vita Flex point of foot, 1-3 times daily
> RAINDROP Technique 2-3 times weekly

Dietary Supplementation:
JuvaPower/Spice, VitaGreen, JuvaTone, ImmuPro, ImmuneTune, Super C, ImmuGel, Rehemogen

NOTE: Avoid citrus juices.

Daily Hepatitis regimen:
- Begin with colon and liver cleanse using Cleaning Trio. After 3 days add JuvaTone, 1-2 tablets 3 times daily
- Super C Chewable: 6 tablets, 3 times daily.

- ImmuPro: Chew 8 tablets at night, 2-4 tablets morning and afternoon.
- VitaGreen: 2-6 capsules, 3 times daily, according to blood type
- Master Formula vitamins: 2-4 tablets, 3 times daily, according to blood type

LIVER CANCER

(See CANCER)

LIVER SPOTS (Senile Lentigenes)

(See also SKIN DISORDERS)

Single Oils:
Idaho tansy

EO Applications:
TOPICAL:
> DILUTE 50-50, apply 2-4 drops over affected area 4 times daily for 2 weeks

LOU GEHRIG'S DISEASE (ALS)

(See NEUROLOGICAL DISORDERS)

LUMBAGO (LOWER BACK PAIN)

(See SPINE INJURIES AND PAIN)

LUNG INFECTIONS

Bronchitis

Bronchitis is characterized by inflammation of the bronchial tube tube lining accompanied by a heavy mucus discharge. Bronchitis can be caused by an infection or exposure to dust, chemicals, air pollution, or cigarette smoke.

When bronchitis occurs regularly over a long periods (i.e. 3 months out of the year for several years) it is known as chronic bronchitis. It can eventually lead to emphysema.

Symptoms:
- Persistent, hacking cough
- Mucus discharge from the lungs
- Difficulty breathing

Avoiding air pollution is an easy way to reduce bronchitis symptoms. In cases where bronchitis is caused by a bacteria or virus, the inhalation of high antimicrobial essential oils may help combat the infection. Heavy mucus may increase after eating foods containing processed sugar or flour.

Single Oils:
Rosemary, *Eucalyptus radiata*, ravensara, thyme, wintergreen, spruce, pine, oregano, helichrysum, tea tree, spearmint, myrtle, Idaho balsam fir

Blends:
Exodus II, ImmuPower, Raven, R.C., Melrose, Thieves, Legacy, Purification, Brain Power

Bronchitis blend:
- 2 drops sage
- 4 drops myrrh
- 5 drops clove
- 6 drops ravensara
- 15 drops frankincense

NOTE: Essential oil blends work especially well in respiratory applications.

EO Applications:
TOPICAL:
> DILUTE according to application code Appendix E). Apply 2-6 drops to neck and chest as needed.
> COMPRESS, warm, on neck, chest and upper back areas 1-3 times daily
> VITA FLEX, on lung points of feet, 2-4 times daily

ORAL:
> GARGLE, hourly, or as needed

INHALATION:
> DIRECT, 5-10 times daily as needed
> DIFFUSION, 15 minutes, 3-10 times daily as needed. Alternate oils/blends each time. Also diffuse at night during sleep
> VAPOR, 2-4 times daily as needed

RETENTION:
> RECTAL, using any of the recommended blends, combine 20 drops with 1 tablespoon olive oil. Insert into rectum with bulb syringe and retain throughout the night. Repeat nightly for 2-3 days.

Dietary Supplementation:
Super C, ImmuPro, ImmuGel, ImmuneTune, Exodus, Cleansing Trio, Fresh Essence +

Pneumonia

(See also THROAT INFECTION)

Single Oils:
Goldenrod, ledum, tea tree, rosemary, thyme, ravensara, Eucalyptus globulus, Eucalyptus radiata, mountain savory, clove, anise, fennel, wintergreen, hyssop, spearmint, frankincense

Blends:
ImmuPower, Thieves, Raven, R.C., Aroma Siez, Sacred Mountain, Melrose, Inspiration, Exodus II

Pneumonia blend:
- 10 drops rosemary
- 8 drops ravensara
- 8 drops frankincense
- 2 drops oregano
- 2 drops peppermint

EO Applications:
TOPICAL:
> DILUTE according to application code (Appendix E). Apply 2-6 drops to neck and chest as needed.
> COMPRESS, warm, on neck, chest and VITA FLEX, on lung points of feet, 2-4 times daily

ORAL:
> GARGLE, hourly, or as needed

INHALATION:
> DIRECT, 5-10 times daily as needed
> DIFFUSION, 15 minutes, 3-10 times daily as needed. Alternate oils/blends each time. Also diffuse at night during sleep
> VAPOR, 2-4 times daily as needed

RETENTION:
> RECTAL, using any of the recommend blends, combine 20 drops with 1 tablespoon olive oil. Insert into rectum with bulb syringe and retain throughout the night. Repeat nightly for 5-6 days.

For long-term chest congestion from welding, smoking, etc., use R.C. and myrtle in hot packs or compresses on chest and back.

The antibacterial and antiviral oils, which are very powerful prophylactic agents for protection against colds, flu, and chest infections, are basil, lavender, hyssop, frankincense, rosemary, bergamot,

Eucalyptus radiata, tea tree, clove, oregano, cistus, thyme, and mountain savory.

Dietary Supplementation:
Super C, Longevity Caps, VitaGreen, ImmuPro, ImmuneTune, Rehemogen, Master Formula Vitamins, AD&E

Oral Care:
Thieves Lozenges, Fresh Essence Plus

Whooping Cough

This is a contagious disease affecting the respiratory system particularly in children. Lungs become infected, as the air passages become clogged with thick mucus. Over the course of several days, the condition worsens, resulting in long coughing bouts (up to 1 minute). The continual coughing makes breathing difficult and labored.

Single Oils:
Rosemary, lavender, lemongrass, thyme, myrtle, petitgrain, nutmeg, oregano, tea tree

Blends:
Thieves, Melrose, Purification, ImmuPower, Raven, R.C.

EO Applications:
TOPICAL:
> DILUTE 20-80, apply 2-4 drops to neck and chest as needed.
> COMPRESS, warm, on neck, chest and upper back areas 1-3 times daily
> VITA FLEX, on lung points of feet, 2-3 times daily

INHALATION:
> DIRECT, 5-10 times daily as needed
> DIFFUSION, 15 minutes, 3-10 times daily as needed. Alternate oils/blends each time. Also diffuse at night during sleep.
> VAPOR, 2-4 times daily as needed

Dietary Supplementation:
Super C, Longevity Caps, VitaGreen, ImmuPro, ImmuneTune, and Rehemogen.

NOTE: Because whooping cough usually affects children, always dilute essential oils in V6 Oil Complex or other cold-pressed vegetable oil before topically applying. Start with low concentrations until response is observed. Diffuse intermittently and observe reaction.

LUPUS

Lupus is an autoimmune disease that has several different varieties:

- *Lupus vulgaris* is characterized by lesions that form on skin. Brownish lesions may form on the face and become ulcerous and form scars.

- Discoid *Lupus erythematosus* is characterized by scaly red patches on the skin and oval or butterfly-shaped lesions on the face. It is milder than the systemic type.

- Systemic *Lupus erythematosus* is more serious than discoid lupus. It inflames the connective tissue in any part of the body, including the joints, muscles, skin, blood vessels, membranes surrounding the lungs and heart, and occasionally the kidneys and brain.

Because lupus is an autoimmune disease, it has been successfully treated using MSM, a form of organic sulfur.

Single Oils:
Cypress, lemongrass

Blends:
ImmuPower, Valor, EndoFlex, Joy, Acceptance, Present Time

Lupus blend:
- 30 drops cypress
- 30 drops lemongrass
- 30 drops EndoFlex

EO Applications:
TOPICAL:
> BODY MASSAGE, once every other day
> RAINDROP Technique, 1-2 times weekly

Lupus daily regimen:
1. BATH SALTS, using EndoFlex, add 30 drops to 1/2 cup Epsom salt or baking soda and add to hot bath. Soak for 30 minutes.
2. VITA FLEX: Massage EndoFlex on bottoms of the feet; follow two hours later with foot massage using Thieves.
3. TOPICAL: Massage 10-15 drops ImmuPower over liver and on feet 2-3 times daily.
4. SULFURZYME: 1-2 Tbsp powder or 5 capsules 1-2 times daily
5. SUPER CAL: 2-3 capsules, 2 times daily
6. IMMUNETUNE: 2-4 capsules 2 times daily
7. ESSENTIALZYME: 2-6 tablets, 2 times daily
8. VITAGREEN: 2-4 capsules, 2 times daily
9. ADRENAL SUPPORT (see ADRENAL GLAND IMBALANCES topic heading)

Dietary Supplementation:
Sulfurzyme, Super Cal, ImmuneTune, Essentialzyme, VitaGreen, Mega Cal

LYME DISEASE AND ROCKY MOUNTAIN SPOTTED FEVER

Viral infection caused by the bite of an infected tick. Lyme disease is caused by the microorganism *Borrelia burgdorferi.*

Singles:
Thyme, oregano, clove, melissa, niaouli, blue cypress

Blends:
PanAway, Melrose, Thieves, Exodus II, ImmuPower

EO Applications:
INGESTION:
> CAPSULE, 00 size, 3 times daily

Dietary Supplementation:
BodyGize, Power Meal, Polyzyme, ImmuPro, ImmuneTune, Wolfberry Crisp, Berry Young Juice, Exodus, Thyromin

Cleansing Trio and JuvaTone for a colon and liver cleanse.

(See also TICK BITES in INSECT BITES)

(See also RHEUMATOID ARTHRITIS)

LYMPHATIC SYSTEM

Essential oils have long been known to aid in stimulating and detoxifying the lymphatic system.

Single Oils:
Ledum, sandalwood, helichrysum, myrtle, grapefruit, lemongrass, cypress, tangerine, orange, tangerine, rosemary

Blends:
Di-Tone, JuvaFlex, JuvaCleanse, EndoFlex, Thieves, Acceptance, R.C., Aroma Life, En-R-Gee, Citrus Fresh

EO Applications:
TOPICAL:

> DILUTE 50-50, massage 2-4 drops on
> sore lymph glands and under arms,
> 2-3 times daily
> RAINDROP Technique weekly or as needed
> COMPRESS, warm, over affected areas
> 1- 2 times daily

Massage oils on sore spots with sensitive lymph glands.

Then apply Cel-Lite Magic and grapefruit or cypress oil, which helps detoxify chemicals stored in body fat.

Lymphatic Cleanse:
- 3 drops cypress
- 1 drop orange
- 2 drops grapefruit

Mix in 1/2 gallon distilled water. Grade B maple syrup may be added. Drink at least two 8 oz. glasses daily.

Dietary Supplementation:
Super C, ImmuGel, Longevity Caps, VitaGreen

Colon and liver cleanse: Cleansing Trio.

Topical Treatment:
Cel-Lite Magic Massage Oil, Morning Start Bath Gel

LYMPHOMA

(See CANCER)

M.C.T. (Mixed Connective Tissue Disease)

(see LUPUS)

M.C.T. is an autoimmune disease similar to lupus in which the connective tissue in the body becomes inflamed and painful. This condition is usually due to poor assimilation of protein and mineral deficiencies.

Single Oils:
Rosemary, *nutmeg*, clove, lemongrass, marjoram, peppermint, wintergreen cypress

Blends:
ImmuPower, Valor, Joy

MCT blend (for aches and discomfort):
- 10 drops basil
- 8 drops wintergreen
- 6 drops cypress
- 3 drops peppermint

EO Applications:
TOPICAL:

> DILUTE 50-50, massage 4-8 drops on
> affected location 2-3 times daily
> VITA FLEX, massage 1-3 drops on liver
> Vita Flex points of the feet
> RAINDROP Technique, weekly or as
> needed.
> MCT/Lupus regimen:
> Rub 2-4 drops of ImmuPower over the
> liver and on liver Vita Flex Points on the
> bottom of the right foot 2-3 times daily.
> This has been reported to help lupus, which
> is similar to M.C.T.

Dietary Supplementation:
ImmuGel, Master Formula, Super C, Super B, VitaGreen, ImmuneTune, ArthroTune, Super Cal, Thyromin

MCT regimen:
1. Avoid acid-ash foods. Instead, use alkaline foods, such as barley or wheat sprouts.

2. VitaGreen: 2-6 capsules, 3 times daily.

3. Use Cleansing Trio to expel toxins. Avoid contact with or use of cigarettes, cleaning products, chemicals and chemical-using industries (auto garages, paint shops, etc.)

4. Build the body:
   - Super C: 1-3 tablets, 3 times daily.
   - Super Cal: 2-4 capsules, 2 times daily.
   - ImmuneTune: 2-4 capsules, 2 times daily.
   - Super B: 1 tablet, 4 times weekly.
   - Master Formula: 3-6 tablets, 2 times daily.
   - ArthroTune: 2-3 capsules, 2 times daily.

MALARIA

Malaria is a serious disease contracted from several species of *Anopheles* mosquitoes. While malaria is largely confined to the continents of Asia and Africa, an increasing number of cases have arisen in North and South America. If not treated, malaria can be fatal.

Symptoms:
- Fever
- Chills
- Anemia

The best defense against malaria is to use insect repellents effective against *Anopheles* mosquitoes. Once a person has contracted the disease, oils such as lemon can help amplify immune response.

Single Oils:
Lemon, thyme, laurel

Topical/Oral Treatment:
Thieves Antiseptic Spray

EO Applications:
INGESTION:
Mix 3-6 drops lemon oil in 1 tsp blue agave syrup and 8 ox. water, shake, and sip regularly when outbreak is impending.

(See INSECT REPELLENT and INSECT BITES)

MALE HORMONE IMBALANCE

As men age, their DHEA and testosterone levels decline. Conversely, levels of dihydrotestosterone (DHT) increase, contributing to prostate enlargement and hair loss. Because pregnenolone is the master hormone from which all hormones are created, men can directly benefit from transdermal pregnenolone creams as a way of jump-starting sagging DHEA levels. Herbs such as saw palmetto and *Pygeum africanum* can prevent the conversion of testosterone into DHT, thereby reducing prostate enlargement and slowing hair loss.

Single Oils:
Rosemary, sage, fennel, ylang ylang, geranium, blue yarrow, clary sage

Blends:
Mister

EO Applications:
INGESTION:
CAPSULE, 0 size, once a day

Dietary Supplementation:
Progen, DHEA, saw palmetto

MEASLES

Single Oils:
Lavender, Roman chamomile, tea tree, clove, thyme, German chamomile

Blends:
ImmuPower

Measles blend:
- 15 drops lavender
- 15 drops Roman chamomile
- 5 drops tea tree

EO Applications:
TOPICAL:
DILUTE 50-50, apply on spots, 3-5 x daily or as needed
BATH SALTS, soak at least 30 minutes in bath daily
Mix 6-9 drops of any of the above essential oils in 8 oz. water, shake well, and use to sponge down patient 1-2 times daily

Dietary Supplementation:
Super C, AD&E, Master Formula Vitamins, Essential Omegas

MEMORY

(See BRAIN DISORDERS)

MENSTRUAL CONDITIONS

Natural hormones such as natural progesterone and pregnenolone are the most effective treatment for menstrual difficulties and irregularities. The most effective method of administration is transdermal delivery in a cream. Just 20 mg applied to the skin twice a day is equivalent to 1000 mg taken internally.

As women reach menopause, progesterone production declines and a state of estrogen dominance often arises. The most commonly prescribed drugs are conjugated estrogens (from horse urine) or synthetic medroxyprogesterone. The molecules in these synthetic hormones are foreign to the human body and can dramatically increase the risk for ovarian and breast cancer with time.

Endometriosis

This occurs when the uterine lining develops on the outer wall of the uterus, ovaries, fallopian tubes, vagina, intestines, or on the abdominal wall. These fragments cannot escape like the normal uterine lining, which is shed during menstruation. Because of this, fibrous cysts often form around the misplaced uterine tissue. Symptoms can include abdominal or back pain during menstruation or pain that often increases after the period is over. Other symptoms may include heavy periods and pain during intercourse.

Single Oils:
Fennel, clary sage

Blends:
Melrose, Thieves

Dietary Supplementation:
ImmuPro, Super C Chewable, PD 80/20, Protec

Topical Treatment:
Prenolone, Prenolone+, Progessence

Regimen:
- Colon and liver cleanse: Cleansing Trio.
- Hot compress of Melrose on the stomach.
- Apply Thieves to bottom of the feet.

Excessive Bleeding

Excessive Bleeding blend:
- 10 drops geranium
- 10 drops helichrysum
- 5 drops cistus

EO Applications:
TOPICAL:
> DILUTE 50-50, apply 4-6 drops to forehead, crown of head, soles of feet, lower abdomen and lower back, 1-3 times daily
> COMPRESS, warm, daily on lower back and abdomen

1/10 tsp. cayenne in 8 oz. warm water may help regulate bleeding during periods.

Hormone Imbalance

(See CHAPTER 11: TOPICAL HORMONE THERAPY)

As women age, their levels of progesterone decline and contribute to osteoporosis, increased risk of breast and uterine cancers, mood swings, depression, and many other conditions. Estrogen levels can also decline and increase women's risk of heart disease. Replacing these declining levels using topically applied progesterone or pregnenolone creams may be the most effective way to replace and boost decline hormone levels. Pregnenolone may be especially effective, as it is the precursor hormone from which the body creates both progesterone and estrogens.

Single Oil:
Geranium, clary sage

Blends:
Mister, Dragon Time, Lady Sclareol, SclarEssence, Transformation

Hormone Balancing blend #1:
- 10 drops basil
- 10 drops marjoram
- 8 drops hyssop
- 4 drops helichrysum
- 6 drops ylang ylang

Hormone Balancing blend #2:
- 5 drops bergamot
- 5 drops geranium

EO Applications:
TOPICAL:
> DILUTE 50-50, apply 4-6 drops to forehead, crown of head, soles of feet, lower abdomen and lower back 1-3 times daily
> VITA FLEX, massage 3-6 drops on reproductive Vita Flex points of feet
> COMPRESS, warm, daily, on lower back or lower abdomen

Dietary Supplementation:
PD80/20

Topical Treatments:
Prenolone, Prenolone+, Progessence, Neurogen

BodyGize and WheyFit contain soy which helps balance hormones and activate (estrogen) receptors. Take BodyGize and WheyFit at least once a day.

Hysterectomy

(See Hormone Imbalance, above)

Single Oils:
Clary Sage

Blends:
Dragon Time, Lady Sclareol, SclarEssence,

Dietary Supplementation:
PD 80/20.

Topical Treatment:
Progessence

Irregular Periods

Blends:
Period regulator blend #1:
- 5 drops peppermint
- 9 drops fleabane
- 16 drops clary sage
- 11 drops sage
- 5 drops jasmine absolute

Period regulator blend #2:
- 10 drops chamomile
- 10 drops fennel

EO Applications:
TOPICAL:
> DILUTE 50-50, apply 4-6 drops to forehead, crown of head, soles of feet, lower abdomen, and lower back 1-3 times daily
> VITA FLEX, massage 3-6 drops on reproductive Vita Flex points of feet, 2-3 times daily
> COMPRESS, warm, daily, on lower back or lower abdomen

Menstrual Cramps

Single Oils:
Clary sage, rosemary, hops, sage, vitex, lavender, Roman chamomile, cypress, tarragon, vetiver, valerian

Blends:
Dragon Time, EndoFlex

Menstrual cramp relief blend:
- 10 drops Dragon Time
- 4 drops hops (*Humulus iupulus*)\

EO Applications:
TOPICAL:
> COMPRESS, warm, over uterus area, 2-3 times weekly
> VITA FLEX, massage 2-4 drops on reproductive Vita Flex points on feet (around ankles), also on lower back and stomach
INGESTION:
> CAPSULE, 0 size, twice daily for 2 weeks prior to menses

Dietary Supplementation:
PD 80/20, VitaGreen, Master Formula HERS

Topical Treatment:
Prenolone, Prenolone+, EndoBalance

When migraine headaches accompany periods, a colon and liver cleanse may reduce symptoms.

Premenstrual Syndrome (PMS)

PMS is one of the most common hormone-related conditions in otherwise healthy women. Women can experience a wide range of symptoms for 10 to 14 days before menstruation, and even 2 to 3 days into menstruation. These symptoms include mood swings, fatigue, headaches, breast tenderness, abdominal bloating, anxiety, depression, confusion, memory loss, sugar cravings, cramps, low back pain, irritability, weight gain, acne, and oily skin and hair. Causes include hormonal, nutritional, psychological, and stress of the Western culture.

Single Oils:
Hops, clary sage, sage, anise seed, fennel, vitex, basil, ylang ylang, rose, neroli, bergamot

Blends:
Dragon Time, Mister, EndoFlex, Exodus II, Acceptance, Aroma Siez, Lady Sclareol, SclarEssence, Transformation

EO Applications:
INHALATION:
> DIRECT, 3-6 times daily
TOPICAL:
> DILUTE 50-50, apply 4-6 drops to forehead, crown of head, soles of feet, lower abdomen and lower back 1-3 times daily

VITA FLEX, massage 2-4 drops on reproductive Vita Flex points of feet
COMPRESS, warm, daily, on lower back or lower abdomen

ORAL:

TONGUE, 1 drop of EndoFlex on the tongue and then hold the tongue against the roof of the mouth, 2-4 times daily

Dietary Supplementation:

Master Formula vitamins, VitaGreen, Super B, Super Cal, Mineral Essence, AD&E, Ultra Young, ImmuneTune, PD 80/20, Thyromin

Topical Treatment:

Prenolone, Prenolone Plus, Progessence

MENTAL FATIGUE

(See Mental Fatigue in FATIGUE heading)

METAL TOXICITY (Aluminum)

(See also HEAVY METALS)

Aluminum is a very toxic metal that can cause serious neurological damage in the human body—even in minute amounts. Aluminum has been implicated in Alzheimer's disease.

People unwittingly ingest aluminum from their cookware, beverage cans, and antacids. Even deodorants have aluminum compounds. The first step toward reducing aluminum toxicity in the body is to avoid these types of aluminum-based products.

Single Oils:

Clove, helichrysum, *Citrus hystrix*

Blends:

Juva Cleanse

EO Applications:
INGESTION:

CAPSULE, 00 size, 2 times daily

TOPICAL:

RAINDROP Technique, weekly

Dietary Supplementation:

Chelex, JuvaTone, Super Cal, ComforTone

MONONUCLEOSIS (Infectious)

(See EPSTEIN-BARR VIRUS)

MORNING SICKNESS

(See NAUSEA or MENSTRUAL CONDITIONS)

MOTION SICKNESS

(See NAUSEA)

MUCUS (Excess)

Many oils are natural expectorants, helping tissues discharge mucus, soft and hard plaque and toxins.

Single Oils:

Frankincense, ledum, lavender, helichrysum, *Eucalyptus radiata*, cypress, lemon, marjoram, myrtle, peppermint, rosemary

Blends:

Di-Tone, 3 Wise Men, Raven., R.C., Purification

Expectorant blend:
- 3 drops marjoram
- 3 drops ledum
- 1 drop lavender

EO Applications:
INHALATION:

DIRECT, 3-5 times daily
DIFFUSION, 20 minutes 3 times daily

INGESTION:

CAPSULE, 0 size, 1 capsule twice a day

TOPICAL:

DILUTE 50-50, apply 2-4 drops on the T4 and T5 thoracic vertebrae (at the neck-to shoulder intersection), 3-5 times daily
VITA FLEX, massage on relevant Vita Flex points on the feet 2-4 times daily

MULTIPLE SCLEROSIS (MS)

(See NEUROLOGICAL DISEASES)

MUMPS (Infectious Parotitis)

An acute, contagious, febrile disease marked by painful swelling and inflammation of the parotid glands and other salivary glands. The causative agent is a paromyxovirus, spread by direct contact, airborne droplets and urine.

Single Oils:
Thyme, melissa, myrrh, blue cypress, wintergreen.

Blends:
Raven, R.C., Thieves, Exodus II

EO Applications:
TOPICAL:
>   DILUTE 50-50, 2-4 drops behind the ears 4 times daily
>   COMPRESS, warm, 1-3 times daily around throat and jaw
>   RAINDROP Technique 1-2 times weekly

INGESTION:
>   CAPSULE, 00 size, 1 capsule twice a day

Dietary Supplementation:
ImmuPro, Super C, Exodus

MUSCLES

Bruised Muscles

(see BRUISING)

To avoid excess blood clotting in a bruised muscle or tissue and increase circulation:

Single Oils:
Clove, German chamomile, helichrysum, wintergreen, cypress, lavender, geranium, peppermint, vetiver, valerian

Blends:
Aroma Siez, Aroma Life, PanAway, Peace & Calming, Ortho Sport, Ortho Ease

E.O. Applications:
TOPICAL:
>   DILUTE 50-50, apply 2-4 drops to bruised area 3 times daily.

Sequence of application for bruise treatment:

General Rules

When selecting oils for injuries, think through the cause and type of injury and select oils for each segment. For instance, whiplash could encompass muscle damage, nerve damage, ligament damage, inflammation, bone injury, and possibly emotion. Select oils for each perceived problem and apply.

When a bruise displays black and blue discoloration and pain, start with helichrysum, wintergreen, Douglas fir, white fir, Idaho balsam fir, or oregano.

Once the pain and inflammation decrease, use cypress, then basil and Aroma Siez to enhance the muscle relaxation.

Follow with peppermint to stimulate the nerves and reduce inflammation. Finish with cold packs.

Dietary Supplementation: ArthroTune, Super Cal, Mineral Essence, Essential Manna

Cramps and Charley Horses

(See also Tight, Spasmed or Torn Muscles)

Magnesium and calcium deficiency may contribute to muscle cramps and charley horses.

Single Oils:
Rosemary, cypress, marjoram, lavender, elemi, German chamomile

Blends:
PanAway, Aroma Siez, Relieve It

E.O. Applications:
TOPICAL:
>   DILUTE 50-50, massage 2-4 drops on cramped muscle 3 times daily.

Dietary Supplementation:
Super Cal, ArthroTune, Mineral Essence, Berry Young Juice, Essential Manna, Mega Cal, BLM

2-3 capsules of ArthroTune, taken each morning and night will help reduce night leg cramps.

Topical Treatment:
Ortho Sport, Ortho Ease

Inflammation Due to Injury

Tissue damage is usually accompanied by inflammation. Reduce inflammation by massaging with anti-inflammatory oils to minimize further tissue damage and speed healing.

Single oils:
Peppermint, spearmint, German chamomile, myrrh, wintergreen, marjoram, clove, Roman chamomile

Blends:
Aroma Siez, PanAway

Muscle Injury blend:
- 12 drops white fir
- 10 drops tea tree
- 8 drops lavender
- 6 drops marjoram
- 3 drops yarrow
- 3 drops spearmint
- 2 drops peppermint

EO Applications:
TOPICAL:
> DILUTE 50-50, massage 2-4 drops on inflamed muscle 3 times daily

Dietary Supplementation:
Super Cal, ArthroTune, Longevity Caps, Mineral Essence, Power Meal, Mega Cal Sulfurzyme, VitaGreen, Ultra Young, BLM

Inflammation Due to Infection

Single Oils:
Ravensara, hyssop, niaouli, blue cypress

EO Application
TOPICAL:
> DILUTE 50-50, massage 2-4 drops on inflamed muscle 3 times daily
> COMPRESS, cold, 1-3 times daily

Dietary Supplementation:
Super Cal, ArthroTune, Longevity Caps, Mineral Essence, Power Meal, Mega Cal Sulfurzyme, VitaGreen, Ultra Young, BLM

For Tired, Fatigued Muscles

Tired muscles may be lacking in minerals such as calcium and magnesium. Super Cal, Essential Manna, Berry Young Delights, and Mineral Essence are excellent sources of both trace and macro minerals and good for all muscle conditions. ArthroTune helps reduce stiffness from sitting for long periods.

Sore Muscles

Single Oils:
Nutmeg, elemi, marjoram, black pepper, basil, spruce, Roman chamomile, wintergreen, rosemary, peppermint

Blends:
Aroma Siez, Peace & Calming, M-Grain

Sore muscle blend #1:
- 4 drops rosemary
- 8 drops juniper
- 8 drops lavender
- 8 drops lemon
- 10 drops wintergreen

Sore muscle blend #2:
- 9 drops cypress
- 8 drops rosemary
- 8 drops lavender
- 2 drops elemi
- 2 drops valerian

EO Applications:
TOPICAL:
> DILUTE 50-50, massage 4-6 drops into sore muscle 3 times daily.
> COMPRESS, warm, 1-3 times daily

Tight, Spasmed or Torn Muscles

Single Oils:
Elemi, wintergreen, Idaho balsam fir, peppermint, basil, white fir, lemongrass, marjoram

Blends:
Aroma Siez, PanAway

Blend for tight muscles:
- 6 drops marjoram
- 4 drops cypress
- 4 drops wintergreen

- 3 drops valerian
- 1 drop helichrysum

Blend for muscle spasms:
- 1-2 drops ravensara
- 4-5 drops Aroma Siez
- 1 drop black pepper

It is usually helpful to alternate cold and hot packs when applying the above essential oil blend to muscles that are in spasm.

Blend for torn muscle:
- 8 drops Idaho balsam fir
- 8 drops sandalwood
- 7 drops Douglas fir
- 5 drops hyssop
- 4 drop lemongrass
- 5 drops helichrysum
- 4 drops wintergreen
- 2 drops vetiver
- 1 drops Idaho tansy

EO Applications:
TOPICAL:
> DILUTE 50-50 in V-6 Mixing Oil, massage 2-6 drops on affected areas. Follow with Ortho Ease Massage Oil.

Muscle Weakness

Single Oils:
Ravensara, Douglas fir, lemongrass, juniper, nutmeg, white fir, Idaho balsam fir

Blends:
En-R-Gee

EO Applications:
TOPICAL:
> DILUTE 50-50, massage 4-6 drops into weak muscle 3 times daily

Dietary Supplementation:
VitaGreen, AminoTech, WheyFit, Longevity Caps, Amino Tech, Power Meal

MUSCULAR DYSTROPHY

Single Oils:
Pine, lavender, marjoram, lemongrass, vetiver, Idaho balsam fir

Blends:
Aroma Siez, Relieve It

EO Applications:
TOPICAL:
> DILUTE 50-50, massage 4-6 drops along spine 3 times daily

Dietary Supplementation:
Essentialzyme, Polyzyme, WheyFit, Power Meal, Essential Omegas, Sulfurzyme, VitaGreen, Mineral Essence, Thyromin, Ultra Young

Topical Treatment:
Ortho Ease, Ortho Sport

NAILS (Brittle or Weak)

Poor or weak nails, often containing ridges, indicate a sulfur deficiency.

Single Oils:
Frankincense, myrrh, lemon

Blends:
Citrus Fresh

EO Applications:
TOPICAL:
> NEAT, 1-3 drops on nails and at base of nails, 3 times per week.

Dietary Supplementation:
Sulfurzyme, Super Cal, Mineral Essence, Mega Cal

Nail strengthening blend:
- 4 drops Wheat Germ Oil
- 4 drops frankincense
- 4 drops myrrh
- 4 drops lemon

Apply 1 drop of the above blend on each nail 2-3 times weekly.

NARCOLEPSY

A chronic ailment consisting of uncontrollable, recurrent attacks of drowsiness and sleep during daytime. May be aggravated by hypothalamus dysregulation or thyroid hormone deficiency.

(see also THYROID)

Single Oils:
Fleabane, rosemary, black pepper, cinnamon bark

Blends:
Brain Power

EO Applications:
INHALATION:
> DIRECT, 4-8 times daily as needed

TOPICAL:
> DILUTE 50-50, apply 1-2 drops on temples, behind ears, back of neck, on forehead, and under nostrils, as needed

Dietary Supplementation:
Mineral Essence, VitaGreen, Thyromin, BrainPower, Ultra Young.

NAUSEA

Patchouli oil contains compounds that are extremely effective in preventing vomiting due to their ability to reduce the gastrointestinal muscle contractions associated with vomiting.[30] Peppermint has also been found to be effective in many kinds of stomach upset, including nausea.

Single Oils:
Peppermint, patchouli, ginger, nutmeg, Idaho tansy

Blends:
Di-Tone

EO Applications:
TOPICAL:
> DILUTE 50-50, massage 1-3 drops behind each ear (mastoids) and over navel 2-3 times hourly.
> COMPRESS, warm, over stomach, as needed

INHALATION:
> DIRECT, 4-6 times hourly as needed

ORAL:
> TONGUE, 1-4 times as needed

Morning Sickness

Single Oils:
Peppermint, spearmint

Blends:
Di-Tone

EO Applications:
TOPICAL:
> DILUTE 50-50, massage 1-3 drops behind each ear (mastoids) and over navel 2-3 times hourly

> COMPRESS, warm, over stomach, as needed

INHALATION:
> DIRECT, 4-6 times hourly as needed

ORAL:
> TONGUE, 1-4 times as needed

Dietary Supplementation: Polyzyme, Essentialzyme

Motion Sickness

Single Oils:
Patchouli, lavender, peppermint, ginger, spearmint

Blends:
Di-Tone, Valor, JuvaFlex, JuvaCleanse

EO Applications:
TOPICAL:
> DILUTE 50-50, massage 1-3 drops behind each ear (mastoids) and over navel 2-3 times hourly
> COMPRESS, warm, over stomach, as needed

INHALATION:
> DIRECT, 4-6 times hourly as needed

ORAL:
> TONGUE, 1-4 times as needed

INGESTION:
> RICE MILK, 1-2 times as needed

Motion Sickness Preventative:
- 4 drops peppermint
- 4 drops ginger
- 1 Tbsp. V6 Oil Complex

Rub 6-10 drops of the above blend on chest and stomach 1 hour before traveling.

Dietary Supplementation: Polyzyme, Detoxzyme, Essentialzyme

NERVE DISORDERS

Nerve disorders usually involve peripheral or surface nerves and include neuritis, neuropathy, neuralgia, Bell's palsy, and carpal tunnel syndrome. In contrast, neurological disorders are usually associated with deep neurological disturbances in the brain, and these conditions include Lou Gehrig's disease, MS, and cerebral palsy. (See NEUROLOGICAL DISEASES)

---

30. Yang, Kinoshita, Koyama, Takahashi, Tai, Nunoura, "Anti-emetic principles of Pogostemon cablin" (Blanco) 1999 *Watanabe Phytomedicine* Vol. 6(2), pp 89-93.

Single Oils:

Peppermint, lavender, cedarwood, German chamomile, Roman chamomile, sage, rosemary, spruce, tangerine, sandalwood

Blends:

Valor, Peace & Calming, Citrus Fresh

General blend for nerve disorders:
- 2 drops peppermint
- 10 drops juniper
- 1 drop geranium
- 8 drops marjoram
- 4 drops helichrysum

EO Applications:
TOPICAL:

NEAT or DILUTE 50-50 as required, apply 2-4 drops to affected area 3-5x daily

Dietary Supplementation:

Super Cal, VitaGreen, Sulfurzyme, Power Meal, Super C, Super B, Mega Cal

Super Cal and Mega Cal provide calcium necessary to maintain nerve signal transmissions along neurological pathways.

Sulfur deficiency is very prevalent in nerve problems. Sulfur requires calcium and vitamin C for the body to metabolize. Super B and Sulfurzyme work well together to help repair nerve damage and the myelin sheath.

Bell's Palsy

A type of neuritis, marked by paralysis on one side of the face and inability to open or close the eyelid.

Single Oils:

Peppermint, helichrysum, juniper

Blends:

Aroma Siez, PanAway, Relieve It

EO Applications:
TOPICAL:

NEAT, massage 1-3 drops on the facial nerve, which is in front and behind the ear and any areas of pain 3-5 times daily until symptoms end.

Dietary Supplementation:

Ultra Young

Carpal Tunnel Syndrome

Nerves pass through a tunnel formed by wrist bones (known as carpals) and a tough membrane on the underside of the wrist that binds the bones together. The tunnel is rigid, so if the tissues within it swell for some reason, they press and pinch the nerves creating a painful condition known as carpal tunnel syndrome. This condition is primarily sports-related or due to activities that involve strenuous or repeated use of wrists. A similar but less common condition can occur in the ankle (tarsal tunnel syndrome), or elbow.

Single Oils:

Peppermint, basil, wintergreen, cypress, marjoram, helichrysum, lemongrass

Blends:

PanAway, Relieve It

Carpal tunnel blend:
- 5 drops wintergreen
- 3 drops cypress
- 1 drop peppermint
- 2 drops marjoram
- 3 drops lemongrass

EO Applications:
TOPICAL:

NEAT or DILUTE 50-50 as required, apply 2-4 drops to affected area 3-5 times daily COMPRESS, cold, on location 2-3 times daily

Dietary Supplementation:

Super C, Super Cal, Mega Cal, BLM, Mineral Essence, Essential Manna

Topical Treatments:

Regenolone, NeuroGen, Ortho Ease, Ortho Sport

Neuralgia

Neuralgia is pain from a damaged nerve. It can occur in the face, spine, or elsewhere. This reoccuring pain can be traced along a nerve pathway. Carpal tunnel syndrome is a specific type of neuralgia. The primary symptom is temporary sharp pain in the peripheral nerve(s).

Single Oils:

Marjoram, helichrysum, peppermint, juniper, nutmeg

Blends:
PanAway, Relieve It, Juva Flex, Peace & Calming

EO Applications:
TOPICAL:
> NEAT or DILUTE 50-50 as required, apply 2-4 drops to affected area 3-5 times daily COMPRESS, cold, on location 2-3 times daily

INHALATION:
> DIRECT, Peace & Calming, 2-4 times daily

Dietary Supplementation:
Ultra Young, Sulfurzyme, Super B, Chelex, PD 80-20, JuvaTone, JuvaPower/Spice

Topical Treatment:
Regenolone, NeuroGen, Ortho Ease, Ortho Sport

Neuritis

Neuritis is a painful inflammation of the peripheral nerves.

It is usually caused by prolonged exposure to cold temperature, heavy-metal poisoning, diabetes, vitamin deficiencies (beriberi and pellagra), and infectious diseases such as typhoid fever and malaria.

Symptoms:
- Pain
- Burning
- Numbness or tingling
- Muscle weakness or paralysis

Single Oils:
Peppermint, lavender, juniper, oregano, thyme, blue yarrow, clove

Blends:
Valor, Aroma Siez, Peace & Calming

EO Applications:
TOPICAL:
> NEAT or DILUTE 50-50 as required, apply 2-4 drops to affected area 3-5 times daily COMPRESS, cold, on location 2-3 times daily

INHALATION:
> DIRECT, Peace & Calming, 2-4 times daily

Dietary Supplementation:
Ultra Young, Sulfurzyme, Super B, Chelex, PD 80-20, JuvaTone, JuvaPower/Spice

Topical Treatment:
Regenolone, NeuroGen, Ortho Ease, Ortho Sport

Neuropathy

Neuropathy refers to actual damage to the peripheral nerves, usually from an auto-immune condition.

Damage to these peripheral nerves (other than spinal or those in the brain), generally starts as tingling in hands and feet and slowly spreads along limbs to the trunk.

Numbness, sensitive skin, neuralgic pain, weakening of muscle power can all develop in varying degrees. Most common causes include complications from diabetes (diabetic neuropathy), alcoholism, vitamin B12 deficiency, tumors, too many pain killers, exposure and absorption of chemicals, metallics, pesticides, and many other causes.

B vitamins and minerals such as magnesium, calcium, potassium, and organic sulfur are important in repairing nerve damage and quenching pain from inflamed nerves.

Fleabane may boost production of pregnenolone and human growth hormone. Pregnenolone aids in repairing damage to the myelin sheath.[31] Juniper also may help in supporting nerve repair.

If paralysis is a problem, a regeneration of up to 60 percent may be possible. If, however, the nerve damage is too severe, treatment may not help. If the damage starts to reverse, there will be pain. Apply a few drops of PanAway neat on location.

Symptoms:
- Tingling or numbness
- Gangrene

Single Oils:
Peppermint, fleabane, juniper, blue yarrow, goldenrod, helichrysum, lemongrass

Blends:
Aroma Siez, PanAway, Peace & Calming

---

31. Baulieu E, Schumacher M, Progesterone as a neuroactive neurosteriod, with special reference to the effect of progesterone on myelination, *Steroids* 2000 Oct-Nov;65(10-11):605-12.

Neuropathy blend #1:
- 10 drops juniper
- 10 drops geranium
- 10 drops helichrysum

Neuropathy blend #2:
- 15 drops geranium
- 10 drops helichrysum
- 6 drops cypress
- 10 drops juniper
- 5 drops peppermint

EO Applications:
TOPICAL:
> NEAT or DILUTE 50-50 as required, apply 2-4 drops to affected area 3-5 times daily
> COMPRESS, cold, on location 2-3 times daily

INHALATION:
> DIRECT, Peace & Calming, 2-4 times daily

Dietary Supplementation:
Super B, Longevity Capsules, Mineral Essence, Essential Omegas, Super Cal, Mega Cal, Super C, VitaGreen, Sulfurzyme, Essential Manna, BodyGize, Ultra Young, Master Formula Vitamins

Topical Treatment:
Regenolone, NeuroGen, Peppermint-Cedarwood Bar Soap

NERVOUS FATIGUE

Nervous fatigue can cause motor skill problems.

Single Oils:
St. John's wort, blue yarrow, juniper, goldenrod, helichrysum, thyme, peppermint

Blends:
Brain Power, Clarity, Peace & Calming, Humility, Hope, Trauma Life

EO Applications:
INHALATION:
> DIRECT, 4-8 times daily as needed

TOPICAL:
> DILUTE 50-50, apply 1-2 drops on temples, behind ears, back of neck , on forehead, and under nostrils, as needed

NERVOUS SYSTEM (Autonomic)

The autonomic nervous system controls involuntary activities such as heartbeat, breathing, digestion, glandular activity, and contraction and dilation of blood vessels.

The autonomic nervous system is composed of two parts that balance and complement each other: the parasympathetic and sympathetic nervous systems.

The sympathetic nervous system has stimulatory effects and is responsible for secreting stress hormones such as adrenaline and noradrenaline.

The parasympathetic nervous system has relaxing effects and is responsible for secreting acetylcholine which slows the heart and speeds digestion.

To Stimulate Parasympathetic Nervous System:

Single Oils:
Lavender, patchouli, rose, marjoram

Blends:
Valor, ImmuPower, Peace & Calming

EO Applications:
INHALATION:
> DIRECT, 1-2 times daily, as needed

INGESTION:
> CAPSULE, 0 size, 1 capsule 2 times daily

TOPICAL:
> RAINDROP Technique, biweekly

To Stimulate Sympathetic Nervous System:

Single Oils:
Peppermint, fennel, grapefruit, ginger, *Eucalyptus radiata*, black pepper

Blends:
Clarity, Brain Power

EO Applications:
INHALATION:
> DIRECT, 1-2 times daily, as needed

INGESTION:
> CAPSULE, 0 size, 1 capsule twice daily

TOPICAL:
RAINDROP Technique, biweekly

Dietary Supplementation:
Power Meal, Super Cal, Sulfurzyme, Ultra Young, Mineral Essence, Mega Cal

NEURITIS, NEUROPATHY, NEURALGIA

(See NERVE DISORDERS)

NEUROLOGICAL DISEASES

ALS (Lou Gehrig's Disease)

Lou Gehrig's Disease is another name for Amyotrophic Lateral Sclerosis (ALS), a degenerative nerve disorder. ALS affects the nerve fibers in the spinal cord which control voluntary movement. Muscles require continuous stimulation by their associated nerves to maintain their tone. Removal or deadening of these nerves results in muscular atrophy. The lack of control forces the muscles to spasm, resulting in twitching and cramps. The sensory pathways are unaffected so feeling is never lost in the afflicted muscles.

Juniper promotes nerve function. Frankincense may help clear the emotions of fear and anger, which is common with people who have these neurological diseases. When these diseases are contracted, people often become suicidal.

Hope, Joy, Gathering, and Forgiveness will help work through the psychological and emotional aspects of the disease.

Single Oils:
Frankincense, helichrysum, oregano, sage, juniper, rosemary, clove, cardamom, vitex.

Blends:
Acceptance, Joy, Gathering, Brain Power, Clarity, Forgiveness

ALS blend:
- 1 drop rosemary
- 1 drop helichrysum
- 1 drop ylang ylang
- 1 drop clove

EO Applications:
INHALATION:
DIRECT, 3-4 times daily
DIFFUSION, 30 minutes, 2-3 times daily
TOPICAL:
DILUTE 50-50, 1-3 drops on brain reflex points on forehead, temples and mastoids (just behind ears). Use a direct pressure application, massaging 6-10 drops of diluted oil from the base of the skull down the neck and down the spine. Put a few drops of the oil on a loofah brush and rub along the spine vigorously. (Always use a natural bristle brush, since the oils may dissolve plastic bristles.)
RAINDROP Technique, 3 times monthly, but use a cold compress instead of a warm one

NOTE: Never use hot packs for neurological problems. Always use cold packs to reduce pain and inflammation. In other words, reduce the temperature of the damaged site.

Dietary Supplementation:
Sulfurzyme, JuvaTone, JuvaPower/Spice, Ultra Young, VitaGreen, Power Meal, Chelex, Chelex, Super Cal, Super C, Super B

Sulfur deficiency is very prevalent in neurological diseases. Sulfur requires calcium and Vitamin C for the body to metabolize. Super B and Sulfurzyme work well together to help repair nerve damage and the myelin sheath.

Huntington's Chorea

Huntington's Chorea is a degenerative nerve disease that generally becomes manifest in middle age. It is marked by uncontrollable body movements, which are followed—and occasionally preceded—by mental deterioration.

(Not to be confused with Sydenham's chorea (often called St. Vitus Dance, chorea minor, or juvenile chorea) which affects children, especially females, usually appearing between between the ages of 7 and 14. The jerking symptoms eventually disappear.)

Single Oils:
Peppermint, juniper, basil

Blends:
Aroma Siez

Nerve blend:
* 5 drops peppermint
* 10 drops juniper
* 3 drops basil
* 5 drops Aroma Siez

EO Applications:
INHALATION:
> DIRECT, 3-4 times daily
> DIFFUSION, 30 minutes, 2-3 times daily

TOPICAL:
> DILUTE 50-50, 1-3 drops on brain reflex points on forehead, temples and mastoids (just behind ears). Use a direct pressure application, massaging 6-10 drops of diluted oil from the base of the skull down the neck and down the spine. Put a few drops of the oil on a loofah brush and rub along the spine vigorously. (Always use a natural bristle brush, since the oils may dissolve plastic bristles.)
> RAINDROP Technique, 3 times monthly, but use a cold compress instead of a warm one.

NOTE: Never use hot packs for neurological problems. Always use cold packs to reduce pain and inflammation. In other words, reduce the temperature of the affected area.

Dietary Supplementation:
Sulfurzyme, JuvaTone, JuvaPower/Spice, Ultra Young, VitaGreen, Power Meal, Rehemogen, Chelex, Super Cal, Super C, Super B, Mega Cal

Multiple Sclerosis (MS)

Multiple Sclerosis is a progressive, disabling disease of the nervous system (brain and spinal cord) in which inflammation occurs in the central nervous system. Eventually, the myelin sheaths protecting the nerves are destroyed, resulting in a slowing or blocking of nerve transmission.

MS is an autoimmune disease, in which the body's own immune system attacks the nerves. Some researchers believe that MS is triggered by a virus, while others make a case that it has a strong genetic or environmental component.

Maintaining MS Status Quo

One of the simplest ways to keep MS symptoms from becoming more severe is to keep the body cool and avoiding any locations or physical activities which heat the body (including hot showers or exercise). Cold baths and relaxed swimming are two of the best activities for relieving symptoms.

Applying heat is the worst thing to do for MS. If an MS patient is experiencing increasingly severe symptoms, lower their body temperature (by up to 3 degrees F) by laying them on a table, covering them with a sheet, ice, shower curtain, and blankets (in that order). Work the feet with oils and watch for benefits.

Symptoms:
* Muscle weakness in extremities
* Deteriorating coordination and balance
* Numbness or prickling sensations
* Poor attention or memory
* Speech impediments
* Incontinence
* Tremors
* Dizziness
* Hearing loss

Single Oils:
Juniper, basil eugenol, helichrysum, geranium, peppermint, thyme, oregano, wintergreen, cypress, marjoram, rosemary

Blends:
Valor, Aroma Siez, Acceptance, Awaken

MS Recipe:
* 10 drops helichrysum
* 10 drops peppermint
* 10 drops rosemary
* 5 drops basil eugenol

EO Applications:
INHALATION:
> DIRECT, 3-4 times daily
> DIFFUSION, 30 minutes, 2-3 times daily

TOPICAL:
> DILUTE 50-50, 1-3 drops on brain reflex points on forehead, temples and mastoids (just behind ears). Use a direct pressure application, massaging 6-10 drops of diluted oil from the base of the skull down

the neck and down the spine. Put a few drops of the oil on a loofah brush and rub along the spine vigorously. (Always use a natural bristle brush, since the oils may dissolve plastic bristles.)

RAINDROP Technique, 3 times monthly, but use a cold compress instead of a warm one.

NOTE: Never use hot packs for neurological problems. Always use cold packs to reduce pain and inflammation. In other words, reduce the temperature of the affected area.

MS Regimen (to be performed daily):

1. Layer neat applications of 4-6 drops of helichrysum, juniper, geranium and peppermint, Raindrop-style, along the spine. Lightly massage oils in the direction of the MS paralysis. For example, if it is in the lower part of the spine, massage down; if it is in the upper part of the spine, massage up. Follow the application with 30 minutes of cold packs (change cold packs as needed).

2. Apply 4-6 drops Valor on the spine. If the MS affects the legs, rub down the spine; if it affects the neck, rub up the spine.

3. Apply 2-3 drops each of cypress and juniper to the back of the neck then cover with 2-3 drops of Aroma Siez.

To to give additional emotional support to the person with MS symptoms, use Acceptance and Awaken. Be patient. Overcoming MS is a long-term endeavor.

Dietary Supplementation:
Sulfurzyme, JuvaTone, JuvaPower/Spice, Ultra Young, VitaGreen, Power Meal, Rehemogen, Chelex, Super Cal, Mega Cal, Super C, Super B

Parkinson's Disease

Parkinson's Disease involves the deterioration of specific nerve centers in the brain and affects more men than women by a ratio of 3:2. The main symptom is tremors, an involuntary shaking of hands, head, or both. Other symptoms include rigidity, slowed movement, and loss of

balance. In many cases these are accompanied by a continuous rubbing together of thumb and forefinger, stooped posture, mask-like face, trouble swallowing, depression, and difficulty performing simple tasks. These symptoms may all be seen at different stages of the disease. The tremors are most severe when the affected part of the body is not in use. There is no pain or other sensation, other than a decreased ability to move. Symptoms appear slowly, in no particular order and may end before they interfere with normal activities. Restoring dopamine levels in the brain can reduce symptoms of Parkinson's. Ultra Young contains a vegetable source of dopamine. Sulfurzyme provides a source of organic sulfur, a vital nutrient for nerve and myelin sheath formation.

Vitex has been shown to reduce the symptoms of Parkinson's disease by 89 percent in animal studies.[32]

Single Oils:
Juniper, peppermint, vitex

Blends:
Peace & Calming, Valor, Juva Cleanse

EO Applications:
INHALATION:
DIRECT, 3-4 times daily
DIFFUSION, 30 minutes, 2-3 times daily
TOPICAL:
DILUTE 50-50, 1-3 drops on brain reflex points on forehead, temples and mastoids (just behind ears). Use a direct pressure application, massaging 6-10 drops of diluted oil from the base of the skull down the neck and down the spine. Put a few drops of the oil on a loofah brush and rub along the spine vigorously. (Always use a natural bristle brush, since the oils may dissolve plastic bristles.)
RAINDROP Technique, 3 times monthly, but use a cold compress instead of a warm one

NOTE: Never use hot packs for neurological problems. Always use cold packs to reduce pain and inflammation. In other words, reduce the temperature of the affected area.

---

32. Gupta M, Mazumder UK, Bhawal SR, "CNS activity of Vitex negundo Linn. in mice," *Indian J Exp Biol* 1999 Feb;37(2):143-6.

Dietary Supplementation:
Sulfurzyme, Ultra Young, Super B, Juva Power, PD80/20, BLM

Juniper promotes nerve function.

NIGHT SWEATS

(See MENSTRUAL CONDITIONS)

Single Oils:
Sage, clary sage, blue yarrow.

Blends:
Mister, EndoFlex, Dragon Time

EO Applications:
TOPICAL:
> DILUTE 50-50, apply 3-5 drops over lower abdomen and back of neck before retiring
> VITA FLEX, apply 2-3 drops to heart, to brain and to liver Vita Flex points on feet

Dietary Supplementation:
Prenolone, Ultra Young, Thyromin.

Topical Treatment:
Dragon Time Bath Gel or Massage Oil

NOSE

Nosebleeds

Nosebleeds usually are not serious. However, if bleeding does not stop in a short time or is excessive or frequent, consult your doctor.

Single Oils:
Helichrysum, geranium, lavender, cypress

Blends:
Nosebleed blend:
- 2 drops helichrysum
- 2 drops lavender
- 2 drops cypress

EO Applications:
TOPICAL:
> NEAT, apply 2-4 drops to the bridge and sides of nose and back of neck. Repeat as needed.

Nosebleed regimen:
Put 1 drop helichrysum, lavender, or cypress on a tissue paper and wrap the paper around a chip of ice about the size of a thumb nail, push it up under the top lip in the center to the base of the nose. Hold from the outside with lip pressure. This usually will stop bleeding in a very short time.

Dry Nose

Single Oils:
Lavender, lemon, peppermint

Dry nose blend:
- 2 drops lavender
- 1 drop myrrh

EO Applications:
INHALATION:
> DIRECT, 3-5 times daily as needed
> DIFFUSION, 20 minutes 3 times daily and before retiring

TOPICAL:
> DILUTE 50-50, apply 1-2 drops to nostril walls with cotton swab twice daily

Nasal Irrigation Regimen:
Rosemary and Melaleuca ericifolia oils can be used in a saline solution for very effective nasal irrigation that clears and decongests sinuses. As recommended by Daniel Pénoël, MD, the saline solution is prepared as follows:

- 12 drops rosemary cineol
- 4 drops tea tree
- 8 tablespoons very fine salt

The essential oils are mixed thoroughly in the fine salt and stored in a sealed container. For each nasal irrigation session, 1 teaspoon of this salt mixture is dissolved into 1 1/2 cups distilled water.

This oils/salt/water solution is then placed in the tank of an oral irrigator to irrigate the nasal cavities, which is done while bending over a sink. This application has brought surprisingly positive results in treating latent sinusitus and other nasal congestion problems.

Dietary Supplementation:
AD&E.

Loss of Smell

(Due to Chronic Nasal Catarrh)

Single Oils:
Basil, peppermint, rosemary, goldenrod, frankincense

EO Applications:
INHALATION:
    DIRECT, 3-5 times daily, or as needed

Dietary Supplementation:
ImmuneTune, Exodus, Power Meal

Polyps (Nasal)

Single Oils:
Citronella

Blends:
Purification

EO Applications:
TOPICAL:
    DILUTE 50-50, carefully apply 1 drop on location inside the nostrils with a cotton swab 1-3 times daily

OBESITY

(see DEPRESSION)

Hormone treatments using natural progesterone (for women) and testosterone (for men) may be one of the most powerful treatments for obesity. In women, progesterone levels drop dramatically after menopause and this can result in substantial weight gain, particularly around the hips and thighs. Using transdermal creams to replace declining progesterone can result in substantial declines in body fat.

Diffusing or directly inhaling essential oils can have an immediate positive impact on moods and appetites. Olfaction is the only sense that can have direct effect on the limbic region of the brain. Studies at the University of Vienna have shown that some essential oils and their primary constituents can stimulate blood flow and activity in the emotional centers of the brain.[33]

Fragrance influences the satiety center in the brain in such a manner that frequent inhalation of pleasing aromas can significantly reduce appetite. Dr. Alan Hirsch, in his landmark studies, showed dramatic weight loss in research subjects using aromas from peppermint oil and vanilla absolute to curb food cravings.[34]

Single Oils:
Peppermint, jasmine absolute, ylang ylang vanilla absolute

Blends:
Joy, Citrus Fresh, Juva Cleanse

Applications:
INHALATION:
    DIRECT, 5-20 times daily or as often as needed

Dietary Supplementation:
BodyGize, Power Meal, ThermaBurn, Juva Power, Amino Tech, WheyFit, BeFit

Topical Treatments:
Progessence, Prenolone, Prenolone+

ORAL CARE (Teeth and Gums)

(see HALITOSIS and Chapter 16: Oral Health Care)

Poor oral hygiene has not only been linked to bad breath (halitosis) but also cardiovascular disease. Some of the same bacteria that populate the mouth have now been implicated in arteriosclerosis.

Essential oils make excellent oral antiseptics, analgesics and anti-inflammatories. Clove essential oil has been used in mainstream dentistry for decades to numb the gums and help prevent infections. Similarly menthol (found in peppermint oil), methyl salycilate (found in wintergreen oil), thymol (found in thyme essential oil) and eucalyptol (found in eucalyptus and rosemary essential oils) are approved OTC drug products for combating gingivitis and periodontal disease.

---

33. Nasel, C. et al. "Functional imaging of effects of fragrances on the human brain after prolonged inhalation." Chemical Senses. 1994;19(4):359-64

34. Hirsch AR. Inhalation of Odorants for Weight Reduction, *Int J Obes*, 1994, page 306

Dental Visits

Prior to visiting the dentist, rub one drop each of helichrysum, clove and PanAway on gums and jaw. Clove may interfere with bonding of crowns so keep it off the teeth if this procedure is planned.

Dental Pain and Infection Control

Single Oils:
Wintergreen, helichrysum, tea tree, *Eucalyptus radiata*, clove, thyme, oregano

Blends:
PanAway, Thieves, R.C.

EO Applications:
TOPICAL:
DILUTE 50-50, apply 1-2 drops on gums and around teeth. Repeat as needed. Just before a tooth extraction, rub 1-2 drops of helichrysum, Thieves and R.C. around the gum area. Rubbing R.C. on gums may also help to bring back feeling after numbness from anesthesia.

Oral Treatments:
Fresh Essence Plus Mouthwash, Dentarome Ultra Toothpaste, Thieves Lozenges, Thieves Antiseptic Spray

Gingivitis & Periodontitis

Periodontal diseases are infections of the gum and bone that hold the teeth in place. Gingivitis affects the upper areas of the gum, where it bonds to the visible enamel, while periodontitis is a more internal infection affecting the gum at the root level of the tooth. In advanced stages, these diseases can lead to painful chewing problems and even tooth loss. Oils such as peppermint, wintergreen, clove, thyme, and eucalyptus can kill bacteria and effectively combat a variety of gum infections.

Single Oils:
Mountain savory, clove, tea tree, peppermint, wintergreen, thyme, oregano

Blends:
Exodus II, Thieves

EO Applications:
ORAL:
GARGLE, up to 10 times daily as needed

Dietary Supplementation:
Super C, Super C Chewable, Dentarome, Dentarome Plus, Fresh Essence Plus Mouthwash, Thieves lozenges

Super C Chewable: Take 1-3 tablets at regular intervals throughout the day.

Oral Treatments:
Fresh Essence Plus Mouthwash, Dentarome Ultra Toothpaste, Thieves Lozenges, Thieves Antiseptic Spray

Bleeding Gums

Single Oils:
Cinnamon, peppermint, mountain savory, wintergreen, myrrh

Blends:
Thieves, Melrose, PanAway

Blend for combatting gum bleeding:
- 2 drops myrrh
- 2 drops thyme
- 1 drop Thieves
- 1 drop Exodus II

EO Applications:
ORAL:
GARGLE, 3-10 times daily, as needed
TOPICAL:
DILUTE 50-50, apply 1-2 drops on gums 2-3 times daily

Dietary Supplementation:
ImmuGel

Oral Hygiene Regimen:

1. Gargle three times daily with Fresh Essence Plus Mouthwash.

2. Brush teeth and gums two times daily with Dentarome Ultra toothpaste.

3. For infection or inflammation, place ImmuGel on a piece of gauze. Roll like a piece of rope place along the gum, and hold in mouth for at least 30 minutes. This works particularly well for leukemia patients because their gums tend to inflame, swell, and become infected.

Mouth Ulcers

Single Oils:
Myrrh, oregano, tea tree

Blends:
Thieves, Exodus II

EO Applications:
ORAL:
GARGLE, 3-10 times daily, as needed
TOPICAL:
DILUTE 50-50, apply 1-2 drops on gums
2 times daily

Oral Hygiene:
Dentarome Ultra Toothpaste, Fresh Essence +
Mouthwash, Thieves lozenges, Thieves
Antiseptic Spray, Immugel

Gargle with Fresh Essence+ Mouthwash or
Thieves Antiseptic Spray. Add 1-2 drops of
Thieves, clove, and Exodus II to strengthen
therapeutic action.

If infection is due to leukemia, saturate a rolled
piece of gauze with ImmuGel and 1-3 drops
Thieves. Place gauze between gums and inner
cheek skin and change gauze pads morning and
evening. Massage abscessed area with 1-2 drops
Thieves.

Teeth Grinding

Single Oils:
Lavender, valerian

Blends:
Peace & Calming

EO Applications:
INHALATION:
DIRECT, 1-3 times daily and before retiring
DIFFUSION, 30 minutes twice a day and
before retiring
TOPICAL:
NEAT, massage 1-3 drops each of lavender
and valerian on bottoms of feet each night
before retiring

Dietary Supplementation:
Mineral Essence

Toothache and Teething Pain

Single Oils:
Clove, wintergreen, German chamomile, tea
tree, Idaho tansy

Blends:
Thieves, Exodus

EO Applications:
TOPICAL:
DILUTE 50-50, apply on affected tooth
and gum area as needed
ORAL:
GARGLE, 4-6 times daily or as needed

Dietary Supplements:
ImmuGel, MegaCal, AD&E

Oral Hygiene:
Thieves Antiseptic Spray, Dentarome Ultra,
Fresh Essence Plus Mouthwash.

NOTE: All essential oils should be diluted 20-80
before being used orally on small children.

OSTEOPOROSIS (Bone Deterioration)

Osteoporosis is primarily caused by four main
factors:

- Progesterone Deficiency
- Lack of Magnesium and boron in diet
- Lack of Vitamin D in diet
- Lack of dietary calcium

Natural progesterone is the single most effective
way to increase bone density in women over age
40. Clinical studies by John Lee, MD, showed
dramatic increases in bone density using just 20
mg of daily topically-applied progesterone

Calcium, magnesium, and boron are a few of the
most important minerals for bone health and are
usually lacking or deficient in most modern diets.
Magnesium is especially important to bone
strength, but most Americans consume only a
fraction of the daily 400 mg daily value needed
for bone health. Calcium and magnesium may not
be adequately metabolized when consumed
because of poor intestinal flora and excess
phytates in the diet (a problem with vegetarians).
Phytates occur in many nuts, grains, and seeds
including rice. Enzymes like phytase are essential
for increasing calcium absorption by liberating
calcium from insoluble phytates complex.

Lack of vitamin D (cholecalciferol) has become epidemic among older people and has contributed to a lack of absorption of calcium in the diet.

Single Oils:
Wintergreen, elemi, spruce, balsam fir, pine, cypress, peppermint, marjoram, rosemary, basil

Blends:
Aroma Siez, Purification, Melrose, Sacred Mountain, Relieve It, PanAway

EO Applications:
TOPICAL:
> DILUTE 50-50, massage 6-10 drops on spine (or area affected) 2-3 times daily

Dietary Supplementation:
Polyzyme, Essentialzyme, Super Cal, Mega Cal, BLM, AlkaLine, AD&E, Mineral Essence, WheyFit, Sulfurzyme, Thyromin, Ultra Young

Topical Treatments:
Prenolone, Prenolone+, Progessence

Super Cal, AlkaLime, and Mineral Essence are all excellent sources of calcium and magnesium which is essential for strong bones. Super Cal not only includes calcium, but also magnesium and boron which are both vital for maintaining bone composition. Mineral Essence is an excellent source magnesium and other trace minerals.

Especially avoid consuming carbonated drinks which can leach calcium out of the body due to their phosphoric acid content.

Ultra Young helps stimulate growth hormone production which can result in much stronger bones.

Studies show that the majority of women that do resistance training 3-4 times a week do not develop osteoporosis.

Topical Treatments:
Prenolone, Prenolone+, EndoBalance

OVARIAN AND UTERINE CYSTS

(See CANCER, MENSTRUAL CONDITIONS)

Single Oils:
Frankincense, geranium, tea tree, oregano, clary age, cypress

Blends:
Melrose, DragonTime, Mister, SclarEssence

Female Cyst blend #1:
- 9 drops frankincense
- 5 drops basil

Female Cyst blend #2:
- 8 drops frankincense
- 8 drops geranium
- 8 drops cypress

EO Applications:
RETENTION:
> TAMPON, nightly for 4 nights.
> NOTE: if irritation occurs, discontinue use for 3 days before resuming use.

TOPICAL:
> COMPRESS, warm, on location, as needed
> VITA FLEX, massage 1-3 drops on the reproductive Vita Flex points, located around the anklebone, on either side of the foot. Work from the ankle bone down to the arch of the foot.

Dietary Supplementation:
Master Formula Hers, PD80/20, Protec

Topical Treatments:
Prenolone, Prenolone+, Progessence

PAIN

One of the most effective essential oils for blocking pain is peppermint. A recent study by in 1994 showed that peppermint oil is extremely effective in blocking calcium channels and substance P, important factors in the transmission of pain signals.[35] Other essential oils also have unique pain-relieving properties, including helichrysum, Idaho balsam fir, and Douglas fir.

MSM, a source of organic sulfur, has also been proven to be extremely effective for killing pain, especially tissue and joint pain. The subject of a

---

35. "Effect of Peppermint and Eucalyptus Oil Preparations on Neurophysiological and experimental algesimetric headache parameters" 1994 Germany Gobel, Schmidt, Soyka Cephalalgia Jun;14(3):228-34; discussion 182.

best-selling book by Dr. Ronald Lawrence and Dr. Stanley Jacobs, MSM is defining the treatment of pain, especially associated with arthritis and fibromyalgia. Sulfurzyme is an excellent source of MSM.

Natural pregnenolone can also blunt pain.

(See ARTHRITIS or HEADACHES)

Bone-Related Pain

Single Oils:
Wintergreen, cypress, fir, spruce, pine, peppermint, helichrysum

Blends:
PanAway, Relieve It

EO Applications:
TOPICAL:
> DILUTE 50-50, 2-4 drops on location as needed
> VITA FLEX, apply to relevant points on feet, repeat as needed

Dietary Supplementation:
Sulfurzyme, Super Cal, Mega Cal, BLM

Topical Treatment:
Ortho Ease, Regenolone, Neurogen

Chronic Pain

To pinpoint the most effective essential oil for quenching pain, it may be necessary to try each of the essential oils in these categories in order to find the one that is most effective for your particular pain situation.

Single Oils:
Peppermint, helichrysum, spruce, wintergreen, ginger, clove, elemi, oregano, Douglas fir, Idaho balsam fir, rosemary

---

How to Use Essential Oils for Pain Control

PanAway is powerful for pain reduction. When applied on location or to the Vita Flex points on the feet, it can act within seconds. Alternate with Relieve It. These 2 blends are powerful combination for deep-tissue pain tas well as bone-related pain.

How MSM Works to Control Pain

When fluid pressure inside cells is higher than outside, pain is experienced. The MSM found in Sulfurzyme equalizes fluid pressure inside cells by affecting the protein envelope of the cell so that water transfers freely in and out.

Blends:
Relieve It, PanAway, Aroma Siez, Release, Sacred Mountain

EO Applications:
TOPICAL:
> DILUTE 50-50, 2-4 drops on location as needed
> COMPRESS, warm, on location as needed
INGESTION:
> CAPSULE, 0 size, 2 times per day

Dietary Supplementation:
Sulfurzyme, Super Cal, ArthroTune, Mega Cal, BLM

Topical Treatment:
Regenolone, Neurogen, Ortho Ease, Morning Start Bath Gel, Ortho Sport, Morning Start, Peppermint-Cedarwood Bar Soap.

Inflammation Pain

(see INFLAMMATION)

Joint Pain:

(See JOINT STIFFNESS and ARTHRITIS)

Muscle-related Pain

Single Oils:
Peppermint, rosemary, marjoram, nutmeg

Blends:
PanAway, Aroma Siez, Relieve It.

EO Applications:
TOPICAL:
> DILUTE 50-50, 2-4 drops on location as needed
> VITA FLEX, apply to relevant points on feet, repeat as needed

Dietary Supplementation:
Sulfurzyme, WheyFit, Mineral Essence,
Super Cal

Topical Treatment:
Ortho Ease, Ortho Sport, Neurogen

Trauma-related Pain

Single Oils:
Sandalwood, geranium

Massage around hairline of the head and tips of the toes.

Trauma pain relief blend:
- 12 drops Idaho balsam fir
- 10 drops tea tree
- 8 drops lavender
- 6 drops marjoram
- 3 drops spearmint
- 2 drops peppermint

Blends:
Trauma Life, Valor, Release

EO Applications:
TOPICAL:
> DILUTE 50-50, 2-4 drops on location, 2-4 times daily. Also massage around hairline and on the tops of the toes.
> COMPRESS, warm, on location as needed

Dietary Supplementation:
Sulfurzyme, Super Cal, Mega Cal

Topical Treatment:
Ortho Ease, Ortho Sport.

Warm compresses help the oils penetrate faster and deeper when applied on location.

PANCREATITIS

Pancreatitis is an inflammation of the pancreas that can be either acute or chronic. Acute pancreatitis can be caused by a sudden blockage in the main pancreatic duct, which results in enzymes becoming backed-up and literally digesting the pancreas unless remedied. Chronic pancreatitis occurs more gradually, with attacks recurring over weeks or months.

Symptoms:
- Abdominal pain
- muscle aches
- vomiting
- abdominal swelling
- sudden hypertension
- jaundice
- rapid weight loss
- fever.

In the case of acute pancreatitis, a total fast for at least 4-5 days is one of the safest and most effective methods of treatment. In the case of infection, fasting should be combined with immune stimulation by using Exodus combined with Vitamin C and B-complex vitamins.

Single Oils:
Geranium, vetiver, peppermint, mountain savory, oregano

Blends:
Exodus II, ImmuPower, Thieves

EO Applications:
RETENTION:
> RECTAL, 3 times per week

TOPICAL:
> RAINDROP Technique, once a week

INGESTION:
> CAPSULE, 0 size, 1 capsule 3 times per week

Dietary Supplementation:
Exodus, ImmuGel, VitaGreen, Super B,
Super C, Essentialzyme

PARASYMPATHETIC NERVOUS SYSTEM

(See NERVOUS SYSTEM-AUTONOMIC)

PARASITES, Intestinal

(See FOOD POISONING)

Many types of parasites use up nutrients, while giving off toxins. This can leave the body depleted, nutritionally deficient, and susceptible to infectious disease.

Using Di-Tone and ParaFree For Parasite Control

The essential oil blend Di-Tone and the liquid supplement ParaFree are excellent for parasite removal.

Di-Tone: Add 6 drops to 1 tsp. V6 Oil Comlex or 4 oz. rice/soy milk and take as a dietary supplement twice a day. Di-Tone can also be diluted in massage oil and applied over abdomen. Or take 25 drops in a capsule 3 times a day for 7 days.

ParaFree (liquid): Take 2-4 droppers in a glass of water 3 times daily for 21 days, then rest for 7 days. Repeat cycle up to three times to achieve desired results.

ParaFree (softgels): Take 5 soft gels 2-3 times daily for 21 days, then rest for 7 days. Repeat up to three times to achieve desired results.

Occasionally parasites can lie dormant in the body and then become active due to ingestion of a particular food or drink. This can result in the appearance and disappearance of symptoms even though parasites are always present.

The parasite, *Cryptosporidium parrum,* may be present in many municipal or tap waters. To remove, water must be distilled or filtered using a .3 micron filter.

Symptoms:
- Fatigue
- Weakness
- Diarrhea
- Gas and bloating
- Cramping
- Nausea
- Irregular bowel movements.

The first step to controlling parasites is beginning a fasting and/or cleansing program. A colon cleanse is particularly important.

Single Oils:
Tarragon, anise seed, Idaho tansy, basil, peppermint, ginger, lemongrass, nutmeg, fennel, juniper, rosewood, tea tree, rosemary

Blends:
Di-Tone, JuvaFlex, JuvaCleanse

Blend for parasite retention enema:
- 10 drops ginger
- 10 drops Di-Tone
- 1 Tbsp. V6 Oil Complex

EO Applications:
INGESTION:
>CAPSULE, 00 size, 3 times per week
>RICE MILK, 1-3 times daily

TOPICAL:
>COMPRESS, warm, over intestinal area, 2 times weekly
>VITA FLEX, daily massage up to 6 drops to the instep area on both feet (small intestine and colon Vita Flex points)

RETENTION:
>RECTAL, use above blend nightly for 7 nights, then rest for 7 nights. Repeat this cycle 3 times to eliminate all stages of parasite development. Alternatively, substitute 2 tbsp liquid ParaFree for the retention blend and retain overnight every other day for a week.

Dietary Supplementation:
Polyzyme, Essentialzyme, ComforTone, ICP, ParaFree, Fresh Essence Plus

Oral Treatments:
Fresh Essence Plus Mouthwash, Dentarome Ultra Toothpaste, Thieves Lozenges

PERIODONTAL DISEASE

(See ORAL CARE)

PERSPIRATION (EXCESSIVE)

Excessive perspiration may indicate adrenal and thyroid problems or diabetes. Sage helps regulate sweating.

Single Oils:
Geranium, rosewood, sage, nutmeg

Blends:
Purification, EndoFlex, En-R-Gee

EO Applications:
TOPICAL:
>DILUTE 20-80, apply 2-4 drops under arms daily

INGESTION:
>CAPSULE, 0 size, 1 capsule twice a day

PH BALANCE

(See Chapter 26) (See ACIDOSIS)

PHLEBITIS - THROMBOSIS

(See CARDIOVASCULAR CONDITIONS)

Phlebitis refers to inflammation of a blood vein. Symptoms include pain and tenderness along the course of the vein, discoloration of the skin, inflammatory swelling, joint pain, and acute edema below the inflamed site.

Natural progesterone is an effective anti-inflammatory.

Single Oils:
Helichrysum, clove, cistus, orange, goldenrod, Idaho tansy, lavender

EO Applications:
INGESTION:
>CAPSULE, 0 size, 1 capsule daily
TOPICAL:
>DILUTE 50-50, apply 5-7 drops on location or over the heart, 3 times daily
>RAINDROP Technique, weekly

Dietary Supplementation:
Essential Omegas, Polyzyme, Essentialzyme, Super Cal, Power Meal, Mega Cal Rehemogen: (3 droppers in water, 3 times daily)

Topical Treatment:
Progessence, Prenolone+

PINKEYE

(See EYE DISORDERS)

PLAQUE

(See CARDIOVASCULAR CONDITIONS)

PLEURISY

Inflammation of the pleura, or outer membranes covering the lungs and the thoracic cavity.

Single Oils:
Ravensara, mountain savory, thyme

Blends:
Raven, R.C., ImmuPower, Exodus II

EO Applications:
TOPICAL:
>DILUTE 20-80, massage 5-7 drops on neck and chest 2-3 times daily
>COMPRESS, warm, on neck, chest and upper back areas, daily
>VITA FLEX, 1-3 drops on lung Vita Flex points of feet daily
>RAINDROP Technique, 1-2 times weekly

Dietary Supplementation:
Exodus, ImmuPro, ImmuneTune, Super C, Ultra Young, Mineral Essence, Sulfurzyme

PNEUMONIA

(See LUNG INFECTIONS)

POLIO

Polio (Poliomylitis) is an acute infectious disease usually manifested in epidemics and caused by a virus. It creates an inflammation of the gray matter of the spinal cord. It is characterized by fever, sore throat, headache, and vomiting, sometimes stiffness of the neck and back. If it develops into the major illness, it can involve paralysis and atrophy of groups of muscles ending in contraction and permanent deformity.

Single Oils:
Frankincense, tea tree, wintergreen, melissa, sandalwood, ravansara, blue cypress

Blends:

Polio blend:
- 2 drops lemon
- 10 drops ylang ylang
- 7 drops frankincense
- 10 drops wintergreen
- 7 drops myrtle
- 8 drops cypress
- 15 drops myrrh
- 10 drops tarragon
- 6 drops sage

Applications:
INGESTION:
>CAPSULE, 0 size, 2 times daily

Dietary Supplementation:
ImmuPro

PREGNANCY

(See also BREASTFEEDING, Postpartum Depression in DEPRESSION, and Diaper Rash and Stretch Marks in SKIN DISORDERS)

Essential oils can be invaluable companions during pregnancy. Oils like lavender and myrrh may help reduce stretch marks and improve the elasticity of the skin. Geranium and Gentle Baby blend have similar effects and can be massaged on the perineum (tissue between vagina and rectum) to lower the risk of tearing or the need for an episiotomy (an incision in the perineum) during birth.

Single Oils:
Lavender, myrrh, geranium, ylang ylang, helichrysum

Blends:
Gentle Baby, Joy, Envision, Valor

Blend for use during labor:
- 4 drops helichrysum
- 2 drops fennel
- 2 drops peppermint
- 5 drops ylang ylang
- 2 drops clary sage

EO Applications:
TOPICAL:
>DILUTE 50-50, massage 2-4 drops on reproductive Vita Flex points on sides of ankles. Apply ONLY after labor has started. Also massage 4-6 drops on lower stomach and lower back.

INHALATION:
>DIFFUSION, diffuse Gentle Baby, Joy or Valor to reduce stress before and after the birth. (Expectant fathers will also find this helps to reduce anxiety while waiting for delivery.)

PROSTATE PROBLEMS

Natural progesterone is one of the best natural remedies for prostate inflammation (BPH) that can obstruct urinary flow and lead to impotence. Transdermal creams are the most effective means of hormone delivery.

Scientists are tracing the higher incidence of hormone-dependent cancers including cancer of the breast, prostate and testes to exposure to endocrine disrupters in the environment.[36] Petrochemical contamination from DDT, PCB, pesticides, the phylate DBP, and synthetic steroids in meat, are all implicated in interfering with hormone receptors, rendering them unable to function properly, eventually leading to cancer.

For prostate problems, peppermint acts as an anti-inflammatory to the prostate. Saw palmetto, Pygeum africanum, and pumpkin seed oil also reduce prostate swelling.[37]

Single Oils:
Oregano, frankincense, myrrh, orange, Idaho balsam fir, cumin, thyme, blue cypress

Blends:
Mister, EndoFlex, Dragon Time, Australian Blue

EO Applications:
TOPICAL:
>DILUTE 20-80, apply 2-4 drops between the rectum and scrotum twice daily. Mister works especially well here
>VITA FLEX, massage 4-6 drops on Vita Flex reproductive points on the feet 2 times daily

RETENTION:
>RECTAL, nightly for 7 days; rest 7 days, then repeat

Dietary Supplementation:
ProGen, Longevity Caps, Protec, ImmuPro, Master Formula HIS, Wolfberry Crisp

Zinc helps reduce prostate swelling. ImmuPro, ProGen, and Master Formula HIS are excellent sources of zinc.

Topical Treatments:
Prenolone, Prenolone +, Progessence

Benign Prostate Hyperplasia (BPH)

Almost all males over age 50 have some degree of prostate hyperplasia, a condition which worsens with age. BPH can severely restrict urine flow and result in frequent, small urinations.

---

36. Skakkebaek NE, "Endocrine disrupters and testicular dysgenesis syndrome," *Horm Res* 2002;57 Suppl 2:43.

37. Zhang X, et al., "Effect of the extracts of pumpkin seeds on the urodynamics of rabbits: an experimental study," *J Tongji Med Univ* 1994:14(4):235-8.

Three herbs which are extremely effective for treating this condition are saw palmetto, pumpkin seed oil, and *Pygeum africanum*. The mineral zinc is also important for normal prostate function and prostate health. The hormone-like activity of some essential oils can support a nutritional regimen to reduce BPH swelling.

Single Oils:
Ledum, frankincense, myrrh, orange, Idaho balsam fir, cumin, tsuga, blue cypress

Blends:
Mister, EndoFlex, Dragon time, Australian Blue

EO Applications:
TOPICAL:
> DILUTE 50-50, 1-3 drops between the rectum and scrotum 1-3 times daily
> VITA FLEX, 1-3 drops on reproductive Vita Flex points on feet, 2 times daily

INGESTION:
> CAPSULE, 00 size, 1 capsule 3 times daily
> RICE MILK, 2-4 times daily

RETENTION,
> RECTAL, 3 times per week, at night

BPH Specific Regimen:
The following regimen reduced PSA (prostate specific antigen) counts 70 percent in 2 months: PSA counts typically rise when BPH occurs.

BPH blend:
- 10 drops frankincense
- 5 drops myrrh
- 3 drops sage

Use the above blend for the following three applications simultaneously:
1. Mix the above amounts of essential oils with 1 tablespoon olive oil and use 3 times weekly as overnight rectal retention enema.
2. Massage 1-3 drops neat on Vita Flex reproductive points on both feet daily
3. Dilute above blend 50-50 with V6 Oil Complex and apply 2-4 drops topically between the rectum and the scrotum daily.

Dietary Supplementation:
ProGen, Master Formula vitamins, Longevity Caps, Protec, ImmuPro, Mineral Essence

Topical Treatments:
Prenolone, Prenolone +, Progessence

Other:
1 oz. Protec with 1-2 drops tsuga essential oil in a rectal retention enema. Retain overnight, 3 times weekly

Prostate Cancer

(See Prostate Cancer in CANCER)

Prostatitis

Prostatitis is an inflammation of the prostate that can present symptoms similar to benign prostate hyperplasia: frequent urinations, restricted flow, etc.

Single Oils:
Rosemary, myrtle, thyme, tsuga, peppermint

Blends:
Mister, Dragon Time, Aroma Siez, Di-Tone

EO Applications:
INGESTION:
> CAPSULE, 0 size, twice daily

RETENTION:
> RECTAL, 3 times per week, at night

TOPICAL:
> DILUTE 20-80, apply 1-3 drops to the area between the rectum and the scrotum daily
> VITA FLEX, massage 4-6 drops on reproductive foot Vita Flex points daily

Dietary Supplementation:
ProGen, Master Formula HIS, Longevity Caps, Protec, ImmuPro, Mineral Essence

Topical Treatment:
Prenolone, Prenolone+, Progessence

PSORIASIS

(See SKIN DISORDERS)

PYORRHEA

(See ORAL CARE)

Essential oils are one of the best treatments against gum diseases such as gingivitis and pyorrhea. Clove oil, for example, is used as a dental disinfectant; and the active principle in clove oil, eugenol, is one of the best-studied germ-killers available.

RADIATION DAMAGE

Many cancer treatments use radiation therapy that can severely damage both the skin and vital organs. Using antioxidant essential oils topically, as well as proper nutrients internally, is helpful in minimizing radiation damage.

Single Oils:
Tea tree, neroli

Blends:
Melrose

EO Applications:
TOPICAL:
> NEAT or DILUTE 50-50, massage 2-4 drops on affected area 1-2 times daily

Dietary Supplementation:
Essential Omegas, AD&E, Super C, Power Meal, ImmuPro, ImmuneTune, Berry Young Juice, Essential Manna

RESTLESS LEG SYNDROME

(See also ATTENTION DEFICIT SYNDROME)

Single Oils:
Valarian, basil, marjoram, lavender, cypress, Roman chamomile, peppermint

Blends:
Peace & Calming, Aroma Siez

EO Applications:
INHALATION:
> DIRECT, 6-8 times daily as needed
> DIFFUSION, 20 minutes, 4 times daily

TOPICAL:
> VITA FLEX Daily, before retiring
> RAINDROP Technique, weekly

Dietary Supplementation:
Mineral Essence, Thyromin, VitaGreen, Mega Cal

RHEUMATIC FEVER

Rheumatic fever results from a *Streptococcus* infection that primarily strikes children (usually before age 14). It can lead to inflammation that damages the heart muscle and valve.

Rheumatic fever is caused by the same genus of bacteria that causes strep throat and scarlet fever. Diffusing essential oils can help reduce the likelihood of contracting the disease. Essential oils such as mountain savory, rosemary, tea tree, thyme, and oregano, have powerful antimicrobial effects.

In cases where a person is already infected, the use of essential oils in the Raindrop Technique may be appropriate.

Single Oils:
Mountain savory, peppermint, thyme, rosemary, tea tree, black pepper, oregano

Blends:
Thieves, Exodus II, ImmuPower

EO Applications:
INHALATION:
> DIFFUSION, 1 hour, 3 times daily

TOPICAL:
> DILUTE 50-50, massage 3-5 drops on bottoms of feet and on carotid artery spots under ear lobes
> RAINDROP Technique, once weekly

Dietary Supplementation:
Exodus, ImmuPro, ImmuneTune, Super C, Sulfurzyme, AD&E, Berry Young Juice, HRT

RINGWORM

(See Ringworm or Athlete's Foot in FUNGAL INFECTIONS)

SALMONELLA

(See FOOD POISONING and INFECTION)

SCABIES

(See also LICE in SKIN DISORDERS)

Scabies are caused by eight-legged insects known as itch mites—tiny parasites the burrow into the skin, usually in the fingers and genital areas. The most common variety, *Sarcoptes scabiei,* can quickly infest other people. Although it only lives six weeks, it continually lays eggs once it digs into the skin.

The most common remedy for scabies and lice is lindane (gamma benzene hexachloride) a highly toxic polychlorinated chemical that is structurally very similar to hazardous banned pesticides such as DDT and chlordane. It is so dangerous that Dr. Guy Sansfacon, head of the Quebec Poison Control Centre in Canada, has requested that lindane be banned.

Natural plant-derived essential oils have the same activity as commercial pesticides but are far safer. Essential oils have been studied for their ability to not only repel insects, but also kill them and their eggs as well. Because many oils are nontoxic to humans, they make excellent treatments to combat scabies infestations.

Single Oils:
Citronella, peppermint, palmarosa, lavandin, *Eucalyptus globulus,* black pepper, ginger

Blends:
Di-Tone, Purification, Peace & Calming

EO Applications:
TOPICAL:
> NEAT, or Dilute 50-50 if needed, apply 2-4 drops on location, 3 times daily
> DILUTE 20-80, massage thoroughly 1 tsp. into scalp at night before retiring. To treat hair or scalp, add 2-4 drops of essential oil to 1 tsp. of shampoo.

Topical Treatment:
Lavender Hair and Scalp Wash, Lemon-Mint Hair and Scalp Wash

SCAR TISSUE

Some essential oils may be valuable for reducing or minimizing the formation of scar tissue:

Single Oils:
Helichrysum, lavender, cypress, elemi, blue yarrow, rose, cistus, myrrh, sandalwood

Blends:
3 Wise Men, Inspiration

Scar prevention blend:
- 4 drops helichrysum
- 6 drops lavender
- 8 drops myrrh
- 2 drops sandalwood

EO Applications:
TOPICAL:
> NEAT, gently apply 2-6 drops over wound or cut daily until healed

Dietary Supplementation:
AD&E, Essential Omegas, Super C, Sulfurzyme, Power Meal, Essential Manna

Topical Application:
Tender Tush Ointment

SCIATICA

(See SPINE INJURIES and PAIN)

SCHIZOPHRENIA

A neurological disease that involves identity confusion. Onset is typically between the late teens and early 30's. Abnormal neurological findings may show a broad range of dysfunction including slow reaction time, poor coordination, abnormalities in eye tracking, and impaired sensory gating. Typically schizophrenia involves dysfunction in one or more areas such as interpersonal relations, work, education, or self-care. Some cases are believed to be caused by viral infection.

Single Oils:
Peppermint, cardamom, cedarwood, vetiver, melissa, frankincense, rosemary

Blends:
Brain Power, Clarity, Valor, M-Grain

EO Applications:
INHALATION:
> DIRECT, 4-6 times daily
TOPICAL:
> RAINDROP Technique, once weekly

Dietary Supplementation:
Mineral Essence, Super Cal, Essential Omegas, Ultra Young, Wolfberry Crisp, Berry Young Juice

SCLERODERMA

Also known as systemic sclerosis, scleroderma is a non-infectious, chronic, autoimmune disease of the connective tissue. Caused by an over-production of collagen, the disease can involve either the skin or internal organs and can be life-threatening. Scleroderma is far more common among women than men.

Single Oils:

Frankincense, Roman chamomile, lavender, patchouli, sandalwood, myrrh

Blends:

Melrose

Scleroderma blend #1:
* 3 drops Roman chamomile
* 3 drops lavender
* 3 drops patchouli

Scleroderma blend #2:
* 4 drops sandalwood
* 4 drops myrrh

EO Applications:
TOPICAL:

DILUTE 50-50, massage 4-6 drops on location 3 times daily. Alternate between blend #1 and blend #2 (above) each day

Dietary Supplementation:

PD 80/20, Cleansing Trio, Essential Omegas, JuvaTone, JuvaPower/Spice, Thyromin, Mineral Essence, Power Meal, Sulfurzyme, Detoxyme

Topical Treatment:

Prenolone

SCOLIOSIS

(See SPINE INJURIES and Chapter 21: Raindrop Technique)

Scoliosis is an abnormal lateral or side-to-side curvature or twist in the spine. It is different from hyperkyphosis (hunchback) or hyperlordosis (swayback) which involve excessive front-to-back accentuation of existing spine curvatures.

While a few cases of scoliosis can be attributed to congenital deformities (such as MS, cerebral palsy, Down's syndrome, or Marfan's syndrome), the vast majority of scoliosis types are of unknown origin.

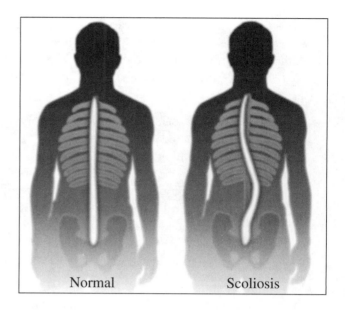

Normal   Scoliosis

Some medical professionals believe that scoliosis may be caused by persistent muscle spasms that pull the vertebrae of the spine out of alignment. Others feel - and there is a growing body of research documenting this hypothesis - that it begins with hard-to-detect inflammation along the spine caused by latent viruses. (See citations in Chapter 21.)

Symptoms:

* When bending forward, the left side of the back is higher or lower than the right side (the patient must be viewed from the rear).

* One hip may appear to be higher or more prominent than the other.

* Uneven shoulders or scapulas (shoulder blades).

* When the arms are hanging loosely, the distance between the left arm and left side is different than the distance between the right arm and right side.

The Raindrop Technique is proving to be one of the most effective therapies for straightening spines misaligned due to scoliosis.

Single Oils:

Oregano, thyme, basil, wintergreen, cypress, marjoram, peppermint.

Blends:

Aroma Siez, PanAway, Valor

EO Applications:
TOPICAL:
RAINDROP Technique, 3-5 times monthly
DILUTE 50-50, as a supplement to
RAINDROP Technique, apply 3-6 drops
along spine daily or as needed

Dietary Supplementation:
Mineral Essence, Super Cal, Essential Manna,
Power Meal, Sulfurzyme

Topical Treatments:
Ortho Ease, Ortho Sport

SCURVY

A condition due to deficiency of vitamin C in the
diet and marked by weakness, anemia, spongy
gums, bleeding of the gums and nose, and a
hardening of the muscles of the calves and legs.

Supplements:
Super C, Super C Chewable, Berry Young
Juice, Power Meal

SEIZURES

Most seizures can be treated by removing all
forms of sugar, artificial colors, and flavors from
diet. Avoid using personal care products with
ammonium-based compounds, such as quater-
niums and polyquaterniums.

(See BRAIN DISORDERS or EPILEPSY)

Single Oils:
Frankincense, sandalwood, melissa, jasmine,
basil

Blends:
Valor, Aroma Siez, Exodus II

EO Applications:
TOPICAL:
DILUTE 50-50, massage 10 drops into
scalp 3 times daily to help reduce risk of
seizure. Supplement with inhalation
therapy below

INHALATION:
DIRECT, 3-5 times daily

Seizure regimen (do all the following):
• Massage 4-6 drops Valor on bottoms of
feet daily

• Diffuse Peace & Calming for 30 minutes
3-4 times daily
• Massage 4-6 drops Joy over heart daily
• Do a Raindrop Technique on spine weekly

Dietary Supplements:
Blue Agave Nectar, Mineral Essence, AD&E,
Master Formula Vitamins, VitaGreen, Super B,
Longevity Caps, Power Meal, Sulfurzyme

SEXUAL DYSFUNCTION

(See IMPOTENCE)

Lack of Libido

Single Oils:
FOR WOMEN: Geranium, ylang ylang, clary
sage, nutmeg, rose, black pepper

(These oils can be inhaled or taken orally as
dietary supplements. Jasmine absolute can also
be used in inhalation therapy or topical use, but
must never be ingested.)

FOR MEN: Myrrh, black pepper, pine, ylang
ylang, ginger, nutmeg, rose

• Ylang Ylang helps balance sexual emotion and
sex drive problems. Its aromatic influence elevates sexual energy and enhances relationships.

• Clary sage can help with lack of sexual desire
particularly with women by regulating and
balancing hormones.

• Nutmeg supports the nervous system to overcome frigidity.

Blends:
Joy, Live with Passion, Sensation, Mister,
Dragon Time, Valor, Lady Sclareol,
SclarEssence, Transformation

Dietary Supplementation:
Ultra Young, Sensation Moisture Cream,
VitaGreen, ProGen, Sulfurzyme

Sulfurzyme provides MSM (sulfur), which can
harmonize libido.

Topical Treatment:
Progessence, Prenolone, Prenolone+, NeuroGen

Excessive Sexual Desire

Single Oils:
Marjoram, lavender, St. John's wort

Blends:
Peace & Calming, Acceptance, Surrender

EO Applications:
INHALATION:
DIRECT, 3-5 times daily
TOPICAL:
DILUTE 50-50, massage 4-6 drops on neck,
shoulders and lower abdomen,
1-3 times daily

Dietary Supplementation:
Mineral Essence, Super B, PD80/20, Mega Cal

Frigidity

Single Oils:
Jasmine absolute, ylang ylang, rose

Blends:
Joy, Valor, Chivalry

EO Applications:
INHALATION:
DIRECT, 3-5 times daily
TOPICAL:
DILUTE 50-50, massage 4-6 drops on neck,
shoulders and lower abdomen, 1-3 times
daily

Topical Treatment:
Progessence, Prenolone, Prenolone+, NeuroGen

SEXUALLY TRANSMITTED DISEASES

(See INFECTIONS)

Herpes Simplex Type II

The Herpes Simplex Virus Type 2, is transmitted by sexual contact and results in sores or lesions. Four to seven days after contact with an infected partner, tingling, burning, or persistent itching usually heralds an outbreak. One or two days later, small pimple-like bumps appear over reddened skin. The itching and tingling continue, and the pimples turn into painful blisters, which burst, bleeding with a yellowish pus. Five to seven days after the first tingling, scabs form, and healing begins.

Antiviral essential oils have generally been very effective in treating herpes lesions and reducing their onset. Oils such as tea tree, melissa, and rosemary have been successfully used for this purpose by Daniel Pénoël, M.D. in his clinical practice. A study at the University of Buenos Aires found that sandalwood essential oil inhibited the replication of Herpes Simplex viruses-1 and -2.[38]

Those with herpes should avoid diets high in the amino acid L-arginine, substituting instead L-lysine. Lysine retards the growth of the virus. Foods such as amaranth are very high in lysine. (Amaranth is used in Essential Manna).

Single Oils:
Melissa, ravensara, tea tree, sandalwood, blue cypress, oregano, thyme, cumin, rosemary

Blends:
Melrose, Thieves, Exodus II, ImmuPower, Purification

Herpes blend #1 (topical):
- 1 drop lavender
- 1 drop tea tree oil

Herpes blend #2 (vaginal):
- 2 drops sage
- 2 drops melissa
- 4 drops ravensara
- 2 drops lavender

EO Applications:
TOPICAL:
NEAT, apply Herpes blend #1 (above) on lesion as soon as it appears. Apply 1-2 drops of neat oil 2-3 times daily, alternating between the above herpes blend and Melrose each day.
RAINDROP Technique, 1-2 treatments
RETENTION:
TAMPON, for vaginal treatment of herpes, use Herpes blend #2 (above), diluted 20-80 in tampon/ pad application nightly. If tampon/pad stings after 5 minutes, remove and change dilution rate to 10-90.

---

38. Benencia F, et al. "Antiviral activity of sandalwood oil against herpes simplex viruses-1 and -2." *Phytomedicine*. 1999;6(2):119-23

Dietary Supplementation:
Exodus, ImmuPro, ImmuneTune, Sulfurzyme, Power Meal, Essential Manna, Super C Chewable, Super B, VitaGreen, Master Formula Vitamins, Cleansing Trio.

Avoid using Ultra Young since this supplement is high in L-arginine.

Topical Treatment:
Thieves Antiseptic Spray, ImmuGel

Genital Warts

Genital warts are a form of viral infection caused by the human papillomavirus (HPV), of which there are more than 60 different types.

One type of HPV virus is among the most common sexually transmitted diseases. Up to 24 million Americans may be currently infected with HPV, usually spread through sexual contact. HPV lives only in genital tissue. HPV can later lead to cervical cancer in women.

Single Oils:
Melissa, oregano, thyme, Idaho tansy, tea tree, *Melaleuca ericifolia,* lavender

Blends:
Melrose, Thieves, ImmuPower

EO Applications:
TOPICAL:
　　　NEAT or DILUTE 50-50, 1-3 drops
　　　2 times daily for 10 days
RETENTION:
　　　TAMPON, nightly

Topical Treatment:
Thieves Antiseptic Spray, ImmuGel, Fresh Essence Plus

Gonorrhea and Syphilis

NOTE: Seek immediate professional medical attention if you suspect you may have either of these diseases.

Single Oils:
Oregano, melissa, thyme, mountain savory, cinnamon

Blends:
Thieves, Exodus II

EO Applications:
INGESTION:
　　　CAPSULE, 00 size, 1 capsule 2 times daily for
　　　15 days

Dietary Supplementation:
Exodus, ImmuPro, Essential Manna

Topical Treatment:
Thieves Antiseptic Spray, ImmuGel

SHINGLES (Herpes Zoster)

(See CHICKEN POX)

SHOCK

Shock can be described as a state of profound depression of the vital processes associated with reduced blood volume and pressure. The blood rushes to the vital organs after trauma.

It may be caused by the sudden stimulation of the nerves and convulsive contraction of the muscles caused by the discharge of electricity. Other causes include sudden trauma, terror, surprise, horror, or disgust.

Symptoms or signs:
- Irregular breathing
- Low blood pressure
- Dilated pupils
- Cold and sweaty skin
- Weak and rapid pulse
- Dry mouth

Any injury that results in the sudden loss of substantial amounts of fluids can trigger shock.

Shock can also be caused by allergic reactions (ana-phylactic shock), infections in the blood (septic shock), or emotional trauma (neurogenic shock).

Shock should be treated by covering the victim with a blanket and elevating the victim's feet unless there is a head or upper torso injury. Inhaling essential oils can also help—especially in cases of emotional shock.

Single Oils: Cardamom, helichrysum, peppermint, tea tree, frankincense, basil, rosemary, sandalwood

Blends:
Clarity, Legacy, Trauma Life, 3 Wise Men, Valor, Harmony, Present Time, Thieves

EO Applications:
INHALATION:
DIRECT, 1-2 drops, as needed
TOPICAL:
DILUTE 50-50, rub 1-2 drops on temples, back of neck, and under nose.

NOTE: When applying essential oil to the temples be careful not to get the oil too close to the eyes.

SINUS INFECTIONS

(See also COLDS and THROAT INFECTIONS)

Nasopharyngitis

Inflammation of the mucous membranes of the back of the nasal cavity where it connects to the throat and the eustachian tubes.

Single Oils:
Eucalyptus radiata, thyme, ravensara

Blends:
Raven, R.C., Thieves, Exodus II

EO Applications:
TOPICAL:
DILUTE 50-50, apply just under jawbone on right and left sides, 4-8 times daily
INHALATION:
DIRECT, 4-8 times daily
ORAL:
GARGLE, 2-5 times daily

Dietary Supplementation:
Super C, Super C Chewable, ImmuPro, ImmuGel, Dentarome Ultra, Fresh Essence Plus Mouthwash, Thieves lozenges, Exodus

Rhinitis

Inflammation of the mucous membranes of the sinus

Single Oils:
Basil, *Eucalyptus radiata*, ravensara, tea tree, Melaleuca ericifolia, peppermint

Blends:
R.C., Melrose, Raven

EO Applications:
INHALATION:
DIRECT, 4-8 times daily
TOPICAL:
NEAT, apply 2-4 drops on forehead and bridge of nose, being careful not to get oils in or near eyes or eyelids. 3-6 times daily

Dietary Supplementation:
Super C, Super C Chewable, Exodus, AD&E, ImmuGel, Dentarome Ultra, Fresh Essence Plus Mouthwash, Thieves lozenges, ImmuPro

Nasal Irrigation Regimen:
Rosemary and tea tree oils can be used in a saline solution for very effective nasal irrigation that clears and decongests sinuses. As recommended by Daniel Pénoël, MD, the saline solution is prepared as follows:

- 12 drops rosemary
- 4 drops Melaleuca ericifolia
- 8 tablespoons very fine salt (salt flower)

The essential oils are mixed thoroughly in the fine salt and kept in a sealable container. For each nasal irrigation session, 1 teaspoon of this salt mixture is dissolved into 1 1/2 cups distilled water. This oils/salt/water solution is then placed in the tank of an oral irrigator to irrigate the nasal cavities, which is done while bending over a sink. This application has brought surprisingly positive results in treating latent sinusitus and other nasal congestion problems.[39]

Sinus Congestion

Single Oils:
Sandalwood, goldenrod, ledum, Idaho balsam fir, ravensara, thyme, *Eucalyptus radiata*, Melaleuca ericifolia, tea tree, peppermint, fennel, rosemary

Blends:
Di-Tone, Raven, R.C., Thieves, Exodus II

EO Applications:
INHALATION:
DIRECT, 3-8 times daily, or as needed
VAPOR, 2-5 times daily, as needed

---

39. Pénoël, Daniel, MD. and Rose Marie, *Natural Home Health Care Using Essential Oils*, Essential Science Publishing, 1998. pp. 166-167

INGESTION:
> SYRUP, 3-6 times daily

ORAL:
> GARGLE, 3-6 times daily

TOPICAL:
> DILUTE 50-50, massage 1-3 drops on each of the following areas: forehead, nose, cheeks, lower throat, chest and upper back, 1-3 times daily
> VITA FLEX, massage 1-3 drops on Vita Flex points on the feet, 2-4 times daily
> RAINDROP Technique, 1-2 times weekly
> BATH SALTS, daily
> Use Nasal Irrigation Regimen: (see Rhinitis)

Dietary Supplementation:
Super C, Super C Chewable, Exodus, AD&E, ImmuGel, Dentarome Ultra, Fresh Essence Plus Mouthwash, Thieves lozenges, ImmuPro

Sinusitis

Essential oils, such as *Eucalyptus radiata* and ravensara strengthen the respiratory system, open the pulmonary tract, and fight respiratory infection.

Single Oils:
Clove, ravensara, myrtle, Melaleuca ericifolia, *Eucalyptus radiata*, *Eucalyptus globulus*, thyme, rosemary, lemon, cypress, lemongrass

Blends:
R.C., Raven, Thieves, Purification, ImmuPower

Sinus blend #1:
• 3 drops *Melaleuca ericifolia*
• 3 drops Raven

Sinus blend #2:
• 10 drops peppermint
• 5 drops *Eucalyptus radiata*
• 2-3 drops tea tree

EO Applications:
INHALATION:
> DIRECT, 3-5 times daily

TOPICAL:
> DILUTE 50-50, apply 1-2 drops to a cotton swab, and swab inside of nostrils 3 times daily. The sinusitis blend is ideal for this method.

ORAL:
> GARGLE, 2-5 times daily
> Use Nasal Irrigation Regimen: (see Rhinitis)

SKIN DISORDERS

(See also BLISTERS and BOILS, LIVER DISORDERS and MENSTRUAL CONDITIONS)

Our skin is our armor and the largest absorbent organ of the body. Protecting the skin environment is essential. Many chemical molecules are too large to be absorbed and lay on the surface of the skin, causing irritation, resulting in rashes, itching, blemishes, flaky and dry skin, dandruff, and allergies. Essential oils are soluble through lipids in the skin and are easily absorbed.

Many skin conditions may be related to dysfunctions of the liver. It may be necessary to cleanse, stimulate, and condition the liver and colon for 30 to 90 days before the skin begins to improve.

Abscesses/Boils:

Skin abscesses are small pockets of pus that collect under the skin. They are usually caused by a bacterial or fungal infection.

A number of essential oils may reduce inflammation and combat infection, helping to bring abscesses/boils to a head, so they can close and heal.

Single Oils:
Tea tree, frankincense, helichrysum, peppermint, lavender, lemon, German chamomile, *Eucalyptus radiata,* rosemary, thyme, mountain savory, palmarosa, patchouli, rosewood, juniper, ravensara, oregano

Blends:
Melrose, Purification, Exodus II, ImmuPower, Thieves, Sacred Mountain

EO Applications:
TOPICAL:
> DILUTE 50-50, apply on location 3-6 times daily

Dietary Supplementation:
JuvaTone, Essential Omegas, Cleansing Trio, AD&E

Tips for Clearing Up Acne

- Eliminate dairy products, fried foods, chemical additives, and sugar from diet.

- Avoid use of makeup or chlorinated water.

- Avoid contact with plastics which may exude estrogenic chemicals.

- Topically apply essential oils such as tea tree to problem areas. Tea tree was shown to be equal to benzoyl peroxide in the treatment of acne, according research published in the *Medical Journal of Australia*.[40]

- Begin a cleansing program with the Cleansing Trio and Sulfurzyme.

Acne

(See Clogged Pores in this section)

Acne results from an excess accumulation of dirt and sebum around the hair follicle and the pores of the skin. This accumulation may be due to an over-production of sebum, an oily substance that is secreted by the sebaceous glands in the hair follicles. As the pores and hair follicles become congested, bacteria begins to feed on the sebum. This leads to inflammation and infection around the hair follicle and the formation of a pimple or a puss-filled blackhead.

One of the most common forms of acne, *Acne vulgaris,* occurs primarily in adolescents due to hormone imbalances which stimulate the creation of sebum.

Acne in adults can be also be caused by hormone balances, as well as use of chlorinated compounds, endocrine system imbalances, or poor dietary practices. Heavy or greasy makeup can also contribute to acne.

Stress may also play a role. According to research conducted by Dr. Toyoda in Japan, acne and other skin problems are a direct result of physical and emotional stress.[41]

Essential oils are outstanding for treating acne because of their ability to dissolve sebum, kill bacteria, and preserve the acid mantle of the skin.

Because essential oils may be slightly drying to the skin when applied undiluted, it may be necessary to dilute them with V6 Oil Complex or grapeseed oil to keep the skin hydrated.

Single Oils:
Tea tree, geranium, vetiver, blue cypress, lavender, patchouli, German or Roman chamomile, rosewood, cedarwood, *Eucalyptus radiata,* orange, clove

Blends:
Melrose, Thieves, Gentle Baby, Purification, JuvaFlex, JuvaCleanse

EO Applications:
TOPICAL:
NEAT or DILUTE 50-50 as required. Gently massage 3-5 drops into oily areas 1-3 times daily. Alternate oils daily for maximum effect

Dietary Supplementation:
Essential Omegas, Power Meal, Mineral Essence, Exodus, Super C, Super C Chewable, Stevia, VitaGreen, Cleansing Trio, Wolfberry Crisp

To resolve acne caused by hormonal imbalance: Ultra Young, Progessence Cream

Topical Treatment:
Mint Satin Scrub, Juniper Satin Scrub, Progessence Cream, Ortho Ease, Melaleuca-Geranium Bar Soap, Lemon-Sandalwood Bar Soap.

Burns

(See BURNS)

Lemongrass and Skin Care

Lemongrass helps clears acne and balances oily skin conditions. Lemongrass is the predominant ingredient in Morning Start Bath and Shower Gel, which can be used to balance the pH of the skin, decongest the lymphatics and stimulate circulation.

---

40. Bassett IB, et al. "A comparative study of tea-tree oil versus benzoyl peroxide in the treatment of acne." *Med J Aust.* 1990;153(8):455-8.

41. Toyoda M, Morohashi M, "Pathenogenesis of acne," *Med Electron Microse* 2001 Mar;34(1):29-40.

Essential oils that help the skin

To rejuvenate and heal skin:
- Rosewood

To prevent and retard wrinkles:
- Lavender, spikenard, and myrrh

To regenerate the skin
- Geranium, helichrysum, and spikenard

To restore skin elasticity
- Rosewood, lavender
- Ylang ylang with lavender

To combat premature aging of the skin
Mix the following recipe into 1 tablespoon of high grade, unperfumed skin lotion and apply on location twice daily.

- 6 drops rosewood
- 4 drops geranium
- 3 drops lavender
- 2 drops frankincense

Chapped, Dry, or Cracked Skin

Single Oils:
Roman chamomile, neroli, rose, cedarwood, palmarosa, sandalwood, lavender, spikenard, myrrh, rosewood

Blends:
Chapped skin blend:
- 1 drop rosewood
- 1 drop patchouli
- 1 drop geranium

Dry skin blend:
- 1 drop rose
- 1 drop Roman chamomile
- 1 drop sandalwood

EO Applications:
TOPICAL:
> DILUTE 20-80 in a quality, unperfumed lotion base or other high grade emolient, skin oil, apply on location as often as needed

Topical Treatment:
Tender Tush Ointment, Sandalwood Moisturizing Cream, Satin Body Lotion, Rose Ointment

Lip Treatment:
Cinnamint Lip Balm

Combine 3-5 drops of essential oils with 1 tsp of Sensation and Genesis Body lotion to create a very effective lotion for rehydrating the skin of chapped hands and maintaining the natural pH balance of the skin.

Alternate oils of rose, Roman chamomile, or sandalwood with body lotion.

Bath and shower gels, such as Dragon Time, Evening Peace, Morning Start, and Sensation, are formulated to help balance the acid mantle of the skin. The AromaSilk Bar Soaps are rich in moisturizers.

Drink at least 8 glasses per day of purified water

Clogged Pores

Single Oils:
Lemon, orange, tea tree, geranium

Blends:
Purification

EO Applications:
TOPICAL:
> NEAT, apply 2-4 drops to affected area and gently remove with cotton ball

Topical Treatment:
AromaSilk, Bar Soaps especially Melaleuca-Rosewood, and Sandalwood Toner. Juniper or Mint Facial Scrub are gentle exfoliators designed to clarify skin and reduce acne. (If their texture is too abrasive for your skin, mix them with Orange Blossom Facial Wash. This is excellent for those with severe or mild acne.)

Spread scrub over face and let dry for perhaps 5 minutes to draw out impurities, pulling and toning the skin at the same time. Put a hot towel over face for greater penetration. Wash off with warm water by gently patting skin with warm face cloth. If you do not have time to let the mask dry, gently massage in a circular motion for 30 seconds, then rinse. Afterwards, apply Sandalwood Moisture Cream or AromaSilk Satin Body Lotion. This also works well underneath foundation makeup.

Diaper Rash

Single Oils:
Lavender, helichrysum, German chamomile cypress

Blends:
Gentle Baby, Clara Derm

EO Applications:
TOPICAL:
> DILUTE 50-50, apply on location 2-4 times daily

Topical Treatment:
Tender Tush Ointment, Lavaderm Cooling Mist, Lavender-Rosewood Bar Soap

Eczema / Dermatitis

(See Psoriasis in this section)

Eczema and dermatitis are both inflammations of the skin and are most often due to allergies, but also can be a sign of liver disease (See LIVER DISORDERS).

Dermatitis usually results from external factors, such as sunburn or contact with poison ivy, metals (wristwatch, earrings, jewelry, etc.). Eczema usually results from internal factors, such as irritant chemicals, soaps and shampoos, allergy to wheat (gluten), etc. In both dermatitis and eczema, skin becomes red, flaky and itchy. Small blisters may form and if broken by scratching, can become infected.

Single Oils:
Lavender, juniper, ledum, *Citrus hystrix*, celery seed, cistus, Roman and German chamomile, geranium, rosewood, thyme

Blends:
JuvaFlex, JuvaCleanse, Purification, Melrose, Gentle Baby

EO Applications:
TOPICAL:
> DILUTE 50-50, apply as needed on location

Dietary Supplementation:
Cleansing Trio, JuvaTone, Rehemogen, Rose Ointment, Juva Power, Detoxyme

Freckles

Single Oils: Idaho tansy.

EO Applications:
TOPICAL:
> DILUTE, 4-6 drops in 1/2 teaspoon of high grade, unperfumed skin lotion. Spread lightly over freckle areas. Use 2-3 times weekly

Fungal Skin Infection

(See FUNGAL INFECTIONS)

Single Oils:
Oregano, lemongrass, tea tree, naiouli, *Melaleuca ericifolia*

Blends:
Melrose, Clara Derm

Antifungal skin blend:
- 10 drops patchouli
- 4 drops lavender
- 2 drops German chamomile
- 5 drops lemon

EO Applications:
TOPICAL:
> DILUTE 50-50, apply on location, 3-5 times daily

Dietary Supplementation:
Cleansing Trio, Mineral Essence, AD&E, Essential Omegas

Topical Treatment: Sandalwood Moisturizer Cream, Rose Ointment

Itching

Itching can be due to dry skin, impaired liver function, allergies, or over-exposure to chemicals or sunlight.

Single Oils:
Peppermint, oregano, lavender, helichrysum, patchouli, nutmeg, German chamomile

Blends:
Aroma Siez, Clara Derm

EO Applications:
TOPICAL:
> DILUTE 50-50, Apply 2-6 drops on location as needed

Dietary Supplementation:
Juva Flex, Essential Omegas, JuvaTone, ComforTone

Topical Treatment:
Tender Tush Ointment

Melanoma

(See CANCER)

Moles

To remove moles: Apply 1-2 drops of oregano neat, directly on the mole, 2-3 times daily.

Poison Oak - Poison Ivy

Single Oils:
Peppermint, *Eucalyptus dives*, German chamomile, lemongrass, lemon, Idaho tansy, tea tree, rosemary, basil

Blends:
Thieves, Purification, Sensation, Melrose, Gentle Baby, R.C., JuvaFlex, JuvaCleanse, Release

EO Applications:
TOPICAL:
> DILUTE 50-50, apply 4-6 drops to affected areas twice daily
> COMPRESS, Cold, apply on affected area, twice daily

Dietary Supplementation:
Master Formula vitamins

Topical Treatment:
Rose Ointment, Stevia, Satin Body Lotion, Morning Start Bath and Shower Gel, Thieves Antiseptic Spray

---

Treating Psoriasis with pH Balance

Psoriasis, eczema, dermatitis, dry skin, allergies, and similar problems indicate an excessive acidic pH in the body. The more acid in the blood and skin, the less therapeutic effect the oils will have. People who have a negative reaction to oils are usually highly acidic. An alkaline balance must be maintained in the blood and skin for the oils to work the best. AlkaLime and VitaGreen are both helpful for this balancing. (See FUNGUS)

Psoriasis

Psoriasis is a non-infectious skin disorder that is marked by skin lesions that can occur in limited areas (such as the scalp) or that can cover up to 80-90 percent of the body.

The overly rapid growth of skin cells is the primary cause of the lesions associated with psoriasis. In some cases, skin cells grow four times faster than normal, resulting in the formation of silvery layers that flake off.

Symptoms:
- Occurs on elbows, chest, knees, and scalp.
- Slightly elevated reddish lesions covered with silver-white scales.
- The disease can be limited to one small patch or can cover the entire body.
- Rashes subside after exposure to sunlight.
- Rashes recur over a period of years.

Single Oils:
Roman chamomile, tea tree, patchouli, helichrysum, rose, German chamomile, lavender

Blends:
Melrose, JuvaFlex, JuvaCleanse

Psoriasis blend:
- 2 drops patchouli
- 2 drops Roman chamomile
- 2 drops lavender
- 2 drops Melrose

EO Applications:
TOPICAL:

NEAT, apply 2-4 drops to affected area twice daily. 6-10 drops can be added to 1 tsp of regular skin lotion and applied daily or as needed
COMPRESS, warm, 3 times weekly
INGESTION:

CAPSULE, 0 size, 1 per day

Dietary Supplementation:
Essential Omegas, Cleansing Trio, AlkaLime, JuvaTone, JuvaPower, Sulfurzyme

Topical Treatment:
Tender Tush Ointment, Rose Ointment

Sagging Skin

Single Oils:
Lavender, helichrysum, patchouli, cypress

Topical Treatment:
Cel-Lite Magic, Boswellia Wrinkle Cream

Skin firming blend (morning):
- 10 drops tangerine
- 10 drops cypress

Skin firming blend (night):
- 8 drops geranium
- 5 drops cypress
- 5 drops helichrysum
- 1 drop peppermint

EO Applications:
TOPICAL:

NEAT or DILUTE 50-50, massage 4-6 drops on affected area twice daily. Use morning blend before dressing in the morning; evening blend before bed at night.

Strength training with weights can help tighten sagging skin.

Skin Ulcers

Single Oils:
Rosewood, clove, helichrysum, Roman chamomile, patchouli, myrrh, lavender

Blends:
Melrose, Purification, Relieve It, 3 Wise Men, Gentle Baby

EO Applications:
TOPICAL:

NEAT or DILUTE 50-50, massage 4-6 drops on affected areas 2 times daily

Dietary Supplementation:
Super C, Exodus, Cleansing Trio

Topical Treatment:
Tender Tush Ointment, AromaSilk Satin Body Lotion, Boswellia Wrinkle Cream

Stretch Marks

Stretch marks are most commonly associated with pregnancy, but can also occur during growth spurts and periods of weight gain.

Single Oils:
Lavender, frankincense, elemi, spikenard, geranium, myrrh

Blends:
Gentle Baby

EO Applications:
TOPICAL:

NEAT or DILUTE 50-50, apply on affected areas 2 times daily

Dietary Supplementation:
Sulfurzyme, Essential Omegas

Topical Treatment:
Tender Tush Ointment, Rose Ointment, A.R.T. Day Activator, A.R.T. Night Reconstructor, A.R.T. Gentle Foaming Cleanser

Vitiligo

A skin disorder marked by patches of skin devoid of skin pigmentation.

Single Oils:
Vetiver, sandalwood, myrrh

Blends:
Purification, Melrose

EO Applications:
TOPICAL:

NEAT, apply 2-4 drops on location, 2 times daily

Wrinkles

Single Oils:
Frankincense, helichrysum, cypress, rose, lavender, ylang ylang, patchouli, sage, geranium, clary sage, rosewood, sandalwood, jasmine, neroli, palmarosa, spikenard

Blends:
Gentle Baby, Sensation

Wrinkle-reducing blend:
- 5 drops sandalwood
- 5 drops helichrysum
- 5 drops geranium
- 5 drops lavender
- 5 drops frankincense

EO Applications:
TOPICAL:
> DILUTE 50-50 in high grade, unperfumed body lotion (AromaSilk Satin Body Lotion) or an emollient vegetable oil and apply on location as needed

NOTE: Be careful not to get lotion or oils near the eyes.

Dietary Supplementation:
Ultra Young, Berry Young Juice, Master Formula vitamins, Thyromin, Stevia

Topical Treatment:
AromaSilk Satin Body Lotion, Rose Ointment, Lavender, Valor and Lemon-Sandalwood Bar Soaps, NeuroGen, Boswellia Wrinkle Cream, Sandalwood Moisture Cream, A.R.T. Day Activator, A.R.T. Night Reconstructor, A.R.T. Gentle Foaming Cleanser

Boswellia wrinkle cream is excellent for dry or prematurely aging skin.

Rose Ointment was developed to feed and rehydrate the skin and to supply nutrients necessary to slow down the aging process. Moreover, it contains no synthetic chemicals which can cause skin irritation.

SLEEP DISORDERS

(See also APNEA, INSOMNIA, or LIVER DISORDERS)

Melatonin is the most powerful natural remedy for restoring both quality and quantity of sleep. It improves the length of the time the body sustains deep, Stage 4 sleep, when the immune system and growth hormone production reaches its maximum. ImmuPro not only contains melatonin, but mineral and polysaccharide complexes to restore natural sleep rhythm and eliminate insomnia.

Single Oils:
Lavender, valerian, goldenrod, marjoram, Roman chamomile, orange

Blends:
Peace & Calming, Surrender, Inspiration, Hope, Humility

EO Applications:
INGESTION:
> CAPSULE, 0 size, 1 per day

INHALATION:
> DIRECT, 1-3 times before bed
> Diffuser: 30 minutes before bed

TOPICAL:
> BATH SALTS, daily, just before bedtime

Dietary Supplementation:
ImmuPro, Essential Omegas, Essentialzyme

SMOKING CESSATION

(See also ADDICTIONS)

Single Oils:
Cinnamon, clove, nutmeg

Blends:
Harmony, JuvaFlex, JuvaCleanse, Peace & Calming, Thieves, Exodus II

EO Applications:
INHALATION:
> DIRECT, whenever the urge for a cigarette arises
> DIFFUSION, 30 minutes, 3 times a day as needed

Dietary Supplementation:
Cleansing Trio, Rehemogen, JuvaTone, Stevia

Cleanse colon and liver with Cleansing Trio and JuvaTone.

JuvaTone, JuvaPower/Spice detoxifies the liver and reduces the cravings for nicotine and caffeine, Take 3 tablets of JuvaTone 3 times daily. amd two tablespoons JuvaPower/Spice daily.

Rehemogen cleanses and detoxifies the blood and works synergistically with JuvaTone and JuvaFlex in rebuilding the liver.

Stevia may also decrease cravings for sugar, tobacco and alcohol.

SNAKE BITES

Single Oils:
Clove

Topical Treatment:
Thieves Antiseptic Spray

EO Applications:
NOTE: Get medical attention immediately.
TOPICAL:
> DILUTE 50-50, Apply 2-3 drops on location every 15 minutes until professional medical help is available

SNORING

Rub 4-6 drops thyme diluted 50-50 on the soles of both feet at bedtime.

SORE THROAT

(See COLDS OR THROAT INFECTION)

SPASTIC COLON

(See DIGESTION PROBLEMS)

SPINA BIFIDA

Spina bifida (SB) is a defect in which the spinal cord of the fetus fails to close during the first month of pregnancy. This results in varying degrees of permanent nerve damage, paralysis in lower limbs, and incomplete brain development.

SB has three different variations:

- The most severe form is Myelomeningocele. The spinal cord and its protective sheath (known as the meninges) protrude from an opening in the spine.

- The next most severe form is Meningocele. Only the meninges protrude from the opening in the spine

- The mildest form is Occulta. It is characterized by malformed vertebrae. Symptoms of this disease range from bowel and bladder dysfunctions to excess build up in the brain of cerebrospinal fluid.

The easiest way to prevent SB is with folic acid supplementation (at least 400 mcg daily), (found in Super B) by all women of child-bearing age.

To Prevent:
Dietary Supplementation:
Master Formula vitamins, Super B, Super C

To Reduce Symptoms:
Single Oils:
Mountain savory, helichrysum, thyme, tea tree

Blends:
Melrose, Thieves, Exodus II

EO Applications:
TOPICAL:
> RAINDROP, weekly
> COMPRESS, warm, 2 times weekly

Dietary Supplementation:
ImmuGel, Essential Omegas, Super B, Super C

SPINE INJURIES AND PAIN

According to numerous chiropractors, the Raindrop Technique using therapeutic-grade essential oils is revolutionizing the treatment of many types of back pain, spine inflammation, and vertebral misalignments. (See chapter 21: RAINDROP TECHNIQUE)

All of the essential oils described in this chapter can be used effectively in a Raindrop Application as well as in traditional massage therapy.

The following essential oils, blends, and supplements and are used for supporting the structural integrity of the spine and reducing discomfort:

Single Oils:
Wintergreen, Douglas fir, spruce, peppermint, marjoram, basil

Chiropractors have found that by applying Valor on the bottom of the feet, spinal manipulations take 60 percent less time and work, and the results last 75 percent longer.

How to Make Your Own High-Powered Massage Oil

Add these formulas to 4 oz. of vegetable or massage oil to create a custom muscle-toning formula.

Massage Oil #1:
- 10 drops wintergreen
- 10 drops balsam fir
- 10 drops marjoram
- 8 drops elemi
- 8 drops vetiver
- 5 drops helichrysum
- 5 drops cypress
- 5 drops peppermint

Massage Oil #2:
- 20 drops wintergreen
- 15 drops marjoram
- 10 drops juniper
- 10 drops cypress
- 6 drops spruce

Blends:
Valor, Aroma Siez, Thieves, ImmuPower, PanAway

EO Applications:
TOPICAL:
DILUTE 50-50, 6-10 drops on location twice a day or as needed
COMPRESS, warm,1-2 times daily (if not inflamed)
RAINDROP Technique, 3 times a month for one month

Dietary Supplements:
Super C, Mineral Essence, Super Cal, WheyFit, Longevity Caps, ArthroTune, MegaCal, BLM

Backache

Single Oils:
Lavender, German chamomile, basil, peppermint, geranium, elemi

Blends:
Backache blend:
- 5 drops clary sage
- 5 drops lavender
- 5 drops chamomile

EO Applications:
TOPICAL:
NEAT, apply 2-4 drops to aching area 1-3 times daily as needed
COMPRESS: warm, if there is no inflammation; cold, if there is inflammation, 1-2 times daily
RAINDROP, weekly for 3 weeks

Topical Treatment: Regenolone, Ortho Sport, Ortho Ease, Peppermint-Cedarwood Bar Soap, Morning Start Bar Soap, Valor Bar Soap, Morning Start Bath Gel

(See MUSCLES)

Calcification of Spine

Single Oils:
Geranium, rosemary, *Eucalyptus radiata*, ravensara, oregano, vetiver, elemi

Blends:
R.C.

EO Applications:
TOPICAL:
RAINDROP Technique, 3 times a month

Dietary Supplementation:
ArthroTune, Sulfurzyme, Super Cal, BLM, MegaCal

Topical Treatment:
Regenolone, Ortho Ease Massage Oil

Herniated Disk / Disk Deterioration

For this situation, it is best to consult a specialist.

For temporary relief until medical attention can be given:

Single Oils:
Helichrysum, basil, thyme, melissa, Idaho balsam fir, spruce, vetiver, valerian

Blends:
Relieve It, PanAway, Aroma Siez

Pointer Technique for Nerve Damage

The "pointer technique" may also be used on the foot Vita Flex points.

If there is nerve damage, apply about 6 drops of peppermint along the spine, starting at the hips and ending at the neck, using Raindrop Technique. Starting at the bottom of the spine, use a small-nosed pointer (about the size of a pencil but with a round end).

Stimulate each vertebra between each rib on the vertebra knuckles all the way up on each side of the spine. Use medium pressure and a rocking motion for 1-10 seconds at each location. Then follow the same procedure once more up the center of the spine directly on each vertebra.

EO Applications:
TOPICAL:
> DILUTE 50-50, apply on location for pain relief
> COMPRESS: Cold, on location as needed
> RAINDROP, weekly (after medical attention). Stimulate vertebrae with the "pointer technique"

Dietary Supplementation:
Sulfurzyme, ArthroTune, Super Cal, BLM, MegaCal

Topical Treatments:
Regenolone, Neurogen, Ortho Sport, Ortho Ease

Lumbago (Lower back pain)

Chronic lower back pain can have many causes, including a damaged or pinched nerve (neuralgia) or a congested colon.

Single Oils:
Marjoram, nutmeg, basil, wintergreen, helichrysum, German chamomile, elemi, peppermint

Blends:
Di-Tone, Relieve It, PanAway

EO Applications:
TOPICAL:
> DILUTE 50-50, 6-10 drops on location twice a day or as needed, Also apply to navel
> VITA FLEX, massage 2-3 drops on stomach and intestine Vita Flex points on the feet
> COMPRESS, warm, 1-2 times daily (if not inflamed)
> RAINDROP Technique, 3 times a month

Dietary Supplementation:
Cleansing Trio, MegaCal, Mineral Essence

Topical Treatments: Regenolone, Neurogen, Ortho Sport and Ortho Ease Massage Oils, Raindrop Technique

Neck Pain and Stiffness

Single Oils:
Basil, marjoram, helichrysum, wintergreen, Douglas fir, Idaho balsam fir, nutmeg, elemi, peppermint

Blends:
Neck stiffness blend:
- 5 drops basil
- 5 drops marjoram
- 3 drops lavender

Neck pain blend:
- 2 drops helichrysum
- 10 drops wintergreen
- 8 drops cypress
- 15 drops basil
- 4 drops peppermint

EO Applications:
TOPICAL:
> DILUTE 50-50, apply 4-6 drops to neck area and massage 1-3 times daily, as needed
> COMPRESS: warm, on neck area, daily or as needed (if no inflammation)

Dietary supplementation:
Mineral Essence, AD&E, MegaCal, BLM

Sciatica

Sciatica is characterized by pain in the buttocks and down the back of the thigh. The pain worsens during coughing, sneezing, or extension or flexion of the back. The pain is caused by pressure on the sciatic nerve as it leaves the spine in the lower pelvic region, due to spinal misalignment, nerve inflammation or both. The sciatic nerve is the largest in the body, with branches throughout the legs and feet, and sciatica pain can be intense and immobilizing.

Acute sciatica has a sudden onset and is usually triggered by a misaligned vertebra pressing against the sciatic nerve due to accident, injury, pregnancy, or inflammation.

Symptoms:
• Lower back pain
• Swelling or stiffness in a leg
• Loss of sensation in a leg
• Muscle wasting in a leg

Sulfurzyme and Super B work well together to help rebuild nerve damage and the myelin sheath.

Single Oils:
Helichrysum, peppermint, nutmeg, thyme, spruce, wintergreen, basil, rosemary, clove, tarragon

Blends:
Aroma Siez, PanAway, Relieve It, Aroma Life

EO Applications:
TOPICAL:
>DILUTE 50-50, 6-10 drops on location twice a day or as needed
>COMPRESS, warm, 1-2 times daily (if not inflamed)
>VITA FLEX, 2-3 drops on Vita Flex points on feet, 2-4 times daily
>RAINDROP Technique, 3 times a month

INGESTION:
>CAPSULE, 0 size, 2 times daily

Dietary Supplementation:
ArthroTune, Sulfurzyme, Super B

Topical Treatments:
Regenolone, Neurogen, Ortho Sport, Ortho Ease

SPRAIN

(See also CONNECTIVE TISSUE)

Single Oils:
Wintergreen, Idaho balsam fir, lemongrass, basil, pine, spruce, cypress, peppermint

Blends:
PanAway, Relieve It, Aroma Siez

EO Applications:
TOPICAL:
>DILUTE 50-50, apply 4-6 drops on location 3-5 times daily
>COMPRESS, cold, on location, 2 times daily

Dietary Supplementation:
Sulfurzyme, Mineral Essence, MegaCal

Topical Treatment:
Regenolone, Prenolone, Ortho Sport

STOMACHACHE

(See DIGESTIVE DISORDERS)

STRESS

Single Oils:
Lavender, chamomile, blue tansy, marjoram, rose, sandalwood, frankincense, cedarwood

Blends:
Humility, Harmony, Valor, Joy

EO Applications:
INHALATION:
>DIRECT, as needed
>DIFFUSION, 30 minutes 1-3 times daily

INGESTION:
>CAPSULE, 0 size, 2 times a day

TOPICAL:
>DILUTE 50-50, apply on temples, neck, and shoulders twice daily, or as needed
>BATH SALTS, daily

Dietary Supplementation:
Super B, Ultra Young, Super C, VitaGreen, Thyromin, Master Formula Vitamins, MegaCal

Topical Treatment:
Ortho Ease, Ortho Sport

STRETCH MARKS

(See SKIN DISORDERS)

STROKE

(See BRAIN DISORDERS)

SUNBURN

(See BURNS)

SYMPATHETIC NERVOUS SYSTEM

(See NERVOUS SYSTEM-AUTONOMIC)

TACHYCARDIA

(See HEART, CARDIOVASCULAR CONDITIONS)

TENDONITIS

(See CONNECTIVE TISSUE)

TEETHING PAIN

(See ORAL CARE)

TEETH GRINDING

(See ORAL CARE)

THROAT INFECTIONS

(See also COLDS, INFECTION, LUNG INFECTIONS, ORAL CARE)

Cough

Single Oils:
Cypress, *Eucalyptus polybractea, Eucalyptus radiata, Eucalyptus globulus,* lemon, frankincense, ravensara, thyme, oregano, peppermint, myrrh, cedarwood

Cough blend #1:
- 6 drops cypress
- 3 drops *Eucalyptus polybractea*

Blends:
Thieves, Melrose, R.C., Raven, Purification, 3 Wise Men, Exodus II, ImmuPower

EO Applications:
INHALATION:
　　DIRECT, 3-6 times daily
　　VAPOR, 2-3 times daily
INGESTION:
　　RICE MILK, 2-4 times daily. It is beneficial to heat the rice milk and sip slowly for more soothing relief.
　　SYRUP, 3-5 times daily
ORAL:
　　TONGUE, 2-6 times daily or as often as needed
　　GARGLE, 4-8 times daily
TOPICAL:
　　DILUTE 50-50, apply 1-3 drops to throat, chest and back of neck 2-4 times daily
　　VITA FLEX, apply 1-3 drops to lung Vita Flex points, 1-3 times daily
　　RAINDROP Technique, weekly

Dietary Supplementation:
Super C, Exodus, ImmuGel, Longevity Caps, VitaGreen, ImmuPro, ImmuneTune, Rehemogen

Mountain savory, ravensara, and thyme applied by Raindrop Technique on the spine are beneficial for any and all chest-related infections.

Topical Treatment:
Thieves Antiseptic Spray

Dry Cough

Mix 2 drops lemon and 3 drops Eucalyptus radiata with 1 tsp. blue agave nectar or maple syrup. Dissolve this mixture into 4 oz. of heated distilled water, and sip slowly. Repeat as often as needed for relief.

Topical Treatment:
Thieves Antiseptic Spray

Laryngitis

Put 1 drop Melrose and 1 drop lemon in 1/2 tsp. blue agave or maple syrup. Hold in back of mouth for 1-2 minutes, then swallow. Repeat as needed.

Topical Treatment:
Thieves Antiseptic Spray

Sore Throat

Single Oils:
Cypress, *Eucalyptus radiata*, lemon, frankincense, ravensara, thyme, oregano, peppermint, myrrh, sage

Blends:
Thieves, Melrose, Raven

Oral Treatment:
Thieves Antiseptic Spray, Fresh Essence Plus, Thieves Lozenges

Sore throat blend #1:
- 2 drops thyme
- 2 drops cypress
- 1 drop *Eucalyptus radiata*
- 1 drop peppermint
- 1 drop myrrh

Sore throat blend #2:
- 2 drops *Eucalyptus globulus*
- 5 drops lemon
- 2 drops wintergreen

Applications:
INHALATION:
>DIRECT, 3-6 times daily
>VAPOR, 2-3 times daily

INGESTION:
>RICE MILK, 2-4 times daily. It is beneficial to heat the rice milk and sip slowly for more soothing relief.
>SYRUP, 3-5 times daily

ORAL:
>TONGUE, 2-6 times daily or as often as needed
>GARGLE, 4-8 times daily

TOPICAL:
>DILUTE 50-50, apply 1-3 drops to throat, chest and back of neck 2-4 times daily
>COMPRESS, warm, on chest area 2-3 times daily
>VITA FLEX, apply 1-3 drops to lung Vita Flex points, 1-3 times daily
>RAINDROP Technique, weekly

Dietary Supplementation:
Super C, Super C Chewable, Thieves lozenges, ImmuPro, Exodus, Longevity Caps

Strep Throat

Single Oils:
Eucalyptus globulus, oregano, thyme, frankincense, myrrh, and mountain savory, white fir, Douglas fir

Dilute 1:1 with vegetable oil and apply 2-4 drops on tongue.

Blends:
Thieves, Exodus II, ImmuPower, Di-Tone, Melrose, Raven

Oral Treatment:
Thieves Antiseptic Spray, Fresh Essence

Strep throat blend:
- 1 drops cinnamon
- 6 drops lavender
- 2 drops hyssop

EO Applications:
INHALATION:
>DIRECT, 3-6 times daily
>VAPOR, 2-3 times daily

INGESTION:
>RICE MILK, 2-4 times daily. It is beneficial to heat the rice milk and sip slowly for more soothing relief.
>SYRUP, 3-5 times daily

ORAL:
>TONGUE, 2-6 times daily or as often as needed
>GARGLE, 4-8 times daily

TOPICAL:
>DILUTE 50-50, apply 1-3 drops to throat, chest and back of neck 2-4 times daily
>COMPRESS, warm, on chest area 2-3 times daily
>VITA FLEX, apply 1-3 drops to lung Vita Flex points, 1-3 times daily
>RAINDROP Technique, weekly

Dietary Supplementation:
ImmuPro, ImmuneTune, Super C, Longevity Caps, Super C Chewable, VitaGreen, Essential Omegas, Rehemogen, Exodus, Cleansing Trio, Thieves Spray, Thieves Lozenges.

Regimen for strep throat:

- ImmuneTune: 2-4 capsules, 3 times daily
- Super C: 2-3 tablets, 3 times daily
- Use Raindrop Technique with ImmuPower and/or Exodus II along sides of spine, weekly
- Gargle every hour with Fresh Essence Plus
- Spray throat with colloidal silver/lemon solution.

Tonsillitis

The tonsils are infection-fighting lymphatic tissues (immune cells) that surround the throat. When these become infected streptococcal bacteria they become inflamed, causing a condition known as tonsillitis.

It became popular in the 1960's and 1970's to have the tonsils removed when they became infected. However, tonsillectomies have become much less frequent as researchers have discovered the important role tonsils play in protecting and fighting infectious diseases and optimizing immune response.

The pharyngeal tonsils located at the back of the throat (known as the adenoids) can also become infected—a condition known as adenitis.

Single Oils:
Clove, tea tree, goldenrod, oregano, mountain savory, ravensara, thyme

Blends:
Exodus II, Thieves, Melrose, Exodus II, ImmuPower

Topical Treatment:
Thieves Antiseptic Spray, Fresh Essence

EO Applications:
INGESTION:
RICE MILK, 2-4 times daily. It is beneficial to heat the rice milk and sip slowly for more soothing relief.
SYRUP, 3-5 times daily
ORAL:
TONGUE, 2-6 times daily or as often as needed
GARGLE, 4-8 times daily

TOPICAL:
DILUTE 50-50, apply 1-3 drops to throat, chest and back of neck 2-4 times daily
COMPRESS, warm, on chest area 2-3 times daily
VITA FLEX, apply 1-3 drops to lung Vita Flex points, 1-3 times daily
RAINDROP Technique, weekly

Dietary Supplementation:
ImmuGel, Super C Chewable, AD&E

THRUSH

(See FUNGAL INFECTIONS)

THYROID PROBLEMS

Located at the base of the neck just below the Adam's apple, the thyroid is the energy gland of the human body. It produces T3 and T4 thyroid hormones that control the body's metabolism. The thyroid also controls other vital functions such as digestion, circulation, immune function, hormone balance, and emotions.

The thyroid gland is actually controlled by the pituitary gland which signals the thyroid when to produce thyroid hormone. The pituitary gland, in turn, is directed by chemical signals sent by the hypothalamus gland which monitors hormone levels in the blood stream.

A lack of thyroid hormone does not necessarily mean that the thyroid is not functioning properly (although in many cases, this may be the case). In some instances, the pituitary may be malfunctioning because of its failure to release sufficient TSH (thyroid stimulating hormone) to spur the thyroid to make thyroid hormone.

Other cases of thyroid hormone deficiency may be due to the hypothalamus failing to release sufficient TRH (thyrotropin releasing hormone).

In cases where thyroid hormone deficiency is caused by a malfunctioning pituitary or hypothalamus, better results may be achieved by using supplements or essential oils that stimulate the pituitary or hypothalamus, such as Ultra Young or Cedarwood.

People with type A blood have more of a tendency to have weak thyroid function.

Hyperthyroid (Graves Disease)

When the thyroid becomes overactive and produces excess thyroid hormone, the following symptoms occur:

Symptoms of hyperthyroidism:
- Anxiety
- Restlessness
- Insomnia
- Premature gray hair
- Diabetes mellitus
- Arthritis
- Vitiligo (loss of skin pigment)

Graves disease, unlike Hashimoto's disease, is an autoimmune disease which results in an excess of thyroid hormone production.

MSM has been studied for its ability to reverse many kinds of autoimmune diseases. MSM is a key component of Sulfurzyme.

Single Oils:
Myrrh, spruce, blue tansy, lemongrass

Blends:
EndoFlex

Supplements:
Sulfurzyme, Essential Omegas, Thyromin, VitaGreen, Mineral Essence

Hypothyroid (Hashimoto's Disease)

(see also HYPOGLYCEMIA)

This condition occurs when the thyroid is underactive and produces insufficient thyroid hormone. Approximately 40 percent of the U.S. population suffers from this disorder to some degree, and these people tend to also suffer from hypoglycemia (low blood sugar).

Hashimoto's disease, like Graves disease, is an autoimmune condition. It affects the thyroid, differently, however, limiting its ability to produce thyroid hormone.

The following symptoms occur:
- Fatigue
- Yeast infections (Candida)
- Lack of energy
- Reduced immune function
- Poor resistance to disease
- Recurring infections

Single Oils:
Ledum, lemongrass, myrtle, peppermint, spearmint, myrrh, clove

Blends:
EndoFlex

EO Applications:
TOPICAL:

DILUTE 50-50, apply 3-5 drops over the thyroid (lower front of the neck on both sides of the trachea), 1-3 times daily
VITA FLEX, apply 1-3 drops on the thyroid Vita Flex points of the feet (located on the inside edge of the ball of the foot, just below the base of the big toe.)

INGESTION:
CAPSULE, 00 size, 1 capsule twice a day

Dietary Supplementation:
Thyromin, VitaGreen, Sulfurzyme, Essential Omegas

TINNITIS (Ringing in Ears)

(See HEARING IMPAIRMENT)

TOOTHACHE

(See ORAL CARE)

TONSILLITIS

(See COLDS AND THROAT INFECTIONS)

TOXEMIA

(See INFECTION)

When toxins or bacteria begin to accumulate in the bloodstream, a condition called toxemia is created. When toxemia occurs during late pregnancy, it is referred to as "preeclampsia."

Single Oils:
Clove, tangerine, orange, cypress

Blends:
Citrus Fresh, Inner Child, Purification

EO Applications:
INGESTION:
> CAPSULE, 00 size, 1 capsule 2 times a day

Dietary Supplementation:
ICP, ComforTone, Exodus, Super C, Berry Young Juice, Essential Manna (rich in potassium).

NOTE: Best results are achieved by eliminating all sugar, white flour, breads, pasta, and fried foods.

TRAUMA (EMOTIONAL)

(See SHOCK)

Emotional trauma can be generated from events that involve loss, bereavement, accidents, or misfortunes. Essential oils, through their ability to tap the emotional and memory center of the brain, may facilitate the processing and release of emotional trauma in a way that minimizes psychological turmoil.

Blends:
Trauma Life, Hope, Forgiveness, Release, Envision, Valor

EO Applications:
TOPICAL:
> DILUTE 50-50, massage 2-4 drops to temples, forehead, crown and shoulders 1-3 times daily

INHALATION:
> DIRECT, 1-3 times daily as needed

Dietary Supplementation:
Essential Omegas, Super C, Mineral Essence

TUBERCULOSIS

(See also LUNG INFECTION)

Tuberculosis (TB) is a highly contagious lung disease caused by *Mycobacterium tuberculosis.* the germs are spread via coughs, sneezes, and physical contact. The most worrisome aspect of this disease is it latency. Those infected may harbor the germ for years, yet display no outward or visible signs of infection. However, when the immune systems become challenged or downregulated due to stress, candida, diabetes, corticosteroid use, or other factors, the bacteria can become reactivated and develop into full-blown TB.

Prior to the 1940's, tuberculosis was one of the leading causes of the death in the United States. After the introduction of anti-TB drugs following World War II, incidences of the disease dwindled. However, the incidence of TB has recently staged a surprising resurgence, with the number of TB cases increasing dramatically since 1984. In 1993 over 25,000 cases of TB were reported.

Because many essential oils have broad-spectrum antimicrobial properties, they can be diffused to prevent the spread of airborne bacteria like *Mycobacterium tuberculosis.* Essential oils and blends such as Thieves, Purification, Raven, R.C., and Sacred Mountain are extremely effective for killing this type of germs.

Many essential oils have also been shown to be immune-stimulating. Lemon oil has been shown to increase lymphocyte production—a pivotal part of the immune system.

Single Oils:
Ravensara, rosemary, lemon, cinnamon, thyme, sandalwood, *Eucalyptus radiata,* clove, oregano, mountain savory, peppermint, spearmint, myrtle, Idaho balsam fir

Blends:
Raven, R.C., Sacred Mountain, Thieves, ImmuPower, Inspiration

EO Applications:
INHALATION:
> DIFFUSION, 1 hour, twice a day and at night.
> DIRECT, 3-5 times daily

TOPICAL:
> DILUTE 50-50, apply 6-10 drops on chest and upper back 1-3 times daily
> COMPRESS, warm, on chest and upper back, twice daily

INGESTION:
> CAPSULE, 00 size, 1 capsule 3 times daily for 10 days

Dietary Supplementation:
ImmuPro, Super C Chewable, Exodus, Longevity Caps, VitaGreen, ImmuneTune, Cleansing Trio

Tuberculosis-specific regimen:

1. Alternate diffusing Raven and R.C. as often as possible during the day

2. Mix the following in 2 Tbsp. V-6 Oil Complex. Insert into rectum with bulb syringe and retain overnight. Do this nightly for 7 nights; rest for 4 nights; then repeat.
   - 2 drops sage
   - 4 drops myrrh
   - 5 drops clove
   - 6 drops ravensara
   - 15 drops frankincense

3. Put 20 drops Raven in a capsule and swallow 3 times daily for 10 days.

4. Rub 4-6 drops Thieves on the bottom of the feet nightly

5. Rub ImmuPower up the spine daily and apply as a compress on back and chest twice a day. Use Raindrop Technique.

6. Take 3-4 capsules Exodus 3 times daily for 21 days. Discontinue use for 7 days before resuming use.

TUMORS

(See CANCER)

TYPHOID FEVER

Typhoid fever is an infectious disease caused by a bacteria known as *Salmonella typhi*. Usually contracted through infected food or water, typhoid is common in lesser-developed countries.

Some people infected with typhoid fever display no visible symptoms of disease, while others become seriously ill. Both people who recover from typhoid fever and those who remain symptomless are carriers for the disease, and can infect others through the bacteria they shed in their feces.

To avoid contracting typhoid fever—especially when traveling overseas—it is essential to drink purified or distilled water and to thoroughly cook foods. Fresh vegetables can be carriers of the bacteria, especially if they have been irrigated with water that has come into contact with human waste.

Symptoms:
- Sustained, high fever (101° to 104° F).
- Stomach pains
- Headache
- Rash of reddish spots
- Impaired appetite
- Weakness

Single Oils:
Ravensara, cinnamon, cassia, peppermint, black pepper, mountain savory, clove, thyme

EO Applications:
TOPICAL:
DILUTE 50-50, massage 4-6 drops on lower abdomen, 2-4 times daily
INGESTION:
CAPSULE, 00 size, 1 capsule 2 times daily for 10 days

Dietary Supplementation:
ImmuPro

ULCERS (Stomach)

(See DIGESTIVE PROBLEMS)

URINARY TRACT/BLADDER INFECTION

(See also KIDNEY DISORDERS)

Infections and inflammation of the urinary tract are caused by bacteria that travel up the urethra. This disorder is more common in women than men because of the woman's shorter urethra. If the infection travels up the ureters and reaches the kidneys, kidney infection can result.

Symptoms:
- Frequent urge to urinate with only a small amount of urine coming out
- Strong smelling urine
- Blood in urine
- Burning or stinging during urination

Bladder infection (known as cystitis or interstitial cystitis) is marked by the following symptoms:

- Tenderness or chronic pain in bladder and pelvic area
- Frequent urge to urinate
- Pain intensity fluctuates as bladder fills or empties
- Symptoms worsen during menstruation

Single Oils:
Oregano, mountain savory, tea tree, thyme, cistus, juniper, rosemary, clove

Blends:
Di-Tone, EndoFlex, R.C., Melrose, Purification, Inspiration, Thieves

EO Applications:
INGESTION:
      CAPSULE, 0 size, 1 capsule 2 times daily
TOPICAL:
      COMPRESS, warm, over bladder, 1-2 times   daily

Dietary Supplementation:
K&B tincture, ImmuPro, AlkaLime

Use K&B tincture (2-3 droppers in distilled water) 3-6 times daily. K & B Tincture helps strengthen and tone weak bladder, kidneys, and urinary tract (see KIDNEY DISORDERS).

Take 1 tsp. of AlkaLime daily, in water only, 1 hour before or after meal.

UTERINE CANCER

(See CANCER)

VAGINAL YEAST INFECTION

(See FUNGAL INFECTIONS or ANTISEPTIC)

Vaginal yeast infections are usually caused from overgrowth of fungi like *Candida albicans*. These *naturally*-occurring intestinal yeast and fungi are normally kept under control by the immune system, but when excess sucrose is consumed or antibiotics are used, these organisms convert from relatively harmless yeast into an invasive, harmful fungus that secretes toxins as part of its life cycle.

Vaginal yeast infections are just one symptom of systemic fungal infestation. While the yeast infection can be treated locally, the underlying problem of systemic candidiasis may still remain unless specific dietary and health practices are used.

Single Oils:
Myrrh, mountain savory, oregano, tea tree, thyme

Blends:
Melrose, 3 Wise Men, Inspiration, Clara Derm

Topical Treatment:
Fresh Essence Plus

EO Applications:
RETENTION:
      TAMPON, 3 times a week, soaked in Fresh Essence Plus

VARICOSE VEINS (SPIDER VEINS)

(See CIRCULATION DISORDERS)

VASCULAR CLEANSING

(See HEAVY METALS and CIRCULATION DISORDERS)

VITILIGO

(See SKIN DISORDERS)

WARTS (GENITAL)

(See SEXUALLY TRANSMITTED DISEASES)

WEST NILE VIRUS

(See INSECT BITES)

WHOOPING COUGH

(See COLDS, FLU, or INFECTION)

WOUNDS, SCRAPES, OR CUTS

(See SKIN DISORDERS and ANTISEPTIC)

When selecting oils to for surface injuries, treat the whole person, not just the cut. Think through the cause and type of injury and select oils for each aspect of the trauma. For instance, a wound could encompass muscle damage, nerve damage, ligament damage, inflammation, infection, bone injury, fever, and possibly an emotion. Therefore, select an oil or blend that treats each of these.

Single Oils:
Lavender, tea tree, rosemary, *Eucalyptus globulus,* cypress, wintergreen, thyme, oregano, German chamomile, lavandin, mountain savory, peppermint

Blends:
Melrose, Purification, Thieves, 3 Wise Men

Topical Treatment:
Thieves Antiseptic Spray, LavaDerm Spray

Bruise and scrape blend (may be used on infants and children):
- 3 drop helichrysum
- 3 drop lavender

Infected cuts blend:
- 7 drops geranium
- 5 drops peppermint
- 10 drops tea tree
- 8 drops orange

EO Applications:
TOPICAL:
    DILUTE 50-50, apply 2-6 drops on location, 1-4 times daily as needed

NOTE: Peppermint may sting when applied to an open wound. To reduce discomfort, dilute with lavender oil or mix in a sealing ointment before applying. When applied to a wound or cut that has a scab, peppermint will soothe, cool, and reduce inflammation in damaged tissue.

Melaleuca alternifolia (Tea tree oil)

During World War II, melaleuca was found to have very strong antibacterial properties and worked well in preventing infection in open wounds. Melrose is a blend containing two types of melaleuca oil, making it an exceptional antiseptic and tissue regenerator.

To reduce bleeding

Single Oils:
Geranium, cypress, helichrysum, lemon, rose, rose hip seed

Blends:
Melrose, Thieves

Wound compress blend:
- 5 drops geranium
- 5 drops lemon
- 5 drops German chamomile

EO Applications:
TOPICAL:
    COMPRESS, cold, 1-2 times until bleeding stops

To reduce scarring:

Single Oils:
Lavender, frankincense, lemongrass, geranium, helichrysum, myrrh, rose hip seed

Blends:
Scar Prevention blend #1:
- 10 drops helichrysum
- 6 drops lavender
- 8 drops lemongrass
- 4 drops patchouli

Scar Prevention blend #2:
- 3 drops lavender
- 3 drops lemongrass
- 3 drops geranium

EO Applications:
TOPICAL:
    DILUTE 50-50, apply 2-4 drops on wound, 2-5 times daily

419

To promote healing:

Single Oils:
Lavender, patchouli, tea tree, neroli, myrrh, helichrysum, sandalwood, Idaho tansy

Blends:
Purification, Melrose

EO Applications:
TOPICAL:
>   DILUTE 50-50, apply 2-4 drops on wound 2-5 times daily.

To disinfect:

Single Oils:
Thyme, tea tree, mountain savory, oregano

Blends:
Melrose, Purification, Thieves, ImmuPower

Applications:
TOPICAL:
>   DILUTE 50-50, apply 2-4 drops on wound 2-5 times daily.

Topical Treatment:
Thieves Antiseptic Spray

First-Aid Spray

- 5 drops lavender
- 3 drops *Melaleuca alternifolia*
- 2 drops cypress

Mix above oils thoroughly in 1/2 teaspoon of salt. Add this to 8 ounces of distilled water and shake vigorously. Put in a spray bottle. Spray minor cuts and wounds before applying bandage. Repeat 2-3 times daily for 3 days. Complete the healing process by applying a drop or two of tea tree oil to the wound daily for the next few days.

WORMS

(See PARASITES)

WRINKLES

(See this heading under SKIN DISORDERS)

YEAST INFECTION

(See HORMONES, VAGINAL YEAST INFECTION, or ANTISEPTIC)

Bibliography

Achanzar WE et al. "Cadmium-induced malignant transformation of human prostate epithelial cells." *Cancer Res.* 2001 Jan 15;61(2):455-8.

Al-Awadi FM, et al. "Studies on the activity of individual plants of an antidiabetic plant mixture." *Acta Diabetol Lat.* 1987;24(1):37-41.

Alderman G, and Elmer H., "Inhibition of Growth and Aflatoxin Production of Aspergillus Parasiticus by Citrus Oils. Z. Leb." *Unt-Forsch* 1976: 353-58.

Aqel MB. "Relaxant effect of the volatile oil of Rosmarinus officinalis on tracheal smooth muscle." *J Ethnopharmacol.* 1991;33(1-2):57-62.

Aruna K., and Sivaramakrishnan V., "Anticarcinogenic Effects of Essential Oils from Cumin, Poppy, and Basil." *Phytotherapy Research* 1996, 577-79.

Aruna, K. and V.M. Sivaramakrishnan. "Anticarcinogenic Effects of the Essential Oils from Cumin, Poppy and Basil." Food Chem Toxicol. 1992;30(11):953-56.

Azizan A, et al. "Mutagenicity and antimutagenicity testing of six chemicals associated with the pungent properties of specific spices as revealed by the Ames Salmonella/microsomal assay." Arch Environ Contam Toxicol. 1995;28(2):248-58.

Barja de Quiroga G, et al. Antioxidant defences and peroxidation in liver and brain of aged rats. Biochemical Journal 272 (1990), 247-250.

Bassett IB, et al. "A comparative study of tea-tree oil versus benzoylperoxide in the treatment of acne." Med J Aust. 1990;153(8):455-8.

Becker, M.D., Robert O. The Body Electric. New York: Wm. Morrow, 1985.

Belaiche, M.D., Paul. Traité de Phytothérapie Et D'Aromathérapie. Paris: Maloine, 1979.

Belvi, Viktor. Aromatherapy. New York: Avon Books, 1993.

Benencia F, et al. "Antiviral activity of sandalwood oil against herpes simplex viruses-1 and -2." Phytomedicine. 1999;6(2):119-23

Bernacchi F et al., In vivo cytogenetic effects of natural humic acid. Mutagenesis. 1996 Sep;11(5):467-9.

Bernardis LL, et al. "The lateral hypothalamic area revisited: ingestive behavior." Neurosci Biobehav Rev. 20(2):189-287 (1996).

Bilgrami KS, et al. "Inhibition of aflatoxin production & growth of Aspergillus flavus by eugenol & onion & garlic extracts." Indian J Med Res. 1992;96:171-5.

Bourre et al., Function of dietary polyunsaturated fatty acids in the nervous system. Prostoglandins, leukotrienes, and essential fatty acids 48 (1993): 5-15.

Bradshaw RH, et al. "Effects of lavender straw on stress and travel sickness in pigs." J Altern Complement Med. 1998;4(3):271-5.

Brodal A. Neurological Anatomy in Relation to Clinical Medicine. New York: Oxford University Press, 1981.

Buchbauer G, et al. "Aromatherapy: evidence for sedative effects of the essential oil of lavender after inhalation." Z Naturforsch [C]. 1991;46(11-12):1067-72.

Burrows, Stanley. Healing for the Age of Enlightenment. Kailua, Hawaii, 1976.

Cai and Wu .Compounds from Syzygium aromaticum possessing growth inhibitory activity against oral pathogens. J Nat Prod. 1996 Oct;59(10):987-90.

Calabrese V, Oxidative stress and antioxidants at skin biosurface: a novel antioxidant from lemon oil capable of inhibiting oxidative damage to the skin. Drugs Exp Clin Res. 1999;25(6):281-7.

Cao G et al., Increases in human plasma antioxidant capacity after consumption of controlled diets high in fruit and vegetables. Am J Clin Nutr. 1998 Nov;68(5):1081-7.

Cao G, et al, Antioxidant capacity in different tissues of young and old rats. Proceedings of the society for Experimental Biology and Medicine 211(1996), 359-365.

Cao G, et al. Automated assay of oxygen radical absorbance capacity with the COBAS FARA II. Clin Chem. 1995 Dec;41(12 Pt 1):1738-44.

Carson CF, et al. "Antimicrobial activity of the major components of the essential oil of Melaleuca alternifolia." J Appl Bacteriol. 1995;78(3):264-9.

Carson et al. Antimicrobial activity of the major components of the essential oil of Melaleuca alternifolia. J Appl Bacteriol. 1995 Mar;78(3):264-9.

Chao et al., Seventy-four Essential Oils Against Streptococcus pneumoniae. Unpublished research, 1998.

Chao, et al., Screening for Inhibitory Activity of Essential Oils on Selected Bacteria, Fungi, and Viruses. Journal of Essential Oil Research, 1997.

Chopra, M.D., Deepak. Quantum Healing. New York: Bantam Books, 1989.

Compendium of Olfactory Research. Edited by Avery N. Gilbert. Dubuque, IA: Kendall Hunt Publishing, 1995.

Concha JM, et al. 1998 William J. Stickel Bronze Award. "Antifungal activity of Melaleuca alternifolia (tea-tree) oil against various pathogenic organisms." J Am Podiatr Med Assoc. 1998;88(10): 489-92

Cornwell S, et al. "Lavender oil and perineal repair." Mod Midwife 1995;5(3):31-3.

Covello et. al. Determination of eugenol in the essence of "Eugenia caryophyllata". Titration in non-aqueous solvent and comparison with other methods of analysis. Boll Chim Farm. 1966 Nov;105(11):799-806.

Cozzi R et al., Desmutagenic activity of natural humic acids: inhibition of mitomycin C and maleic hydrazide mutagenicity. Mutat Res. 1993 Mar;299(1):37-44.

Cox et al. The mode of antimicrobial action of the essential oil of Melaleuca alternifolia (tea tree oil). J Appl Microbiol. 2000 Jan;88(1):170-5.

Crowell P. Prevention and therapy of cancer by dietary monoterpenes. J Nutr. 1999 Mar;129(3):775S-778S.

Dakhil MA, Morsy TA. The larvicidal activities of the peel oils of three citrus fruits against Culex pipiens. J Egypt Soc Parasitol. 1999 Aug;29(2):347-52.Dalvi et al. Effect of peppermint oil on gastric emptying in man: a preliminary study using a radiolabelled solid test meal.Indian J Physiol Pharmacol. 1991 Jul;35(3):212-4.

Darom, David. Beautiful Plants of the Bible. Israel: Palphot, Ltd.

Deans SG, et al, Natural antioxidants from aromatic and medicinal plants. In Role of Free Radicals in Biological Systems, pp. 159-165 (1993a) [J Feher, A Blazovics, B Matkovics and M Mezes, editors]. Budapest: Akademiai Kiado.

Delaveau P, et al. "Neuro-depressive properties of essential oil of lavender." C R Seances Soc Biol Fil. 1989;183(4):342-8.

Dember WN, et al., Olfactory Stimulation and Sustained Attention, Compendium of Olfactory, (Avery N. Gilbert, Editor) pp. 39-46.

Didry N, et al. "Activity of thymol, carvacrol, cinnamaldehyde and eugenol on oral bacteria." Pharm Acta Helv. 1994;69(1):25-8.

Diego MA, et al. "Aromatherapy positively affects mood, EEG patterns of alertness and math computations." Int J Neurosci. 1998 Dec;96 (3-4):217-24.

Dolara P, et al. "Analgesic effects of myrrh." Nature. 1996 Jan 4;379(6560):29.

Doss, Besada. The Story of Abu Simbel. Essex, England: Longman Group UK Limited, 1973.

Dunn C, et al. "Sensing an improvement: an experimental study to evaluate the use of aromatherapy, massage and periods of rest in an intensive care unit." J Adv Nurs. 1995;21(1):34-40.

Dwivedi C, et al. "Chemopreventive effects of sandalwood oil on skin papillomas in mice." Eur J Cancer Prev. 1997;6(4):399-401.

Elisabetsky et al. Anticonvulsant properties of linalool in glutamate-related seizure models. Phytomedicine. 1999 May;6(2):107-13.

Elkins Rita, "Blue/Green Algae." Pleasant Grove, UT. 1995.

Elson CE, et al. "Impact of lemongrass oil, an essential oil, on serum cholesterol." Lipids. 1989;24(8):677-9.

Fang, H.J., et al. "Studies on the chemical components and anti-tumour action of the volatile oils from Pelargonium graveoleus." Yao Hsueh Hsueh Pao. 1989;24(5):366-71.

Faoagali JL, et al. "Antimicrobial effects of melaleuca oil." Burns. 1998;24(4):383. No abstract available.

Farag et. al. Acute hepatic damage in rats impairs metharbital metabolism. Pharmacology. 1987;34(4):181-91.

Farag et al., Antioxidant activity of some spice essential oils on linoleic acid oxidation in aqueous media. JAOCS June 1989;66: 792-799.

Farag et al., Inhibitory effects of individual and mixed pairs of essential oils on the oxidation and hydrolysis of cottonseed oil and butter. FASC, 1989; 40: 275-279.

Farag et al., Safety evaluation of thyme and clove essential oils as natural antioxidants. Afr J Agr Sci. 1991;18: 169-175,

Farag, Ph.D., Radwan S. "Safety Evaluation of Thyme and Clove Essential Oils as Natural Antioxidants." African Journal of Agricultural Sciences, Vol. 18, No. 1. Gisa, Egypt: Cairo University, 1991.

Fleming, T., Ed. PDR for Herbal Medicines, Medical Economics Company, Inc., Montvale, NJ (1998).

Fyfe L, et al. "Inhibition of Listeria monocytogenes and Salmonella enteriditis by combinations of plant oils and derivatives of benzoic acid: the development of synergistic antimicrobial combinations." Int J Antimicrob Agents. 1997;9(3):195-9.

Garrison, Omar. Tantra: The Yoga of Sex. New York: Harmony Books, 1964.

Gattefossé, René-Maurice. Gattefossé's Aromatherapy. Saffron Walden, UK: C.W. Daniel & Co., 1993.

Ghelardini et al. Local anaesthetic activity of the essential oil of Lavandula angustifolia. Planta Med. 1999 Dec;65(8):700-3

Gobel et al. Effect of peppermint and eucalyptus oil preparations on neurophysiological and experimental algesimetric headache parameters. Cephalalgia. 1994 Jun;14(3):228-34; 182.

Gobel H, et al. "Effect of peppermint and eucalyptus oil preparations on neurophysiological and experimental algesimetric headache parameters." Cephalalgia. 1994; 14(3):228-34.

Grassmann J, Schneider D, Weiser D, Elstner EF. Antioxidative effects of lemon oil and its components on copper induced oxidation of low density lipoprotein. Arzneimittelforschung. 2001 Oct;51(10):799-805.

Guenther, Ernest. The Essential Oils. Florida: Malabar, 1950.

Guillemain J, et al. "Neurodepressive effects of the essential oil of Lavandula angustifolia Mill." Ann Pharm Fr. 1989;47(6):337-43.

Gumbel, D. Principles of Holistic Therapy with Herbal Essences, Haug International, Brussels, Belgium (1993)

Halliwell B & Gutteridge JMC, Free Radicals in Biology and Medicine, 2nd Edition. (1989), Oxford: Clarendon Press.

Hakim IA, Harris RB, Ritenbaugh C. Citrus peel use is associated with reduced risk of squamous cell carcinoma of the skin. Nutr Cancer. 2000;37(2):161-8.

Hammer KA, et al. "In vitro susceptibilities of lactobacilli and organisms associated with bacterial vaginosis to Melaleuca alternifolia (tea tree) oil." Antimicrob Agents Chemother. 1999;43(1):196.

Hammer KA, et al. "Susceptibility of transient and commensal skin flora to the essential oil of Melaleuca alternifolia (tea tree oil)." Am J Infect Control. 1996;24(3):186-9.

Harmon, D, Aging: a theory based on free radical and radiation chemistry. J. Gerontology 11, (1956): 298-300.

Harmon, D, Free radical theory of aging: Effect of free radical inhibitors on the mortality rate of male LAFmice. J. Gerontology 23 (1968): 476-482.

Harmon, D, Free radical theory of aging: Effect of the amount and degree of unsaturation of dietary fat on mortality rate. J. Gerontology 26 (1971): 451-457.

Hasan HA, et al. "Inhibitory effect of spice oils on lipase and mycotoxin production." Zentralbl Mikrobiol. 1993;148(8):543-8.

Hausen BM, et al. "Comparative studies of the sensitizing capacity of drugs used in herpes simplex." Derm Beruf Umwelt. 1986;34(6):163-70.

Hay IC, et al. "Randomized trial of aromatherapy. Successful treatment for alopecia areata." Arch Dermatol. 1998; 134(11):1349-52.

Hayes AJ, Markovic B. Toxicity of Australian essential oil Backhousia citriodora (Lemon myrtle). Part 1. Antimicrobial activity and in vitro cytotoxicity. Food Chem Toxicol. 2002 Apr;40(4):535-43.

Hayflick, L. How and Why We Age. Ballantine Books, New York, 1994.

Hirsch, Alan. "Inhalation of 2 acetylpyridine for weight reduction." Chemical Senses 18:570 (1993).

Hirsch, Alan. A Scentsational Guide to Weight Loss. Rockport, MA: Element, 1997.

Hoffer BJ, Olson L, and Palmer MR Toxic effects of lead in the developing nervous system: in oculo experimental models. Environ Health Perspect. 1987 Oct;74:169-75.

Hudak A et al., The favorable effect of humic acid based complex micro-element preparations in cadmium exposure. Orv Hetil. 1997 Jun 1;138 (22):1411-6.

Inhibition of growth and aflatoxin production of Aspergillus parasiticus by citrus oils. Z Lebensm Unters Forsch. 1976 Apr 28;160(4):353-8.

Inouye S, et al. "Antisporulating and respiration-inhibitory effects of essential oils on filamentous fungi." Mycoses. 1998;41(9-10):403-10.

Inouye S, et al., Inhibitory effect of essential oils on apical growth of Aspergillus fumigatus by vapour contact. Mycoses. 2000;43(1-2):17-23.

Inouye S, Takizawa T, Yamaguchi H. Antibacterial activity of essential oils and their major constituents against respiratory tract pathogens by gaseous contact. J Antimicrob Chemother. 2001 May;47(5):565-73.

Jayashree T, et al. "Antiaflatoxigenic activity of eugenol is due to inhibition of lipid peroxidation." Lett Appl Microbiol. 1999; 28(3):179-83.

Jones MM and Basinger MA. Restrictions on the applicability of mixed ligand chelate therapy (MLC) in acute cadmium intoxication. Res Commun Chem Pathol Pharmacol. 1979 Jun;24(3):525-31.

Juergens UR, et al. "The anti-inflammatory activity of L-menthol compared to mint oil in human monocytes in vitro: a novel perspective for its therapeutic use in inflammatory diseases." Eur J Med Res. 1998; 3(12):539-45.

Kaplan RJ & Greenwood CE, Dietary saturated fatty acids and brain function. Neurochemistry Research 23, (1989)615-626.

Kim HM, et al. "Lavender oil inhibits immediate-type allergic reaction in mice and rats." J Pharm Pharmacol. 1999;51(2):221-6.

Komori T, Fujiwara R, Tanida M, Nomura J. Application of fragrances to treatments for depression Nihon Shinkei Seishin Yakurigaku Zasshi. 1995 Feb;15(1):39-42

Kucera LS, et al. "Antiviral activities of extracts of the lemon balm plant." Ann NY Acad Sci. 1965 Jul 30;130(1):474-82.

Kulieva ZT. "Analgesic, hypotensive and cardiotonic action of the essential oil of the thyme growing in Azerbaijan." Vestn Akad Med Nauk SSSR. 1980;(9):61-3.

Lachowicz KJ, et al. "The synergistic preservative effects of the essential oils of sweet basil (Ocimum basilicum L.) against acid-tolerant food microflora." Lett Appl Microbiol. 1998;26(3):209-14.

LaDoux, M.D., Joseph. Rationalizing Thoughtless Emotions. Insight, Sept. 1989.

LaLonde RT and Xie S. Glutathione and N-acetylcysteine inactivations of mutagenic 2(5H)-furanones from the chlorination of humics in water. Chem Res Toxicol. 1993 Jul-Aug;6(4): 445-51. Nature. 1978 Sep 28;275(5678):311-3.

Lamptey MS & Walker BL, A possible dietary role for linolenic acid in the development of the young rat. Journal of Nutrition 106, (1976) 86-93.

Lantry LE, et al. "Chemopreventive effect of perillyl alcohol on 4-(methylnitrosamino)-1-(3-pyridyl)-1-butanone induced tumorigenesis in (C3H/HeJ X A/J)F1 mouse lung." J Cell Biochem Suppl. 1997;27:20-5.

Larrondo JV, et al. "Antimicrobial activity of essences from labiates." Microbios. 1995; 82(332): 171-2.

Lis-Balchin, M., et al. "Antimicrobial activity of Pelargonium essential oils added to a quiche filling as a model food system." Lett Appl Microbiol. 1998;27(4):207-10.

Lis-Balchin, M., et al. "Comparative antibacterial effects of novel Pelargonium essential oils and solvent extracts." Lett Appl Microbiol. 1998;27(3): 135-41.

Lopez-Bote et. al. Effect of dietary administration of oil extracts from rosemary and sage on lipid oxidation in broiler meat. Br Poult Sci. 1998 May;39(2):235-40.

Lorenzetti BB, et al. "Myrcene mimics the peripheral analgesic activity of lemongrass tea." J Ethnopharmacol. 1991;34(1):43-8.

Mahmood N, et al. "The anti-HIV activity and mechanisms of action of pure compounds isolated from Rosa damascena." Biochem Biophys Res Commun. 1996;229(1):73-9.

Mailhebiau, Philippe. La Nouvelle Aromathérapie. Editions. France: Jakin, 1994.

Mangena T, et al. "Comparative evaluation of the antimicrobial activities of essential oils of Artemisia afra, Pteronia incana and Rosmarinus officinalis on selected bacteria and yeast strains." Lett Appl Microbiol. 1999;28(4):291-6.

Masquelier, J. Radical Scavenging Effect of Proanthocyanidins. Paris, 1986.

Maury, Marguerite. The Secret and Life of Youth. Saffon Waldon, UK: C.W. Daniels & Co., 1995.

McGuffin, M., et al. Botanical Safety Handbook, CRC Press, Boca Raton, FL (1997)

Meeker HG, et al. "The antibacterial action of eugenol, thyme oil, and related essential oils used in dentistry." Compendium. 1988;9(1):32, 34-5, 38 passim.

Meunier, Christiane. Lavandes & Lavandins. Aix-en-Provence, France: Chaudoreille, 1985.

Michie, C.A., et al. "Frankincense and myrrh as remedies in children." J R Soc Med. 1991;84(10): 602-5.

Miltner et al. Emotional qualities of odors and their influence on the startle reflex in humans. Psychophysiology. 1994 Jan;31(1):107-10.

Miyake Y et al., Identification of coumarins from lemon fruit (Citrus limon) as inhibitors of in vitro tumor promotion and superoxide and nitric oxide generation. J Agric Food Chem. 1999 Aug;47(8):3151-7.

Modgil R, et al. "Efficacy of mint and eucalyptus leaves on the physicochemical characteristics of stored wheat against insect infestation." Nahrung. 1998;42(5):304-8.

Moleyar V, et al. "Antibacterial activity of essential oil components." Int J Food Microbiol. 1992;16(4): 337-42.

Momchilova, A. M. 330 Years of Bulgarian Rose Oil. Sofia, Bulgaria, 1994.

Montagna, F. J. HDR Herbal Desk Reference Kendall/Hunt Publishing Company, Dubuque, IA (1979).

Motomura N, Sakurai A, Yotsuya Y. Reduction of mental stress with lavender odorant. Percept Mot Skills. 2001 Dec;93(3):713-8.

Murray, M. Encyclopedia of Nutritional Supplements, Prima Publishing, Rocklin, CA (1996).

Nagababu E, et al. "The protective effects of eugenol on carbon tetrachloride induced hepatotoxicity in rats." Free Radic Res. 1995;23(6):617-27.

Naidu KA. "Eugenol--an inhibitor of lipoxygenase-dependent lipid peroxidation." Prostaglandins Leukot Essent Fatty Acids. 1995;53(5):381-3.

Nakamoto K, et al. "In vitro effectiveness of mouthrinses against Candida albicans." Int J Prosthodont. 1995;8(5):486-9.

Nasel, C. et al. "Functional imaging of effects of fragrances on the human brain after prolonged inhalation." Chemical Senses. 1994;19(4):359-64

Nenoff P, et al. "Antifungal activity of the essential oil of Melaleuca alternifolia (tea tree oil) against pathogenic fungi in vitro." Skin Pharmacol. 1996;9(6):388-94.

Neuringer M & Connor WE, N-3 fatty acids in the brain and retina: evidence for their essentiality. Nutrition Reviews 44, 285-294.

Niazi, H. The Egyptian Prescription. Cairo, Egypt: Elias Modern Press, 1988.

Nikolaevskii VV, et al. "Effect of essential oils on the course of experimental atherosclerosis." Patol Fiziol Eksp Ter. 1990; (5):52-3.

Nishijima H, et al. "Mechanisms mediating the vasorelaxing action of eugenol, a pungent oil, on rabbit arterial tissue." Jpn J Pharmacol. 1999 Mar;79(3):327-34.

Nordenstrom, Bjorn. Biologically Closed Circuits. Sweden.

Okuyama H, Minimum requirements of n-3 and n-6 essential fatty acids for the function of the central nervous system and for the prevention of chronic disease. Proceedings of the Society for Experimental Biology and Medicine 200, (1992) 174-176.

Olson L, et al., Some toxic effects of lead, other metals and antibacterial agents on the nervous system--animal experiment models. Acta Neurol Scand Suppl. 1984;100:77-87.

Osterberg R and Mortensen K. The growth of fractal humic acids: cluster correlation and gel formation. Radiat Environ Biophys. 1994;33(3):269-76.

Panizzi L, et al. "Composition and antimicrobial properties of essential oils of four Mediterranean Lamiaceae." J Ethnopharmacol. 1993;39(3):167-70.

Pattnaik S, et al. "Antibacterial and antifungal activity of ten essential oils in vitro." Microbios. 1996;86(349):237-46.

Pedersen, M. Nutritional Herbology, A Reference Guide to Herbs, Wendell W. Whitman Company, Warsaw, IN (1998)

Pénoël, Daniel. Natural Home Health Care Using Essential Oils. Salem, UT: Essential Science Publishing, 1998.

Pénoël, M.D., Daniel and Pénoël, R.-M., Natural Home Health Care Using Essential Oils. La Drome, France: Editions Osmobiose, 1988.

Pénoël, M.D., Daniel and Pierre Franchomme. L'aromathérapie exactement. Limoges, France: Jollois, 1990.

Plato. Chronicles 156 E.

Pourgholami M.H. et.al. Evaluation of the anticonvulsant activity of the essential oil of Eugenia caryophyllata in male mice. J Ethnopharmacol. 1999 Feb;64(2):167-71.

Privitera, James. Silent Clots. Covina, CA: 1996

Ramadan W. et. al. Oil of bitter orange: new topical antifungal agent. Int J Dermatol. 1996 Jun;35(6):448-9.

Recsan Z, et al, Effect of essential oils on the lipids of the retina in the aging rat: a possible therapeutic use. J Ess Oil Res 9, (1997) 53-56.

Reddy AC, et al. "Effect of curcumin and eugenol on iron-induced hepatic toxicity in rats." Toxicology 1996;107(1):39-45.

Reddy AC, et al. "Studies on anti-inflammatory activity of spice principles and dietary n-3 polyunsaturated fatty acids on carrageenan-induced inflammation in rats." Ann Nutr Metab. 1994;38(6): 349-58.

Reddy BS, et al. "Chemoprevention of colon carcinogenesis by dietary perillyl alcohol." Cancer Res. 1997;57(3):420-5.

Restick, M.D., Richard. The Brain. New York: Random House, 1991.

Riede UN et al., Collagen stabilization induced by natural humic substances. Arch Orthop Trauma Surg. 1992;111(5):259-64.

Rompelberg CJ, et al. "Antimutagenicity of eugenol in the rodent bone marrow micronucleus test." Mutat Res. 1995;346(2):69-75.

Rompelberg CJ, et al. "Effect of short-term dietary administration of eugenol in humans" Hum Exp Toxicol. 1996;15(2):129-35.\

Rompelberg et al. Antimutagenicity of eugenol in the rodent bone marrow micronucleus test. Mutat Res. 1995 Feb;346(2):69-75.

Rotstein et al., Effects of aging on the composition and metabolism of docosahexaenoate-containing lipids of retina. Lipids. 1987 Apr;22(4):253-60.

Russin, et al. Inhibition of rat mammary carcinogenesis by monoterpenoids. Carcinogenesis. 1989 Nov;10(11):2161-4.

Ryan PB, Huet N, and MacIntosh DL. Longitudinal Investigation of Exposure to Arsenic, Cadmium, and Lead in Drinking Water. Environ Health Perspect. 2000 Aug;108(8):731-735.

Sato T et al., Adsorption of mutagens by humic acid. Sci Total Environ. 1987 Apr;62:305-10. Sato T et al., Mechanism of the desmutagenic effect of humic acid. Mutat Res. 1987 Feb;176(2):199-204.

Ryman, Daniele. Aromatherapy: The Complete Guide to Plant and Flower Essences for Health and Beauty. New York: Bantam Books, 1993.

Saeed SA, et al. "Antithrombotic activity of clove oil." JPMA J Pak Med Assoc. 1994;44(5):112-5.

Safe Shopper's Bible: A Consumer's Guide to Nontoxic Household Products, Cosmetics, and Food." Macmillan, New York, NY (1995).

Samman MA, et al. "Mint prevents shamma-induced carcinogenesis in hamster cheek pouch." Carcinogenesis. 1998;19(10):1795-801.

Schrauzer GN. Anticarcinogenic effects of selenium. Cell Mol Life Sci. 2000 Dec;57(13-14):1864-73.

Schreuder M. Private communication with Brunswick Laboratories, Warcham, MA.
March 21, 2001.

Schubert J and Derr SK. Mixed ligand chelate therapy for plutonium and cadmium poisoning.

Schubert J, Riley EJ, and Tyler SA. Combined effects in toxicology-a rapid systematic testing procedure: cadmium, mercury, and lead. J Toxicol Environ Health. 1978 Sep-Nov;4(5-6):763-76.

Scott BL & Bazan NG, Membrane docosahexaenoate is supplied to the developing brain and retina by the liver. Proceedings of the National Academy of sciences USA 86, (1989) 2903-2907.

Shapiro S, et al. "The antimicrobial activity of essential oils and essential oil components towards oral bacteria." Oral Microbiol Immunol. 1994;9(4): 202-8.

Sharma JN, et al. "Suppressive effects of eugenol and ginger oil on arthritic rats." Pharmacology. 1994;49(5):314-8.

Shirota S, et al. "Tyrosinase inhibitors from crude drugs." Biol Pharm Bull. 1994; 17(2):266-9.

Siurein S A. Effects of essential oil on lipid peroxidation and lipid metabolism in patients with chronic bronchitis]. Klin Med (Mosk). 1997;75 (10):43-5.

Socci DJ, et al, Chronic antioxidant treatment improves the cognitive performance in aged rats. Brain Research 693, (1995) 88-94.

Srivastava KC. "Antiplatelet principles from a food spice clove." Prostaglandins Leukot Essent Fatty Acids. 1993;48(5):363-72.

Steinman, David and Samuel S. Epstein. "The Safe Shopper's Bible: A Consumer's Guide to Nontoxic Household Products, Cosmetics, and Food" MacMillan, New York, NY (1995)

Steinmetz et. al.,Transmission and scanning electronmicroscopy study of the action of sage and rosemary essential oils and eucalyptol on Candida albicans. Mycoses. 1988 Jan;31(1):40-51.

Stubbs CD & Smith AD, The modification of mammalian membrane polyunsturated fatty acid composition in relation to membrane fluidity and function. Biochimica et Biophysica Acta 779, (1984)89-137.

Sukumaran K, et al. "Inhibition of tumour promotion in mice by eugenol." Indian J Physiol Pharmacol. 1994;38(4):306-8.

Syed TA, et al. "Treatment of toenail onychomycosis with 2% butenafine and 5% Melaleuca alternifolia (tea tree) oil in cream." Trop Med Int Health. 1999;4(4):284-7.

Sysoev NP. "The effect of waxes from essential-oil plants on the dehydrogenase activity of the blood neutrophils in mucosal trauma of the mouth." Stomatologiia 1991;70(1):12-3.

Takacsova M, et al. "Study of the antioxidative effects of thyme, sage, juniper and oregano." Nahrung. 1995;39(3):241-3.

Tantaoui-Elaraki A, et al. "Inhibition of growth and aflatoxin production in Aspergillus parasiticus by essential oils of selected plant materials." J Environ Pathol Toxicol Oncol. 1994;13(1):67-72.

Terpstra AH, Lapre JA, de Vries HT, Beynen AC.The hypocholesterolemic effect of lemon peels, lemon pectin, and the waste stream material of lemon peels in hybrid F1B hamsters. Eur J Nutr. 2002 Feb;41(1):19-26.

The Bible. King James Version. Books from Old and New Testament.

Tisserand, R. and T. Balacs Essential Oil Safety, Churchill Livingstone, New York, NY (1996).

Tiwari BK, et al. "Evaluation of insecticidal, fumigant and repellent properties of lemongrass oil." Indian J Exp Biol. 1966;4(2):128-9.

Tovey ER, et al. "A simple washing procedure with eucalyptus oil for controlling house dust mites and their allergens in clothing and bedding." J Allergy Clin Immunol. 1997; 100(4):464-6.

Tyler, V. E. Herbs of Choice Pharmaceutical Products Press, Binghamton, NY (1994).

Tyler, V. E. The Honest Herbal, Lubrect & Cramer, Ltd., Port Jervis, NY (1995).

Ulmer et. al., [Chronic obstructive bronchitis. Effect of Gelomyrtol forte in a placebo-controlled double-blind study]. Fortschr Med. 1991 Sep 20;109(27):547-50.

Unnikrishnan MC, et al. "Tumour reducing and anticarcinogenic activity of selected spices." Cancer Lett. 1990;51(1):85-9.

Valnet, Jean. Robert Tisserand, ed. "The Practice of Aromatherapy." Healing Arts Press, Rochester, VT (1990).

Veal L. The potential effectiveness of essential oils as a treatment for headlice, Pediculus humanus capitis. Complement Ther Nurs Midwifery. 1996 Aug;2(4):97-101.

Vernet-Maury E, et al. "Basic emotions induced by odorants: a new approach based on autonomic pattern results." J Auton Nerv Syst. 1999;75 (2-3): 176-83.

Visser SA. Some biological effects of humic acids in the rat. Acta Biol Med Ger. 1973;31(4):569-81.

Visser SA. Effect of humic substances on mitochondrial respiration and oxidative phosphorylation. Sci Total Environ. 1987 Apr;62:347-54.

Wagner J, et al. "Beyond benzodiazepines: alternative pharmacologic agents for the treatment of insomnia." Ann Pharmacother. 1998;32(6):680-91.

Wahnon R, et al, Age and membrane fluidity. Mechanisms of Aging and Development 50, (1989) 249-255.

Wan J, et al. "The effect of essential oils of basil on the growth of Aeromonas hydrophila and Pseudomonas fluorescens." J Appl Microbiol. 1998;84(2):152-8.

Wang, L.G., et al. "Determination of DNA topoisomerase II activity from L1210 cells--a target for screening antitumor agents." Chung Kuo Yao Li Hsueh Pao. 1991;12(2):108-14.

Wattenberg L.W. et. al. Inhibitory effects of 5-(2-pyrazinyl)-4-methyl-1,2-dithiol-3-thione (Oltipraz) on carcinogenesis induced by benzo[a]pyrene, diethylnitrosamine and uracil mustard. Carcinogenesis. 1986 Aug;7(8):1379-81.

Weyers W, et al. "Skin absorption of volatile oils. Pharmacokinetics." Pharm Unserer Zeit. 1989; 18(3):82-6.

Wie MB, et al. "Eugenol protects neuronal cells from excitotoxic and oxidative injury in primary cortical cultures." Neurosci Lett. 1997: 4;225(2):93-6.

Yamada K, et al. "Anticonvulsive effects of inhaling lavender oil vapour." Biol Pharm Bull. 1994;17(2):359-60.

Yamamoto N, et al, Effects of dietary alpha-linolenate/linolenate balance of brain lipid composition and learning ability of rats. Journal of Lipid Research 28, (1987) 144-151.

Yamasaki K, et al. "Anti-HIV-1 activity of herbs in Labiatae." Biol Pharm Bull. 1998;21(8):829-33.

Yang, K.K. et al., "Antiemetic principles of Pogostemon cablin (Blanco) Benth." Phytomedicine 1999, 6(2): 89-93.

Youdim KA, et al. "Beneficial effects of thyme oil on age-related changes in the phospholipid C20 and C22 polyunsaturated fatty acid composition of various rat tissues." Biochim Biophys Acta. 1999;1438(1): 140-6.

Yokota H, et al., Suppressed mutagenicity of benzo[a]pyrene by the liver S9 fraction and microsomes from eugenol-treated rats. Mutat Res. 1986 Dec;172(3):231-6.

Youdim KA, Deans SG et al., Beneficial effects of thyme oil on age-related changes in the phospholipid C20 and C22 polyunsaturated fatty acid composition of various rat tissues. Biochim Biophys Acta. 1999 Apr 19;1438(1):140-6.

Youdim KA, Deans SG., Dietary supplementation of thyme (Thymus vulgaris L.) essential oil during the lifetime of the rat: its effects on the antioxidant status in liver, kidney and heart tissues. Mech Aging Dev. 1999 Sep 8;109(3):163-75.

Youdim KA, et al., Effect of thyme oil and thymol dietary supplementation on the antioxidant status and fatty acid composition of the aging rat brain. Br J Nutr. 2000 Jan;83(1):87-93.

Young, D. Gary. An Introduction to Young Living Essential Oils. Payson, UT, 2001.

Young, Robert O. Sick and Tired. Alpine, UT, 1977.

Yousef, R.T. and G.G. Tawil. "Antimicrobial activity of volatile oils." Pharmazie 1980; 35(11);798-701

Zanker KS, et al. "Evaluation of surfactant-like effects of commonly used remedies for colds." Respiration. 1980;39(3):150-7.

Zheng GQ, et al. Sesquiterpenes from clove (Eugenia caryophyllata) as potential anticarcinogenic agents. J Nat Prod. 1992 Jul;55(7):999-1003.

APPENDIX A

Examples of AFNOR /ISO Standards

Clary sage

AFNOR/ISO European and World Standards
for Therapeutic-Grade
Salvia sclarea
Gas Chromatograph profile 4.10

CONSTITUENTS	Traditional	Crushed Green
Linalyl acetate		
min %	62	56
max %	78	70.5
Linalol		
min %	6.5	13
max %	13.5	24
Sclareol		
min %	.4	.4
max %	2.6	2.6
δ-germacrene		
min %	1.5	1.2
max %	12	7.5
α-terpineol		
min %	traces	1
max %	1.2	5

Clove

AFNOR/ISO Standards for Therapeutic-Grade
Syzygium aromaticum
Gas Chromatograph profile 4.8

CONSTITUENTS	Min %	Max %
Eugenol	80	92
B-caryophyllene	4	17
Eugenyl acetate	.2	4

Basil

AFNOR/ISO Standards for Therapeutic-Grade
Basilicum ocimum
Gas Chromatograph profile 4.8

CONSTITUENTS	Min %	Max %
Methyl chavicol	75	85
1,8 cineol	1	3.5
Trans-beta ocimene	.9	2.8
Linalol	.50	.30
Methyl eugenol	.3	2.5
Terpinen-4-ol	.20	.60
Camphor	.15	.50

Cypress

AFNOR/ISO Standards for Therapeutic-Grade
Cupressus sempervirens
Gas Chromatograph profile 4.11

CONSTITUENTS	Min %	Max %
α-pinene	40	65
δ-3-carene	12	25
limonene	1.8	5
α-Terpenyl acetate	1	4
Myrcene	1	3.5
Cedrol	.8	7
β-pinene	.5	3
D-germacrene	.5	3
Terpinen-4-ol	.2	2

Lavender

AFNOR/ISO Standards for Therapeutic-Grade

Lavandula angustifolia

Gas Chromatograph profile 4.10

CONSTITUENTS	Min %	Max %
Linalol	25	38
Linalyl acetate	25	45
cis-β-ocimene	4	10
trans-β-ocimene	1.5	6
terpinen-4-ol	2	6
Lavendulyl acetate	2	—
Lavendulol	.3	—
β-phellandrene	traces	.5
α-terpineol	—	1
Octanone-3	traces	2
Camphor	traces	.5
Limonene	—	.5
1,8 cineole	—	1

Roman chamomile

AFNOR/ISO Standards for Therapeutic-Grade

Chamaemelum nobilis

Gas Chromatograph profile 4.10

CONSTITUENTS	Min %	Max %
Isobutyl angelate + Isoamyl methacrylate	30	45
Isoamyl angelate	12	22
Methyl allyl angelate	6	10
2-methyl butyl angelate	3	7
Isoamyl isobutyrate	3	5
Trans-pino-carveol	2	5
Isobutyl n-butyrate	2	9
α-pinene	1.5	5
Pinocarvone	1.3	4
Isobutyl methacrylate	1	3
2-methyl butyl methacrylate	.5	1.5

Eucalyptus globulus

AFNOR/ISO European and World Standards for Therapeutic-Grade

Eucalyptus globulus

Gas Chromatograph profile 4.11

CONSTITUENTS	Pure Essential Oil		Rectified Essential Oil	
	crushed raw	traditional	70%-75%	80%-85%
1,8 cineol				
min %	48	58	70	80
α-Pinene				
min %	10	20	Traces	Traces
max %	20	22	20	12
Aromadendrene				
min %	6	1	—	—
max %	10	5	traces	traces
Limonene				
min %	2	1	2	2
max %	4	8	15	15
p-cymene				
min %	1	1	1	1
max %	3	5	6	10
trans-pinocarveol				
min %	1	1	traces	traces
max %	4	5	10	6
Globulol				
min %	.5	.5	—	—
max %	2.5	1.5	traces	traces

Appendix B

Food "Ash" pH

Alfalfa Grass	+29.3	Cauliflower	+3.1	Juice, natural fruit	-8.7
Almond	+3.6	Cayenne Pepper	+18.8	Juice, white sugar	
Apricot	-9.5	Celery	+13.3	sweetened fruit	-33.4
Artichokes	+1.3	Cheese, Hard	-18.1	Kamut Grass	+27.6
Asparagus	+1.1	Cherry, Sour	+3.5	Ketchup	-12.4
Avocado (protein)	+15.6	Cherry, Sweet	-3.6	Kohlrabi	+5.1
Banana, Ripe	-10.1	Chia, sprouted	+28.5	Lecithin, pure (soy)	+38.0
Banana, Unripe	+4.8	Chicken	-18.0 to -22.0	Leeks (bulbs)	+7.2
Barley Grass	+28.7	Chives	+8.3	Lemon, fresh	+9.9
Barley malt syrup	-9.3	Coconut, fresh	+0.5	Lentils	+0.6
Beans, French cut	+11.2	Coffee	-25.1	Lettuce	+2.2
Beans, Lima	+12.0	Comfrey	+1.5	Lettuce, Fresh cabbage	+14.1
Beans, White	+12.1	Corn oil	-6.5	Lettuce, Lamb's	+4.8
Beef	-34.5	Cranberry	-7.0	Limes	+8.2
Beer	-26.8	Cream	-3.9	Liquor	-28.6 to -38.7
Beet sugar	-15.1	Cucumber, fresh	+31.5	Liver	-3.0
Beet, fresh red	+11.3	Cumin	+1.1	Macadamia Nuts	-11.7
Biscuit, White	-6.5	Currant	-8.2	Mandarin Orange	-11.5
Blueberry	-5.3	Currant, Black	-6.1	Mango	-8.7
Borage	+3.2	Currant, Red	-2.4	Margarine	-7.5
Brazil Nuts	-0.5	Dandelion	+22.7	Marine Lipids	+4.7
Bread, Rye	-2.5	Date	-4.7	Mayonnaise	-12.5
Bread, White	-10.0	Dog grass	+22.6	Meats, Organ	-3.0
Bread, whole-grain	-4.5	Eggs	-18.0 to -22.0	Milk sugar	-9.4
Bread, whole-meal	-6.5	Endive, fresh	+14.5	Milk, Homogenized	-1.0
Brussels Sprouts	-1.5	Fennel	+1.3	Millet	+0.5
Buckwheat groats	+0.5	Fig juice powder	-2.4	Molasses	-14.6
Butter	-3.9	Filbert	-2.0	Mustard	-19.2
Buttermilk	+1.3	Fish, Fresh Water	-11.8	Nut soy (Soaked,	
Cabbage, Green,		Fish, Ocean	-20.0	then air dried)	+26.5
December harvest	+4.0	Flax seed oil	-1.3	Olive Oil	+1.0
Cabbage, Green,		Flax seed	+3.5	Onion	+3.0
March harvest	+2.0	Fructose	-9.5	Orange	-9.2
Cabbage, Red	+6.3	Garlic	+13.2	Oysters	-5.0
Cabbage, Savoy	+4.5	Gooseberry, Ripe	-7.7	Papaya	-9.4
Cabbage, White	+3.3	Grapefruit	-1.7	Peach	-9.7
Cantaloupe	-2.5	Grapes, Ripe	-7.6	Peanuts	-12.8
Caraway	+2.3	Hazelnut	-2.0	Pear	-9.9
Carrot	+9.5	Honey	-7.6	Peas, fresh	+5.1
Cashews	-9.3	Horseradish	+6.8	Peas, ripe	+0.5

Pineapple	-12.6	Shave grass	+21.7	Tangerine	-8.5
Pistachios	-16.6	Sorrel	+11.5	Tea (Black)	-27.1
Plum, Italian	-4.9	Soy beans, (cooked,		Tofu	+3.2
Plum, yellow	-4.9	then ground)	+12.8	Tomato	+13.6
Pork	-38.0	Soy Flour	+2.5	Turbinado	-9.5
Potatoes, stored	+2.0	Soy Sprouts	+29.5	Turnip	+8.0
Primrose	+4.1	Soybeans, fresh	+12.0	Veal	-35.0
Pumpkin	-5.6	Spelt	+0.5	Walnuts	-8.0
Quark	-17.3	Spinach		Watercress	+7.7
Radish, Sprouted	+28.4	(other than March)	+13.1	Watermelon	-1.0
Radish, Summer black	+39.4	Spinach, March harvest	+8.0	Wheat Germ	-11.4
Radish, White (spring)	+3.1	Straw grass	+21.4	Wheat Grass	+33.8
Raspberry	-5.1	Strawberry	-5.4	Wheat	-10.1
Red radish	+16.7	Sugar cane juice,		Wine	-16.4
Rhubarb stalks	+6.3	dried (Sucanat)	-9.6	Zucchini	+5.7
Rice syrup, brown	-8.7	Sugar Cane, Refined			
Rice, brown	-12.5	(white)	-17.6		
Rose Hips	-15.5	Sunflower Oil	-6.7		
Rutabaga	+3.1	Sunflower Seeds	-5.4		
Sesame seeds	+.5	Sweeteners, artificial	-26.5		

Reference:
Young, Robert O. *Sick and Tired.*
Alpine, UT, 1977.

The determination of whether a food is acid or
alkaline is not gauged by its pH, but the pH of its
residue or metabolism.

APPENDIX C

Essential Oils Certified as GRAS or Food Additives by the FDA

Oil				Oil				Oil			
Anise	GRAS	FA		Laurus nobille	GRAS	FA		Thyme	GRAS	FA	
Angelica	GRAS	FA		Lavender	GRAS	FA		Tsuga	GRAS	FA	FL
Basil	GRAS	FA		Lavindin	GRAS	FA		Valerian	GRAS	FA	FL
Bergamot	GRAS	FA		Lemon	GRAS	FA		Vetiver	GRAS	FA	
Cajeput		FA		Lemongrass	GRAS	FA		Wintergreen		FA	
Cardamom		FA		Lime	GRAS	FA		Yarrow		FA	
Carrot Seed		FA		Mandarin	GRAS	FA		Ylang ylang	GRAS	FA	
Cassia	GRAS	FA		Marjoram	GRAS	FA					
Cedarwood		FA		Melaleuca alternifolia		FA		**Blends**			
Celery Seed	GRAS	FA		Mountain Savory		FA		Abundance	GRAS		
Chamomile, Roman	GRAS	FA		Melissa	GRAS	FA		Believe		FA	
Chamomile, German	GRAS	FA		Myrrh	GRAS	FA	FL	Citrus Fresh	GRAS		
Cinnamon bark & leaf	GRAS	FA		Myrtle	GRAS	FA		Christmas Spirit	GRAS		
Cistus		FA		Neroli	GRAS	FA		Di-Tone	GRAS		
Citronella	GRAS	FA		Nutmeg	GRAS	FA		EndoFlex	GRAS		
Citrus rinds	GRAS	FA		Onycha (Styrax benzoin)	GRAS	FA		Gratitude		FA	
Clary Sage	GRAS	FA		Orange	GRAS	FA		Joy	GRAS		
Clove	GRAS	FA		Oregano	GRAS	FA		Juva Cleanse	GRAS		
Coriander	GRAS	FA		Palmarosa	GRAS	FA		Juva Flex	GRAS		
Cumin	GRAS	FA		Patchouli	GRAS	FA	FL	Longevity	GRAS		
Dill	GRAS	FA		Pepper	GRAS	FA		Thieves	GRAS		
Eucalyptus globulus	GRAS	FA	FL	Peppermint	GRAS	FA		M-Grain	GRAS		
Elemi	GRAS	FA	FL	Petitgrain	GRAS	FA		Purification	GRAS		
Fennel	GRAS	FA		Pine	GRAS	FA	FL	Relieve It	GRAS		
Fir, Balsam		FA		Rosemary Cineol	GRAS	FA		Sacred Mountain	GRAS		
Frankincense	GRAS	FA	FL	Rose	GRAS	FA		White Angelica	GRAS		
Galbanum	GRAS	FA	FL	Rosewood		FA					
Geranium	GRAS	FA		Savory	GRAS	FA					
Ginger	GRAS	FA		Sage	GRAS	FA					
Goldenrod	GRAS			Sandalwood	GRAS	FA	FL				
Grapefruit	GRAS	FA		Spearmint	GRAS	FA					
Helichrysum	GRAS	FA		Spikenard		FA					
Hyssop	GRAS	FA		Spruce	GRAS	FA	FL				
Jasmine	GRAS	FA		Tangerine	GRAS	FA					
Juniper	GRAS	FA		Tarragon	GRAS	FA					

CODE:

FA	FDA-approved food additive
FL	Flavoring agent
GRAS	Generally regarded as safe

Appendix D

Bible References

Cedarwood

Leviticus 14:51—"And he shall take the cedar wood, and the hyssop, and the scarlet, and the living bird, and dip them in the blood of the slain bird, and in the running water, and sprinkle the house seven times:"

Leviticus 14:52—"And he shall cleanse the house with the blood of the bird, and with the running water, and with the living bird, and with the cedar wood, and with the hyssop, and with the scarlet."

Numbers 19:6—"And the priest shall take cedar wood, and hyssop, and scarlet, and cast [it] into the midst of the burning of the heifer."

Numbers 24:6—"As the valleys are they spread forth, as gardens by the river's side, as the trees of lign aloes which the Lord hath planted, [and] as cedar trees beside the waters."

2 Samuel 5:11—"And Hiram king of Tyre sent messengers to David, and cedar trees, and carpenters, and masons: and they built David an house."

2 Samuel 7:2—"That the king said unto Nathan the prophet, See now, I dwell in an house of cedar, but the ark of God dwelleth within curtains."

2 Samuel 7:7—"In all [the places] wherein I have walked with all the children of Israel spake I a word with any of the tribes of Israel, whom I commanded to feed my people Israel, saying, Why build ye not me an house of cedar?"

1 Kings 4:33—"And he spake of trees, from the cedar tree that [is] in Lebanon even unto the hyssop that springeth out of the wall: he spake also of beasts, and of fowl, and of creeping things, and of fishes."

1 Kings 5:6—"Now therefore command thou that they hew me cedar trees out of Lebanon; and my servants shall be with thy servants: and unto thee will I give hire for thy servants according to all that thou shalt appoint: for thou knowest that [there is] not among us any that can skill to hew timber like unto the Sidonians."

1 Kings 5:8—"And Hiram sent to Solomon, saying, I have considered the things which thou sentest to me for: [and] I will do all thy desire concerning timber of cedar, and concerning timber of fir."

1 Kings 5:10—"So Hiram gave Solomon cedar trees and fir trees [according to] all his desire."

1 Kings 6:9—"So he built the house, and finished it; and covered the house with beams and boards of cedar."

1 Kings 9:11—"([Now] Hiram the king of Tyre had furnished Solomon with cedar trees and fir trees, and with gold, according to all his desire,) that then king Solomon gave Hiram twenty cities in the land of Galilee."

2 Kings 19:23—"By thy messengers thou hast reproached the Lord, and hast said, With the multitude of my chariots I am come up to the height of the mountains, to the sides of Lebanon, and will cut down the tall cedar trees thereof, [and] the choice fir trees thereof: and I will enter into the lodgings of his borders, [and into] the forest of his Carmel."

1 Chronicles 22:4—"Also cedar trees in abundance: for the Zidonians and they of Tyre brought much cedar wood to David."

2 Chronicles 1:15—"And the king made silver and gold at Jerusalem [as plenteous] as stones, and cedar trees made he as the sycomore trees that [are] in the vale for abundance."

2 Chronicles 2:8—"Send me also cedar trees, fir trees, and algum trees, out of Lebanon: for I know that thy servants can skill to cut timber in Lebanon; and behold, my servants [shall be] with thy servants,"

2 Chronicles 9:27—"And the king made silver in Jerusalem as stones, and cedar trees made he as the sycomore trees that [are] in the low plains in abundance."

Ezra 3:7—"They gave money also unto the masons, and to the carpenters; and meat, and drink, and oil, unto them of Zidon, and to them of Tyre, to bring cedar trees from Lebanon to the sea of Joppa, according to the grant that they had of Cyrus king of Persia."

Isaiah 41:19—"I will plant in the wilderness the cedar, the shittah tree, and the myrtle, and the oil tree; I will set in the desert the fir tree, [and] the pine, and the box tree together:"

Ezekiel 17:3—"And say, Thus saith the Lord God; A great eagle with great wings, longwinged, full of feathers, which had divers colours, came unto Lebanon, and took the highest branch of the cedar:"

Ezekiel 17:22—"Thus saith the Lord God; I will also take of the highest branch of the high cedar, and will set [it]; I will crop off from the top of his young twigs a tender one, and will plant [it] upon an high mountain and eminent:"

Ezekiel 17:23—"In the mountain of the height of Israel will I plant it: and it shall bring forth boughs, and bear fruit, and be a goodly cedar: and under it shall dwell all fowl of every wing; in the shadow of the branches thereof shall they dwell."

Zechariah 11:2—"Howl, fir tree; for the cedar is fallen; because the mighty are spoiled: howl, O ye oaks of Bashan; for the forest of the vintage is come down."

Cinnamon

Revelation 18:13—"And cinnamon, and odours, and ointments, and frankincense, and wine, and oil, and fine flour, and wheat, and beasts, and sheep, and horses, and chariots, and slaves, and souls of men."

Fir

1 Kings 6:15—"And he built the walls of the house within with boards of cedar, both the floor of the house, and the walls of the ceiling: [and] he covered [them] on the inside with wood, and covered the floor of the house with planks of fir."

1 Kings 6:34—"And the two doors [were of] fir tree: the two leaves of the one door [were] folding, and the two leaves of the other door [were] folding."

1 Kings 9:11—"([Now] Hiram the king of Tyre had furnished Solomon with cedar trees and fir trees, and with gold, according to all his desire,) that then king Solomon gave Hiram twenty cities in the land of Galilee."

2 Kings 19:23—"By thy messengers thou hast reproached the Lord, and hast said, With the multitude of my chariots I am come up to the height of the mountains, to the sides of Lebanon, and will cut down the tall cedar trees thereof, [and] the choice fir trees thereof: and I will enter into the lodgings of his borders, [and into] the forest of his Carmel."

2 Chronicles 2:8—"Send me also cedar trees, fir trees, and algum trees, out of Lebanon: for I know that thy servants can skill to cut timber in Lebanon; and, behold, my servants [shall be] with thy servants."

2 Chronicles 3:5—"And the greater house he cieled with fir tree, which he overlaid with fine gold, and set thereon palm trees and chains."

Psalms 104:17—"Where the birds make their nests: [as for] the stork, the fir trees [are] her house."

Song Of Solomon 1:17—"The beams of our house [are] cedar, [and] our rafters of fir."

Isaiah 14:8—"Yea, the fir trees rejoice at thee, [and] the cedars of Lebanon, [saying], Since thou art laid down, no feller is come up against us."

Isaiah 37:24—"By thy servants hast thou reproached the Lord, and hast said, By the multitude of my chariots am I come up to the height of the mountains, to the sides of Lebanon; and I will cut down the tall cedars thereof, [and] the choice fir trees thereof: and I will enter into the height of his border, [and] the forest of his Carmel."

Isaiah 41:19—"I will plant in the wilderness the cedar, the shittah tree, and the myrtle, and the oil tree; I will set in the desert the fir tree, [and] the pine, and the box tree together:"

Isaiah 55:13—"Instead of the thorn shall come up the fir tree, and instead of the brier shall come up the myrtle tree: and it shall be to the Lord for a name, for an everlasting sign [that] shall not be cut off."

Isaiah 60:13—"The glory of Lebanon shall come unto thee, the fir tree, the pine tree, and the box together, to beautify the place of my sanctuary; and I will make the place of my feet glorious."

Ezekiel 27:5—"They have made all thy [ship] boards of fir trees of Senir: they have taken cedars from Lebanon to make masts for thee."

Ezekiel 31:8—"The cedars in the garden of God could not hide him: the fir trees were not like his boughs, and the chestnut trees were not like his branches; nor any tree in the garden of God was like unto him in his beauty."

Hosea 14:8—"Ephraim [shall say], What have I to do any more with idols? I have heard [him], and observed him: I [am] like a green fir tree. From me is thy fruit found."

Nahum 2:3—"The shield of his mighty men is made red, the valiant men [are] in scarlet: the chariots [shall be] with flaming torches in the day of his preparation, and the fir trees shall be terribly shaken."

Zechariah 11:2—"Howl, fir tree; for the cedar is fallen; because the mighty are spoiled: howl, O ye oaks of Bashan; for the forest of the vintage is come down."

Frankincense

Leviticus 2:15—"And thou shalt put oil upon it, and lay frankincense thereon: it [is] a meat offering."

Leviticus 2:16—"And the priest shall burn the memorial of it, [part] of the beaten corn thereof, and [part] of the oil thereof, with all the frankincense thereof: [it is] an offering made by fire unto the Lord."

Leviticus 5:11—"But if he be not able to bring two turtledoves, or two young pigeons, then he that sinned shall bring for his offering the tenth part of an ephah of fine flour for a sin offering; he shall put no oil upon it, neither shall he put [any] frankincense thereon: for it [is] a sin offering"

Leviticus 6:15—"And he shall take of it his handful, of the flour of the meat offering, and of the oil thereof, and all the frankincense which [is] upon the meat offering, and shall burn [it] upon the altar [for] a sweet savour, [even] the memorial of it, unto the Lord."

Leviticus 24:7—"And thou shalt put pure frankincense upon [each] row, that it may be on the bread for a memorial, [even] an offering made by fire unto the Lord."

Numbers 5:15—"Then shall the man bring his wife unto the priest, and he shall bring her offering for her, the tenth [part] of an ephah of barley meal; he shall pour no oil upon it, nor put frankincense thereon; for it [is] an offering of jealousy, an offering of memorial, bringing iniquity to remembrance."

1 Chronicles 9:29—"[Some] of them also [were] appointed to oversee the vessels, and all the instruments of the sanctuary, and the fine flour, and the wine, and the oil, and the frankincense, and the spices."

Nehemiah 13:5—"And he had prepared for him a great chamber, where aforetime they laid the meat offerings, the frankincense, and the vessels, and the tithes of the corn, the new wine, and the oil, which was commanded [to be given] to the Levites, and the singers, and the porters; and the offerings of the priests."

Nehemiah 13:9—"Then I commanded, and they cleansed the chambers: and thither brought I again the vessels of the house of God, with the meat offering and the frankincense."

Song Of Solomon 3:6—"Who [is] this that cometh out of the wilderness like pillars of smoke, perfumed with myrrh and frankincense, with all powders of the merchant?"

Song Of Solomon 4:6—"Until the day break, and the shadows flee away, I will get me to the mountain of myrrh, and to the hill of frankincense."

Song Of Solomon 4:14—"Spikenard and saffron; calamus and cinnamon, with all trees of frankincense; myrrh and aloes, with all the chief spices:"

Matthew 2:11—"And when they were come into the house, they saw the young child with Mary his mother, and fell down, and worshiped him: and when they had opened their treasures, they presented unto him gifts; gold, and frankincense, and myrrh."

Revelation 18:13—"And cinnamon, and odours, and ointments, and frankincense, and wine, and oil, and fine flour, and wheat, and beasts, and sheep, and horses, and chariots, and slaves, and souls of men."

Hyssop

Leviticus 14:49—"And he shall take to cleanse the house two birds, and cedar wood, and scarlet, and hyssop:"

Leviticus 14:51—"And he shall take the cedar wood, and the hyssop, and the scarlet, and the living bird, and dip them in the blood of the slain bird, and in the running water, and sprinkle the house seven times:"

Leviticus 14:52—"And he shall cleanse the house with the blood of the bird, and with the running water, and with the living bird, and with the cedar wood, and with the hyssop, and with the scarlet:"

Numbers 19:6—"And the priest shall take cedar wood, and hyssop, and scarlet, and cast [it] into the midst of the burning of the heifer."

Numbers 19:18—"And a clean person shall take hyssop, and dip [it] in the water, and sprinkle [it] upon the tent, and upon all the vessels, and upon the persons that were there, and upon him that touched a bone, or one slain, or one dead, or a grave:"

1 Kings 4:33—"And he spake of trees, from the cedar tree that [is] in Lebanon even unto the hyssop that springeth out of the wall: he spake also of beasts, and of fowl, and of creeping things, and of fishes."

Psalms 51:7—"Purge me with hyssop, and I shall be clean: wash me, and I shall be whiter than snow."

John 19:29—"Now there was set a vessel full of vinegar: and they filled a spunge with vinegar, and put [it] upon hyssop, and put [it] to his mouth."

Hebrews 9:19—"For when Moses had spoken every precept to all the people according to the law, he took the blood of calves and of goats, with water, and scarlet wool, and hyssop, and sprinkled both the book, and all the people."

Myrrh

Esther 2:12—"Now when every maid's turn was come to go in to king Ahasuerus, after that she had been twelve months, according to the manner of the women, (for so were the days of their purifications accomplished, [to wit], six months with oil of myrrh, and six months with sweet odours, and with [other] things for the purifying of the women;)"

Psalms 45:8—"All thy garments [smell] of myrrh, and aloes, [and] cassia, out of the ivory palaces, whereby they have made thee glad."

Proverbs 7:17—"I have perfumed my bed with myrrh, aloes, and cinnamon."

Song Of Solomon 1:13—"A bundle of myrrh [is] my wellbeloved unto me; he shall lie all night betwixt my breasts."

Song Of Solomon 3:6—"Who [is] this that cometh out of the wilderness like pillars of smoke, perfumed with myrrh and frankincense, with all powders of the merchant?"

Song Of Solomon 4:6—"Until the day break, and the shadows flee away, I will get me to the mountain of myrrh, and to the hill of frankincense."

Song Of Solomon 4:14—"Spikenard and saffron; calamus and cinnamon, with all trees of frankincense; myrrh and aloes, with all the chief spices:"

Song Of Solomon 5:1—"I am come into my garden, my sister, [my] spouse: I have gathered my myrrh with my spice; I have eaten my honeycomb with my honey; I have drunk my wine with my milk: eat, O friends; drink, yea, drink abundantly, O beloved."

Song Of Solomon 5:5—"I rose up to open to my beloved; and my hands dropped [with] myrrh, and my fingers [with] sweet smelling myrrh, upon the handles of the lock."

Song Of Solomon 5:13—"His cheeks [are] as a bed of spices, [as] sweet flowers: his lips [like] lilies, dropping sweet smelling myrrh."

Matthew 2:11—"And when they were come into the house, they saw the young child with Mary his mother, and fell down, and worshiped him: and when they had opened their treasures, they presented unto him gifts; gold, and frankincense, and myrrh."

Mark 15:23—"And they gave him to drink wine mingled with myrrh: but he received [it] not."

John 19:39—"And there came also Nicodemus, which at the first came to Jesus by night, and brought a mixture of myrrh and aloes, about an hundred pound [weight]."

Myrtle

Zechariah 1:8—"I saw by night, and behold a man riding upon a red horse, and he stood among the myrtle trees that [were] in the bottom; and behind him [were there] red horses, speckled, and white."

Zechariah 1:10—"And the man that stood among the myrtle trees answered and said, These [are they] whom the Lord hath sent to walk to and fro through the earth."

Zechariah 1:11—"And they answered the angel of the Lord that stood among the myrtle trees, and said, We have walked to and fro through the earth, and, behold, all the earth sitteth still, and is at rest."

Spikenard

Song of Solomon 4:14—"Spikenard and saffron; calamus and cinnamon, with all trees of frankincense, myrrh and aloes, with all chief spices."

Mark 14:3—"And being in Bethany in the house of Simon the leper, as he sat at meat, there came a woman having an alabaster box of ointment of spikenard very precious; and she brake the box, and poured [it] on his head."

John 12:3—"Then took Mary a pound of ointment of spikenard, very costly, and anointed the feet of Jesus, and wiped his feet with her hair: and the house was filled with the odour of the ointment."

APPENDIX E

Essential Oil Application Codes

Application Codes

NEAT = straight, undiluted
Dilution usually NOT required; suitable for all but the most sensitive skin. Safe for children over 2 years old.

PHOTO = Photosensitizing
Avoid using on skin exposed to direct sunlight or UV rays (i.e. sunlamps, tanning beds, etc.)

50-50 = Dilute 50-50
Dilution recommended at 50-50 (1 part essential oils to 1 part vegetable or massage oil) for topical and internal use, especially when used on sensitive areas — face, neck, genital area, underarms, etc. Keep out of reach of children.

20-80 = Dilute 20-80
Always dilute 20-80 (1 part essential oils to 4 parts vegetable or massage oil) before applying to the skin or taking internally. Keep out of reach of children.

Single Oils

Angelica	PHOTO	50-50
Anise		50-50
Basil		50-50
Bergamot	PHOTO	50-50
Benzoin		50-50
Cajeput		50-50
Cedar, Western Red		50-50
Cardemom		50-50
Carrot Seed		NEAT
Cassia		**20-80**
Celery Seed		NEAT
Cedarwood		NEAT
Chamomile, German		NEAT
Chamomile, Roman		NEAT
Cinnamon Bark		**20-80**
Cistus		NEAT
Citronella		50-50
Citrus Hystrix	PHOTO	50-50
Clary Sage		50-50
Clove		**20-80**
Coriander		50-50
Cumin		50-50
Cypress		50-50
Davana		NEAT
Dill		50-50
Elemi		NEAT
Eucalyptus dives		50-50
Eucalyptus globulus		50-50
Eucalyptus polybractea		50-50
Eucalyptus radiata		50-50

Fennel		NEAT
Fir, Douglas		50-50
Fir, Idaho Balsam		50-50
Fir, White		50-50
Fleabane		50-50
Frankincense		50-50
Galbanum		NEAT
Geranium		50-50
Ginger		50-50
Goldenrod		50-50
Grapefruit	PHOTO	50-50
Helichrysum		50-50
Hyssop		**20-80**
Jasmine		NEAT
Juniper		50-50
Laurus nobilis		50-50
Lavandin		50-50
Lavender		NEAT
Ledum		NEAT
Lemon	PHOTO	50-50
Lemongrass		**20-80**
Lime	PHOTO	50-50
Mandarin		50-50
Manuka		NEAT
Marjoram		50-50
Melaleuca ericifolia		50-50
Melissa		NEAT
Mountain Savory		50-50
Myrrh		NEAT
Myrtle		50-50

Neroli	NEAT	Sandalwood	NEAT
Niaouli	50-50	Spearmint	50-50
Nutmeg	50-50	Spikenard	NEAT
Orange	PHOTO 50-50	Spruce	50-50
Oregano	**20-80**	Tangerine	PHOTO 50-50
Palmarosa	50-50	Tansy	50-50
Patchouli	NEAT	Tansy, Blue	NEAT
Pepper, Black	50-50	Tarragon	50-50
Peppermint	50-50	Tea Tree	50-50
Petitgrain	NEAT	Thyme	**20-80**
Pine	50-50	Tsuga	50-50
Ravensara	50-50	Valerian Root	NEAT
Rose	NEAT	Vetiver	NEAT
Rosemary CT cineol	50-50	Wintergreen	50-50
Rosemary CT verbenon	50-50	Yarrow	NEAT
Rosewood	NEAT	Ylang Ylang	NEAT
Sage	50-50		

Blends

Abundance	50-50	Into The Future	NEAT
Acceptance	NEAT	Joy	PHOTO .... NEAT
Aroma Life	NEAT	Juva Cleanse	NEAT
Aroma Siez	50-50	JuvaFlex	50-50
Australian Blue	NEAT	Lady Sclareol	50-50
Awaken	NEAT	Legacy	**20-80**
Believe	50-50	Live With Passion	NEAT
Brain Power	NEAT	Longevity	**20-80**
Chivalry	50-50	Magnify Your Purpose	NEAT
Christmas Spirit	50-50	Melrose	50-50
Citrus Fresh	50-50	Mister	NEAT
Clarity	NEAT	Motivation	NEAT
Di-Tone	NEAT	M-Grain	50-50
Dragon Time	NEAT	PanAway	50-50
Dream Catcher	NEAT	Peace & Calming	NEAT
EndoFlex	NEAT	Present Time	NEAT
En-R-Gee	50-50	Purification	NEAT
Envision	NEAT	R.C.	NEAT
Evergreen Essence	50-50	R.C.	50-50
Exodus II	50-50	Release	50-50
Forgiveness	NEAT	Relieve It	50-50
Gathering	NEAT	Sacred Mountain	NEAT
Gentle Baby	NEAT	SARA	NEAT
Gratitude	50-50	SclarEssence	50-50
Grounding	NEAT	Sensation	NEAT
Harmony	NEAT	Surrender	NEAT
Highest Potential	50-50	Thieves	**20-80**
Hope	NEAT	3 Wise Men	NEAT
Humility	NEAT	Transformation	PHOTO 50-50
ImmuPower	50-50	Trauma Life	NEAT
Inner Child	NEAT	Valor	NEAT
Inspiration	NEAT	White Angelica	PHOTO .... NEAT

APPENDIX F

ORAC Research

A test recently developed by USDA researchers at Tufts University in Boston, Massachussetts, has been able to identify the highest known antioxidant foods. Known as ORAC (oxygen radical absorbance capacity), this test is the first of its kind to measure both time and degree of free-radical inhibition.

All antioxidant capacity measures are estimated by Ferric Reducing Power and are expressed as micromole Trolox equivalent (TE) per 100 grams, accurate to plus or minus 5%

Essential Oils Antioxidant Capacity

Clove	1,078,700
Myrrh	379,800
Citronella	312,000
Coriander	298,300
Fennel	238,400
Clary Sage	221,000
German Chamomile	218,600
Cedarwood	169,000
Rose	160,400
Nutmeg	158,100
Longevity (Blend)	151,100
Marjoram	139,905
Melissa	134,300
Ylang Ylang	130,000
Palmarosa	127,755
Rosewood	113,200
Manuka	106,200
Wintergreen	101,800
Geranium	101,000
Ginger	99,300
Bay Laurel	98,900
Eucalyptus citriodora	83,000
Cumin	82,400
Black Pepper	79,700
Vetiver	74,300
Petitgrain	73,600
Blue Cypress	73,100
Citrus hystrix	69,200
Douglas Fir	69,000

EO list continued on next page

Foods Antioxidant Capacity

Berry Young Juice	3,604
Blueberries	2,400
Kale	1,770
Noni Juice	1,712
Xango Juice	1,644
Strawberries	1,540
Spinach	1,260
Raspberries	1,220
Brussels sprouts	980
Plums	949
Broccoli florets	890
Beets	840
Oranges	750
Red Grapes	739
Red Bell Peppers	710
Cherries	670
Yellow corn	400
Eggplant	390
Limu Juice	305
Carrots	210

Blue Tansy 68,800
Goldenrod 61,900
Melaleuca ericifolia 61,100
Blue Yarrow 55,900
Spikenard 54,800
Basil 54,000
Patchouli 49,400
White Fir 47,900
Tarragon 37,900
Cajeput 37,600
Peppermint 37,300
Cardamom 36,500
Dill 35,600
Celery Seed 30,300
Fleabane (Canadian) 26,700
Mandarin 26,500
Lime 26,200
Galbanum 26,200
Myrtle 25,400
Cypress 24,300
Grapefruit 22,600
Hyssop 20,900
Balsam Fir 20,500
Niaouli 18,600
Thyme 15,960
Oregano 15,300
Cassia 15,170
Sage 14,800
Mountain Savory 11,300
Cinnamon Bark 10,340
Tsuga 7,100
Valarian 6,200
Cistus 3,860
Eucalyptus globulous 2,410
Orange 1,890
Lemongrass 1,780
Helichrysum 1,740
Ravensara 890
Lemon 660
Frankincense 630
Spearmint 540
Lavender 360
Rosemary 330
Juniper 250
Roman chamomille 240
Sandalwood 160

APPENDIX G

Flash Points for Essential Oils

Single Oils

Angelica	111°F
Anise	>200°F
Basil	177°F
Bergamot	149°F
Buplevere	108°F
Cajeput	116°F
Calamus	194°F
Canadian Red Cedar	145°F
Cardamom	154°F
Carrot Seed	144°F
Cassia	152°F
Cedar Leaf	142°F
Cedarwood	>200°F
Chamomile, German	>200°F
Chamomile, Mixta	144°F
Chamomile, Roman	150°F
Cinnamon Bark	179°F
Cistus	114°F
Citronella	147°F
Clary Sage	190°F
Clove	>200°F
Coriander	153°F
Cumin	142°F
Cypress	103°F
Cypress, Blue	>200°F
Davana	>200°F
Dill	150°F
Elemi	114°F
Eucalyptus Citriodora	176°F
Eucalyptus Dives	149°F
Eucalyptus Globulus	114°F
Eucalyptus Polybractea	112°F
Eucalyptus Radiata	130°F
Fennel	168°F
Fir	104°F
Fir, Idaho Balsam	118°F
Fir, Douglas	103°F
Fir, White	107°F

Fleabane	118°F
Frankincense	102°F
Galbanum	104°F
Geranium	181°F
Ginger	168°F
Goldenrod	118°F
Grapefruit	133°F
Helichrysum	150°F
Hyssop	158°F
Inula	>200°F
Jasmine	>200°F
Juniper	104°F
Laurel	142°F
Lavandin	168°F
Lavender	157°F
Ledum	147°F
Lemon	109°F
Lemongrass	181°F
Lime	109°F
Mandarin	113°F
Marjoram	149°F
Melaleuca ericifolia	127°F
Melissa	189°F
Mountain Savory	170°F
Mugwort	162°F
Myrrh	>200°F
Myrtle	100°F
Niaouli (MQV)	168°F
Nutmeg	110°F
Orange	142°F
Oregano	168°F
Palmarosa	199°F
Patchouli	>200°F
Black Pepper	112°F
Peppermint	172°F
Petitgrain	150°F
Pine	103°F
Ravensara	124°F
Rose	156°F
Rosemary	116°F

Rosemary Verbanon	103°F	Exodus II	165°F
Rosewood	178°F	Forgiveness	172°F
Sage	146°F	Gathering	142°F
Sage Lavender	108°F	Gentle Baby	170°F
Sandalwood	>200°F	Gratitude	115°F
Spearmint	149°F	Grounding	134°F
Spikenard	193°F	Harmony	144°F
Spruce	102°F	Highest Potential	155°F
Tamanu	>200°F	Hope	142°F
Tangerine	115°F	Humility	194°F
Tansy, Blue	137°F	ImmuPower	132°F
Tansy, Idaho	168°F	Inner Child	131°F
Tarragon	148°F	Inspiriation	153°F
Tea Tree	157°F	Into The Future	152°F
Thyme	162°F	Joy	146°F
Tsuga	103°F	Juva Cleanse	135°F
Valerian	112°F	JuvaFlex	165°F
Vetiver	>200°F	Legacy	131°F
Wintergreen	191°F	Live with Passion	170°F
Yarrow	172°F	Longevity	137°F
Ylang Ylang	>200°F	M-Grain	159°F
		Magnify Your Purpose	163°F
		Melrose	137°F

Blends

		Mister	155°F
Abundance	144°F	Motivation	131°F
Acceptance	66°F	PanAway	187°F
Aroma Life	142°F	Peace and Calming	128°F
Aroma Siez	157°F	Present Time	142°F
Australian Blue	150°F	Purification	132°F
Awaken	164°F	Raven	127°F
Believe	129°F	R.C.	119°F
Brain Power	152°F	Release	209°F
Chivalry	135°F	Relieve It	123°F
Christmas Spirit	125°F	Sacred Mountain	124°F
Citrus Fresh	125°F	SARA	185°F
Clarity	156°F	Sensation	181°F
Di-Tone	163°F	Surrender	131°F
Dragon Time	171°F	Thieves	144°F
Dream Catcher	142°F	3 Wise Men	186°F
EndoFlex	149°F	Trauma Life	133°F
En-R-Gee	121°F	Valor	143°F
Envision	122°F	White Angelica	180°F

APPENDIX H

Key Scientific Research on Essential Oils

Scientific Research List

1. "Effect of a Diffused Essential Oil Blend on Bacterial Bioaerosols"

2. "Screening for Inhibitory Activity of Essential Oils on Selected Bacteria, Fungi, and Viruses"

3. "Antibacterial Properties of Plant Essential Oils"

4. "Influence of Some Spice Essential Oils on *Aspergillus parasiticus* Growth and Production of Aflatoxins in a Synthetic Medium"

5. "Antioxidant Activity of Some Spice Essential Oils on Linoleic Acid Oxidation in Aqueous Media"

6. "Antimicrobial Activity of Some Egyptian Spice Essential Oils"

7. "Antimicrobial Properties of Spices and Their Essential Oils"

8. "The Antimicrobial Activity of Essential Oils and Essential Oil Components Towards Oral Bacteria"

9. "Anticarcinogenic Effects of the Essential Oils From Cumin, Poppy and Basil"

10. "Effects of Essential Oil on Lipid Peroxidation and Lipid Metabolism in Patients with Chronic Bronchitis"

11. "Effect of Essential Oils on the Course of Experimental Atherosclerosis"

12. "Inhibition of Growth and Aflatoxin Production in *Aspergillus parasiticus* by Essential Oils of Selected Plant Materials"

13. "Odors and Learning"

14. "Weight Reduction through Inhalation of Odorants"

15. "Anti-inflammatory Activity of *Passiflora incarnata* L. in Rats"

16. "Medroxyprogesterone Interferes with Ovarian Steroid Protection Against Coronary Vasospasm"

17. "Methyl-Sulfonyl-Methane (M.S.M.): A Double-Blind Study of Its Use in Degenerative Arthritis"

18. "Chemopreventive Effect of Perillyl Alcohol on 4-(methylnitrosamino)-1-(3-pyridyl)-1-buta-none Induced Tumorigenesis in (C3H/HeJ X A/J)F1 Mouse Lung"

19. "Chemoprevention of Colon Carcinogenesis by Dietary Perillyl Alcohol"

Abstracts

1. Effect of a Diffused Essential Oil Blend on Bacterial Bioaerosols

Author: S.C. Chao, D. G. Young, and C.J. Oberg

Journal: Journal of Essential Oil Research 10, 517-523 (Sept/Oct 1998)

Location: Weber State University, Ogden, UT

Conclusion: Diffusion of the oil blend, Thieves, can significantly reduce the number of aerosol-borne bacteria.

Abstract: A proprietary blend of oils (named Thieves) containing cinnamon, rosemary, clove, eucalyptus, and lemon was tested for its antibacterial activity against airborne *Micrococcus luteus*, *Pseudomonas aeruginosa*, and *Staphylococcus aureus*. The bacteria cultures were sprayed in an enclosed area, and Thieves was diffused for a given amount of time. There was an 82 percent reduction in *M. luteus* bioaerosol, a 96 percent reduction in the *P. aeruginosa* bioaerosol, and a 44 percent reduction in the *S. aureus* bioaerosol following 10 minutes of exposure.

2. Screening for Inhibitory Activity of Essential Oils on Selected Bacteria, Fungi, and Viruses

Author: S.C. Chao, D.G. Young, and C.J. Oberg

Journal: Journal of Essential Oil Research

Location: Weber State University, Ogden, UT

Conclusion: Many essential oils were demonstrated to have antimicrobial.

Abstract: 45 essential oils were tested for their inhibitory effect against bacteria, yeast, molds, and two bacteriophage. Of the oils tested, all oils showed inhibition compared to controls. Cinnamon bark and tea tree essential oils showed an inhibitory effect against all the test organisms and phage. Other oils with broad ranges of inhibition included lemongrass, mountain savory, Roman chamomile, rosewood, and spearmint.

3. Antibacterial properties of plant essential oils

Author: S. G. Deans, G. Ritchie

Journal: International Journal of Food Microbiology 5, 165-180 (1987)

Location: Scotland Agricultural College

Conclusion: Many essential oils have antibacterial properties.

Abstract: Fifty plant essential oils were tested in different concentrations for antibacterial activity against 25 genera of bacteria. The ten most antibacterial oils were: angelica, bay, cinnamon, clove, thyme, almond, marjoram, pimento, geranium, and lovage.

4. Influence of Some Spice Essential Oils on Aspergillus parasiticus Growth and Production of Aflatoxins in a Synthetic Medium

Author: R. S. Farag, Z. Y. Daw, S. H. Abo-Raya

Journal: Journal of Food Science, Vol 54, No. 1, 74-76 (1989)

Location: Cairo University, Giza, Egypt

Conclusion: Essential oils of thyme, cumin, clove, caraway, rosemary, and sage all possess antifungal properties.

Abstract: The essential oils of thyme, cumin, clove, caraway, rosemary, and sage were tested for antifungal properties. The essential oils completely inhibited growth of fungal mycelium and aflatoxin production. The oils from most effective to least effective were: thyme > cumin > clove > caraway > rosemary > sage. The basic components of these oils were determined by gas-liquid chromatography to be: thyme—thymol, cumin—cumin aldehyde, clove—eugenol, caraway—carvone, rosemary —borneol, and sage—thujone.

5. Antioxidant Activity of Some Spice Essential Oils on Linoleic Acid Oxidation in Aqueous Media

Author: R. S. Farag, A.Z.M.A. Badei, F. M. Hewedi, G.S.A. El-Baroty

Journal: JAOCS, Vol. 66, No. 6 (June 1989)

Location: Cairo University, Giza, Egypt

Conclusion: Essential oils of caraway, clove, cumin, rosemary, sage, thyme possess antioxidant activity on linoleic acid oxidation.

Abstract: Essential oils of caraway, clove, cumin, rosemary, sage and thyme were examined for antioxidant activity in linoleic acid. These oils were all found to have an antioxidant effect which increased when their concentrations were increased. The effectiveness of these essential oils on linoleic acid oxidation was in the following order: caraway, sage, cumin, rosemary, thyme, clove.

6. Antimicrobial Activity of Some Egyptian Spice Essential Oils

Author: R.S. Farag, Z. Y. Daw, F. M. Hewedi, G.S.A. El-Baroty

Journal: Journal of Food Protection, Vol. 52 (September 1989)

Location: Cairo University, Giza, Egypt

Conclusion: Essential oils of sage, rosemary, caraway, cumin, clove, and thyme were shown to have antimicrobial properties.

Abstract: Essential oils of sage, rosemary, caraway, cumin, clove, and thyme were studied for their antibacterial effects. The minimum inhibitory concentration for each essential oil was also determined. Various essential oils were inhibitory at extremely low concentrations (0.25-12 mg/ml). Gram-positive bacteria were shown to be more sensitive to the essential oils than were gram-negative. Thyme and cumin oils had stronger antimicrobial activity than the other oils. The chemical structures of compounds in the essential oils were related to the antimicrobial activity.

7. Antimicrobial Properties of Spices and Their Essential Oils

Author: L. R. Beuchat

Journal: Nat. Antimicrob. Syst. Food Preserv. 167-79 (1994)

Location: University of Georgia, Griffin, Georgia

Conclusion: Many spices and herbs possess antimicrobial properties against various bacteria, yeasts, and molds.

Abstract: Many spices and herbs possess antimicrobial actions. These include plants of the genus *Allium*, such as onions and garlic; spices such as thyme, oregano, savory, sage, cinnamon, clove, vanilla, and others. Microbes inhibited by these herbs and spices include gram-positive and gram-negative bacteria, yeasts, and molds.

8. The Antimicrobial Activity of Essential Oils and Essential Oil Components Towards Oral Bacteria

Author: S. Shapiro, A. Meier, B. Guggenheim

Journal: Oral Microbiology and Immunology 1994: 202-208 (Copyright Munksgaard 1994)

Location: University of Zurich, Switzerland

Conclusion: Essential oils of tea tree, peppermint, and sage showed potent antimicrobial action against anaerobic oral activity.

Abstract: Antimicrobial activity of some essential oils on anaerobic oral bacteria was analyzed. The most potent essential oils tested were Australian tea tree oil, peppermint oil, and sage oil. Thymol and eugenol were the most potent oil components.

9. Anticarcinogenic Effects of the Essential Oils From Cumin, Poppy and Basil

Author: K. Aruna, V. M. Sivaramakrishnan

Journal: Phytotherapy Research, Vol. 10, 577-580 (1996)

Location: Cancer Institute (W.I.A.) Adyar Madras, India

Conclusion: Essential oils of cumin, poppy, and basil all possess potent anticarcinogenic properties.

Abstract: Essential oils of cumin, poppy, and basil were assessed for anticarcinogenic properties. The activity of glutathione-S-transferase, a carcinogen-detoxifying enzyme, was increased by over 78 percent in the stomach, liver, and esophagus of Swiss mice when they were treated with cumin, poppy, and basil essential oils.

10. Effects of Essential Oil on Lipid Peroxidation and Lipid Metabolism in Patients with Chronic Bronchitis

Author: S. A. Siurin

Journal: Klinicheskaia Meditsina, 75(10):43-5 (1997)

Location: Scientific Group NII of Pulmonology, Monchegorsk, Russia.

Conclusion: Lavender essential oil aids in normalizing lipid levels.

Abstract: Essential oils were tested in 150 patients with chronic bronchitis for their effects on lipid peroxidation and lipid metabolism. Essential oils of rosemary, basil, fir, eucalyptus, and lavender were found to have antioxidant effect and lavender was found to normalize lipid levels.

11. Effect of Essential Oils on the Course of Experimental Atherosclerosis

Author: V. V. Nikolaevskii, N. S. Kononova, A. I. Pertsoviskii, I.F. Shinkarchuk

Journal: Patologicheskaia Fiziologiia i Eksperimentalnaia Terapiia (5):52-3 (Sep-Oct 1990)

Conclusion: Inhalation of lavender and monarda essential oils reduces cholesterol content in the aorta of rabbits, providing an angioprotective effect.

Abstract: Lavender, monarda, and basil essential oils were tested in rabbits for their effect on atherosclerosis. When inhaled, lavender and monarda essential oils did not affect blood cholesterol content, but reduced cholesterol content in the aorta. These oils provide a heart-protective effect.

12. Inhibition of Growth and Aflatoxin Production in Aspergillus parasiticus by Essential Oils of Selected Plant Materials

Author: A. Tantaoui-Elaraki, L. Beraoud

Journal: Journal of Environmental Pathology, Toxicology and Oncology;13(1):67-72 (1994)

Location: Hassan II Institute for Agriculture and Veterinary Medicine, Rabat-Instituts, Morocco

Conclusion: Several essential oils (cinnamon, thyme, oregano, and cumin) were shown to have strong antifungal properties.

Abstract: Essential oils of cinnamon, thyme, oregano, cumin, curcumin, ginger, lemon, and orange were tested on *Aspergillus parasiticus* for antifungal properties. The most inhibitory essential oils were cinnamon, thyme, oregano, and cumin.

13. Odors and Learning

Author: A. R. Hirsch, M.D., L. H. Johnston, M.D.

Journal: J. Neurol Orthop Med Surg 17:119-126 (1996)

Location: Smell & Taste Research Foundation, Chicago, Illinois, USA

Conclusion: Pleasant odors increased performance of individuals on cognitive tasks.

Abstract: This study assessed the effects of hedonically positive odors on performance of cognitive tasks. Results indicate that normally performing subjects completed a cognitive task an average 17 percent faster on subsequent trials when a pleasing odor was present. Further studies are desirable to determine if odors would be useful in general education and education of those with learning disabilities.

14. Weight Reduction through Inhalation of Odorants

Author: A. R. Hirsch, M.D., R. Gomez

Journal: Annals of Clinical and Laboratory Science (Official Journal of the Association of Clinical Scientists) Volume 24 September-October Number 5

Location: Smell & Taste Research Foundation, Chicago, Illinois, USA

Conclusion: Use of aroma inhalers aided study volunteers in weight loss over a 6-month period.

Abstract: To measure the role of olfaction in weight loss, odorant inhalers were given to 3,193 overweight volunteers. Study participants were instructed to inhale odorants 3 times in each nostril whenever hunger occurred. Average weight loss was 2.1 percent body weight per month. These results suggest inhalation of odorants may induce sustained weight loss over a 6-month period.

15. Anti-inflammatory Activity of Passiflora incarnata L. in Rats

Author: F. Borrelli, L. Pinto, A. A. Izzo, N. Mascolo, F. Capasso, V. Mercati, E. Toja, G. Autore

Journal: Phytotherapy Research, Vol. 10, S104-S106 (1996)

Location: University of Naples, Naples, Italy

Conclusion: *Passiflora incarnata* extract was found to have anti-inflammatory activity in rats.

Abstract: Ethanolic extract of *Passiflora incarnata* (passion flower) was tested for anti-inflammatory activity in rats. The extract significantly inhibited swelling and inflammation.

16. Medroxyprogesterone Interferes with Ovarian Steroid Protection Against Coronary Vasospasm

Author: K. Miyagawa, J. Rosch, F. Stanczyk, K. Hermsmeyer

Journal: Nature Medicine, Vol. 3 (3); (March 1997)

Location: Oregon Health Sciences University, Beaverton, Oregon

Conclusion: Progesterone was found to cause less risk of cardiovascular disease than medroxyprogesterone, a synthetic progesterone.

Abstract: Progesterone and medroxyprogesterone, a synthetic progesterone, were tested on rhesus monkeys. Medroxyprogesterone was found to cause an increased risk of cardiovascular disease compared to progesterone.

17. Methyl-Sulfonyl-Methane (M.S.M.) A Double-Blind Study of Its Use in Degenerative Arthritis

Author: R. M. Lawrence

Journal: Preliminary correspondence, not yet published

Location: UCLA School of Medicine, Los Angeles, CA

Conclusion: MSM helps patients with degenerative arthritis in pain management.

Abstract: A double-blind study was conducted on patients suffering from degenerative joint disease. After 6 weeks, patients given MSM showed an 82 percent improvement in pain on average. MSM is a safe, non-toxic method of managing pain.

18. Chemopreventive Effect of Perillyl Alcohol on 4-(methylnitrosamino)-1-(3-pyridyl)-1-butanone Induced Tumorigenesis in (C3H/HeJ X A/J)F1 Mouse Lung

Author: L. E. Lantry, Z. Zhang, F. Gao, K. A. Crist, Y. Wang, G. J. Kelloff, R. A. Lubet, M. You

Journal: Journal of Cellular Biochemistry Supplement; 27:20-5 (1997)

Location: Medical College of Ohio, Toledo, OH.

Conclusion: Perillyl alcohol possesses chemopreventive effects in a mouse lung tumor experiment.

Abstract: Perillyl alcohol, a naturally occurring monoterpene found in lavender, cherries, and mint was given to laboratory mice which were then exposed to carcinogens. Perillyl-treated mice had a 22 percent reduction in tumor incidence compared to non-treated mice. Perillyl alcohol is an effective chemopreventive compound in mouse lung tumors.

19. Chemoprevention of Colon Carcinogenesis by Dietary Perillyl Alcohol

Author: B. S. Reddy, C. X. Wang, H. Samaha, R. Lubet, V. E. Steele, G. J. Kelloff, C. V. Rao

Journal: Cancer Research 1;57(3): 420-5 (1997 Feb)

Location: American Health Foundation, Valhalla, NY

Conclusion: Perillyl alcohol is shown to have chemopreventive activity in colon cancer in lab rats.

Abstract: Perillyl alcohol, a monoterpene found in lavender, was administered to rats which were then given azoxymethane (AOM), an agent causing colon carcinogenesis. Perillyl alcohol inhibited the incidence of adenocarcinomas of the colon and small intestine as compared to the control.

APPENDIX I

Five Key Groups of Essential Oil Compounds

Hydrogen
Carbon
Oxygen

Phenylpropanoids
C6 with C3 sidechain (Phenylalanine unit)

Eugenol	Cinnamic acid
Eugenol acetate	p-courmaric acid
Anethole	gingerol
Cinnamaldehide	myristicin

Monoterpenes
C10 (2 Isoprene units)

borneol	linalol
bornyl acetate	linalyl acetate
camphene	d-/l-limponene
camphor	menthofuran
car-3-ene	menthol
carvacrol	menthone
carvone	menthyl acetate
1,8 cineol (eucalyptol)	α/β-myrcene
geranial/neral (citral)	β-ocimene
citronellal	α/β phellanderene
α/β-citronellal	α/β-pinene
cuminaldehyde	sabinene
p-cymene	piperitone
dipentene	terpinene
fenchone	thujone
geraniol	thymol
nerol	thymyl acetate
geranyl acetate	verbenone
	γ-terpinene

Sesquiterpenes
C15 (3 isoprenes units)

α/β-bisabolol	α/β-vetivol
β/δ-cadinene	α-ylangene
α/β-caryophyllene	α-zingiberene
α-copaene	ledol
α-curcumene	longifolene
eudesmol	nerolidol
farnesene	patchoulol
germacrene B + D	α/β-santalene
himachalol	α/β-santalol
himachalene	

Diterpenes
C20 (4 isoprene unite)

Sclareol
carnosol

Triterpenes
C30 (6 Isoprene units)

ginsenoside
glycyrrhizin

Sesquiterpene Content of Selected Essential Oils

Cedarwood 98%	Patchouli 71%	German Chamomile 47%
Vetiver 97%	Myrrh 62%	Spikenard 36%
Sandalwood 90%	Ginger 59%	Galbanum 11%
Black Pepper 74%	Vitex 50%	Frankincense 8%

APPENDIX J

Glossary of Medical Actions

alopecia: baldness, loss of hair

allopathic: refers to conventional contemporary medical approaches using prescription drugs to provide symptom relief in the treatment of illness

amenorrhea: absence of menstruation

anabolism: the creation of body tissue—the opposite of catabolism—usually from other nutrients or components

anesthetic: loss of feeling or sensation; substance which causes such a loss

analgesic: remedy or agent which deadens or relieves pain

anthelmintic: substance unfriendly to worms and parasites; a vermifuge; destroys, expels intestinal worms

anodyne: stills pain and quiets disturbed feelings

antibiotic: prevents the growth of, or destroys bacteria

anticatarrhal: agent which helps remove excess catarrh (excess mucous secreted by inflamed mucous membranes) from the body

anti-emetic: agent which reduces the incidence and severity of nausea or vomiting

antihistamine: counteracts the effects of histamine (which produces capillary dilation and, in larger doses, hemoconcentration)

anti-inflammatory: reduces inflammation

antilithic: prevents the formation of a calculus or stone

antimicrobial: agent which resists or destroys pathogenic micro-organisms

antineuralgic: relieves or reduces nerve pain

antioxidant: natural or synthetic substances that help inhibit destructive oxygen- and free radical-induced deterioration (oxidation) of substances and tissues in the body.

antipruritic: relieves or prevents itching.

antipyretic: reduces fever; see febrifuge

antisclerotic: prevents the hardening of tissue

antiseptic: destroys and prevents the development of microbes

antispasmodic: prevents and eases spasms or convulsions

antitoxic: antidote or treatment that counteracts the effects of poisons and toxins

antitussive:	relieves coughs
antiviral:	inhibits the growth of virus
aperient:	mild laxative
astringent:	causes contraction of organic tissues
bechic:	anything that relieves or cures coughs; or refers to coughs
calmative:	a sedative
carcinogen:	substance or agent which produces or creates cancer
cardiotonic:	having a stimulating effect on the heart
carminative:	agent which prevents the formation of gas (flatulence) in the intestinal system typically to relieve pain due to colic or cramping.
catabolism:	the breaking down of tissue or material within the body. Digestion is a catabolic process.
cathartic:	purgative, capable of causing a violent purging or catharsis of the body
cellulite:	accumulation of toxic matter in the form of fat in the tissue
cholagogue:	stimulates the secretion and flow of bile into the duodenum
choleretic:	aids excretion of bile by the liver, so there is a greater flow of bile
cicatrisant:	agent which promotes healing by the formation of scar tissue
cutaneous:	pertaining to the skin
cytophylactic:	referring to cytophylaxis: the process of increasing the activity of leucocytes in defense of the body against infection
cytotoxic:	toxic to all cells
demulcent:	agent which protects mucous membranes and allays irritation
diuretic:	aids production of urine, promotes urination, increases flow
edema:	a painless swelling caused by fluid retention beneath the skin's surface
emetic:	induces vomiting
emmenagogue:	induces or assists menstruation
emollient:	softens and soothes skin
enteritis:	inflammation of the mucous membrane of the intestine
expectorant:	promotes the removal of mucous from the respiratory system
febrifuge:	combats fever
fungicidal:	prevents and combats fungal infection
germicidal:	destroys germs or microorganisms such as bacteria
halitosis:	offensive breath
hemostatic:	arrests bleeding
hepatic:	relating to the liver, tones and aids its function
hypertensive:	agent which raises blood pressure

hypnotic: causing sleep

hypocholesterolemia: lowering the cholesterol content of the blood

hypotensive: agent which lowers blood pressure

laxative: promotes evacuation of the bowels

lipolytic: causing lipolysis, the chemical disintegration or splitting of fats

microbe: a minute living organism, especially pathogenic bacteria, viruses, etc.

mucolytic: dissolving or breaking down mucous

narcotic: substance which induces sleep; intoxicating or poisonous in large doses

neat: term used for describing the application of essential oil without dilution in a carrier oil

nervine: strengthening and toning to the nervous and nervous system

nephritis: inflammation of the kidneys

neuralgia: a stabbing pain along a nerve pathway

neurasthenia: nervous exhaustion

olfaction: the sense of smell

ophthalmia: inflammation of the eye, a term usually applied to conjunctivitis

otitis: inflammation of the ear

pathogenic: causing or producing disease pruritis: itching

psychosomatic: the manifestation of physical symptoms resulting from a mental state

restorative: agent that helps strengthen and revive the body systems

rhinitis: inflammation of the mucous membrane of the nose

rubefacient: reddening the skin, an agent that reddens the skin by producing hyperemia

soporific: substance which induces sleep

spasmolytic: antispasmodic

stomachic: digestive aid and tonic; improving the appetite

styptic: astringent agent which stops or reduces external bleeding

sudorific: agent which causes sweating

thrombosis: the formation of a blood clot (thrombus)

topical application: refers to applying something directly to the exterior surface of the skin; not internal.

vasoconstrictor: agent which causes narrowing of the blood vessels

vasodilator: agent which causes dilation of the blood vessels

vermifuge: expels intestinal worms

vesicant: causing blistering to the skin

vulnerary: agent which helps heal wounds and sores by external application

APPENDIX K
Common and Botanical Plant Names

Botanical Name First:

Abies balsamea . . . . .Balsam Fir	*Cuminum cyminum* . . . . .Cumin
Abies concolor .White Fir	*Cupressus sempervirens* . . . . .Cypress
Achillea millefolium . . . . .Yarrow	*Cymbopogon flexuosus* . . . . .Lemongrass
Acorus calamus . . . . .Calamus	*Cymbopogon nardus* . . . . .Citronella
Anethum graveolens . . . . .Dill	*Daucus carota* . . . . .Carrot Seed
Angelica archangelica . . . . .Angelica	*Elettaria cardamomum* . . . . .Cardamom
Aniba rosaeodora . . . . .Rosewood	*Eucalyptus citriodora* . . . . . .Eucalyptus citriodora
Apium graveolens . . . . .Celery Seed	*Eucalyptus dives* . . . . .Eucalyptus dives
Artemisia dracunculus . . . . .Tarragon	*Eucalyptus globulus* . . . . .Eucalyptus globulus
Boswellia carteri . . . . .Frankincense	*Eucalyptus polybractea* . . .Eucalyptus polybractea
Callitris intratropica . . . . .Blue cypress	*Eucalyptus radiata* . . . . .Eucalyptus radiata
Cananga odorata . . . . .Ylang Ylang	*Ferula gummosa* . . . . .Galbanum
Canarium luzonicum . . . . .Elemi	*Foeniculum vulgare* . . . . .Fennel
Cedrus atlantica . . . . .Cedarwood	*Gaultheria procumbens* . . . . .Wintergreen
Chamaemelum nobile . . . . . .Chamomile (Roman)	*Helichrysum italicum* . . . . .Helichrysum
Cinnamomum cassia . . . . .Cassia	*Hyssopus officinalis* . . . . .Hyssop
Cinnamomum verum . . . . .Cinnamon Bark	*Jasminum officinale* . . . . .Jasmine
Cistus ladanifer .Cistus	*Juniperus communis* . . . . .Juniper
Citrus aurantifolia . . . . .Lime	*Juniperus osteosperma* . . . . .Juniper
Citrus aurantium . . . . .Neroli	*Laurus nobilis* . . . . .Bay Laurel
Citrus aurantium . . . . .Orange	*Lavandula angustifolia* . . . . .Lavender
Citrus bergamia . . . . .Bergamot	*Lavandula x hybrida* . . . . .Lavandin
Citrus limon . . . . .Lemon	*Ledum groenlandicum* . . . . .Ledum
Citrus nobilis . . . . .Tangerine	*Leptospormum scoparium* . . . . .Manuka
Citrus reticulata . . . . .Mandarin	*Matricaria recutita* . . . . .Chamomile (German)
Citrus x paradisi . . . . .Grapefruit	*Melaleuca alternifolia* . . . . .Tea Tree
Commiphora myrrha . . . . .Myrrh	*Melaleuca ericifolia* . . . . .Melaleuca ericifolia
Conyza canadensis . . . . .Fleabane	*Melaleuca leucadendra* . . . . .Cajeput
Coriandrum sativum . . . . .Coriander	*Melaleuca quinquenervia* . . . . .Niaouli

457

Melissa officinalis . . . . .Melissa

Mentha spicata . . . . .Spearmint

Mentha piperita . . . . .Peppermint

Myristica fragrans . . . . .Nutmeg

Myrtus communis . . . . .Myrtle

Nardostachys jatamansi . . . . .Spikenard

Ocimum basilicum . . . . .Basil

Origanum compactum . . . . .Oregano

Origanum majorana . . . . .Marjoram

Pelargonium graveolens . . . . .Geranium

Picea mariana .Spruce

Pimpinella anisum . . . . .Anise

Pinus sylvestris . . . . .Pine

Piper nigrum . . . . Black Pepper

Pogostemon cablin . . . . Patchouli

Pseudotsuga menziesii . . . . .Douglas Fir

Ravensara aromatica . . . . .Ravensara

Rosa damascena . . . . .Rose

Rosmarinus officinalis CT 1,8 cineol . . . . .Rosemary

Salvia officinalis . . . . .Sage

Salvia sclarea . . . . .Clary Sage

Santalum album . . . . .Sandalwood

Satureja montana . . . . .Mountain Savory

Solidago canadensis . . . . .Goldenrod

Syzygium aromaticum . . . . .Clove

Tanacetum annuum . . . . .Blue Tansy

Tanacetum vulgare . . . . .Tansy

Thuja plicata . . . . .Western Red Cedar

Thymus vulgaris CT linalol . . . . . . .Thyme Linalol

Thymus vulgaris CT thymol . . . . .Thyme

Tsuga canadensis . . . . .Tsuga

Valeriana officinalis . . . . .Valerian

Vetiveria zizanioides . . . . .Vetiver

Vitex negundo . . . . .Vitex

Zingiber officinale . . . . .Ginger

Common Name First:

Angelica . . . .*Angelica archangelica*

Anise . . . .*Pimpinella anisum*

Balsam Fir . . . .*Abies balsamea*

Basil . . . .*Ocimum basilicum*

Bay Laurel . . . .*Laurus nobilis*

Bergamot . . . .*Citrus bergamia*

Black Pepper . . . .*Piper nigrum*

Blue cypress . . . .*Callitris intratropica*

Blue Tansy . . . .*Tanacetum annuum*

Cajeput . . . .*Melaleuca leucadendra*

Calamus . . . .*Acorus calamus*

Cardamom . . . .*Elettaria cardamomum*

Carrot Seed . . . .*Daucus carota*

Cassia . . . .*Cinnamomum cassia*

Cedarwood . . . .*Cedrus atlantica*

Celery Seed . . . .*Apium graveolens*

Chamomile (German) . . . .*Matricaria recutita*

Chamomile (Roman) . . . . . .*Chamaemelum nobile*

Cinnamon Bark . . . .*Cinnamomum verum*

Cistus . . . .*Cistus ladanifer*

Citronella . . . .*Cymbopogon nardus*

Clary Sage . . . .*Salvia sclarea*

Clove . . . .*Syzygium aromaticum*

Coriander . . . .*Coriandrum sativum*

Cumin . . . .*Cuminum cyminum*

Cypress . . . .*Cupressus sempervirens*

Dill . . . .*Anethum graveolens*

Douglas Fir . . . .*Pseudotsuga menziesii*

Elemi . . . .*Canarium luzonicum*

Eucalyptus dives . . . .*Eucalyptus dives*

Eucalyptus citriodora . . . . . .*Eucalyptus citriodora*

Eucalyptus globulus . . . .*Eucalyptus globulus*

Eucalyptus polybractea . . .*Eucalyptus polybractea*
Eucalyptus radiata . . . .*Eucalyptus radiata*
Fennel . . . .*Foeniculum vulgare*
Fleabane . . . .*Conyza canadensis*
Frankincense . . . .*Boswellia carteri*
Galbanum . . . .*Ferula gummosa*
Geranium . . . .*Pelargonium graveolens*
Ginger . . . .*Zingiber officinale*
Goldenrod . . . .*Solidago canadensis*
Grapefruit . . . .*Citrus x paradisi*
Helichrysum . . . .*Helichrysum italicum*
Hyssop . . . .*Hyssopus officinalis*
Jasmine . . . .*Jasminum officinale*
Juniper . . . .*Juniperus communis*
Juniper . . . .*Juniperus osteosperma*
Bay Laurel . . . .*Laurus nobilis*
Lavandin . . . .*Lavandula x hybrida*
Lavender . . . .*Lavandula angustifolia*
Ledum . . . .*Ledum groenlandicum*
Lemon . . . .*Citrus limon*
Lemongrass . . . .*Cymbopogon flexuosus*
Lime . . . .*Citrus aurantifolia*
Mandarin . . . .*Citrus reticulata*
Manuka . . . .*Leptospormum scoparium*
Marjoram . . . .*Origanum majorana*
Melaleuca ericifolia . . . .*Melaleuca ericifolia*
Melissa . . . .*Melissa officinalis*
Mountain Savory . . . .*Satureja montana*
Myrrh . . . .*Commiphora myrrha*
Myrtle . . . .*Myrtus communis*
Neroli . . . .*Citrus aurantium*
Niaouli . . . .*Melaleuca quinquenervia*
Nutmeg . . . .*Myristica fragrans*
Orange . . . .*Citrus aurantium*
Oregano . . . .*Origanum compactum*
Peppermint . . . .*Mentha piperita*
Pine . . . .*Pinus sylvestris*
Patchouli . . . .*Pogostemon cablin*

Ravensara . . . .*Ravensara aromatica*
Rose . . . .*Rosa damascena*
Rosemary . . . .*Rosmarinus officinalis CT 1, 8 cineol*
Rosewood . . . .*Aniba rosaeodora*
Sage . . . .*Salvia officinalis*
Sandalwood . . . .*Santalum album*
Spearmint . . . .*Mentha spicata*
Spikenard . . . .*Nardostachys jatamansi*
Spruce . . . .*Picea mariana*
Tangerine . . . .*Citrus nobilis*
Tansy . . . .*Tanacetum vulgare*
Tarragon . . . .*Artemisia dracunculus*
Tea Tree . . . .*Melaleuca alternifolia*
Thyme . . . .*Thymus vulgaris CT thymol*
Thyme Linalol . . . .*Thymus vulgaris CT linalol*
Tsuga . . . .*Tsuga canadensis*
Valerian . . . .*Valeriana officinalis*
Vetiver . . . .*Vetiveria zizanioides*
Vitex . . . .*Vitex negundo*
Western Red Cedar . . . .*Thuja plicata*
White Fir . . . .*Abies concolor*
Wintergreen . . . .*Gaultheria procumbens*
Yarrow . . . .*Achillea millefolium*
Ylang Ylang . . . .*Cananga odorata*

459

APPENDIX L

Plant Parts Used to Distill Essential Oils

Wood/Bark/Stems
Balsam fir
Blue cypress
Buddah wood
Cedarwood (Himalyan)
Cinnamon
Cypress
Douglas fir
Emerald cypress
Jade cypress
Juniper
Lemon myrtle
Pine
Rosewood
Sandalwood
Spruce
Tsuga
Western red cedar
White fir

Root
Ginger
Patchouli
Valarian
Vetiver

Seed
Anise
Coriander
Fennel
Nutmeg

Leaves/Stems
Basil
Cassia
Cistus
Dill
Elemi
Eucalyptus dives
Eucalyptus globulus
Eucalyptus polybractea
Eucalyptus radiata
Hyssop
Laurus noblis
Ledum
Lemongrass
Manuka
Marjoram
Tea Tree
Melaleuca ericifolia
Melissa
Mountain savory
Myrtle
Oregano
Peppermint
Petitgrain
Ravensara
Rosemary
Sage
Spearmint
Spikenard
Tarragon
Thyme
Vitex
Wintergreen

Flowering tops
Clary sage
Geranium
German chamomile
Goldenrod
Helichrysum
Lavender
Roman chamomile
Tansy

Flower
Jasmine *(absolute)*
Neroli *(absolute)*
Rose
Ylang ylang

Gum/Resin
Frankincense
Galbanum
Myrrh
Styrax benzoin

Fruit/Rind
Bergamot
Black pepper
Clove
Grapefruit
Lemon
Mandarin
Orange
Tangerine

APPENDIX M

Ningxia Wolfberry Research

Long History in China

In the early 1980s, a group of researchers from the Natural Science Institute began studying a region on the West Elbow Plateau of the Yellow River in Inner Mongolia where people lived to be over 100 years old—10 to 20 years longer than the average person in the region. The inhabitants shared one trait that distinguished them from others. They were predominantly vegetarian and regularly consumed wolfberries. Moreover, the people who consumed this fruit lived free of common degenerative diseases like arthritis, cancer, and diabetes.

Both the Ningxia wolfberry (also known as *Lycium barbarum* by botanists and as the goji berry by native Chinese) and ginseng *(Panax ginseng)* have been highly regarded for centuries as the foremost nutritional and therapeutic plants in China. In fact, the Chinese hold a strong belief that human life might be extended significantly by using either of these herbs for an extended period. Unfortunately, ginseng is considered too strong for continuous use, and large amounts may not be suitable for people with high blood pressure or heart disease. On the other hand, the wolfberry is much milder, with no known risk from continuous use.

Some 17 different varieties of wolfberry have been identified. However, only one – the Ningxia cultivar – has been shown to possess the extraordinary nutrient and anti-oxidant content to support greater longevity. Until recently the Ningxia wolfberry was grown only on the Yellow River in the Ningxia Province of China, but it has been successfully transplanted and cultivated at the Young Living farm in Mona, Utah

18 Amino Acids and 21 Trace Minerals

In 1988, the Beijing Nutrition Research Institute conducted detailed chemical analyses and nutritional composition studies of the dried wolfberry fruit. The Ningxia wolfberry contained over 18 amino acids, 21 trace minerals, more protein than bee pollen, more vitamin C than oranges, and nearly as much beta carotene as carrots.

Perhaps this is why the Chinese have traditionally attributed so many benefits to the wolfberry, claiming it protects liver function, replenishes vital essences, improves visual acuity, and lowers blood pressure and cholesterol. The Ningxia wolfberry was also said to strengthen muscles and bones, stimulate the heart, and work as an aid to treat diabetes and impotence.

Strongest Antioxidant Known

According to a new test known as ORAC (Oxygen Radical Absorbance Capacity), developed by USDA researchers at Tufts University, The Ningxia Wolfberry is the highest known antioxidant food, possessing an unmatched ability to absorb injurious free radicals that attack the body and contribute to cancer and aging.

Developed by Dr. Guohua Cao at the USDA Human Nutrition Research Center on Aging at Tufts University, the ORAC test is one of the most sensitive and reliable methods for measuring the ability of antioxidants to absorb oxygen radicals. It is the only test to combine both time and degree of inhibition of free radicals.

Strongest Known Antioxidant Foods

	ORAC
Ningxia wolfberry	25,300
Prunes	5,770
Blueberries	2,400
Kale	1,770
Strawberries	1,540
Spinach	1.260
Raspberries	1,220
Beets	840
Oranges	750

Oxygen Radical Absorbance Capacity (ORAC) of 3.5 oz.

Since the early 1980s, the Ningxia wolfberry has been the subject of a number of important clinical studies—including several published by the State Scientific and Technological Commission in China. These studies have documented the antioxidant and immune-stimulating properties of the Chinese wolfberry.

From July 1982 to January 1984, the Ningxia Institute of Drug Inspection conducted a pharmacological experiment using multi-index screening (Register No. 870303). Their conclusion was:

> The fruits and pedicels of the Ningxia wolfberry were effective in increasing white blood cells, protecting the liver, and relieving hypertension. The alcoholic extract of wolfberry fruits inhibited tumor growth in mice by 58 percent, and the protein of wolfberry displayed an insulin-like action that was effective in promoting fat decomposition and reducing blood sugar.

Another clinical experiment by the Ningxia Institute (Register No. 870306, October 1982 to May 1985) studied the effects of Ningxia wolfberry on the immune, physiological, and biochemical indexes of the blood of aged volunteers. The results indicated that the wolfberry caused the blood of older people to noticeably revert to a younger state.

Can the Ningxia Wolfberry Boost Immune Function?

According to a report of the State Scientific and Technological Commission of China, the Ningxia wolfberry contains compounds known as lycium polysaccharides, which appear to be highly effective in promoting immunity. This conclusion was supported in a number of clinical trials.

In one study on a group of cancer patients, the wolfberry triggered an increase in both lymphocyte transformation rate and white blood cell count (measures of immune function). In another study involving a group of 50 people with lower-limit white blood cell counts, the Ningxia wolfberry increased phagocytosis and the titre of serum antibodies (another index of immune function). Unhealthy levels of titre of serum antibodies have long been associated with Chronic Fatigue Syndrome (also known as Epstein-Barr). Does this mean that the wolfberry could be used as a weapon against Epstein-Barr? The possibilities are intriguing.

In another study, consumption of Ningxia wolfberry led to a strengthening of immunoglobulin A levels (an index of immune function). Because the decline of immunoglobulin A is one of the signs of aging, an increase in these levels suggests that the wolfberry may enable injured DNA to better repair itself and ward off tissue degeneration.

Is the Ningxia Wolfberry a Powerful Antioxidant?

As we grow older, the levels of lipid peroxide in our blood increase, while levels of health-protecting antioxidants, like superoxide dismutase (SOD), decrease. In a clinical study of people who consumed doses of wolfberry, SOD in the blood increased by a remarkable 48 percent while hemoglobin increased by 12 percent. Even better, lipid peroxide levels dropped by an astonishing 65 percent.

Does the Ningxia Wolfberry Protect Eyesight?

A test was conducted on the effects of wolfberry on eyesight. Twenty-seven people were tested and showed a dramatic improvement in both dark adaptation and vitamin A and carotene content of their serum (measures of eyesight acuity).

More recent studies in the 1990s lend additional scientific support, as summarized below:

Abstracts

1. Use of Wolfberry *(Lycium barbarum* polysaccharides*)* to Treat Cancer

Author: G. W. Cao, W. G. Yang, P. Du

Journal: Chunghua Chung Lui Tsa Chih 16 (Nov. 1994): 428-31

Location: Second Military Medical University, Shanghai

Conclusion: *Lycium barbarum* polysaccharides can be used as an adjuvant in the treatment of cancer.

Abstract: Seventy-nine advanced cancer patients were treated with a combination of LAK/IL-2* and *Lycium barbarum* polysaccharides. Patients treated with only LAK/IL-2 showed a response rate of only 16 percent, while those treated with both LAK/IL-2 and *Lycium barbarum* polysaccharides showed a response rate of 40.9 percent. Moreover, the mean remission in the *Lycium barbarum* group lasted significantly longer. *Lymphokine-activated natural killer cells (LAK) and interleukin 2 (IL-2).

2. The Role of Lycium barbarum Polysaccharide as an Antioxidant

Author: X. Zhang

Journal: Chung Kuo Chung Yao Tsa Chih 18 (Feb. 1993): 110-2, 128

Location: Beijing Military Hospital

Conclusion: The effects of free radicals on cells can be prevented and reversed by incubation with either *Lycium barbarum* polysaccharide or superoxide dismutase.

Abstract: Researchers incubated cells (Xenopus Oocytes) in a solution containing a free-radical-producing system for 6 hours. The changes in the electrical profile of the cell membranes were determined using a microelectrode electrophysiological technique. The results showed that *Lycium barbarum* polysaccharide prevented and reversed free radical damage to the cells.

3. Protective Action of *Lycium barbarum* on Hydrogen Peroxide-induced Lipid Peroxidation

Author: B. Ren, Y. Ma, Y. Shen, B. Gao

Journal: Chung Kuo Chung Yao Tsa Chih 20 (May 1995): 303-4

Location: Ningxia Medical College, Yinchuan

Conclusion: *Lycium barbarum* protects red blood cell membranes against lipid peroxidation.

Abstract: Hydrogen peroxide (H_2O_2), a powerful promoter of oxidative damage, was used to promote lipid peroxidation of the red blood cell membranes of rats. Dried *Lycium* berries showed the greatest protective effect against H_2O_2 damage, followed by *Lycium barbarum* polysaccharide.

4. Effects of Lycium barbarum on the Attachment and Growth of Human Gingival Cells to Root Surfaces

Author: B. Liu

Journal: Chung Kuo Chung Yao Tsa Chih 27 (May 1992): 159-61, 190

Location: College of Stomatology, Fourth Medical University, Xian

Conclusion: *Lycium barbarum* improved the attachment and growth of human gingival cells to root surfaces.

Abstract: A dose of 1.25 mg/ml *Lycium barbarum* was used to stimulate the in vitro attachment of human gingival fibrobasts to the surfaces of dental roots. In response to *Lycium barbarum* exposure, cells on diseased root surfaces increased in quantity, exhibited better growth and distribution. *Drynaria* displayed similar effects but was not as potent as the *Lycium barbarum*.

APPENDIX N

Stevia Research

Stevia: Safe, Non-caloric Supersweet Supplement with Health-giving Properties

For over 1600 years, the natives of Paraguay in South America have used this intensely sweet herb as a health agent and sweetener. Known as *Stevia rebaudiana* by botanists and yerba dulce (honey leaf) by the Guarani Indians, stevia has been incorporated into many native medicines, beverages, and foods for centuries. The Guarani used stevia separately or combined with herbs like yerba mate and lapacho.

Fifteen times sweeter than sugar, stevia was introduced to the West in 1899, when M. S. Bertoni discovered natives using it as a sweetener and medicinal herb. However, stevia never gained popularity in Europe or the United States and was only gradually adopted by several countries throughout Far East Asia.

With Japan's ban on the import of synthetic sweeteners in the 1960's, stevia began to be seriously researched by the Japanese National Institute of Health as a natural sugar substitute. After almost a decade of studies examining the safety and antidiabetic properties of the herb, Japan became a major producer, importer, and user of stevia. Japanese food companies began including stevia in hundreds of products, and eventually stevia use spread through Asia. Stevioside, the super sweet glycoside derived from stevia that is 300 times sweeter than sugar, was even used to sweeten Diet Coke sold in Japan.

Even though stevia is still relatively unknown in the United States, it has gained widespread popularity as a low-calorie sweetener throughout South America and Asia. Both the stevia leaf and stevioside are used in Taiwan, China, Korea, and Japan, with many of these same countries growing and harvesting large amounts of the raw herb.

In 1994, the U.S. Food and Drug Administration permitted the importation and use of stevia as a dietary supplement. However, its adoption by American consumers as a noncaloric sweetener has been very slow because the FDA does not currently permit stevia to be marketed as a food additive. This means that stevia cannot be sold as a sweetener (all sweeteners are classified as food additives by the FDA). Moreover, stevia faces fierce opposition by both the artificial sweetener (aspartame) and sugar industries in the U.S.

Stevia, however, is more than just a non-caloric sweetener. Several modern clinical studies have documented the ability of stevia to lower and balance blood sugar levels, support the pancreas and digestive system, protect the liver, and combat infectious microorganisms. (Oviedo et al., 1971; Suzuki et al., 1977; Ishit et al., 1986; Boeckh, 1986; Alvarez, 1986.)

In one study, Oviedo et. al. showed that oral administration of a stevia leaf extract reduced blood sugar levels by over 35 percent. Another study conducted by Suzuki et al. documented similar results. Clearly, these and other clinical evaluations indicate that stevia holds significant promise for the treatment of diabetes.

APPENDIX O

MSM Research

MSM: A New Solution for Arthritis, Allergies, and Pain

MSM (Methylsulfonylmethane) is a natural sulfur-bearing nutrient that occurs widely in nature (found in everything from mother's breast milk to fresh vegetables). It is an exceptional source of nutritional sulfur—a mineral that is vital to protein synthesis and sound health.

Why is sulfur so important to the body? Because sulfur is a mineral which, like vitamin C, is constantly being used up and depleted. When we fail to replenish our reserves of nutritional sulfur, we become more vulnerable to disease and degenerative conditions. Some possible signs of sulfur deficiency are:

- Poor nail and hair growth
- Eczema
- Dermatitis
- Poor muscle tone
- Acne / Pimples
- Gout
- Rheumatism
- Arthritis
- Weakening of nervous system
- Constipation
- Impairment of mental faculties
- Lowered libido

MSM is more than just another essential nutrient. According to research compiled by Ronald Lawrence, Ph.D., M.D., and Stanley Jacob, M.D., MSM represents a safe, natural solution for chronic headaches, back pain, tendonitis, fibromyalgia, rheumatism, arthritis, athletic injuries, muscle spasms, asthma, and allergies.

In a book entitled, *The Miracle of MSM,* available through Essential Science Publishing, both Dr. Jacobs and Dr. Lawrence discuss how MSM has benefited

hundred of patients. A UCLA neuropsychiatrist, Dr. Lawrence is convinced that MSM will revolutionize how millions of people deal with inflammatory autoimmune diseases like rheumatism, asthma, bursitis, and tendonitis, as well as autoimmune diseases like arthritis, lupus, scleroderma, and allergies.

Other doctors have also seen their patients dramatically improve using 2 to 4 grams of MSM daily. According to David Blyweiss, M.D., of the Institute of Advanced Medicine in Lauderhill, Florida, many patients experience a 50 percent improvement in their arthritis symptoms, along with less fatigue, better sleep, and better ability to exercise.

Dr. Lawrence has also used MSM to improve the condition of patients who were virtually crippled with arthritis and back pain. One patient was able to get out of bed for the first time after just two weeks on MSM. And after two months of MSM use, he could walk to the grocery store.

Another of Dr. Lawrence's patients was a 70-year-old woman who was suffering from severe arthritis. In this case, MSM actually postponed the need for double knee replacement. In fact, after only two months on oral MSM, she was walking again with much less pain and stiffness.

Numerous other MSM users have experienced results equivalent to cortisone—but without side effects like immune suppression, fluid retention, and weakness.

According to Stanley Jacobs, M.D., there may be no pharmaceutical back pain therapy better—or safer—than MSM. "MSM has an important role to play in the nonsurgical treatment of back pain," he said. "I have seen several hundred patients for back pain secondary to osteoarthritis, disc degeneration, spinal misalignments, or accidents. For such pain-related conditions, MSM is usually beneficial."

"I have been recommending MSM for more than six months," said Richard Shaefer, a chiropractor from Wheeling, Illinois. "The results have been excellent. I consistently see major reduction in pain and inflammation in arthritic joints, along with improved range of motion. I can't think of a single individual who isn't getting some kind of positive effect."

MSM may have other benefits aside from its pain and inflammation-reducing properties. Numerous patients have reported a surge in energy levels along with thicker hair, nails, and skin. Some have even reported a softening or disappearance of scar tissue.

One user reported a marked increase in stamina and energy after starting on MSM. "For a long while I have had the blahs," complained Lou Salyer of Tucson, Arizona. "I had no stamina. I had to force myself to get things done around the house. After two days on MSM, it was like a blast of energy. I am amazed at how much I get done now."

MSM may also do much more than relieve pain. "Prior to taking MSM (30 grams a day for 20 years), I would have a cold or flu two or three times a year," stated Dr. Jacobs. "Since I've been taking MSM, I've not had a single cold or the flu. I can't say that MSM prevented my cold or the flu, but it is a fascinating observation."

MSM contains an exceptionally bioavailable source of sulfur, one of the most neglected minerals needed by the human body. Carl Pfeiffer, M.D., Ph.D., a world-renowned expert on nutritional medicine, agrees, "Sulfur is the forgotten essential element."

Found in such foods as garlic and asparagus, the sulfur within MSM is a critical part of the amino acids cysteine and methionine, which form the building blocks of the nails, hair, and skin. Sulfur is also found in therapeutic mineral baths and hot springs that have brought relief to arthritis sufferers for centuries.

MSM is very closely related to DMSO, a powerful pain reliever that was the subject of a *60 Minutes* report in April, 1980. DMSO has been approved by the FDA for interstitial cystitis, a painful urinary tract condition.

The Youth Nutrient

Of particular importance is MSM's ability to equalize water pressure inside the cells—a considerable benefit for those plagued with bursitis, arthritis, and tendonitis. These kinds of inflammatory outbreaks are created when the water pressure inside the cells jumps past the pressure outside the cells, creating pressure and pain. MSM acts as a sort of cellular safety valve, affecting the protein envelope of the cell so that water transfers freely in and out of the cell. The result: rapid relief and less damage to tissues. And because it elasticizes the hold between the cells, MSM can restore flexibility to inflamed tissues.

When our bodies grow older and are chronically shortchanged of key minerals like sulfur and MSM, the bonds between our cells become increasingly rigid and brittle—a condition that can lead to a loss in skin flexibility and contribute to skin wrinkles. The internal manifestations of this cellular brittleness are far less visible but have a far greater negative impact on the body. MSM's ability to reintroduce flexibility into cell structures, therefore, can have widespread restorative affects.

APPENDIX P

FOS Research

FOS: Supernutrient Documented to Rebuild Intestinal Flora, Improve mineral absorption, and more.

- Minimal impact on blood sugar levels
- Glycemic index of 0
- Ideal sweetener for diabetics.
- Increases populations of beneficial bifidobacteria in the colon
- Reduces populations of harmful bacteria, such as *Clostridium perfringens*
- Improves calcium and magnesium absorption
- Improves liver function

A naturally sweet, indigestible fiber derived from chicory roots, FOS (fructooligosaccharides) are one of the best-documented, natural nutrients for promoting the growth of *Lactobacilli* and *bifidobacteria* bacteria, a key to sound health. FOS has also been clinically studied for its ability to increase magnesium and calcium absorption, lower blood glucose, cholesterol, and LDL levels, and to inhibit production of the reductase enzymes that can contribute to cancer. Because FOS can increase magnesium absorption, it can also lead to lowered blood pressure and better cardiovascular health.

FOS is one of the most powerful prebiotics to be researched in the last decade (a "prebiotic" feeds intestinal flora; a "probiotic" adds more actual cultures to existing intestinal flora). The subject of over 100 clinical studies, FOS is one of the best-documented natural nutrients for improving the healthy balance of bacteria in intestines and stimulating the growth of the beneficial *bifidobacteria*—also called "friendly flora"—that reside in the colon.

How important to good health are these so-called "friendly flora" that populate our intestines? They are our front-line defense against invading disease-causing organisms, combating premature aging caused by the toxin-producing bacteria and fungi that reside in our intestines.

FOS Builds Up Friendly Flora

Subjects	Dose g/day	Duration	Fecal *Bifidobacteria* # bacteria (log) per gram		Reference
9	1	14	9.8	10.2	Tokunaga, 92
9	3	14	9.9	10.4	Tokunaga, 92
9	5	14	9.7	10.3	Tokunaga, 92
20	12.5	12	7.9	9.1	Bouhnik, 93
38	8	14	5.2	6.2	Rochat, 94
12	4	25	9.5	9.8	Buddington, 96
			Start of Study	End of Study	

Seven Reasons Why *Bifidobacteria* Are Vital to Health

1. They produce substances that stop the growth of harmful, toxic gram-negative and positive bacteria in the intestines (Kawase 1982, Rasic 1983, Gibson and Wang 1994a&b).

2. They occupy space on the intestinal wall that could be populated by pathogenic organisms. When *Bifidobacteria* increase in numbers, they crowd out invasive toxin-generating microorganisms.

3. They slow down the production of damaging protein breakdown products, such as ammonia. This lowers blood ammonia levels that can be toxic to the human body (Bezkoravainy et al., 1989).

4. They produce B vitamins and folic acid (Nishizawa 1960, Liescher 1961).

5. They produce digestive enzymes, like phosphatases and lysozymes (Kawase 1982, Minagawa 1970).

6. They stimulate the immune system and promote immune attack against cancer cells (Mitsuoka 1980, Sekine et al., 1985).

FOS Raises Magnesium Absorption by over 75%

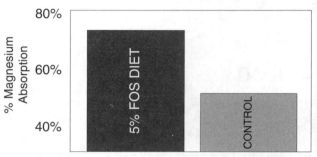

After 10-13 days on 5% FOS diet

FOS Raises Calcium Absorption by over 20%

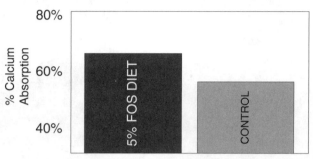

After 10-13 days on 5% FOS diet

7. They increase the absorption of essential minerals magnesium and calcium. As we age, magnesium levels in the body decline, contributing to high blood pressure and diabetes.

Technically a fiber rather than a sugar, FOS is totally unlike conventional sugars because it feeds the beneficial *bifidobacteria* while selectively starving the parasitical yeast, fungi, and bacteria that contribute to disease. Most toxin-producing microorganisms in the intestines are unable to use FOS as food. Conventional sugars, like sucrose and lactose on the other hand, work in just the opposite fashion: they tend to feed harmful bacteria more readily than it feeds beneficial bacteria.

Increases Mineral Absorption

Besides building up the beneficial bacteria in the body, FOS has also been shown to improve blood sugar control, liver function, and calcium and magnesium absorption.

A 1997 animal study conducted at the Nutritional Research Center in Japan found that a 5 percent FOS diet increased magnesium and calcium absorption substantially. A 1998 Showa University study, obtained similar results (Ohta et al., 1998, 1997, 1995; Morohashi et al., 1998).

Magnesium is one of the most important nutrients we obtain from our diet, being involved in over 300 enzyme reactions in the body. As we age, our magnesium levels drop markedly, which creates a deficiency that increases the risk of angina, atherosclerosis, cardiac arrhythmias, depression,

and diabetes (Schauss, 1998; Jansson, 1981). A study conducted by National Research Council of Canada showed that long-term marginal magnesium deficiency can reduce the life span of laboratory animals by almost 40 percent (Heroux et al., 1977).

Liver Health

FOS also improves liver health. A 1999 Louvain Catholic University study found that a 10 percent diet of FOS can protect against fat accumulating in the liver and lower both blood glucose and insulin levels.

Virtually No Effect on Blood Sugar Levels

FOS may be the ideal nutrient for diabetics. Because FOS is an indigestible sugar, it triggers no spikes in blood sugar levels the way sucrose and glucose do. About 40 to 60 percent as sweet as sugar, FOS is found in low quantities in many types of foods. However, to obtain just a quarter teaspoon of FOS from foods in your diet, you would have to consume 13 bananas, 16 tomatoes, or 16 onions. Chicory roots have one of the highest amounts of FOS of any plant, and most natural FOS supplements are commercially derived from water-extraction of the roots.

Recommended Dosages

To obtain the best results from FOS, daily intake should range between 5 and 10 grams a day. Dosages above 15 grams may cause gas or intestinal cramping from excess bifidobacteria populations.

APPENDIX Q

Comparative Antimicrobial Activity of Essential Oils and Antibiotics

The following are test data comparing the antimicrobial ability between essential oils (cinnamon and oregano) and antibiotics (penicillin and ampicillin). The method is disk diffusion and the results are the mean value of three replicates.

These preliminary data indicate that essential oils of cinnamon and oregano are comparable with penicillin and ampicillin in inhibitory activity against *E. coli and Staphylococcus aureus*.

Material	Loading amount (µl)*	*Escherichia coli* zone of inhibition (cm)	*Staphylococcus aureus* zone of inhibition (cm)
Penicillin	3	0	3.2
	6	0	3.4
	8	0	3.6
	12	0	3.6
Ampicillin	3	1.9	2.6
	6	2.1	2.6
	8	2.5	2.7
	12	2.6	2.8
Cinnamon	3	2.4	2.4
	6	2.8	2.8
	8	-	3.0
	12	3.0	3.2
Oregano	3	2.6	3.2
	6	3.3	3.6
	8	-	3.6
	12	3.3	3.8

*The concentration of penicillin = 1.76 unit / µl
The concentration of ampicillin = 5 µg / µl

APPENDIX R

Chlorine and Trihalomethanes Research

Chlorine is one of the most reactive and toxic elements known to man. When put in the public water supply as a disinfectant, it creates disinfection byproducts (DBP) that can cause cancer, birth defects, and spontaneous abortions.

Besides being used in the water supply, chlorine is also chemically bonded in the manufacture of numerous industrial chemicals.

Many toxic herbicides, fungicides, and insecticides are created by attaching one or more chlorine molecules to a carbon skeleton. Once ingested or inhaled, chlorinated chemicals leach into the fat cells and become trapped.

Some of the most common and toxic of these chemicals include a quartet of chlorinated carcinogenic chemicals known as trihalomethanes (THMs): chloroform, bromoform, bromodichloromethane, and chlorobromomethane. These trihalomethanes are created when chlorine reacts with naturally occurring organic matter in raw water.

THMs are very volatile—this means they can be inhaled during bathing as well as consumed in potable water. Showering, washing dishes, and flushing a toilet can also contaminate the air with trihalomethanes.

Once inhaled or ingested, THMs accumulate in the fat cells—the same way dioxins do. Once trapped inside the body, they chemically bind with and damage DNA.

A California Department of Health study surveyed 5,144 pregnant women to determine the effects of THMs in the drinking water (Waller et al., 1998). They measured levels of THMs from water tests of public utilities, and matched these against the study group.

They found that pregnant women who consumed more than 5 glasses of water a day containing more than 75 ppb (parts per billion) had double the risk of spontaneous abortion.

Women who drank less water or who drank water with lower levels of THMs had substantially lower risk of miscarriage. Women who drank filtered water also had significantly lower risk of miscarriage.

Researchers at the University of North Carolina at Chapel Hill also examined the link between THMs and miscarriages in populations living throughout central North Carolina (Savitz et al., 1995). They found that women who suffered the highest exposure to THM in the drinking water had almost triple the risk of miscarriage.

Another study conducted by the U.S. Department of Health and Human Services examined the effect of THMs in the water supply of 75 towns throughout the state of New Jersey (Bove et al., 1995). When scientists compared levels of THMs to the frequency of birth defects, they found that women who consumed water exceeding 80 ppb THMs had triple the risk of giving birth to infants with neural tube defects.

The authors suggested that one of the reasons for this may be due to the fact that vitamin B12 may be disrupted in the body due to chloroform, a common THM.

Another statewide study in New Jersey also linked THMs in drinking water to a doubled risk of neural tube defects (Klotz et al., 1998).

An even larger epidemiological study by the National Institute of Public Health in Norway surveyed the effects of chlorinated water on 141,077 infants born in Norway between 1993 and 1995 (Magnus et al., 1999). Researchers found that the higher the chlorine content of the water and the higher the organic matter in the water, the higher the risk for birth defects including cardiac defects, respiratory tract defects, and urinary tract defects.

Murray S. Malcolm, M.D., a public health physician in New Zealand, spearheaded a country-wide study that examined the role of THMs in triggering birth defects and cancer. He concluded, "A quarter of all bladder, colon, rectal cancers, and birth defects may be preventable by reducing disinfection byproducts (i.e., THMs) exposure" (Malcolm et al., 1999; Wellington School of Medicine, New Zealand).

APPENDIX S

Body Systems Chart

Product Type Key:

S	Essential Oil Single	**E**	Essential Waters
B	Essential Oil Blend	**F**	Powergize Fitness
D	Dietary Supplement	**O**	Oral Care
P	Personal Care/Hair and Skin		
L	Lotions/Creams/Massage Oils		
G	Bath and Shower Gels/Soaps		

Product	Product Type	Nervous System	Cardiovascular System	Respiratory System	Digestive/Elimination	Immune/Anti-infectious	Glandular/Hormonal	Emotional Balance	Muscle & Bone	Anti Aging	Oral Hygiene	Skin and Hair
Abundance	B			●		●		●				
Acceptance	B	●						●				
A D & E	D	●				●						
AlkaLime	D		●		●				●			
Amino Tech	F								●			
Angelica	S	●						●				
Animal Scents Pet Shampoo	G											●
Animal Scents Pet Ointment	L											●
Anise	S				●					●		
Aroma Life	B		●									
Aroma Siez	B			●					●			
AromaSilk Lavender Volume Wash	P											●
AromaSilk Lavender Volume Rinse	P											●
AromaSilk Lemon-Sage Clarifying Wash	P											●
AromaSilk Lemon-Sage Clarifying Rinse	P											●
AromaSilk Rosewood Moisturizing Wash	P											●
AromaSilk Rosewood Moisturizing Rinse	P											●
ArthroTune	D								●			
A.R.T. Day Activator	P											●
A.R.T. Night Reconstructor	P											●
A.R.T. Gentle Foaming Cleanser	P											●

Product Type Key:

S Essential Oil Single   **E** Essential Waters
B Essential Oil Blend   **F** Powergize Fitness
D Dietary Supplement   **O** Oral Care
P Personal Care/Hair and Skin
L Lotions/Creams/Massage Oils
G Bath and Shower Gels/Soaps

Product

Product	Product Type	Nervous System	Cardiovascular System	Respiratory System	Digestive/Elimination	Immune/Anti-infectious	Glandular/Hormonal	Emotional Balance	Muscle & Bone	Anti Aging	Oral Hygiene	Skin and Hair
Australian Blue	B							●				
Awaken	B							●				
Basil	S		●						●			
Basil Essential Water	E								●			
Bath Gel Base	G											●
Be-Fit	F								●			
Bergamot	S				●			●				●
Berry Young Juice	F					●				●		
BLM Capsules	D								●			
BLM Powder	D								●			
Blue Agave Nectar	F						●		●			
Body Gize	D				●	●			●			
Boswellia Wrinkle Crème	P									●		●
Brain Power	B	●						●				
Cajeput	S		●	●								
CarboZyme	D				●							
Cardamom	S				●							
CardiaCare	D		●									
Carrot Seed Oil	S	●	●									●
Cassia	S		●		●					●	●	
Cedar Essential Water	E							●				●
Cedar, Canadian Red	S			●				●				●
Cedar, Western Red	S											●
Cedarwood	S	●		●								
Cel-Lite Magic	L											●
Celery Seed	S				●							
Chamomile Moisturizing Bar Soap	G											●
Chamomile, German	S	●						●				●
Chamomile, German Essential Water	E	●										●
Chamomile, Roman	S	●						●				●

Product Type Key:

S Essential Oil Single
B Essential Oil Blend
D Dietary Supplement
P Personal Care/Hair and Skin
L Lotions/Creams/Massage Oils
G Bath and Shower Gels/Soaps

E Essential Waters
F Powergize Fitness
O Oral Care

Product	Product Type	Nervous System	Cardiovascular System	Respiratory System	Digestive/Elimination	Immune/Anti-infectious	Glandular/Hormonal	Emotional Balance	Muscle & Bone	Anti Aging	Oral Hygiene	Skin and Hair
Chelex	D				●							
Chivalry	B							●				
Christmas Spirit	B	●	●					●				
Cinnamint Lip Balm	P											●
Cinnamon Bark	S					●						
Cistus	S					●				●		
Citronella	S								●			●
Citrus Fresh	B					●		●				
Citrus Hystrix	S						●	●				
ClaraDerm Spray	P											●
Clarity	B	●						●				
Clary Sage	S						●					
Clary Sage Essential Water	E						●					●
Clove	S		●	●	●	●				●	●	
ComforTone	D				●	●						
Coriander	S				●		●					
Cortistop, Women's	D						●					
Cumin	S				●	●						
Cypress	S		●							●		
Cypress, Blue	S					●						
Dentarome	O										●	
Dentarome Plus	O										●	
Dentarome Ultra	O		●								●	
Detoxzyme Capsules	D				●	●						
Di-Tone	B				●							
Dill	S				●							
Dragon Time	B						●	●				
Dragon Time Bath Gel	G						●	●				
Dream Catcher	B							●				
Elemi	S											●

479

Product Type Key:

S Essential Oil Single
B Essential Oil Blend
D Dietary Supplement
P Personal Care/Hair and Skin
L Lotions/Creams/Massage Oils
G Bath and Shower Gels/Soaps

E Essential Waters
F Powergize Fitness
O Oral Care

Product	Product Type	Nervous System	Cardiovascular System	Respiratory System	Digestive/Elimination	Immune/Anti-infectious	Glandular/Hormonal	Emotional Balance	Muscle & Bone	Anti Aging	Oral Hygiene	Skin and Hair
En-R-Gee	D	●						●				
EndoFlex	B						●					
Envision	B							●				
Essentialzyme	D				●				●			
Essential Manna	D				●	●			●			
Essential Omegas	D	●	●									●
Eucalyptus citriodora	S			●								
Eucalyptus Essential Water	E			●				●	●			
Eucalyptus globulus	S			●					●		●	
Eucalyptus polybrachta	S			●								
Eucalyptus radiata	S			●								●
Evening Peace Bath Gel	G											●
Evergreen Essence	B							●				
Exodus	D					●						
Exodus II	B					●						
Fennel	S				●		●					
Fir, Douglas	S			●					●			
Fir, White	S			●				●	●	●		
Fir, White Essential Water	E											●
Fleabane, Canadian (Conyza)	S		●				●					
Forgiveness	B							●				
Frankincense	S	●				●		●		●		●
Fresh Essence Plus	O				●						●	
Galbanum	S					●						
Gathering	B							●				
Genesis Lotion	L											●
Gentle Baby	B							●				●
Geranium	S								●			●
Ginger	S	●			●							
Goldenrod	S		●				●					

Product Type Key:

S   Essential Oil Single
B   Essential Oil Blend
D   Dietary Supplement
P   Personal Care/Hair and Skin
L   Lotions/Creams/Massage Oils
G   Bath and Shower Gels/Soaps

E   Essential Waters
F   Powergize Fitness
O   Oral Care

Product	Product Type	Nervous System	Cardiovascular System	Respiratory System	Digestive/Elimination	Immune/Anti-infectious	Glandular/Hormonal	Emotional Balance	Muscle & Bone	Anti Aging	Oral Hygiene	Skin and Hair
Grapefruit	S		●							●		
Grounding	B							●				
Harmony	B							●				
Helichrysum	S		●						●			
Highest Potential	B							●				
Hope	B							●				
H₂Oils, Lemon	D			●				●				
H₂Oils, Lemon/Grapefruit	D			●				●				
H₂Oils, Lemon/Orange	D			●				●				
H₂Oils, Peppermint	D			●				●				
HRT	D		●									
Humility	B							●				
Hyssop	S	●	●	●								
ICP	D		●		●							
Idaho Balsam Fir	S	●			●		●					
ImmuGel	D					●						
ImmuneTune	D					●				●		
ImmuPower	B					●						
ImmuPro	D					●						
Inner Child	B							●				
Inspiration	B							●				
Into the Future	B							●				
Jasmine (Absolute)	S						●	●				
Joy	B							●				
Juniper	S				●			●				
Juniper Essential Water	E							●	●			●
JuvaFlex	B				●			●				
JuvaTone	D				●	●						
Juva Cleanse	B				●					●		
Juva Power	D				●					●		

Product Type Key:

S Essential Oil Single
B Essential Oil Blend
D Dietary Supplement
P Personal Care/Hair and Skin
L Lotions/Creams/Massage Oils
G Bath and Shower Gels/Soaps

E Essential Waters
F Powergize Fitness
O Oral Care

Product	Product Type	Nervous System	Cardiovascular System	Respiratory System	Digestive/Elimination	Immune/Anti-infectious	Glandular/Hormonal	Emotional Balance	Muscle & Bone	Anti Aging	Oral Hygiene	Skin and Hair
Juva Spice	D				●					●		
K & B	D				●							
KidScents Bath Gel	G											●
KidScents Lotion	L											●
KidScents Shampoo	P											●
KidScents Toothpaste	O										●	
Lady Sclareol	B						●	●				
Laurel nobilus	S			●	●	●						
LavaDerm Cooling Mist	P							●				●
Lavandin	S		●	●					●			
Lavender	S	●	●					●				●
Lavender Essential Water	E	●										●
Lavender-Rosewood Moisturizing Bar Soap	G											●
Lavender Volume Hair & Scalp Wash	P											●
Lavender Volume Nourishing Rinse	P											●
Ledum	S				●	●				●		●
Legacy	B							●				
Lemon	S			●	●	●				●		
Lemon-Sage Clarifying Hair & Scalp Wash	P											●
Lemon-Sage Clarifying Nourishing Rinse	P											●
Lemon-Sandalwood Cleansing Bar Soap	G											●
Lemongrass	S					●			●			
Lime	S			●	●	●				●		
Live with Passion	B	●						●				
Longevity	B									●		
Longevity Essential Oil Caps	D		●							●		
Lipozyme	D				●							
M-Grain	B	●										
Magnify Your Purpose	B	●						●				
Mandarin	S				●					●		●

Product Type Key:

S Essential Oil Single
B Essential Oil Blend
D Dietary Supplement
P Personal Care/Hair and Skin
L Lotions/Creams/Massage Oils
G Bath and Shower Gels/Soaps

E Essential Waters
F Powergize Fitness
O Oral Care

Product	Product Type	Nervous System	Cardiovascular System	Respiratory System	Digestive/Elimination	Immune/Anti-infectious	Glandular/Hormonal	Emotional Balance	Muscle & Bone	Anti Aging	Oral Hygiene	Skin and Hair
Marjoram	S		●						●			
Massage Oil Base	L								●			●
Master Formula vitamins	D	●	●			●		●				
Mega Cal	D		●						●			
Melaleuca alternifolia	S			●		●			●			●
Melaleuca ericifolia	S			●								●
Melaleuca-Geranium Moisturizing Bar Soap	G											●
Melaleuca quinquenervia	S			●					●			
Melissa	S						●			●		●
Melissa Essential Water	E	●										●
Melrose	B			●								●
Mineral Essence	D	●	●			●	●	●	●			
Mighty Mist	D									●		
Mister	B						●					
Morning Start Shower Gel	G											●
Morning Start Moisturizing Bar Soap	G							●				●
Motivaton	B	●						●				
Mountain Essence Essential Water	E			●								●
Mountain Savory	S					●						
Mugwort	S				●							
Myrrh	S	●				●	●					●
Myrtle	S			●	●		●		●			
Neroli	S					●						●
NeuroGen	L	●						●	●			
Niaouli	S			●								
Nutmeg	S	●					●	●				
Onycha	S		●					●				
Orange	S				●	●				●		●
Orange Blossom Facial Wash	P											●
Oregano	S			●		●			●	●		

Product Type Key:

S Essential Oil Single
B Essential Oil Blend
D Dietary Supplement
P Personal Care/Hair and Skin
L Lotions/Creams/Massage Oils
G Bath and Shower Gels/Soaps

E Essential Waters
F Powergize Fitness
O Oral Care

Product	Product Type	Nervous System	Cardiovascular System	Respiratory System	Digestive/Elimination	Immune/Anti-infectious	Glandular/Hormonal	Emotional Balance	Muscle & Bone	Anti Aging	Oral Hygiene	Skin and Hair
Ortho Sport	L								●			
Ortho Ease	L								●			●
Palmarosa	S		●				●					●
PanAway	B	●							●			
ParaFree Liquid and Softgel	D				●	●						
Patchouli	S											●
PD 80/20	D						●	●	●			
Peace & Calming	B	●						●				
Pepper, Black	S	●			●							
Peppermint	S	●		●	●				●		●	●
Peppermint-Cedarwood Moisturizing Bar Soap	G								●			●
Peppermint Essential Water	E				●				●		●	●
Petitgrain	S							●				
Pine	S			●				●				
PolyZyme	D				●				●	●		
Power Meal	F		●		●	●			●			
Prenolone	L	●					●	●	●	●		
Prenolone +	L	●					●	●	●	●		
Present Time	B							●				
ProGen	D						●					
Progessence	L						●			●		
Protec	D						●			●		
Purification	B				●			●				●
R.C.	B			●								●
Ravensara	S			●		●						
RC	B			●								
Regenolone	L	●					●		●			●
Rehemogen	D		●		●							
Relaxation	B							●				●
Release	B							●				

Product Type Key:

S Essential Oil Single
B Essential Oil Blend
D Dietary Supplement
P Personal Care/Hair and Skin
L Lotions/Creams/Massage Oils
G Bath and Shower Gels/Soaps

E Essential Waters
F Powergize Fitness
O Oral Care

Product	Product Type	Nervous System	Cardiovascular System	Respiratory System	Digestive/Elimination	Immune/Anti-infectious	Glandular/Hormonal	Emotional Balance	Muscle & Bone	Anti Aging	Oral Hygiene	Skin and Hair
Relieve It	B								●			
Rose	S							●				●
Rose Ointment	P											●
Rosemary (CT cineol)	S		●		●			●				
Rosewood	S											●
Rosewood Moisturizing Hair & Scalp Wash	P											●
Rosewood Moisturizing Nourishing Rinse	P											●
Sacred Mountain	B							●				
Sacred Mountain Bar Soap for Oily Skin	G							●				●
Sage	S				●	●						
Sandalwood	S	●						●	●			●
Sandalwood Moisture Crème	P											●
Sandalwood Toner	P											●
SARA	B							●				
Satin Body Lotion	L											●
Satin Facial Scrub-Juniper	P											●
Satin Facial Scrub-Mint	P											●
Sclar Essence	B/D				●		●					
Sensation	B							●	●			
Sensation Bath and Shower Gel	G											●
Sensation Hand and Body Lotion	L											●
Sensation Massage Oil	L											●
Spearmint	S				●			●				
Spearmint Essential Water	E										●	●
Spikenard	S							●				●
Spruce	S	●		●				●				
Stevia Extract	D		●		●	●						
Sulfurzyme Capsules or Powder	D	●				●				●	●	●
Sunsation Suntan Oil	L											●
Super B	D	●	●						●			

485

Product Type Key:

S	Essential Oil Single	**E**	Essential Waters
B	Essential Oil Blend	**F**	Powergize Fitness
D	Dietary Supplement	**O**	Oral Care
P	Personal Care/Hair and Skin		
L	Lotions/Creams/Massage Oils		
G	Bath and Shower Gels/Soaps		

Product

Product	Product Type	Nervous System	Cardiovascular System	Respiratory System	Digestive/Elimination	Immune/Anti-infectious	Glandular/Hormonal	Emotional Balance	Muscle & Bone	Anti Aging	Oral Hygiene	Skin and Hair
Super C	D			●		●				●		
Super C Chewable	D					●				●		
Super Cal	D	●	●					●	●			
Surrender	B	●						●				
Tangerine	S					●		●		●		●
Tansy, Blue	S	●										
Tansy, Idaho	S					●						
Tansy, Idaho Essential Water	P											●
Tarragon	S	●			●							
Tender Tush Ointment	P											●
Tea Tree	S			●							●	
ThermaBurn	D							●				
ThermaMist	D				●			●				
Thieves	B					●				●	●	
Thieves Cleaner	P					●						
Thieves Cleansing Bar Soap	G											●
Thieves Cleansing Spray	P					●						
Thieves Lozenges	O			●							●	
Thieves Wipes	P					●						
3 Wise Men	B							●				
Thyme	S					●			●	●		
Thyme Essential Water	E				●						●	●
Thyromin	D						●					
Trauma Life	B							●				
Transformation	B	●						●	●			
Tsuga	S		●	●								
UltraSeptic Spray	P										●	●
Ultra Young	D					●	●			●		
Ultra Young +	D					●	●			●		
V-6 Mixing Oil	L								●			●

Product Type Key:

S Essential Oil Single
B Essential Oil Blend
D Dietary Supplement
P Personal Care/Hair and Skin
L Lotions/Creams/Massage Oils
G Bath and Shower Gels/Soaps

E Essential Waters
F Powergize Fitness
O Oral Care

Product	Product Type	Nervous System	Cardiovascular System	Respiratory System	Digestive/Elimination	Immune/Anti-infectious	Glandular/Hormonal	Emotional Balance	Muscle & Bone	Anti Aging	Oral Hygiene	Skin and Hair
Valerian	S	●										
Valor	B	●						●	●			●
Valor Moisturizing Bar Soap	P	●										●
Vetiver	S	●					●	●				●
VitaGreen	D	●	●		●	●		●				
WheyFit	F								●	●		
White Angelica	B							●				
Wintergreen	S								●			
Wolfberry Crisp Bars	F				●	●			●	●		
Wolfberry Eye Creme	P									●		●
Yarrow	S					●	●					●
Yarrow, Blue	S						●	●				
Ylang Ylang	S		●				●	●				

APPENDIX T

Single Oil Data

Single Oil Name	Botanical Name	Safety Data	Products containing Single Oil
Angelica	*Angelica archangelica* (Umbelliferae)	GRAS, FA, P, PH, DS	Awaken, Forgiveness, Grounding, Harmony, Live with Passion, Surrender
Anise	*Pimpinella anisum* (Umbelliferae)	GRAS, FA, DS	Awaken, Di-Tone, Dream Catcher, ICP, Essentialzyme, ParaFree, Power Meal, Polyzyme, Detoxzyme, Lipozyme, ComforTone
Basil	*Ocimum basilicum* (Labiatae)	GRAS, FA, E+, CH, P+, SI, DS	Aroma Siez, Clarity, M-Grain ArthroTune, Super Cal
Bergamot	*Citrus bergamia* (Rutaceae)	GRAS, FA, SI, DS, CH+	Awaken, Chivalry, Clarity, Forgiveness, Gentle Baby, Harmony, Joy, White Angelica, Progessence, Genesis Lotion, Prenolone, Prenolone+, Regenolone, NeuroGen, Rosewood Shampoo/ Conditioner, Dream Catcher, Dragon Time Bath Gel, Evening Peace Bath Gel
Blue Cypress	*Callitris intratropica*		Brain Power, Highest Potential
Cajeput	*Melaleuca leucadendra* (Myrtaceae)	SI	
Calamus	*Acorus calamus* (Araceae)	SI, P+, CH+	Exodus II
Cardamom	*Elettaria cardamomum* (Zingiberaceae)	GRAS, FA, DS SI	Clarity, Transformation
Carrot Seed Oil	*Daucus carota* (Umbelliferae)	GRAS, FA, DS	Rose Ointment
Cassia	*Cinnamomum cassia* (Lauraceae)	GRAS, FA, DS, P, CH, SI+	Exodus II, Oils of Ancient Scripture
Cedar, Canadian Red	*Thuja plicata* (Cupressaceae)		KidScents Lotion
Cedar, Western Red	*Thuja plicata* (Cupressaceae)	SI	Evergreen Essence

Single Oil Name	Botanical Name	Safety Data	Products containing Single Oil
Cedarwood	*Cedrus atlantica* (Pinaceae)		Australian Blue, Brain Power, SARA, Grounding, Highest Potential, Inspiration, Into the Future, Oils of Ancient Scripture, KidScents Lotion, Live with Passion, Sacred Mountain, Sacred Mountain Bar Soap, Peppermint-Cedarwood Bar Soap, Cel-Lite Magic
Celery Seed		P, SI, DS	JuvaCleanse
Chamomile (German/Blue)	*Matricaria chamomilla/recutita* (Compositae)	GRAS, FA, DS	EndoFlex, Surrender, K&B Tincture, JuvaTone, ComforTone
Chamomile (Roman)	*Chamaemelum nobile* (Compositae)	GRAS, FA, DS	Awaken, Chivalry, Clarity, Forgiveness, Gentle Baby, Harmony, Joy, JuvaFlex, Surrender, M-Grain, Motivation, Genesis Lotion, Lemon Sage Shampoo/Conditioner, Sandalwood Toner, Satin Body Lotion, Wolfberry Eye Creme, Dragon Time Bath Gel, Evening Peace Bath Gel, Chelex Tincture, K&B Tincture, Tender Tush Ointment, Rehemogen Tincture, Clara Derm
Cinnamon Bark	*Cinnamomum verum* (Lauraceae)	GRAS, FA, DS, P, SI+, CH	Abundance, Christmas Spirit, Exodus II, Gathering, Highest Potential, Magnify Your Purpose, Oils of Ancient Scripture, Thieves, Cinnamint Lip Balm, Thieves Bar Soap, ImmuGel, Mineral Essence, Carbozyme, Fresh Essence Plus, Dentarome Plus/Ultra Toothpaste, Thieves Antiseptic Spray, Thieves Wipes, Thieves Household Cleaner
Cistus	*Cistus ladanifer* (Cistaceae)	FA	ImmuPower, ImmuneTune, KidScents Lotion
Citronella	*Cymbopogon nardus* (Gramineae)	GRAS, FA, DS, P, SI	Purification, Sunsation Suntan Oil
Citrus Hystrix		DS, SI, PH, CH	Trauma Life
Clary Sage	*Salvia sclarea* (Labiatae)	GRAS, FA, P, DS	Into the Future, Live with Passion, Progessence, Lavender Shampoo/Conditioner, Prenolone, Prenolone+, Rosewood Shampoo/Conditioner, Dragon Time EO/Bath Gel/Massage Oil, EveningPeace Bath Gel, SclarEssence Cel-Lite Magic, Cortistop WOMEN Lady Sclareol, Transformation

Single Oil Name	Botanical Name	Safety Data	Products containing Single Oil
Clove	*Syzygium aromaticum* (Myrtaceae)	GRAS, FA, DS, A, SI+	Abundance, BLM Capsules & Powder, Carbozyme, En-R-Gee, ImmuPower, Longevity, Longevity Caps, Melrose, PanAway, Thieves, Dentarome Plus/Ultra Toothpaste, Kidscent Toothpaste, Fresh Essence Plus, Thieves Bar Soap, K&B Tincture, Essential Omegas, ImmuGel, Essentialzyme, ParaFree, AromaGuard Stick Deodorant, Thieves Antiseptic Spray, Thieves Wipes, Thieves Household Cleaner
Coriander	*Coriandrum sativum L.* (Umbelliferae)	GRAS, FA,DS	
Cumin	*Cuminus cyminum* (Umbelliferae)	GRAS, FA, DS, SI	ImmuPower, Protec, ParaFree, Detoxzyme
Cypress	*Cupressus sempervirens* (Cupressaceae)		Aroma Life, Aroma Siez, RC, H-R-T Tincture, Cel-Lite Magic, ArthroTune, BodyGize, Power Meal, Super Cal
Davana	*Artemisia pallens* (Compositae)		Trauma Life
Dill	*Anethum graveolens* (Umbelliferae)	GRAS, FA, DS, E	
Elemi	*Canarium luzonicum* (Burseraceae)		Ortho Sport
Eucalyptus citriodora	*Eucalyptus citriodora* (Myrtaceae)		RC
Eucalyptus dives	*Eucalyptus dives* (Myrtaceae)	SI, P	
Eucalyptus globulus	*Eucalyptus globulus* (Myrtaceae)	FA, FL, DS	RC, Fresh Fresh Essence Plus Mouthwash, Dentarome Plus/Ultra Toothpaste, Chelex Tincture, Ortho Sport
Eucalyptus polybractea	*Eucalyptus polybractea* (Myrtaceae)		
Eucalyptus radiata	*Eucalyptus radiata* (Myrtaceae)		RC, Thieves, AromaGuard Stick Deodorant, Thieves Bar Soap, Carbozyme, Thieves Antiseptic Spray, Dentarome Plus/Ultra Toothpaste, Fresh Essence Plus Mouthwash, Thieves Wipes, Thieves Household Cleaner
Fennel	*Foeniculum vulgare* (Umbelliferae)	GRAS, FA, DS, E, P	Di-Tone, JuvaFlex, Mister, Progessence, Detoxzyme, Lipozyme, Prenolone, Prenolone+, Dragon Time EO/Bath Gel/Massage Oil, K&B Tincture, ICP, SclarEssence Essentialzyme, ParaFree, Power Meal, ProGen, Cortistop WOMEN

Single Oil Name	Botanical Name	Safety Data	Products containing Single Oil
Fir, Douglas	*Pseudotsuga menziesii* (Pinaceae)	SI	Regenolone
Fir, Idaho Balsam	*Abies grandis* (Pinaceae)	FA, FL, SI, DS	Gratitude, BLM Powder & Capsules, Sacred Mountain, Believe, En-R-Gee, Sacred Mountain Bar Soap, Transformation
Fir, White	*Abies grandis* (Pinaceae)	SI	Arthrotune, ImmuneTune, AromaGuard Stick Deodorant, Evergreen Essence, Grounding, Australian Blue, Into the Future
Fleabane	*Conyza canadensis* (Compositae)		Progessence, ProMist, ThermaBurn, Ultra Young, Ultra Young Plus, Cortistop WOMEN
Frankincense	*Boswellia carteri* (Burseraceae)	FA, FL, DS	Abundance, Acceptance, Awaken, Believe, Brain Power, Chivalry, Clara Derm, Exodus II, Forgiveness, Gathering, Harmony, Humility, ImmuPower, Gratitude, Inspiration, Into the Future, Longevity, Oils of Ancient Scripture, 3 Wise Men, Trauma Life, Valor, Valor Bar Soap, Boswellia Wrinkle Creme, Protec, Wolfberry Eye Creme, Exodus, ThermaBurn, Cortistop WOMEN, Tender Tush Ointment, A.R.T Day Activator, A.R.T. Night Reconstructor, A.R.T Gentle Foaming Cleanser
Galbanum	*Ferula gummosa* (Umbelliferae)	FA, FL, DS	Chivalry, Exodus II, Gathering, Gratitude Highest Potential, Oils of Ancient Scripture
Geranium	*Pelargonium graveolens* (Geraniaceae)	GRAS, FA, DS, FL	Acceptance, Chivalry, Clarity, EndoFlex, Envision, Forgiveness, Gathering, Lady Sclareol, Highest Potential, Gentle Baby, Harmony, Humility, Joy, JuvaFlex, Release, SARA, Trauma Life, White Angelica, AromaGuard Stick Deodorant, Boswellia, Wrinkle Creme, Progessence, Genesis Lotion, Lemon-Sage Shampoo/Conditioner, Prenolone, Prenolone+, Rosewood Shampoo/Conditioner, KidScents Lotion, Satin Body Lotion, Wolfberry Eye Creme, Dragon Time Bath Gel, Evening Peace Bath Gel, Melaleuca-Geranium Bar Soap, K&B Tincture, JuvaTone, KidScents Liquid Soap

Single Oil Name	Botanical Name	Safety Data	Products containing Single Oil
Ginger	*Zingiber officinale* (Zingiberaceae)	GRAS, FA, DS, A, PH	Abundance, Di-Tone, Live with Passion, ComforTone, ICP, Mint Condition, Magnify Your Purpose, Lipozyme
Goldenrod	*Solidago canadensis* (Asteraceae)	DS	
Grapefruit	*Citrus x paradisi* (Rutaceae)	GRAS, FA, DS	Citrus Fresh, Cel-Lite Magic Bodygize, Power Meal, ProMist, Super C, ThermaMist
Helichrysum	*Helichrysum italicum* (Compositae)	GRAS, FA, DS	Aroma Life, Brain Power, Forgiveness, Awaken, JuvaFlex, JuvaCleanse, Live with Passion, M-Grain, PanAway, Trauma Life, Chelex Tincture, ArthroTune, CardiaCare, Clara Derm
Hyssop	*Hyssopus officinalis* (Labiatae)	GRAS, FA, DS, E+, HBP+, P+	Chivalry, Exodus II, Harmony, ImmuPower, Relieve It, White Angelica, Exodus, Oils of Ancient Scripture
Jasmine (Absolute)	*Jasminum officinale* (Oleaceae)		Awaken, Chivalry, Clarity, Dragon Time, Forgiveness, Gentle Baby, Harmony, Highest Potential, Inner Child, Joy, Lady Sclareol, Into the Future, Live with Passion, Lavender Shampoo/Conditioner, Genesis Lotion, Satin Body Lotion, Dragon Time Bath Gel/Massage, Evening Peace Bath Gel, Sensation EO/Lotion/Bath Gel/Message Oil
Juniper	*Juniperus osteosperma* and/or *J. scopulorum* (Cupressaceae)	GRAS, FA, DS SI	Awaken, Di-Tone, Dream Catcher, En-R-Gee, Grounding, Hope, Into the Future, 3 Wise Men, NeuroGen, Cel-Lite Magic,Ortho Ease, Morning Start Bath Gel, Morning Start Bar Soap, K&BTincture, Lipozyme, Arthro Tune
Laurel	*Laurus nobilis* (Lauraceae)	GRAS, FA, DS, SI	Exodus, ParaFree
Lavandin	*Lavandula x hybrida* (Labiatae)	GRAS, FA, DS,	Purification, Release

Single Oil Name	Botanical Name	Safety Data	Products containing Single Oil
Lavender	*Lavandula angustifolia* CT linalol (Labiatae)	GRAS, FA, DS	Aroma Siez, Awaken, Brain Power, RC, Chivalry, Envision, Forgiveness, Gentle Baby, Harmony, Gathering, Highest Potential, M-Grain, Mister, Motivation, SARA, Surrender, Trauma Life, ProGen LavaDerm Cooling Mist, AromaGuard Stick Deodorant, Lavender Shampoo/ Conditioner, Tender Tush Ointment, Orange Blossom Facial Wash, Sunsation Suntan Oil, Sandalwood Moisture Creme, Wolfberry Eye Creme, Juniper Satin Scrub, Lavender Rosewood Bar Soap, Dragon Time EO/Bath Gel/Massage Oil Relaxation Massage Oil, Clara Derm
Ledum	*Ledum groenlandicum* (Ericaceae)	DS	JuvaCleanse
Lemon	*Citrus limon* (Rutaceae)	GRAS, FA, DS, PH, SI	Chivalry, Citrus Fresh, Clarity, Thieves, Forgiveness, Gentle Baby, Harmony, Joy, RC, Surrender, Genesis Lotion, Lavender Shampoo/Conditioner, Lemon-Sage Shampoo/Conditioner, KidScents Shampoo, Orange Blossom Facial Wash, Dragon Time Bath Gel, Evening Peace Bath Gel, AromaGuard Stick Deodorant, Thieves Bar Soap, Lemon-Sandalwood Bar Soap, H-R-T Tincture, AlkaLime, AminoTech, Bodygize, CardiaCare, Carbozyme, ImmuGel, ImmuneTune, JuvaTone, MegaCal, Mineral Essence, Power Meal, Super C, Super C Chewable, WheyFit, VitaGreen, KidScents Detangler, Dentarome Plus/Ultra Toothpaste, Fresh Essence Plus Mouthwash, Thieves Antiseptic Spray, Thieves Wipes, Thieves Household Cleaner, Transformation, A.R.T. Gentle Foaming Cleanser
Lemongrass	*Cymbopogon flexuosus* (Gramineae)	GRAS, FA, DS, CH, SI+	ICP, Di-Tone, En-R-Gee, Inner Child, Purification, NeuroGen, Sunsation Suntan Oil, Morning Start Bath Gel, Morning Start Bar Soap, Ortho Ease, Ortho Sport, Bodygize, Be-Fit, Lipozyme, VitaGreen
Lime	*Citrus aurantifolia* (Rutaceae)	GRAS, FA, DS, PH+	Lemon-Sage Shampoo/Conditioner AlkaLime, Super C, AminoTech, Master Formula Children's

Single Oil Name	Botanical Name	Safety Data	Products containing Single Oil
Mandarin	*Citrus reticulata* (Rutaceae)	GRAS, FA, DS, PH	Awaken, Citrus Fresh, Joy, Dragon Time Bath Gel, Master Formula Children's, Super C, Bodygize
Marjoram	*Origanum majorana* (Labiatae)	GRAS, FA, DS, P	Aroma Life, Aroma Siez, Dragon Time, M-Grain, RC, Dragon Time Bath Gel, Ortho Ease, Ortho Sport ArthroTune, CardiaCare, Super Cal
Melaleuca ericifolia (formerly Rosalina)	*Melaleuca ericifolia* (Myrtaceae)		Melaleuca-Geranium Bar Soap
Melissa	*Melissa officinalis* (Labiatae)	GRAS, FA, DS	Brain Power, Forgiveness, Hope, Humility, Live with Passion, White Angelica, VitaGreen
Mountain Savory	*Satureja montana* (Labiatae)	GRAS, FA, DS, CH, SI+	ImmuPower, Surrender
Mugwort		GRAS, FA, DS P, CH	Comfortone
Myrrh	*Commiphora myrrha* (Burseraceae)	FA, FL, DS	Abundance, Chivalry, Exodus II, Protec, Gratitude, Hope, Humility, Oils of Ancient Scripture, 3 Wise Men, White Angelica, Boswellia Wrinkle Creme, Rose Ointment, Sandalwood Moisture Creme, Sandalwood Toner, Thyromin Clara Derm
Myrtle	*Myrtus communis* (Myrtaceae)	FA, FL, DS	EndoFlex, Inspiration, Mister, Purification, RC, JuvaTone, ProGen, ThermaBurn, Thyromin
Neroli	*Citrus aurantium bigaradia* (Rutaceae)	GRAS, FA, DS	Acceptance, Awaken, Humility, Inner Child, Live with Passion, Present Time
Niaouli	*Melaleuca quinquenervia* (Myrtaceae)		Melrose, AromaGuard Stick Deodorant
Nutmeg	*Myristica fragrans* (Myristicaceae)	GRAS, FA, DS, SI, E, P, CH+	EndoFlex, En-R-Gee, Magnify Your Purpose, Royal Essence Tincture, Be-Fit, ParaFree, Power Meal, ThermaBurn
Onycha	*Styrax benzoin* (Styracaceae)		Oils of Ancient Scripture
Orange	*Citrus aurantium* (Rutaceae)	GRAS, FA, DS, PH	Abundance, Christmas Spirit, Chivalry, Citrus Fresh, Envision, Harmony, Inner Child, Peace & Calming, SARA, Bodygize, Essential Omegas, ImmuneTune, ImmuPro, Lady Sclareol, Mighty Vites, Longevity, Longevity Caps, Power Meal, Super C, Wolfberry Bar

Single Oil Name	Botanical Name	Safety Data	Products containing Single Oil
Oregano	*Origanum compactum* (Labiatae)	GRAS, FA, DS, SI+	ImmuPower, Regenolone, Ortho Sport Massage Oil, ImmuGel
Palmarosa	*Cymbopogon martinii* (Gramineae)	GRAS, FA, DS	Awaken, Chivalry, Clarity, Forgiveness, Gentle Baby, Harmony, Joy, Genesis Lotion, Rose Ointment, Dragon Time Bath Gel, Evening Peace Bath Gel
Patchouli	*Pogostemon cublin* (Labiatae)	FA, FL, DS	Abundance, Di-Tone, Live with Passion, Magnify Your Purpose, Peace & Calming, Orange Blossom Facial Wash, Lipozyme, Rose Ointment
Pepper (black)	*Piper nigrum* (Piperaceae)	GRAS, FA, DS, SI	Dream Catcher, En-R-Gee, Relieve It, Cel-Lite Magic, ArthroTune
Peppermint	*Mentha piperita* (Labiatae)	GRAS, FA, DS, SI+, HB,P, CH+	Aroma Siez, Clarity, Di Tone, M-Grain, Mister, PanAway, Raven, RC, Relieve It, AromaGuard Stick Deodorant, Cinnamint Lip Balm, Mint Condition Dentarome Plus/Ultra Toothpaste, Detoxzyme, Fresh Essence Plus Mouthwash, Lipozyme, Peppermint Satin Scrub MINT, NeuroGen, Regenolone, Satin Body Lotion, Morning Start Bath Gel, Peppermint-Cedarwood Bar Soap, Morning Start Bar Soap, Ortho Ease, Ortho Sport, Relaxation Massage Oil, Polyzyme, BLM Powder, Cortistop WOMEN, ComforTone, Thyromin, SclarEssence Satin Scrub, Essential Manna (Carob Mint), Essentialzyme, Transformation, Mineral Essence, Pro-Gen, ProMist, ThermaMist
Petitgrain	*Citrus aurantium* (Rutaceae)	GRAS, FA, DS	
Pine	*Pinus sylvestris* (Pinaceae)	FA, FL, SI, DS	Evergreen Essence, Grounding, RC, Lemon-Sage Shampoo/Conditioner, ImmuneTune
Pine, Ponderosa	*Pinus ponderosa* (Pinaceae)	SI	Evergreen Essence
Ravensara	*Ravensara aromatica* (Lauraceae)		ImmuPower, Respiratory S, ImmuneTune
Rose	*Rosa damascena* (Rosaceae)	GRAS, FA, DS,	Awaken, Chivalry, Envision, Forgiveness, Gathering, Gentle Baby, Harmony, Joy, Humility, Highest Potential, SARA, Trauma Life, White Angelica, Rose Ointment

Single Oil Name	Botanical Name	Safety Data	Products containing Single Oil
Rosemary	*Rosmarinus officinalis* CT cineol (Labiatae)	GRAS, FA, DS, E+, HBP, P+ CH+	Clarity, En-R-Gee, JuvaFlex, Melrose, Purification, Thieves, Morning Start Bath Gel, VitaGreen, AromaGuard Stick Deodorant, Thieves Bar Soap, Morning Start Bar Soap, Chelex Tincture, Rehemogen Tincture, Sandalwood Moisture Creme, Be-Fit, Carbozyme, ComforTone, Polyzyme, ICP, ImmuGel, JuvaTone, Orange Blossom Facial Wash, Fresh Essence Plus Mouthwash, Thieves Antiseptic Spray, Thieves Wipes, Thieves Household Cleaner, Transformation, Dentarome Plus/Ultra Toothpaste
Rosewood	*Aniba rosaeodora* (Lauraceae)		Acceptance, Awaken, Believe, Chivalry, Clarity, Forgiveness, Gentle Baby, Joy, Gratitude, Harmony, Humility, Valor, Inspiration, Magnify Your Purpose, White Angelica, Genesis Lotion, Rose Ointment, AromaGuard Stick Deodorant, Rosewood Shampoo/Conditioner, KidScents Lotion, Sandalwood Moisture Creme, Sandalwood Toner, Satin Body Lotion, Wolfberry Eye Creme, Dragon Time Bath Gel, Evening Peace Bath Gel, Sensation EO/Lotion/Bath Gel/Massage Oil, Lavender Rosewood Bar Soap, Valor Bar Soap, H-R-T Tincture, Relaxation Massage Oil, Lady Sclareol, Tender Tush Ointment
Sage	*Salvia officinalis* (Labiatae)	GRAS, FA, DS, E+, P+, CH+	Chivalry, EndoFlex, Envision, Magnify Your Purpose, Mister, Protec, Lemon Sage Shampoo/Conditioner, Dragon Time Massage Oil/Bath Gel, K&B Tincture, Progen
Sage Lavender	*Salvia lavandulifolia*		Awaken, Chivalry, Harmony, Lady Sclareol, SclarEssence

Single Oil Name	Botanical Name	Safety Data	Products containing Single Oil
Sandalwood	*Santalum album* (Santalaceae)	FA, FL, DS	Acceptance, Awaken, Brain Power, Chivalry, Dream Catcher, Forgiveness, Gathering, Harmony, Highest Potential, Inner Child, Inspiration, Live with Passion, Magnify Your Purpose, Oils of Ancient Scripture, Release, 3 Wise Men, Trauma Life, White Angelica, Boswellia Wrinkle Creme, Rosewood Shampoo/ Conditioner, Sandalwood Moisture Creme, Sandalwood Toner, Satin Body Lotion, Evening Peace Bath Gel, Lemon-Sandalwood Bar Soap, Ultra Young, Ultra Young Plus, Tender Tush Ointment, Lady Sclareol, A.R.T Day Activator, A.R.T Gentle Foaming Cleanser, A.R.T Night Reconstructor
Spearmint	*Mentha spicata* (Labiatae)	GRAS, FA, DS SI, CH+	Citrus Fresh, EndoFlex, Cinnamint Lip Balm, Fresh Essence Plus Mouthwash, Relaxation Massage Oil, Mint Condition, ProMist, ThermaBurn, ThermaMist, Thyromin
Spikenard	*Nardostachys jatamansi* (Valerianaceae)		Exodus II, Humility, Exodus, Oils of Ancient Scripture
Spruce	*Picea mariana* (Pinaceae)	FA, FL, DS SI	Abundance, Christmas Spirit, Chivalry, Envision, Gathering, Grounding, Harmony, Hope, Highest Potential, Inner Child, Inspiration, Motivation, Present Time, RC, Relieve It, Sacred Mountain, Surrender, 3 Wise Men, Trauma Life, Valor, White Angelica, Sacred Mountain Bar Soap, Valor Bar Soap, ArthroTune
Tangerine	*Citrus nobilis* (Rutaceae)	GRAS, FA, DS SI, PH	Awaken, Citrus Fresh, Dream Catcher, Inner Child, Peace & Calming, Bodygize, Relaxation Massage Oil, ComforTone KidScents Detangler, KidScents Shampoo
Tansy, Blue	*Tanacetum annum* (Compositae)		Acceptance, Australian Blue, Awaken, Dream Catcher, Highest Potential, JuvaFlex, Peace & Calming, Release, SARA, Valor, Dragon Time Bath Gel, Evening Peace Bath Gel, Valor Bar Soap, JuvaTone, Tender Tush Ointment
Tansy, Idaho	*Tanacetum vulgare* (Compositae)	E+, P+. CH+	Awaken, ImmuPower, Into the Future, ParaFree, KidScents Shampoo, Lady Sclareol

Single Oil Name	Botanical Name	Safety Data	Products containing Single Oil
Tarragon	*Artemisia dracunculus* (Compositae)	GRAS, FA, DS, E+, P+, CH+	Di-Tone, ComforTone, ICP, Essentialzyme, Lipozyme, KidScents Detangler
Tea Tree	*Melaleuca alternifolia* (Myrtaceae)		Melrose, Purification, AromaGuard Stick Deodorant, Rose Ointment, Sunsation Suntan Oil, Melaleuca-Geranium Bar Soap, Rehemogen Tincture, ParaFree Clara Derm
Thyme, Red	*Thymus vulgaris* (Labiatae)	GRAS, FA, DS, HBP, M, CH	Longevity, Longevity Caps, Kidscent Toothpaste, ImmuGel, ParaFree, Rehemogen, Ortho Ease
Tsuga	*Tsuga canadensis* (Pinaceae)	SI+	
Valerian	*Valeriana officinalis* (Valerianaceae)	FA, FL, DS	Trauma Life
Vetiver	*Vetiveria zizanoides* (Gramineae)	FA, FL, DS	Fresh Essence Plus Mouthwash, Lady Sclareol, Melaleuca-Geranium Bar Soap, Ortho Ease, Ortho Sport, ParaFree
Wintergreen	*Gaultheria procumbens* (Ericaceae) *Betula alleghaniensis*	E+, P+, CH+ A	PanAway, Dentarome Plus/Ultra Toothpaste Regenolone, Be-Fit, Super Cal, ArthoTune, Rosewood Shampoo/Conditioner, BLM Capsules & Powder, Ortho Ease, Ortho Sport
Yarrow	*Achillea millefolium* (Compositae)		Dragon Time, Mister, Dragon Time Massage Oil, Prenolone/Prenolone+, ProGen
Ylang Ylang	*Cananga odorata* (Annonaceae)	GRAS, FA, DS,	Aroma Life, Awaken, Chivalry, Clarity, Dream Catcher, Forgiveness, Gathering, Gentle Baby, Gratitude, Grounding, Harmony, Humility, Australian Blue Highest Potential, Inner Child, Joy, Motivation, Peace & Calming, Present Time, Release, Sacred Mountain, SARA, White Angelica, Boswellia Wrinkle Creme, Progessence, Genesis Lotion, Lemon Sage Shampoo/Conditioner, Prenolone/Prenolone+, Satin Body Lotion, CardiaCare, Sensation EO/Lotion/Bath Gel/Massage Oil, Dragon Time Bath Gel/Massage Oil, Evening Peace Bath Gel, Sacred Mountain Bar Soap, H-R-T Tincture, Relaxation Massage Oil, Lady Sclareol

Safety Data Legend:

A   Anti-coagulant – May enhance the effects of blood thinners; avoid using with Aspirin, heparin, Warfarin, etc)

CH   Do not use on children younger than 18 months of age

CH+   Do not use on children younger than 5 years of age

DS   Dietary supplement

E   Use with **caution** if susceptible to **epilepsy** (small amounts or in dilution)

E+   **Avoid** if susceptible to **epilepsy** (can trigger a seizure)

FA   Food additive

FL   Flavoring agent

GRAS Generally regarded as safe

HBP   Use with **caution** if dealing with **high blood pressure** (small amounts)

HBP+ **Avoid** if dealing with **high blood pressure**

P   Use with **caution** during pregnancy

P+   **Avoid** during pregnancy

PH   **Photosensitivity** – direct exposure to sunlight within 24 hours after use could cause dermatitis (test first)

PH+   **Extreme Photosensitivity** – direct exposure to sunlight after use within 72 hours can cause severe dermatitis (avoid exposing affected area of skin to direct sunlight for 48-72 hours)

SI   Could possibly result in **skin irritation** (dilution may be necessary)

SI+   Can cause **extreme skin irritation** (dilution highly recommended)

APPENDIX U

Oil Blends Data

Blend Name	Single Oil Contents	Safety Data	Uses/Application Areas
Abundance	Myrrh, Cinnamon Bark, Patchouli, Orange, Clove, Ginger, Spruce, Frankincense	SI, CH	Diffuse; wrists, ears, neck, face; wallet/purse; painting; direct inhalation
Acceptance	Geranium, Blue Tansy, Frankincense, Sandalwood, Neroli, Rosewood (Carrier: Almond Oil)		Diffuse; liver, heart, chest, face, ears, neck, thymus, wrists; sacral chakra; direct inhalation
Aroma Life	Cypress, Marjoram, Helichrysum, Ylang Ylang (Carrier: Sesame Seed Oil)		Heart; Vita Flex heart points, under left ring finger, under left ring toe, above left elbow, neck; spine; direct inhalation
Aroma Siez	Basil, Marjoram, Lavender, Peppermint, Cypress	SI, CH	Muscles; neck; heart; Vita Flex points; full body massage; bath; direct inhalation
Australian Blue	Blue Cypress, Ylang Ylang Cedarwood, Blue Tansy, White Fir		Diffuse; chest, heart, forehead, neck, temples, wrists; direct inhalation
Awaken	Lemon, Mandarin, Bergamot, Ylang Ylang, Rose, Rosewood, Geranium, Palmarosa, Roman Chamomile, Jasmine, Hyssop, Frankincense, Sandalwood, Helichrysum, Juniper, Blue Tansy, Tangerine, Black Pepper, Anise Neroli, Spruce, Lavender, Orange, Angelica, Sage Lavender (Carrier: Almond Oil)	PH	Diffuse; chest, heart, forehead, neck, temples, wrists; full body massage; bath
Believe	Idaho Balsam Fir, Rosewood, Frankincense		Diffuse; heart, forehead, neck, temples, wrists; bath; direct inhalation
Brain Power	Cedarwood, Sandalwood, Frankincense, Melissa, Australian Blue Cypress, Lavender, Helichrysum		Diffuse; neck, throat, nose; inside of cheeks, wrists; direct inhalation

Blend Name	Single Oil Contents	Safety Data	Uses/Application Areas
Chivalry	Spruce, Rosewood, Blue Tansy, Frankincense, Mandarin, Bergamot, Lemon, Ylang Ylang, Rose, Palmarosa, Roman Chamomile, Jasmine, Hyssop, Lavender, Orange, Sandalwood, Angelica, Sage Lavender, Idaho Balsam Fir, Myrrh, Galbanum	SI	Diffuse; crown; neck, wrists; direct inhalation
Christmas Spirit	Orange, Cinnamon Bark, Spruce	SI, CH	Diffuse; crown; neck, wrists; heart, temple; bath; direct inhalation
Citrus Fresh	Orange, Tangerine, Mandarin, Grapefruit, Lemon, Spearmint	SI, PH DS	Diffuse; ears, heart, wrists; neck, wrists; full body massage; bath; purify drinking water
Clarity	Basil, Cardamom, Rosemary cineol, Peppermint, Rosewood, Geranium, Lemon, Palmarosa, Ylang Ylang, Bergamot, Roman Chamomile, Jasmine	SI, P, PH+, CH, DS	Diffuse; forehead, neck, temples, wrists, neck; bath direct inhalation
Di-Tone	Tarragon, Ginger, Peppermint, Juniper, Anise, Fennel, Lemongrass, Patchouli	SI, P, E, CH+, DS	Vita Flex points, compress ankles; stomach; abdomen, bottom of throat; direct inhalation
Dragon Time	Clary Sage, Fennel, Lavender, Jasmine, Yarrow, Marjoram	P	Vita Flex points; diffuse; abdomen, lower back, location direct inhalation
Dream Catcher	Sandalwood, Bergamot, Ylang Ylang, Juniper, Blue Tansy, Tangerine, Black Pepper, Anise	PH	Diffuse; forehead, eye brows, temples, ears, throat chakra; neck, wrists; bath; direct inhalation
EndoFlex	Spearmint, Sage, Geranium, Myrtle, Nutmeg, German Chamomile (Carrier: Sesame Seed Oil)	SI, E, CH	Thyroid, kidneys, liver, pancreas, glands; Vita Flex points; direct inhalation
En-R-Gee	Rosemary cineol, Juniper, Nutmeg, Idaho Balsam Fir, Black Pepper, Lemongrass, Clove	SI, E	Diffuse; wrists, ears, neck, temples, feet; full body massage; direct inhalation
Envision	Spruce, Sage, Rose, Geranium, Orange, Lavender	HBP, E, P	Vita Flex points; diffuse; wrists, temples; bath; massage direct inhalation
Evergreen Essence	Colorado Blue Spruce, Ponderosa Pine, Pine, Red Fir Cedar, White Fir, Black Pine Piñon Pine, Lodge Pole Pine	SI	Diffuse; forehead, heart, temples, neck, thymus, direct inhalation

Blend Name	Single Oil Contents	Safety Data	Uses/Application Areas
Exodus II	Cinnamon Bark, Cassia, Calamus, Myrrh, Hyssop, Frankincense, Spikenard, Galbanum (Carrier: Olive Oil)	SI+, P+, CH+	Diffuse; Direct Inhale; Chest, ears, wrist, spine, (Raindrop style); VitaFlex direct inhalation
Forgiveness	Frankincense, Sandalwood, Lavender, Melissa, Angelica, Helichrysum, Rose, Rosewood, Geranium, Lemon, Palmarosa, Ylang Ylang, Bergamot, Roman Chamomile, Jasmine (Carrier: Sesame Seed Oil)		Diffuse; navel, heart, ears, wrists; direct inhalation
Gathering	Galbanum, Frankincense, Sandalwood, Lavender, Cinnamon Bark, Rose, Spruce, Geranium, Ylang Ylang		Diffuse; forehead, heart, temples, neck, thymus, face, chest; direct inhalation
Gentle Baby	Geranium, Rosewood, Palmarosa, Lavender, Roman Chamomile, Ylang Ylang, Rose, Lemon, Bergamot, Jasmine		Diffuse; ankles, lower back, abdomen, feet, face, neck; massage; bath; direct inhalation direct inhalation
Gratitude	Idaho Balsam Fir, Frankincense, Rosewood, Myrrh, Galbanum Ylang Ylang		Diffuse; ears; chest, heart, temples, neck, feet, wrists direct inhalation
Grounding	Juniper, Angelica, Ylang Ylang, Cedarwood, Pine, Spruce, White Fir	SI	Diffuse; brain stem, back of neck, sternum, temples direct inhalation
Harmony	Hyssop, Spruce, Lavender, Frankincense, Geranium, Ylang Ylang, Orange, Sandalwood, Angelica, Sage Lavender, Rose, Rosewood, Lemon, Palmarosa, Bergamot, Roman Chamomile, Jasmine	P, E+, HBP, PH	Diffuse; Vita Flex points; ears, feet, heart; energy meridians, crown direct inhalation
Highest Potential	Galbanum, Frankincense, Sandalwood, Lavender, Cinnamon Bark, Rose, Spruce, Geranium, Ylang Ylang, Blue Cypress, Cedarwood, Blue Tansy, White Fir, Jasmine		Diffuse; ears; chest, heart, temples, wrists, neck, feet; direct inhalation
Hope	Melissa, Myrrh, Juniper, Spruce (Carrier: Almond Oil)		Diffuse; ears; chest, heart, temples, solar plexus, neck, feet, wrists; direct inhalation
Humility	Geranium, Ylang Ylang, Frankincense, Spikenard, Myrrh, Rose, Rosewood, Melissa, Neroli (Carrier: Sesame Seed Oil)		Diffuse; heart, neck, temples; direct inhalation

Blend Name	Single Oil Contents	Safety Data	Uses/Application Areas
ImmuPower	Cistus, Frankincense, Hyssop, Ravensara, Mountain Savory, Oregano, Clove, Cumin, Idaho Tansy	SI, P, E, CH	Diffuse; throat, chest, spine, feet; thymus; neck, under arms direct inhalation
Inner Child	Orange, Tangerine, Jasmine, Ylang Ylang, Spruce, Sandalwood, Lemongrass, Neroli	PH, SI	Diffuse; navel, chest, temples nose; direct inhalation
Inspiration	Cedarwood, Spruce, Rosewood, Sandalwood, Frankincense, Myrtle, Mugwort		Diffuse; temples, crown, shoulders, back of neck direct inhalation
Into the Future	Frankincense, Jasmine, Clary Sage, Juniper, Idaho Tansy, White Fir, Orange, Cedarwood, Ylang Ylang, White Lotus (Carrier: Almond Oil)		Diffuse; bath; heart, wrists neck; compress; full body massage; direct inhalation
Joy	Lemon, Mandarin, Bergamot, Ylang Ylang, Rose, Rosewood, Geranium, Palmarosa, Roman Chamomile, Jasmine	PH, CH	Diffuse; heart, ears, neck, thymus, temples, forehead, wrists; bath; compress; massage; direct inhalation
Juva Cleanse	Helichrysum, Celery Seed, Ledum	CH+	Take 1 capsule size 0 1-2 times daily
JuvaFlex	Fennel, Geranium, Rosemary cineol, Roman Chamomile, Blue Tansy, Helichrysum (Carrier: Sesame Seed Oil)	SI	Vita Flex points; feet, spine, liver; full body massage direct inhalation
Lady Sclareol	Rosewood, Vetiver, Geranium, Orange, Clary Sage, Ylang Ylang, Sandalwood, Sage Lavender Jasmine (absolute), Idaho Tansy	P, CH	Apply 2-4 drops to Vita Flex Points
Legacy	(See LEGACY in Blend section for complete list of 91 single oils)	SI, CH	Diffuse; forehead, wrists, sternum, feet; neck; direct inhalation
Live with Passion	Melissa, Helichrysum, Clary Sage, Cedarwood, Angelica, Ginger, Neroli, Sandalwood, Patchouli, Jasmine		Diffuse; Wrists, temples, chest, forehead; neck, bath; direct inhalation
Longevity	Clove, Orange, Thyme Frankincense	DS, CH+	Take 1 capsule size 00 1-2 x daily
M-Grain	Basil, Marjoram, Lavender, Peppermint, Roman Chamomile, Helichrysum	SI, CH	Diffuse; forehead, crown shoulders, neck, temples; Vita Flex points; massage direct inhalation
Magnify Your Purpose	Sandalwood, Nutmeg, Patchouli, Rosewood, Cinnamon Bark, Ginger, Sage	E, P, SI, CH	Vita Flex points; feet, wrists, temples; diffuse; bath; massage direct inhalation

Blend Name	Single Oil Contents	Safety Data	Uses/Application Areas
Melrose	Melaleuca (Alternifolia & Quinquenervia), Rosemary cineol, Clove	SI	Topically on location diffuse; forehead, liver; direct inhalation
Mister	Sage, Fennel, Lavender, Myrtle, Yarrow, Peppermint (Carrier: Sesame Seed Oil)	P+, E, CH	Vita Flex points; ankles, lower pelvis, prostate (dilute); compress; direct inhalation
Motivation	Roman Chamomile, Ylang Ylang, Spruce, Lavender		Diffuse; chest, neck; solar plexus, sternum, feet, navel, ears; wrists, palms; direct inhalation
PanAway	Wintergreen, Helichrysum, Clove, Peppermint	SI, CH	Apply on location of pain; Vitaflex feet; direct inhalation
Peace & Calming	Tangerine, Orange, Ylang Ylang, Patchouli, Blue Tansy	PH	Diffuse; navel, nose, neck, feet; bath; wrists; direct inhalation
Present Time	Neroli, Spruce, Ylang Ylang (Carrier: Almond Oil)		Thymus; neck, forehead direct inhalation
Purification	Citronella, Lemongrass, Rosemary cineol, Melaleuca, Lavandin, Myrtle	SI	Diffuse; Vita Flex points; ears, feet, temples; on location of injury; direct inhalation
Raven	Ravensara, Eucalyptus radiata, Peppermint, Wintergreen, Lemon	SI, CH	Diffuse; compress; Vita Flex points; lungs, throat; pillow; suppository; direct inhalation
R.C.	Eucalyptus (E. globulus, E. radiata, E. australiana, E. citriodora), Myrtle, Marjoram, Pine, Cypress, Lavender, Spruce, Peppermint	CH	Compress; diffuse; chest, back, feet; sinuses, nasal passages; ears, neck, throat; massage; direct inhalation
Release	Ylang Ylang, Lavandin, Geranium, Sandalwood, Blue Tansy (Carrier: Olive Oil)		Compress on liver; ears, feet, Vita Flex points; wrists
Relieve It	Spruce, Black Pepper, Hyssop, Peppermint	SI, P, E, HBP, CH	Apply on location of pain; direct inhalation; Raindrop Technique
Sacred Mountain	Spruce, Ylang Ylang, Cedarwood Idaho Balsam Fir	SI	Diffuse; solar plexus, brain stem, crown, neck ears, thymus, wrists; direct inhalation
SARA	Blue Tansy, Rose, Lavender, Geranium, Orange, Cedarwood, Ylang Ylang, White Lotus (Carrier: Almond Oil)		En-R-Gee centers; Vita Flex points; temples, nose; places of abuse; direct inhalation
SclarEssence	Clary Sage, Peppermint, Sage Lavender, Fennel	DS, P+, CH	1-10 drops in capsule with VO, Ingest 1 capsule daily as needed
Sensation	Rosewood, Ylang Ylang, Jasmine		Diffuse; apply on location; massage; bath; direct inhalation

Blend Name	Single Oil Contents	Safety Data	Uses/Application Areas
Surrender	Lavender, Roman Chamomile, German Chamomile, Angelica, Mountain Savory, Lemon, Spruce	SI, DS	Forehead, rim of ears, nape of neck, chest, solar plexus; bath direct inhalation
Thieves	Clove, Lemon, Cinnamon Bark, Eucalyptus radiata, Rosemary cineol	SI+, P, CH	Diffuse; feet, throat, stomach, intestines; thymus, under arms; direct inhalation
3 Wise Men	Sandalwood, Juniper, Frankincense, Spruce, Myrrh (Carrier: Almond Oil)		Diffuse; crown of head; neck, forehead, solar plexus, thymus direct inhalation
Transformation	Lemon, Peppermint, Sandalwood, Clary Sage, Frankincense, Idaho Balsam Fir, Rosemary, Cardamom	P, PH, CH	Diffuse or apply to Vita Flex points
Trauma Life	Citrus Hystrix, Davana, Geranium, Spruce, Helichrysum, Rose, Sandalwood, Frankincense, Lavender, Valerian		Diffuse; spine; feet, chest, ears, neck, forehead direct inhalation
Valor	Spruce, Rosewood, Blue Tansy, Frankincense (Carrier: Almond Oil)		Feet; diffuse; heart, wrists, solar plexus, neck to thymus, spine; direct inhalation
White Angelica	Geranium, Spruce, Myrrh, Ylang Ylang, Hyssop, Bergamot, Melissa, Sandalwood, Rose, Rosewood (Carrier: Almond Oil)	PH	Diffuse; shoulders, crown, chest, ears, neck, forehead, wrists; bath; direct inhalation; compress

Safety Data Legend:

A	Anti-coagulant – May enhance the effects of blood thinners
CH	Do not use on children younger than 18 months of age
CH+	Do not use on children younger than 5 years of age
DS	Dietary supplement
E	Use with **caution** if susceptible to **epilepsy** (small amounts or in dilution)
E+	**Avoid** if susceptible to **epilepsy** (can trigger a seizure)
FA	Food additive
FL	Flavoring agent
GRAS	Generally regarded as safe
HBP	Use with **caution** if dealing with **high blood pressure** (small amounts)
HBP+	**Avoid** if dealing with **high blood pressure**
P	Use with **caution** during pregnancy
P+	**Avoid** during pregnancy
PH	**Photosensitivity** – direct exposure to sunlight within 24 hours after use could cause dermatitis (test first)
PH+	**Extreme Photosensitivity** – direct exposure to sunlight after use within 72 hours can cause severe dermatitis (avoid exposing affected area of skin to direct sunlight for 48-72 hours)
SI	Could possibly result in **skin irritation** (dilution may be necessary)
SI+	Can cause **extreme skin irritation** (dilution highly recommended)

Index